# Pocket Guide
# to Evaluations
# of Drug Interactions

## NOTICE

This publication does not purport to include all reported drug interactions. All expressions of opinion and statements presented in this publication concerning the incidents and severity of possible drug interactions, as well as recognition, side effects, and treatment of such interactions, represent the consensus of the staff and consultants of First DataBank and the American Pharmaceutical Association Scientific Review Panel.

This book is intended for use by health professionals, and it should not be used by anyone who does not have such specialized training. The book can serve to assist the practitioner, but it is not a substitute for professional knowledge, judgment, training, and experience.

The inclusion in this publication of the drug in respect to which patent or trademark rights may exist shall not be deemed, and is not intended as, a grant of, or authority to exercise, any right or privilege protected by such patent or trademark. All such rights and privileges are vested in the patent or trademark owner, and no other person may exercise the same without express permission, authority, or license secured from such patent or trademark owner.

# Pocket Guide to Evaluations of Drug Interactions

Editors
**Frederic J. Zucchero, M.A., R.Ph.**
**Mark J. Hogan, Pharm.D.**
**Christine D. Sommer, Pharm.D.**

Assistant Editor
**John Patrick Curran, R.Ph., PA-C**

FOURTH EDITION
AMERICAN PHARMACEUTICAL ASSOCIATION
WASHINGTON, D.C.

**Managing Editor:** Julian I. Graubart
**Abstractors:** Daniel H. Albrant, Pharm.D.,
Jeann Lee Gillespie, Pharm.D.,
and Susan Moss Marks, R.Ph.
**Production Coordinator:** Mary A. Burns
**Graphic Artist:** Claire Purnell Graphic Design
**Indexer:** Suzanne R. Peake

ISBN 1-58212-030-7

ISSN 1521-8392

Printed in Canada

Copyright © 2002, American Pharmaceutical Association, 2215 Constitution Avenue, N.W., Washington, D.C. 20037-2985. http://www.aphanet.org. All rights reserved.

*No part of this publication may be reproduced, stored in a retrieval system, or transmitted, in any form or by any means, electronic, mechanical, photocopying, recording, or otherwise, without prior written permission from the publisher.*

To comment on this book via e-mail, send your message to the publisher at aphabooks@mail.aphanet.org.

---

**How to Order This Book**

By phone: **800-878-0729** – VISA®, MasterCard®, and American Express® cards accepted.

# Table of Contents

*Evaluations of Drug Interactions* Directory .................... vi
How to Use *Pocket Guide to Evaluations of Drug Interactions* .... vii

*Chapter One*
  Analgesic drug interactions: narcotics, nonnarcotics, nonsteroidal anti-inflammatory agents, and agents for gout. ....... 1

*Chapter Two*
  Anesthetic and neuromuscular blocking agents' drug interactions ............................................. 25

*Chapter Three*
  Antiarrhythmic drug interactions ........................... 45

*Chapter Four*
  Anticoagulant drug interactions. ........................... 69

*Chapter Five*
  Anticonvulsant drug interactions ......................... 103

*Chapter Six*
  Antidepressant drug interactions......................... 136

*Chapter Seven*
  Antihypertensive drug interactions....................... 162

*Chapter Eight*
  Anti-infective drug interactions........................... 179

*Chapter Nine*
  Antineoplastic drug interactions.......................... 216

*Chapter Ten*
  Antipsychotic and antianxiety drug interactions ........... 230

*Chapter Eleven*
  Beta-adrenergic blocking agents' drug interactions ........ 259

*Chapter Twelve*
  Cardiac glycoside drug interactions...................... 273

*Chapter Thirteen*
  Diuretic drug interactions ............................... 291

*Chapter Fourteen*
  Hypoglycemic drug interactions ......................... 301

*Chapter Fifteen*
  Sedative-hypnotic drug interactions...................... 316

*Chapter Sixteen*
  Vitamin/nutrient/food drug interactions .................. 326

*Chapter Seventeen*
  Xanthine drug interactions .............................. 336

*Chapter Eighteen*
  Miscellaneous drug interactions ......................... 356

Appendices
  A. Related drugs ....................................... 390
  B. Code 1 interactions................................... 399

Index..................................................... 403

# Evaluations of Drug Interactions Directory

## Editors

Frederic J. Zucchero, M.A., R.Ph.
Adjunct Instructor in Pharmacy Practice
St. Louis College of Pharmacy
Medical Director
First DataBank–St. Louis
rick_zucchero@firstdatabank.com

Mark J. Hogan, Pharm.D.
Adjunct Instructor in Pharmacy Practice
St. Louis College of Pharmacy
General Manager
First DataBank–St. Louis
mark_hogan@firstdatabank.com

Christine D. Sommer, Pharm.D.
Adjunct Instructor in Pharmacy Practice
St. Louis College of Pharmacy
Associate Director, Medical Affairs
First DataBank–St. Louis
christine_sommer@firstdatabank.com

## Assistant Editor

John Patrick Curran, R.Ph., PA-C
Adjunct Instructor in Pharmacy Practice
St. Louis College of Pharmacy
Clinical Pharmacist
First DataBank-St. Louis
pat_curran@firstdatabank.com

## Consulting Contributors

Bruce Alexander, Pharm.D.; Jerry L. Bauman, Pharm.D.; Rebecca S. Finley, Pharm.D., M.S.; Jerry L. Frazier, Pharm.D.; William R. Garnett, Pharm.D.; Pamela D. Garzone, Ph.D.; Norman L. Katz, Ph.D., R.Ph.; John Loomis, Pharm.D.; David L. Lourwood Jr., Pharm.D., BCPS; Kenneth Rockwell Jr., Pharm.D., M.S.; Philip J. Rogers, BPharm, Ph.D., MRPharmS, ACPP; Terrence L. Schwinghammer, Pharm.D.; Jon J. Tanja, M.S., FASCP; Stanley S. Weber, Pharm.D., FASHP, BCPP

## American Pharmaceutical Association Scientific Review Panel

Daniel H. Albrant, Pharm.D.; Ann B. Amerson, Pharm.D.; Connie Lee Barnes, Pharm.D.; Ruth Ann Calloway, R.Ph., M.S.; Mark A. Chamberlain, Pharm. D.; Joanne M. Yasuda, Pharm.D.

# How to Use *Pocket Guide to Evaluations of Drug Interactions*

### Chapter Assignments

Each monograph is assigned a chapter based upon classification and pharmacologic effect. The first drug listed in the monograph heading is the drug whose pharmacologic effect was altered by the second drug. If the affected drug is not assigned a chapter, the monograph is placed in the therapeutic chapter of the other agent. For drug interactions in which neither of the two involved agents has an assigned chapter, the monographs are listed in Chapter 18 (Miscellaneous Drug Interactions) and alphabetized by the drug whose pharmacologic action is altered.

### Drug Interaction Monographs

Most monographs contain eight concise pieces of information:
1. The **title** of the monograph by generic name of the interacting drugs
2. A **significance code** based on the interaction's potential harm to the patient and its frequency and predictability
3. A statement on the interaction's **potential effects**\*
4. Patient management **recommendations** for the healthcare professional to consider with respect to the interaction
5. A **summary** of studies in the literature
6. A discussion of pharmacologically, pharmacokinetically, or chemically **related drugs** to either of the interacting drugs (see Appendix A for a complete list of the agents in a specific related drug class)
7. A comment on the postulated **mechanism** for the drug interaction
8. A cross reference to the more **detailed information** found in *Evaluations of Drug Interactions*, which is paginated by section, followed by page, followed by subpage (e.g., 5/40.05 refers to section 5, page 40, subpage 05).

### Significance Codes

Each drug-drug interaction monograph has been assigned a significance code based on three major factors: potential harm to the patient, frequency and predictability of occurrence, and degree and quality of documentation. The significance code is to be considered applicable only to the agents that appear in the monograph title. The related drugs that are mentioned are not given a significance code.

Code 1.
Highly clinically significant—Drug interactions that are of great potential harm to the patient, that are predictable or frequent, and that are well documented (see Appendix B for list of Code 1 interactions)

Code 2.
Moderately clinically significant—Drug interactions that are of moderate potential harm to the patient, that are less predictable or frequent, and that lack complete documentation

---

\* Older monographs in *Evaluations of Drug Interactions* lack this statement, and so it is missing in the corresponding monographs of the *Pocket Guide*.

Code 3.
Minimally clinically significant—Drug interactions that are of little potential harm to the patient, that have variable predictability or occur infrequently, and that have little documentation

Code 4.
Not clinically significant—Drug interactions in which documentation may be based on theoretical considerations, the effects are not clinically significant, and no adverse effects are expected

# Chapter One

# Analgesic Drug Interactions:

## Narcotics, Nonnarcotics, Nonsteroidal Anti-inflammatory Agents, and Agents for Gout

Analgesic

## Acetaminophen-Alcohol, Ethyl
**Significance:** 3—minimally clinically significant
**Potential Effects:** Chronic alcohol ingestion may potentiate acetaminophen toxicity.
**Recommendations:** Chronic alcohol abusers should be cautioned about enhancement of acetaminophen toxicity by alcohol.
**Summary:** The risk of acetaminophen-induced hepatotoxicity may be potentiated by chronic, heavy alcohol consumption; however, contrasting data are available. An acute ingestion of alcohol and chronic alcohol intake may protect against hepatotoxicity.
**Related Drugs:** There are no drugs related to acetaminophen or alcohol.
**Mechanism:** Acetaminophen is metabolized and oxidized to a reactive toxic metabolite, inactivated by conjugation with glutathione. Alcohol may deplete glutathione stores.
**Detailed Information:** See *EDI*, 1/0.01

## Acetaminophen-Charcoal
**Significance:** 3—minimally clinically significant
**Recommendations:** Activated charcoal should be given as soon as possible after an acute acetaminophen overdose to reduce the absorption of acetaminophen. However, if charcoal is not used for acetaminophen overdose, the administration of these agents should be separated by as much time as possible.
**Summary:** There are data to show that activated charcoal significantly reduces the absorption of acetaminophen.
**Related Drugs:** There are no drugs related to acetaminophen.
**Mechanism:** Activated charcoal adsorbs acetaminophen in the gastrointestinal tract, limiting its absorption.
**Detailed Information:** See *EDI*, 1/0.10

## Acetaminophen-Isoniazid
**Significance:** 3—minimally clinically significant
**Potential Effects:** Isoniazid decreased the clearance of acetaminophen which may lead to hepatotoxicity.
**Recommendations:** The use of concurrent isoniazid and acetaminophen should be approached with caution. Hepatic function should be monitored for signs of acetaminophen hepatotoxicity.
**Summary:** Isoniazid decreases the clearance of acetaminophen and can cause severe hepatotoxicity.
**Related Drugs:** There are no drugs related to acetaminophen or isoniazid.
**Mechanism:** With large doses of acetaminophen, the metabolic pathways become saturated, leading to the formation of a toxic intermediate. A hepatic enzyme has been shown to catalyze this toxic intermediate and this enzyme is induced by isoniazid.
**Detailed Information:** See *EDI*, 1/0.15

## Acetaminophen-Oral Contraceptive Agents
**Significance:** 3—minimally clinically significant
**Potential Effects:** Oral contraceptive agents may increase the metabolism of acetaminophen.
**Recommendations:** It is not known if larger doses of acetaminophen would be required in women receiving oral contraceptive agents.
**Summary:** Oral contraceptive agents have been shown to increase the metabolism of acetaminophen.
**Related Drugs:** There were no differences found in the pharmacokinetics of acetaminophen with women taking conjugated estrogens. There are no drugs related to acetaminophen.

**Mechanism:** The acetaminophen glucuronide metabolite was increased in women taking oral contraceptive agents.
**Detailed Information:** See *EDI*, 1/0.21

## Acetaminophen-Phenobarbital

**Significance:** 3—minimally clinically significant
**Potential Effects:** Phenobarbital enhances the metabolism of acetaminophen. This enhancement may lead to increased acetaminophen induced hepatic damage because of the depletion of enzymes that inactivate the toxic metabolite.
**Recommendations:** The concurrent use of these agents need not be avoided. However, some patients may be at a greater risk of developing hepatotoxicity.
**Summary:** The concurrent administration of acetaminophen and phenobarbital may result in an increased risk of hepatotoxicity and hepatic necrosis. However, conflicting data are available.
**Related Drugs:** Primidone has shown to increase the clearance of acetaminophen and decrease its half-life and area-under-curve. A similar interaction may be expected to occur between acetaminophen and other barbiturates. There are no drugs related to acetaminophen.
**Mechanism:** Phenobarbital may increase the formation of acetaminophen's toxic metabolite, normally inactivated by conjugation with glutathione. Excessive metabolite formation may deplete glutathione.
**Detailed Information:** See *EDI*, 1/0.23

## Acetaminophen-Phenytoin

**Significance:** 2—moderately clinically significant
**Potential Effects:** Concurrent use may result in increased acetaminophen clearance and depletion of glutathione stores, leading to potential acetaminophen toxicity.
**Recommendations:** No specific precautions are required; however, patients may be at a greater risk of developing hepatotoxicity should acetaminophen overdose occur. Treatment of acetaminophen poisoning in patients receiving phenytoin may need to be modified.
**Summary:** Concurrent administration of acetaminophen and phenytoin may result in an increased clearance and reduced bioavailability of acetaminophen, potentially increasing the formation of a toxic acetaminophen metabolite, making patients taking phenytoin more prone to develop hepatotoxicity after an acetaminophen overdose.
**Related Drugs:** A similar interaction may occur between acetaminophen and the other hydantoin anticonvulsants. There are no drugs related to acetaminophen.
**Mechanism:** Phenytoin may increase the metabolism of acetaminophen by causing a marked induction of oxidation and glucuronidation, leading to the formation of acetaminophen's toxic metabolite, normally inactivated by conjugation. This metabolite binds covalently to hepatic tissue macromolecules and can cause oxidative stress, tissue damage, or necrosis.
**Detailed Information:** See *EDI*, 1/0.30

## Acetaminophen-Propranolol

**Significance:** 3—minimally clinically significant
**Potential Effects:** Propranolol may decrease the metabolism of acetaminophen leading to increased levels.

## Analgesic

**Recommendations:** The concurrent use of these agents need not be avoided in patients with normal hepatic function. Patients with decreased hepatic function should be carefully monitored for increased acetaminophen levels if these agents are used concurrently.

**Summary:** There are data to show that acetaminophen concentrations were increased with concurrent propranolol. However, contrasting data have shown propranolol to have no significant effect on acetaminophen metabolism.

**Related Drugs:** Other beta-blocking agents that are hepatically metabolized may be expected to interact with acetaminophen. There are no drugs related to acetaminophen.

**Mechanism:** Propranolol may inhibit the oxidation and glucuronidation pathways in the liver, leading to the reduction in the clearance of acetaminophen.

**Detailed Information:** See *EDI*, 1/0.35

## Acetaminophen-Ranitidine

**Significance:** 3—minimally clinically significant

**Potential Effects:** Coadministration of acetaminophen and ranitidine may result in an increase in acetaminophen plasma concentrations.

**Recommendations:** Caution should be used when coadministering acetaminophen and ranitidine. Acetaminophen should be given at least one hour after ranitidine administration to avoid an increase in acetaminophen plasma concentrations.

**Summary:** Coadministration of acetaminophen and ranitidine may result in an increase in acetaminophen plasma concentrations.

**Related Drugs:** No significant changes in acetaminophen pharmacokinetics have been documented when given with cimetidine; however, changes in acetaminophen pharmacokinetics were noted when it was administered one hour after cimetidine. It is not known if a similar interaction would occur between acetaminophen and other $H_2$ receptor antagonists. There are no drugs related to acetaminophen.

**Mechanism:** Ranitidine and cimetidine have been shown *in vitro* to be weak inhibitors of acetaminophen glucuronyltransferase activity. Ranitidine may inhibit metabolism of acetaminophen, causing an increase in peak plasma levels.

**Detailed Information:** See EDI, 1/0.40

## Acetaminophen-Sulfinpyrazone

**Significance:** 3—minimally clinically significant

**Potential Effects:** Sulfinpyrazone may increase the toxic effects of acetaminophen on the liver, especially in cases of acetaminophen overdose.

**Recommendations:** Avoid using these agents together. If they are used together, liver function should be monitored.

**Summary:** Sulfinpyrazone has been reported to increase the clearance of acetaminophen and reduce its half-life. The increased clearance may lead to a depletion of hepatic glutathione, leading to hepatic necrosis.

**Related Drugs:** Probenecid reduces the hepatic formation of acetaminophen glucuronide. There are no drugs related to acetaminophen.

**Mechanism:** Sulfinpyrazone enhances the elimination of acetaminophen, leading to the formation of acetaminophen's toxic metabolite, normally inactivated by conjugation with glutathione. Excessive metabolite formation may deplete glutathione.

**Detailed Information:** See *EDI*, 1/0.50

## Analgesic

### Acetaminophen-Terfenadine

**Significance:** 2—moderately clinically significant

**Potential Effects:** Concurrent administration of terfenadine with high dose acetaminophen administration may result in increased terfenadine levels and cardiotoxicity.

**Recommendations:** Concurrent use of terfenadine and large doses of acetaminophen should be approached with caution.

**Summary:** In a single case report, concomitant administration of terfenadine and acetaminophen resulted in Torsades de Pointes, a serious ventricular arrhythmia.

**Related Drugs:** Although documentation is lacking, a similar reaction would be expected to occur between large doses of acetaminophen and astemizole. Increased serum levels of loratadine may also be expected; however, elevated levels of loratadine have not been shown to produce Torsades de Pointes. Cetirizine is excreted mostly as unchanged drug; lack of metabolism suggests that this agent is unlikely to interact like terfenadine or astemizole.

**Mechanism:** The formation of the N-acetyl-p-aminobenzoquinone imine from acetaminophen has been shown to inhibit the cytochrome $P450_{3A4}$ isozyme. It is postulated that high dose acetaminophen administration resulted in accumulation of terfenadine and Torsades de Pointes.

**Detailed Information:** See *EDI*, 1/0.63

### Alfentanil-Erythromycin

**Significance:** 2—moderately clinically significant

**Potential Effects:** Erythromycin inhibits the metabolism of alfentanil, resulting in increased levels.

**Recommendations:** Caution should be used if alfentanil is administered to patients maintained on erythromycin. The dose of alfentanil may need to be decreased or the use of alfentanil may need to be avoided.

**Summary:** A study has shown that the clearance of alfentanil is decreased by erythromycin.

**Related Drugs:** A like interaction may occur between alfentanil and other macrolide antibiotics. Whether an interaction would occur between erythromycin and narcotic analgesics is unknown.

**Mechanism:** This interaction may occur as a result of competitive inhibition of alfentanil by erythromycin.

**Detailed Information:** See *EDI*, 1/0.65

### Alfentanil-Fluconazole

**Significance:** 3—minimally clinically significant

**Potential Effects:** Concurrent fluconazole may decrease alfentanil clearance and increase alfentanil-induced subjective effects.

**Recommendations:** Patients should be carefully monitored for changes in alfentanil serum levels and drug effects with concurrent use of fluconazole. The dose of alfentanil may need to be adjusted.

**Summary:** Concurrent intravenous or oral fluconazole may decrease alfentanil clearance, increase alfentanil mean elimination half-life, and increase alfentanil-induced respiratory depression.

**Related Drugs:** Serum methadone peak and trough concentrations increased when given with fluconazole. A similar interaction may occur between fluconazole and other narcotic analgesics. It is not known whether an interaction would occur between other imidazole antifungal agents and narcotic analgesics.

## Analgesic

**Mechanism:** Alfentanil is metabolized by cytochrome $P450_{3A}$ isoenzymes (predominately by cytochrome $P450_{3A4}$) and fluconazole is a fairly strong inhibitor of cytochrome $P450_{3A}$ isoenzymes; therefore, it is postulated that fluconazole may inhibit alfentanil metabolism.
**Detailed Information:** See *EDI*, 1/0.67

## Allopurinol-Aluminum Hydroxide

**Significance:** 3—minimally clinically significant
**Potential Effects:** Aluminum hydroxide may decrease the absorption of allopurinol. This may lead to a decrease in allopurinol action, resulting in increased uric acid levels.
**Recommendations:** Patients should be advised to take aluminum hydroxide at least three hours after taking allopurinol because this was shown to circumvent the interaction.
**Summary:** Receiving concurrent allopurinol and aluminum hydroxide for high uric acid and phosphate concentrations will not decrease uric acid levels. When administration times were separated, uric acid levels were shown to decrease.
**Related Drugs:** All antacids may alter the pharmacokinetics of allopurinol. There are no drugs related to allopurinol.
**Mechanism:** Aluminum hydroxide may decrease the gastrointestinal absorption of allopurinol by changing gastrointestinal transit time or pH, or by binding or chelating allopurinol.
**Detailed Information:** See *EDI*, 1/0.70

## Allopurinol-Probenecid

**Significance:** 3—minimally clinically significant
**Recommendations:** The concurrent administration of allopurinol and probenecid need not be avoided. However, this regimen should be used cautiously in patients with impaired renal function because of the danger of urate or urate precursors forming in the kidney. Fluid intake should be maintained at a level of 3L/day in all patients taking these drugs. Alkalinization of the urine may also be desirable as a means of promoting and ensuring adequate uric acid clearance through the kidney.
**Summary:** Concurrent use of allopurinol and probenecid may decrease the effectiveness of allopurinol.
**Related Drugs:** A similar interaction can expect to occur with sulfinpyrazone. There are no drugs related to allopurinol.
**Mechanism:** Allopurinol may inhibit the metabolism of probenecid and probenecid may increase the renal excretion of oxypurinol (alloxanthine), resulting in a decrease in the inhibition of uric acid production.
**Detailed Information:** See *EDI*, 1/1.00

## Aspirin-Acetazolamide

**Significance:** 2—moderately clinically significant
**Potential Effects:** The concurrent use of these agents may result in acetazolamide or salicylate toxicity.
**Recommendations:** If concomitant administration is necessary, patients should be monitored for increased acetazolamide and/or salicylate serum levels or toxicity. One or both agents may need to be discontinued.
**Summary:** Concurrent administration of aspirin and acetazolamide leads to a decrease in clearance and plasma protein binding, and an increase in unbound acetazolamide. There are also reports of severe salicylate intoxication and the development of severe acid-base imbalance.

## Analgesic

**Related Drugs:** The concurrent administration of aspirin and dichlorphenamide may result in salicylate intoxication. An interaction may be expected to occur between acetazolamide and other salicylates. An interaction may not occur with aspirin and methazolamide.

**Mechanism:** Aspirin may inhibit the plasma protein binding of acetazolamide, inhibiting its renal tubular secretion. For salicylate intoxication, the interaction may result from metabolic acidemia, increasing the salicylate available.

**Detailed Information:** See *EDI*, 1/2.10

## Aspirin-Alcohol, Ethyl

**Significance:** 2—moderately clinically significant

**Recommendations:** The combination of alcohol and aspirin should be avoided in patients predisposed to gastrointestinal disease. Concurrent use does not appear to present a significant problem in normal subjects. Predisposed patients requiring an analgesic may use acetaminophen or buffered aspirin. Patients receiving aspirin for its hematologic (antiplatelet) effects should be cautioned about the potential hazards of concurrent alcohol use.

**Summary:** Aspirin or alcohol alone will disrupt the gastric mucosal barrier. Alcohol potentiates the erosive effects of aspirin resulting in increased fecal blood loss and may prolong bleeding time.

**Related Drugs:** A similar interaction does not occur with buffered salicylate products, choline salicylate, and diflunisal. Other salicylates have been found to effect clotting factor synthesis and are irritating to the gastric mucosa.

**Mechanism:** Aspirin breaks down the normal gastric mucosal barrier, resulting in injury and irritation to the gastrointestinal mucosa. Aspirin effects hemostasis and potentiates the prolonged bleeding time associated with aspirin therapy.

**Detailed Information:** See *EDI*, 1/3.00

## Aspirin-Aluminum Hydroxide, Magnesium Hydroxide

**Significance:** 2—moderately clinically significant

**Recommendations:** Patients should be counseled before initiating, switching, or discontinuing antacid use while on high dose salicylate therapy, since different antacids affect salicylate levels to varying degrees because of differing extents of urinary alkalinization. Patients using enteric-coated products should be advised not to ingest antacids simultaneously to avoid premature drug release from this particular dosage form.

**Summary:** Salicylate levels decrease following the concurrent administration of an antacid preparation containing aluminum hydroxide and magnesium hydroxide.

**Related Drugs:** A similar interaction is expected to occur with magnesium trisilicate, sodium bicarbonate, calcium carbonate, and salicylate preparations. There is conflicting data regarding the levels of salicylates with diflunisal.

**Mechanism:** The decreased serum salicylate concentration is attributed to an increase in urine alkalinity and an increase in gastric pH, effecting the delivery of the salicylate to the gastric area or a decreased gastric transit time.

**Detailed Information:** See *EDI*, 1/5.00

## Aspirin-Charcoal

**Significance:** 3—minimally clinically significant

**Recommendations:** Because of aspirin's rapid absorption, it has been recommended that activated charcoal be given as soon as possible in an acute aspirin overdose. A 10:1 ratio of activated charcoal to aspirin has also been recommended. However, if charcoal is not used for aspirin overdose, it may be advisable to separate the administration of aspirin and charcoal by as much time as possible.

**Summary:** Concomitant administration of activated charcoal and aspirin significantly reduces the gastrointestinal absorption of aspirin.

**Related Drugs:** A like interaction is expected with other salicylates.

**Mechanism:** Activated charcoal adsorbs aspirin in the gastrointestinal tract, limiting its absorption.

**Detailed Information:** See *EDI*, 1/6.10

## Aspirin-Dipyridamole

**Significance:** 3—minimally clinically significant

**Potential Effects:** Dipyridamole may decrease the metabolism of aspirin resulting in increased levels.

**Recommendations:** The clinical significance of this interaction has not been determined. Aspirin levels may need to be monitored during concurrent therapy with dipyridamole.

**Summary:** There are data to show that dipyridamole causes an increase in the peak concentration and area-under-curve of unchanged aspirin.

**Related Drugs:** It is not known if dipyridamole would interact with other salicylates. There are no drugs related to dipyridamole.

**Mechanism:** Dipyridamole may decrease the deacetylation of aspirin, resulting in increased levels.

**Detailed Information:** See *EDI*, 1/6.30

## Aspirin-Ginkgo

**Significance:** 3—minimally clinically significant

**Potential Effects:** The addition of *Ginkgo biloba* to the therapy of a patient maintained on aspirin may result in increased bleeding times and possible hemorrhagic complications.

**Recommendations:** Caution should be observed if *Ginkgo biloba* is added to the therapy of a patient maintained on aspirin. Patients should be monitored for increased bleeding times and hemorrhagic complications.

**Summary:** The addition of *Ginkgo biloba* extract to the regimen of a patient maintained on aspirin may result in spontaneous bleeding and hemorrhagic complications.

**Related Drugs**: It is not known whether an interaction would occur between the other platelet aggregation inhibitors and *Ginkgo biloba* extract.

**Mechanism:** Although the mechanism of this interaction is not known, the terpenoid ginkgolide B, a component of *Ginkgo biloba,* has been shown to be a potent inhibitor of platelet-activating factor which is necessary for platelet aggregation. The long-term use of this extract was associated with subdural hematomas and increased bleeding time.

**Detailed Information:** See *EDI*, 1/6.50

Analgesic

## Aspirin-Griseofulvin

**Significance:** 3—minimally clinically significant

**Potential Effects:** The addition of griseofulvin to an aspirin regimen may result in decreased plasma salicylate levels.

**Recommendations:** It is recommended that an alternative nonsteroidal anti-inflammatory agent be used if possible. However, if concurrent aspirin and griseofulvin therapy is necessitated, the doses of griseofulvin and aspirin could be staggered and the salicylate serum concentration should be carefully monitored. The dose of aspirin may need to be adjusted.

**Summary:** There are data to show concurrent administration of aspirin and griseofulvin resulted in a marked decrease in the salicylate serum concentrations.

**Related Drugs:** It is unknown whether an interaction would occur between griseofulvin and other salicylates. There are no drugs related to griseofulvin.

**Mechanism:** The mechanism of this interaction is not known; however, the most probable mechanism involves the interference of aspirin absorption by griseofulvin.

**Detailed Information:** See *EDI*, 1/6.60

## Aspirin-Methylprednisolone

**Significance:** 2—moderately clinically significant

**Potential Effects:** Methylprednisolone may decrease salicylate levels, possibly by increasing the glomerular filtration rate.

**Recommendations:** Although serum salicylate levels may decrease with concurrent methylprednisolone therapy, the decrease appears to be transient. However, salicylate levels should be closely monitored since an increased dosage of aspirin may be necessary if the decrease in levels persists. Also, it is important to be aware of significantly increased salicylate levels when the corticosteroid dosage is decreased or discontinued.

**Summary:** There are data to show that plasma concentrations of salicylate decrease and clearance increases with concomitant methylprednisolone or prednisone. This may lead to unwarranted increases in the dosage of aspirin.

**Related Drugs:** A similar interaction is expected with dexamethasone, triamcinolone, methylprednisolone and other corticosteroids.

**Mechanism:** Corticosteroids have been shown to increase the glomerular filtration rate, and the decreased salicylate concentrations may be the result of an increase in salicylate clearance induced by prednisone.

**Detailed Information:** See *EDI*, 1/7.00

## Aspirin-Nitroglycerin

**Significance:** 3—minimally clinically significant

**Recommendations:** Although the clinical effects of the interaction may not be significant, physicians should be aware that nitroglycerin's vasodilatory and hemodynamic effects may be altered by the concomitant administration of aspirin.

**Summary:** There are data to show that aspirin increases the amount of nitroglycerin absorbed and the peak concentration of nitroglycerin.

**Related Drugs:** A similar interaction is expected with aspirin and other salicylates and with nitroglycerin and other nitrate derivatives.

**Mechanism:** Aspirin may increase the amount of nitroglycerin absorbed through vasodilation or it may modify the effect of nitroglycerin.

**Detailed Information:** See *EDI*, 1/8.10

## Analgesic

### Aspirin-Oral Contraceptive Agents
**Significance:** 3—minimally clinically significant
**Potential Effects:** The effect of aspirin may be decreased by the short-term use of oral contraceptive agents.
**Recommendations:** Patients on chronic aspirin therapy who are taking oral contraceptive agents for a short time may require a temporary increase in the aspirin dosage.
**Summary:** There are data to show that a low dose estrogen contraceptive agent significantly reduces the pharmacokinetics of aspirin.
**Related Drugs:** A similar interaction may be expected to occur between oral contraceptive agents and other salicylates.
**Mechanism:** Oral contraceptive agents may induce the metabolism of aspirin.
**Detailed Information:** See *EDI*, 1/8.21

### Codeine-Quinidine
**Significance:** 2—moderately clinically significant
**Potential Effects:** The concurrent administration of codeine and quinidine may result in a decrease in the pharmacologic effects of codeine.
**Recommendations:** Patients receiving concurrent therapy with codeine and quinidine should be observed for decreased effectiveness of codeine. An alternative analgesic, such as morphine, may need to be considered.
**Summary:** Concurrent administration of codeine and quinidine may result in a decrease in the pharmacologic effects of codeine. Studies show that this decrease is significant in patients who are extensive metabolizers of debrisoquine.
**Related Drugs:** Dihydromorphine levels decreased when quinidine was given with dihydrocodeine, but no significant changes in dihydrocodeine's pharmacologic effects were observed. Pretreatment with diphenoxylate has resulted in a decrease in the $C_{max}$ and an increase in the $T_{max}$ of quinidine; the effects of quinidine on diphenoxylate have not been evaluated. Quinidine caused no significant changes in the pharmacologic effects of hydrocodone or oxycodone, despite some alterations in pharmacokinetic parameters.
**Mechanism:** It is believed that quinidine inhibits the O-demethylation of codeine to its active metabolite, morphine, at the cytochrome $P450_{2D6}$ isoenzyme.
**Detailed Information:** See *EDI*, 1/8.23

### Colchicine-Cyclosporine
**Significance:** 2—moderately clinically significant
**Potential Effects:** Concurrent use of cyclosporine and colchicine may result in elevated cyclosporine blood levels, nephrotoxicity, and myopathy.
**Recommendations:** Patients maintained on a cyclosporine regimen should be carefully monitored for changes in cyclosporine serum levels and renal status if colchicine is added to therapy. The dose of cyclosporine may need to be decreased or colchicine may need to be discontinued. In patients with familial Mediterranean fever in whom colchicine is required, an alternative immunosuppressant agent may be required.
**Summary:** Coadministration of cyclosporine and colchicine may result in an elevation of cyclosporine blood levels, nephrotoxicity, and myopathy.
**Related Drugs:** There are no drugs related to cyclosporine or colchicine.

# Analgesic

**Mechanism:** Colchicine may increase cyclosporine absorption or decrease hepatic metabolism, resulting in increased cyclosporine levels, although the exact mechanism is unknown.
**Detailed Information:** See *EDI*, 1/8.24

## Diclofenac-Cyclosporine

**Significance:** 2—moderately clinically significant
**Potential Effects:** The concurrent use of these agents may result in a decreased renal function.
**Recommendations:** Monitor renal function closely if these agents are used together. Diclofenac may need to be discontinued.
**Summary:** Decreased renal function resulted when diclofenac was added to the therapy of a patient maintained on cyclosporine. Renal function did not respond to lowering the cyclosporine dose.
**Related Drugs:** Sulindac, ketoprofen, mefanamic acid, naproxen and piroxicam have been reported to cause a similar interaction with cyclosporine. Although documentation is lacking, a similar interaction may be expected to occur between cyclosporine and the other nonsteroidal anti-inflammatory agents based on pharmacologic similarity and the proposed mechanism. It is unknown if there is a similar interaction between tacrolimus and nonsteroidal anti-inflammatory agents.
**Mechanism:** It has been suggested that nonsteroidal anti-inflammatory drugs may enhance cyclosporine nephrotoxicity by inhibiting prostaglandin synthesis. It has been postulated that nonsteroidal anti-inflammatory drugs may enhance the toxic effects of cyclosporine independent of any change in cyclosporine level.
**Detailed Information:** See *EDI*, 1/8.25

## Fenoprofen-Phenobarbital

**Significance:** 3—minimally clinically significant
**Potential Effects:** Phenobarbital may increase the metabolism of fenoprofen, resulting in decreased effects.
**Recommendations:** Although the concurrent use of these agents need not be avoided, it is prudent to be aware of the possibility of this interaction as the dose of fenoprofen may need to be increased.
**Summary:** There are data to show that phenobarbital decreases the area-under-curve and increases the elimination rate constant of fenoprofen.
**Related Drugs:** A similar interaction may occur between phenobarbital and other NSAIAs and between fenoprofen and other barbiturates. The concurrent use of phenylbutazone and phenobarbital may reduce the half-life of phenylbutazone.
**Mechanism:** Phenobarbital may increase the metabolism of fenoprofen by inducing the hepatic microsomal enzymes responsible for its metabolism.
**Detailed Information:** See *EDI*, 1/8.30

## Fentanyl-Propranolol

**Significance:** 3—minimally clinically significant
**Potential Effects:** Propranolol decreases the first pass extraction of fentanyl by the lungs, resulting in increased systemic availability.
**Recommendations:** Monitor patients for increased effects of fentanyl if coadministered with propranolol.
**Summary:** There are data to show that coadministration of propranolol and fentanyl may lead to an increased entry of fentanyl into the systemic circulation.

## Analgesic

**Related Drugs:** It is not known whether an interaction would occur between propranolol and other narcotic analgesics or between fentanyl and other beta blocking agents.

**Mechanism:** The mechanism for this interaction is not known. Data are available to show that propranolol can alter the amount of fentanyl which accumulates in the lungs.

**Detailed Information:** See *EDI*, 1/8.35

## Gold Sodium Thiomalate-Naproxen

**Significance:** 2—moderately clinically significant

**Potential Effects:** Concurrent use of these agents may result in pneumonitis.

**Recommendations:** One or both agents should be discontinued if pneumonitis develops.

**Summary:** There are data to show that concurrent gold sodium thiomalate and naproxen have resulted in toxic pneumonitis.

**Related Drugs:** It is not known whether an interaction would occur between gold sodium thiomalate and other NSAIAs. A similar interaction may be expected between naproxen and other gold compounds.

**Mechanism:** Gold sodium thiomalate inhibits the lymphocyte proliferation and naproxen may cause additional immunosuppressive effects. Gold compounds may have an inhibitory effect on cell-mediated immune response and naproxen may have an additive effect.

**Detailed Information:** See *EDI*, 1/8.37

## Gold Sodium Thiomalate-Tobacco

**Significance:** 3—minimally clinically significant

**Recommendations:** Further studies are needed to determine whether there is a similar effect on the uptake of gold by other cells, particularly monocytes, since the effect of gold on the function of the monocytes appears to be an important aspect of the antirheumatic activity of gold complexes. Therefore, no special precautions appear necessary at this time.

**Summary:** There are data to show that tobacco-smoking patients using gold sodium thiomalate have higher erythrocyte gold concentrations and lower plasma gold concentrations than nonsmokers.

**Related Drugs:** Evidence shows that tobacco smoking raised erythrocyte gold concentrations in patients receiving auranofin. A similar interaction may occur between tobacco smoking and the injectable gold compound, aurothioglucose.

**Mechanism:** Tobacco smokers have elevated concentrations of thiocyanate and cyanide which form complexes with gold. Gold also binds to albumin and in erythrocytes.

**Detailed Information:** See *EDI*, 1/8.41

## Ibuprofen-Baclofen

**Significance:** 3—minimally clinically significant

**Potential Effects:** Ibuprofen may cause a decrease in the clearance of baclofen, leading to toxicity.

**Recommendations:** Patients should be monitored for acute renal insufficiency and signs of baclofen toxicity (e.g., confusion, disorientation, bradycardia, hypothermia) when baclofen is administered with ibuprofen.

**Summary:** There are data to show that ibuprofen potentiates baclofen toxicity and increases serum blood urea nitrogen and creatinine levels.

Analgesic

**Related Drugs:** A similar interaction may occur between baclofen and other NSAIAs. There are no drugs related to baclofen.

**Mechanism:** Acute renal insufficiency secondary to ibuprofen therapy may result in a decreased clearance of baclofen and baclofen toxicity.

**Detailed Information:** See *EDI*, 1/8.43

## Indomethacin-Aluminum Hydroxide

**Significance:** 3—minimally clinically significant

**Potential Effects:** Aluminum hydroxide may reduce the rate and extent of indomethacin absorption.

**Recommendations:** Although the concurrent use of these agents need not be avoided, it may be best to separate their administration by as much time as possible.

**Summary:** Aluminum hydroxide may reduce the rate and extent of indomethacin absorption.

**Related Drugs:** Due to conflicting results, it is difficult to determine if an interaction would occur between indomethacin and other antacids or between aluminum hydroxide and other NSAIAs.

**Mechanism:** Aluminum hydroxide may adsorb indomethacin or indomethacin may form an insoluble aluminum salt.

**Detailed Information:** See *EDI*, 1/8.50

## Indomethacin-Aspirin

**Significance:** 3—minimally clinically significant

**Recommendations:** Because concurrent administration of these agents offers no therapeutic advantage over higher doses of either drug alone, concurrent use is not recommended. However, the clinical significance of this interaction appears to be minimal, and concomitant use need not be avoided.

**Summary:** There are data to show that large doses of aspirin may decrease the serum levels of indomethacin.

**Related Drugs:** Sodium salicylate has been shown to interact with other NSAIAs. Documentation is lacking regarding an interaction between indomethacin and other salicylates.

**Mechanism:** The mechanism is not fully known; however, aspirin decreases the bioavailability of oral indomethacin.

**Detailed Information:** See *EDI*, 1/9.00

## Indomethacin-Cimetidine

**Significance:** 3—minimally clinically significant

**Potential Effects:** Cimetidine may decrease indomethacin levels.

**Recommendations:** Indomethacin and cimetidine may be given together since the therapeutic effectiveness of indomethacin was not shown to be affected.

**Summary:** There are data to show that patients who receive indomethacin and cimetidine have a decreased plasma concentration, urinary excretion and metabolites of indomethacin.

**Related Drugs:** Because of conflicting data, it is difficult to determine if an interaction would occur between cimetidine and other NSAIAs or between indomethacin and other $H_2$-receptor antagonists.

**Mechanism:** Cimetidine may decrease the absorption of indomethacin.

**Detailed Information:** See *EDI*, 1/10.01

## Analgesic

### Indomethacin-Nitroglycerin
**Significance:** 3—minimally clinically significant

**Recommendations:** When administered orally, indomethacin does not appear to adversely alter the beneficial effect of nitroglycerin on exercise tolerance in patients with stable angina of effort. Currently no information is available concerning the concomitant administration of these drugs in patients with unstable angina or myocardial infarction. If the drugs are coadministered, these latter patients should be observed for a possible reduction in anginal threshold and/or myocardial ischemia.

**Summary:** There are data to show that indomethacin reduces the vasodilator effect of nitroglycerin. However, all data do not support this.

**Related Drugs:** A similar interaction may occur between indomethacin and other nitrate derivatives and between nitroglycerin and other NSAIAs.

**Mechanism:** Nitroglycerin may stimulate the synthesis and release of prostacyclin and other prostaglandins which may be responsible for its vasodilatory effect. Indomethacin inhibits prostaglandin synthesis.

**Detailed Information:** See *EDI*, 1/10.10

### Indomethacin-Phenylpropanolamine
**Significance:** 2—moderately clinically significant

**Recommendations:** If indomethacin and phenylpropanolamine are to be used together, the patient's blood pressure should be monitored frequently within the first hour after both agents are administered. If a hypertensive episode should occur, phentolamine has been used to successfully reduce the blood pressure.

**Summary:** There are data to show that taking a preparation containing phenylpropanolamine may lead to the development of serious hypertension.

**Related Drugs:** There are no documented reports involving phenylpropanolamine and other NSAIAs. It may be possible that other sympathomimetics and other NSAIAs may interact similarly.

**Mechanism:** Phenylpropanolamine is an indirect-acting sympathomimetic possessing vasoconstrictive activity, and indomethacin may suppress the synthesis of the prostaglandins which normally reduces blood pressure by vasodilatation.

**Detailed Information:** See *EDI*, 1/11.00

### Indomethacin-Probenecid
**Significance:** 2—moderately clinically significant

**Potential Effects:** Probenecid may increase indomethacin levels, which may lead to an increase in side effects.

**Recommendations:** The use of these agents together need not be avoided. However, if increased side effects occur, the indomethacin dose may need to be decreased.

**Summary:** The administration of probenecid can reduce the plasma clearance and elevate the plasma levels of indomethacin.

**Related Drugs:** A similar interaction has been shown to occur between probenecid and ketoprofen and probenecid and naproxen and may be expected to occur between probenecid and other NSAIAs. It is unknown whether sulfinpyrazone interacts similarly with indomethacin.

**Mechanism:** Probenecid reduces nonrenal and possibly the biliary clearance of indomethacin. Probenecid may inhibit the glucuronidation of ketoprofen and renal excretion of ketoprofen conjugates.

**Detailed Information:** See *EDI*, 1/13.00

## Analgesic

### Meperidine-Chlorpromazine
**Significance:** 2—moderately clinically significant
**Recommendations:** The combination of meperidine and chlorpromazine is widely used as an operative premedicant. The dose of meperidine should be reduced by 25% to 50% when given with phenothiazines.
**Summary:** Chlorpromazine potentiates the sedative, hypotensive, and respiratory depressant effects of meperidine.
**Related Drugs:** Other phenothiazines, thioxanthenes, butyrophenones, dihydroindolones, and dibenzoxazepines may interact with meperidine. Fentanyl, hydromorphone and oxymorphone have been shown to interact with other phenothiazines. A similar interaction may occur with other narcotics.
**Mechanism:** Chlorpromazine increases the rate of appearance of normeperidine, a toxic metabolite of meperidine. Promethazine decreases the metabolism and prolongs the half-life of narcotic analgesics.
**Detailed Information:** See *EDI*, 1/15.00

### Meperidine-Phenelzine
**Significance:** 1—highly clinically significant
**Potential Effects:** Concurrent use of these agents may result in potentially fatal CNS excitation or depression.
**Recommendations:** Concurrent use of these agents should be avoided. If the interaction occurs, IV corticosteroids may be beneficial. This interaction may occur several days after phenelzine is discontinued.
**Summary:** Concomitant use of meperidine and phenelzine may result in excitatory and depressant effects on the CNS leading to deep coma and death.
**Related Drugs:** Pargyline, tranylcypromine, isocarboxazid, furazolidone and procarbazine have been reported to interact with meperidine. Dextromethorphan has interacted with phenelzine resulting in death. The administration of propoxyphene with phenelzine has resulted in sedation and somnolence. Nalorphine has reportedly enhanced depression. All narcotics should be used cautiously in the presence of MAO inhibitors.
**Mechanism:** Although the mechanism is not specifically known, the combination of meperidine and MAO inhibitors has been shown to increase serotonin. MAO inhibitors also act as enzyme inhibitors, allowing accumulation of toxic levels of the agent.
**Detailed Information:** See *EDI*, 1/17.00

### Meperidine-Phenobarbital
**Significance:** 3—minimally clinically significant
**Recommendations:** If increased sedation occurs or analgesic efficacy decreases following concurrent administration of phenobarbital and meperidine, the dosage of one or both agents should be adjusted accordingly.
**Summary:** The use of phenobarbital causes an increase in the clearance of meperidine, an increase in the cumulative excretion of normeperidine, and a decrease in the cumulative urinary excretion of meperidine.
**Related Drugs:** A similar interaction has been shown to occur with methadone and phenobarbital. The administration of propoxyphene has resulted in an increase in phenobarbital levels. Due to conflicting data, it is difficult to determine if an interaction would occur between phenobarbital and other narcotic analgesics. A similar interaction may be expected to occur between meperidine and other barbiturates.

## Analgesic

**Mechanism:** Phenobarbital induces the hepatic metabolism of meperidine, resulting in an increased formation of normeperidine.
**Detailed Information:** See *EDI*, 1/18.10

## Meperidine-Phenytoin

**Significance:** 3—minimally clinically significant
**Recommendations:** Oral doses of meperidine generate greater amounts of normeperidine than equal analgesic IV doses. Therefore, IV doses may be preferable to oral dosing in those receiving phenytoin. Also, to gain satisfactory analgesia, patients on long-term phenytoin therapy may require more frequent and larger doses of meperidine when phenytoin is being used concurrently.
**Summary:** The use of phenytoin may result in an increased clearance and plasma concentration of meperidine and a decreased elimination half-life and bioavailability.
**Related Drugs:** A similar interaction may occur between meperidine and other hydantoin anticonvulsants. An interaction may occur with other narcotic analgesics.
**Mechanism:** The probable mechanism of the increased elimination of meperidine may be due to the enhanced metabolism by phenytoin.
**Detailed Information:** See *EDI*, 1/19.00

## Methadone-Ammonium Chloride

**Significance:** 3—minimally clinically significant
**Recommendations:** It may be best to measure steady-state plasma levels in patients complaining of withdrawal symptoms during concurrent ammonium chloride. This interaction may be useful in the treatment of methadone intoxication, since the total body clearance of methadone can be increased by approximately 50% by lowering urinary pH to 5.1.
**Summary:** There are data to show that concurrent administration of methadone and ammonium chloride causes an increase in the renal clearance of methadone.
**Related Drugs:** Since all narcotics are excreted unchanged to some extent, an interaction between ammonium chloride and the other narcotics is expected to occur. Other agents that acidify the urine may also interact with methadone.
**Mechanism:** The renal clearance of methadone is highly influenced by urinary pH and the clearance will increase as the pH decreases. Above a pH of 6, metabolism is the main route of elimination.
**Detailed Information:** See *EDI*, 1/20.10

## Methadone-Diazepam

**Significance:** 3—minimally clinically significant
**Potential Effects:** Diazepam may increase the effects of methadone.
**Recommendations:** The concurrent use of methadone and diazepam need not be avoided; however, patients should be monitored for possible enhancement of methadone effects and respiratory depression when receiving concurrent diazepam.
**Summary:** There are data to show that the concurrent use of methadone and diazepam has resulted in an increase in pupillary constriction and scores on a subjective opioid effects rating scale.
**Related Drugs:** Propoxyphene has been shown to alter the pharmacokinetics of agents related to diazepam. There are data to show that meperidine given with diazepam or diazepam's related agents has resulted in a depressed respiratory rate. It is difficult to determine whether a similar effect would occur with diazepam and other narcotic analgesics or between methadone and other benzodiazepines.

Analgesic

**Mechanism:** The mechanism of this interaction is unknown; however, coadministration of methadone and diazepam does not result in altered pharmacokinetics of either agent.
**Detailed Information:** See *EDI*, 1/21.00

## Methadone-Didanosine

**Significance:** 3—minimally clinically significant
**Potential Effects:** The addition of methadone to a regimen including didanosine may decrease the absolute oral bioavailability of didanosine.
**Recommendations:** Concomitant use of didanosine and methadone should be used with caution. If it is deemed necessary to administer both medications, an adjustment of the dose of didanosine may be required.
**Summary:** Adding methadone to a regimen including didanosine may decrease the absolute oral bioavailability of didanosine, reducing the didanosine AUC and $C_{max}$ by 63% and 66%, respectively.
**Related Drugs:** Adding methadone to regimens including stavudine or zidovudine has resulted in decreased bioavailability of these two agents. Withdrawal symptoms developed after zidovudine was given to a patient stabilized on a levomethadone maintenance program, necessitating an increase in levomethadone dosage. It is not known whether an interaction would occur between methadone and other nucleoside analogue reverse transcriptase inhibitors or between didanosine and the other narcotics.
**Mechanism:** A methadone-induced delay in gastric motility may result in decreased rate and extent of didanosine and stavudine absorption, allowing greater opportunity for enzymes or acids to catalyze degradation of the antiretrovirals. Additional studies are needed to determine the exact mechanism. Methadone was shown to inhibit the formation of the primary metabolite of zidovudine in an *in vitro* study of human liver microsomes.
**Detailed Information:** See *EDI*, 1/8.27

## Methadone-Nevirapine

**Significance:** 2—moderately clinically significant
**Potential Effects:** Concurrent use of nevirapine and methadone resulted in decreased methadone serum levels.
**Recommendations:** Patients undergoing methadone maintenance should be monitored for symptoms of opiate withdrawal if nevirapine is added to their medication regimen. With concurrent methadone and nevirapine, the patient should be monitored for the possibility of methadone overdose if nevirapine is discontinued from concurrent therapy.
**Summary:** Concurrent use of nevirapine and methadone may result in decreased methadone serum levels, possibly causing withdrawal symptoms, and necessitating an increase in methadone dosage.
**Related Drugs:** Similar effects were noted when patients on methadone maintenance received nelfinavir and when they received ritonavir; no interaction has been observed with saquinavir or indinavir. Conversely, ritonavir appears to have caused a decrease in fentanyl clearance in one patient.
**Mechanism:** Nevirapine is metabolized through the cytochrome $P450_{3A4}$ isoenzyme and also induces its own metabolism. Methadone is also metabolized by the cytochrome $P450_{3A4}$ isoenzyme; therefore, when coadministered, nevirapine may induce the metabolism of methadone, leading to decreased serum levels and subsequent withdrawal symptoms.
**Detailed Information:** See *EDI*, 1/22.50

## Analgesic

### Methadone-Rifampin
**Significance:** 2—moderately clinically significant
**Potential Effects:** The addition of rifampin to the therapy of a patient maintained on methadone may result in an increase in methadone oral clearance and decreased serum levels, resulting in withdrawal symptoms.
**Recommendations:** In those patients receiving methadone, antituberculosis therapy with isoniazid should be well tolerated. However, rifampin alone or rifampin plus isoniazid may offer desirable therapeutic benefits. In those cases, methadone dosage may need to be increased within several days of beginning cotherapy.
**Summary:** Patients maintained on methadone in a maintenance program for addiction may experience withdrawal symptoms when rifampin therapy is instituted. Methadone plasma concentrations may be decreased by 33% to 68% in patients receiving concomitant rifampin compared with patients on nonrifampin regimens.
**Related Drugs:** Although documentation is lacking regarding a similar interaction with the other narcotics or between methadone and rifabutin, because of pharmacologic similarity an interaction may be expected to occur.
**Mechanism:** Rifampin decreased methadone plasma concentrations, increased the urinary excretion of methadone's major metabolite, and increased the oral clearance of methadone by fourfold. These results suggest that rifampin induces the hepatic metabolism of methadone. However, there was no consistent change in the methadone half-life, indicating that other mechanisms may be involved.
**Detailed Information:** See *EDI,* 1/23.00

### Morphine-Amitriptyline
**Significance:** 3—minimally clinically significant
**Potential Effects:** Concurrent use of these agents may result in enhanced analgesia.
**Recommendations:** Concurrent use of these agents may increase morphine levels, and this may be beneficial in some patients, although not consistently. Choice of a tricyclic antidepressant should be based on clinical evaluation.
**Summary:** There are data to show that amitriptyline significantly increases the bioavailability of morphine. Amitriptyline and other tricyclic antidepressants may enhance the analgesic effect of morphine. However, there are contrasting data to show that tricyclic antidepressants do not produce analgesia.
**Related Drugs:** Because of conflicting results, it is difficult to determine if an interaction would occur between amitriptyline and other narcotics or between morphine and other tricyclic antidepressants.
**Mechanism:** The increased analgesic effect may be due to the synergy produced by the two agents in a common neural circuit. The metabolism of desipramine may also be inhibited by methadone.
**Detailed Information:** See *EDI,* 1/24.10

### Morphine-Cimetidine
**Significance:** 2—moderately clinically significant
**Recommendations:** A severe interaction may occur with the concurrent use of these agents. If respiratory depression or other CNS side effects develop, the narcotic dose may need to be decreased or the drug may need to be discontinued. In one report, naloxone successfully reversed the CNS effects. However, no cause and effect relationship for an interaction has been established, and these agents need not be routinely avoided.

## Analgesic

**Summary:** There are data to show that the administration of cimetidine and morphine have led to serious CNS side effects. This interaction may be exacerbated in patients with pre-existing breathing disorders.

**Related Drugs:** A similar interaction may occur between cimetidine and other narcotic analgesics. Documentation is lacking regarding an interaction between morphine and other $H_2$-receptor antagonists.

**Mechanism:** Cimetidine may potentially exaggerate the effect of morphine by competitive inhibition, by reducing hepatic clearance and blood flow, or by preventing hepatic microsomal oxidation.

**Detailed Information:** See *EDI*, 1/25.00

## Morphine-Cyclosporine

**Significance:** 2—moderately clinically significant

**Potential Effects:** The concurrent administration of cyclosporine and morphine may result in the development of severe neurologic symptoms.

**Recommendations:** Cyclosporine may increase morphine's neuropsychosis symptoms (e.g., anxiety, aphasia, amnesia, severe confusion). Cyclosporine may also lessen withdrawal symptoms in morphine-dependent patients. Patients should be monitored closely for adverse events when administering these agents concurrently. There have been no reports of an increased incidence of graft rejection with the concurrent use of morphine and cyclosporine; however, further studies are needed.

**Summary:** Concurrent administration of cyclosporine and morphine resulted in the development of severe neurologic symptoms. It has been suggested that cyclosporine may have caused a decreased excitation threshold of the neuronal cell, thereby potentiating the dysphoric effect of morphine or causing the neuropsychiatric manifestation. Studies in mice have shown that cyclosporine is capable of attenuating the severity of morphine withdrawal upon naloxone administration.

**Related Drugs:** The analgesic effects of morphine, methadone, and fentanyl increased in animals that lack *P*-glycoprotein; therefore, *P*-glycoprotein may limit the access of these drugs to the brain. Meperidine and morphine-6-glucuronide effects were not increased. Morphine, morphine-6-glucuronide, methadone, meperidine, and loperamide are *P*-glycoprotein substrates in *in vitro* cell culture systems. It is not known whether an interaction would occur between cyclosporine and the other narcotics.

**Mechanism:** *P*-glycoprotein may limit the bioavailability of some opiates in the brain and spinal cord; therefore, administration of *P*-glycoprotein inhibitors, such as cyclosporine, might increase the sensitivity of the CNS to these opiates. If the immune system function is altered, the CNS opiate activity may be modulated. One study suggests that cyclosporine affects the CNS directly because it was shown that an immune system was not needed in mice to attenuate morphine withdrawal with coadministration of cyclosporine.

**Detailed Information:** See *EDI*, 1/28.50

## Morphine-Metoclopramide

**Significance:** 3—minimally clinically significant

**Potential Effects:** Metoclopramide may increase the sedation effects of oral extended release morphine.

**Recommendations:** Metoclopramide may increase the sedation and decrease the time to onset of sedation of morphine. Patients should be monitored for increased sedation when administering these agents concurrently.

## Analgesic

**Summary:** There are data to show that the administration of morphine and metoclopramide may lead to a faster onset of action of morphine and increased levels of sedation.

**Related Drugs:** It is not known if a similar interaction would occur between metoclopramide and other narcotics. There are no drugs related to metoclopramide.

**Mechanism:** Metoclopramide increases gastric emptying; therefore, the rate of morphine absorbed may be increased and the time to peak concentration decreased.

**Detailed Information:** See *EDI*, 1/26.10

## Naproxen-Alendronate

**Significance:** 2—moderately clinically significant

**Potential Effects:** Concurrent administration of alendronate and naproxen may result in synergistic gastric ulceration.

**Recommendations:** Caution is advised with the concurrent administration of bisphosphonates and nonsteroidal anti-inflammatory agents. The patient should be carefully monitored for increased gastric irritation and possible ulceration.

**Summary:** Concurrent administration of alendronate and naproxen resulted in synergistic gastric ulceration.

**Related Drugs:** Two studies in animal models demonstrated that the combination of a bisphosphonate and indomethacin caused an increase in the severity and incidence of gastric lesions when compared to indomethacin alone. An interaction may be expected to occur between other bisphosphonates and NSAIAs, although documentation is lacking.

**Mechanism:** Ulceration may be caused in part by bisphosphonate local irritation of the mucosa, along with the synergistic effects of the NSAIA.

**Detailed Information:** See EDI, 1/26.30

## Naproxen-Cholestyramine

**Significance:** 3—minimally clinically significant

**Potential Effects:** Cholestyramine may delay the absorption of naproxen.

**Recommendations:** Any potential interaction may be avoided by administering naproxen two hours prior to or four to six hours after cholestyramine.

**Summary:** There are data to show that cholestyramine delays the absorption of naproxen and there may be a delay in pain relief before steady-state concentrations of naproxen are achieved.

**Related Drugs:** The half-life of tenoxicam and piroxicam were reduced when coadministered with cholestyramine. Phenylbutazone absorption was shown to be delayed by cholestyramine. Cholestyramine has been shown to delay the absorption of acidic drugs. A similar interaction may occur between naproxen and other anion exchange resins.

**Mechanism:** As the pH of the surrounding fluid becomes more basic, more naproxen is adsorbed to the resin and the resin slows the rate of absorption of naproxen.

**Detailed Information:** See *EDI*, 1/27.00

## Oxyphenbutazone-Methandrostenolone

**Significance:** 3—minimally clinically significant

**Recommendations:** When oxyphenbutazone is administered concurrently with methandrostenolone, and possibly other anabolic steroids, the resulting increased serum oxyphenbutazone levels

## Analgesic

may increase the risk of adverse reactions. Patients receiving both agents should be monitored closely for oxyphenbutazone-induced toxicity.

**Summary:** When oxyphenbutazone and methandrostenolone are concurrently administered, serum oxyphenbutazone levels may be elevated.

**Related Drugs:** Because of conflicting results, it is difficult to determine whether an interaction would occur between sulfinpyrazone and methandrostenolone. A similar interaction may occur with other anabolic steroids and oxyphenbutazone.

**Mechanism:** Inhibition of oxyphenbutazone metabolism and the displacement of oxyphenbutazone from its binding site on serum albumin are the proposed mechanisms in this interaction.

**Detailed Information:** See *EDI,* 1/29.00

### Phenylbutazone-Charcoal

**Significance:** 3—minimally clinically significant

**Recommendations:** It has been recommended that activated charcoal be administered as soon as possible after an acute phenylbutazone overdose to significantly reduce the absorption of phenylbutazone. However, if charcoal is not being used for phenylbutazone overdose, it may be advisable to separate the administration of phenylbutazone and charcoal by as much time as possible.

**Summary:** The absorption of phenylbutazone was greatly reduced with the concurrent administration of phenylbutazone.

**Related Drugs:** Oxyphenbutazone may interact similarly with activated charcoal. There are no drugs related to charcoal.

**Mechanism:** Charcoal adsorbs phenylbutazone and prevents its absorption.

**Detailed Information:** See *EDI,* 1/30.10

### Phenylbutazone-Desipramine

**Significance:** 3—minimally clinically significant

**Recommendations:** Data on the clinical effects of this interaction are not available. Since both drugs are normally administered on a long-term basis and since only the rate, rather than the extent, of phenylbutazone absorption seems to be affected, the clinical significance may be minor. Patients may be monitored for possible decreased phenylbutazone effect if concurrent tricyclic antidepressant therapy is indicated.

**Summary:** Concurrent administration of phenylbutazone and desipramine has resulted in reduced plasma levels of phenylbutazone. This may lead to a diminished therapeutic effect of phenylbutazone.

**Related Drugs:** Oxyphenbutazone absorption is decreased by desipramine. Imipramine has been shown to decrease phenylbutazone absorption. It is unknown whether other tricyclic antidepressants or tetracyclic antidepressants will produce the same effect, but agents with significant anticholinergic effect may be expected to exert a similar effect.

**Mechanism:** Gastrointestinal absorption of phenylbutazone is inhibited or delayed from an anticholinergic inhibition of gastric emptying.

**Detailed Information:** See *EDI,* 1/31.00

### Phenylbutazone-Misoprostol

**Significance:** 3—minimally clinically significant

**Potential Effects:** Enhanced phenylbutazone-induced neurological side effects may result.

## Analgesic

**Recommendations:** Neurological side effects should be monitored with concurrent administration of phenylbutazone and misoprostol. Phenylbutazone may need to be discontinued.

**Summary:** There are data to show that the concurrent administration of phenylbutazone and misoprostol results in enhanced neurological side effects.

**Related Drugs:** There are no drugs related to misoprostol. It is not known whether an interaction would occur between misoprostol and other NSAIAs.

**Mechanism:** The mechanism of this interaction is unknown.

**Detailed Information:** See *EDI*, 1/33.00

### Probenecid-Clofibrate

**Significance:** 3—minimally clinically significant

**Recommendations:** Although the clinical significance was not determined, it is important to monitor patients and use a lower dose of clofibrate when necessary.

**Summary:** The concurrent use of probenecid and clofibrate has been shown to cause a reduction in renal and metabolic clearance of clofibric acid (metabolite of clofibrate), leading to an increase in the therapeutic and toxic effects of clofibrate.

**Related Drugs:** There are no drugs related to clofibrate. An interaction may occur between clofibrate and sulfinpyrazone.

**Mechanism:** The decrease in clofibric acid binding may be caused by direct displacement from plasma protein binding sites. Through competitive inhibition, probenecid may inhibit the formation of clofibric acid glucuronide, leading to accumulation of the glucuronide in the plasma with subsequent hydrolysis to clofibric acid.

**Detailed Information:** See *EDI*, 1/35.00

### Probenecid-Penicillamine

**Significance:** 3—minimally clinically significant

**Recommendations:** The concurrent use of these agents is contraindicated in hyperuricemic cystinuric patients. However, the clinical significance of this interaction was not determined in patients receiving penicillamine for reasons other than cystinuria. Therefore, these patients should be observed for a decreased effect of penicillamine.

**Summary:** There are data to show that the coadministration of these agents has resulted in increased cystine excretion and decreased cystine-penicillamine mixed disulfide excretion in the urine, reducing the beneficial effects of penicillamine.

**Related Drugs:** There are no drugs related to penicillamine. It is not known if sulfinpyrazone would interact with penicillamine.

**Mechanism:** The mechanism of the interaction is unknown.

**Detailed Information:** See *EDI*, 1/36.10

### Propoxyphene-Alcohol, Ethyl

**Significance:** 2—moderately clinically significant

**Recommendations:** It is unlikely that moderate amounts of alcohol and the usual doses of propoxyphene will result in a serious adverse reaction. However, patients should be advised about the dangers associated with concurrent ingestion of therapeutic doses of propoxyphene and large amounts of alcohol or excessive amounts of propoxyphene with any amount of alcohol. Naloxone has been used successfully to reverse propoxyphene-induced respiratory depression.

**Summary:** Concurrent ingestion of propoxyphene and alcohol may result in dangerous respiratory and CNS depression.

**Related Drugs:** An interaction may occur between alcohol and other narcotic analgesics.

**Mechanism:** Alcohol has been shown to increase the systemic availability of propoxyphene and lower the minimum lethal blood concentration of propoxyphene.

**Detailed Information:** See *EDI*, 1/37.00

## Propoxyphene-Amphetamine

**Significance:** 3—minimally clinically significant

**Recommendations:** The use of amphetamines and other indirect acting sympathomimetics for the treatment of propoxyphene-induced CNS depression is not recommended. Naloxone, a narcotic antagonist, has been shown to be effective in controlling both respiratory depression and convulsive seizures following propoxyphene overdoses and has not been shown to have proconvulsant activity.

**Summary:** Amphetamines, which may be used to treat propoxyphene-induced CNS depression, may increase the seizure potential of propoxyphene.

**Related Drugs:** A similar interaction is expected to occur with other indirect-acting sympathomimetics and propoxyphene. A like interaction is expected to occur with other narcotic analgesics and amphetamines.

**Mechanism:** Amphetamines produce CNS stimulation by indirectly increasing the release of norepinephrine and by impeding its neuronal reuptake.

**Detailed Information:** See *EDI*, 1/39.00

## Propoxyphene-Charcoal

**Significance:** 3—minimally clinically significant

**Recommendations:** It has been recommended that activated charcoal be used as adjunct therapy in an acute propoxyphene overdose to adsorb any propoxyphene remaining in the stomach. A specific narcotic antagonist such as naloxone should be administered to counteract any respiratory depression or convulsions caused by an overdose of propoxyphene. However, if charcoal is not being used for propoxyphene overdose, the administration of the two agents should be separated by as much time as possible.

**Summary:** There are data to show that activated charcoal significantly reduces plasma levels of propoxyphene.

**Related Drugs:** Documentation is lacking regarding a similar interaction between charcoal and the other narcotic analgesics.

**Mechanism:** Activated charcoal adsorbs propoxyphene in the gastrointestinal tract, limiting its absorption.

**Detailed Information:** See *EDI*, 1/40.10

## Propoxyphene-Orphenadrine

**Significance:** 4—not clinically significant

**Recommendations:** Although it may be prudent to be aware of a possible interaction, the concurrent use of these agents need not be avoided. If CNS effects do occur, they are probably caused by either agent alone or by an additive effect and may require a reduction in the dose or discontinuation of one or both agents.

**Summary:** An alleged interaction with the concurrent use of these agents cannot be substantiated. The CNS effects observed were similar to those reported for either agent alone.

## Analgesic

**Related Drugs:** A lack of interaction may be expected between orphenadrine and other narcotic analgesics, as well as between propoxyphene and other anti-parkinsonian anticholinergics.
**Mechanism:** The mechanism is unknown, but may be due to the combined effect on the central nervous system by both drugs.
**Detailed Information:** See *EDI*, 1/41.00

### Sulfinpyrazone-Aspirin

**Significance:** 2—moderately clinically significant
**Recommendations:** Aspirin and other salicylates, especially in high doses, should be avoided in patients taking sulfinpyrazone for its uricosuric effect.
**Summary:** There are data to show that aspirin antagonizes the uricosuric activity of sulfinpyrazone and sulfinpyrazone-induced uric acid excretion may be significantly inhibited by large doses of aspirin. However, contrasting data have shown that aspirin significantly increases the plasma clearance of sulfinpyrazone.
**Related Drugs:** Sodium salicylate has been shown to interact in a similar manner with sulfinpyrazone. A like interaction is expected to occur with other salicylates. Phenylbutazone has been shown to block the uricosuric action of large amounts of aspirin and vice versa. Oxyphenbutazone and probenecid may interact with aspirin.
**Mechanism:** Sulfinpyrazone and salicylates compete for common binding sites on plasma proteins and prevent sulfinpyrazone from reaching its site of action.
**Detailed Information:** See *EDI*, 1/43.00

### Sulfinpyrazone-Niacin

**Significance:** 3—minimally clinically significant
**Recommendations:** Patients should be monitored for a possible decrease in the uricosuric activity of sulfinpyrazone. Niacin may need to be discontinued if this occurs.
**Summary:** The concurrent use of sulfinpyrazone and niacin may inhibit the uricosuric action of sulfinpyrazone.
**Related Drugs:** There are no drugs related to niacin. An interaction may occur between niacin and probenecid.
**Mechanism:** It is not known if niacin interferes with the mechanism of action of sulfinpyrazone or if it is from the hyperuricemia that is a common side effect of niacin.
**Detailed Information:** See *EDI*, 1/45.00

### Sulfinpyrazone-Probenecid

**Significance:** 4—not clinically significant
**Recommendations:** The data concerning this drug interaction are inconclusive; therefore, no particular action need be taken. However, concurrent use might be avoided because the possible benefits of such therapy would be negligible.
**Summary:** There are data to show that the concurrent use of sulfinpyrazone and probenecid may produce an increase in uric acid secretion.
**Related Drugs:** There is no documentation of a similar interaction between probenecid and phenylbutazone or its metabolite oxyphenbutazone.
**Mechanism:** Probenecid blocks the renal tubular secretion of sulfinpyrazone and its major active metabolite.
**Detailed Information:** See *EDI*, 1/47.00

# Chapter Two

# Anesthetic and Neuromuscular Blocking Agents' Drug Interactions

## Anesthetic

### Bupivacaine-Diazepam

**Significance:** 3—minimally clinically significant

**Potential Effects:** Administration of diazepam prior to bupivacaine administration may result in increased serum levels of bupivacaine.

**Recommendations:** Patients receiving diazepam premedication prior to use of epidural bupivacaine should be closely monitored for an increase in the pharmacologic effects of bupivacaine. The dose of bupivacaine may have to be adjusted.

**Summary:** There are data to indicate that administration of diazepam will alter bupivacaine pharmacokinetics, resulting in increased levels of bupivacaine.

**Related Drugs:** An interaction may occur between bupivacaine and the other benzodiazepines, which undergo phase I metabolism. The other local anesthetics would be expected to interact similarly with diazepam.

**Mechanism:** Diazepam may inhibit the metabolism of bupivacaine, which has the same route of metabolism.

**Detailed Information:** See *EDI*, 2/0.01

### Bupivacaine-Ritodrine

**Significance:** 2—moderately clinically significant

**Potential Effects:** Concurrent use of these agents may result in beta adrenergic stimulation of the heart, resulting in hypotension and tachycardia.

**Recommendations:** Caution should be used with patients who have received ritodrine for preterm labor when an anesthetic is to be used during cesarean section. Anesthesia may have to be deferred to allow the betamimetic effects of ritodrine to subside. Patient's cardiac status should be closely monitored.

**Summary:** There are data to show that coadministration of bupivacaine and ritodrine has resulted in ventricular tachycardia, fibrillation and hypotension, necessitating cardiopulmonary resuscitation.

**Related Drugs:** A similar interaction can be expected to occur with other local anesthetic agents and ritodrine. There are no drugs related to ritodrine.

**Mechanism:** While the mechanism of this interaction is unknown, it is thought that unopposed beta-adrenergic stimulation of the heart occurred as a result of the residual effects of ritodrine and the sympathetic blockade of bupivacaine.

**Detailed Information:** See *EDI*, 2/0.03

### Enflurane-Isoniazid

**Significance:** 3—minimally clinically significant

**Recommendations:** If a patient receiving isoniazid is given enflurane anesthesia, renal function should be monitored, since enflurane induced nephrotoxicity may occur as a result of elevated serum fluoride levels induced by isoniazid in some patients.

**Summary:** There are data to show that administration of isoniazid and the use of enflurane anesthesia resulted in significantly elevated serum fluoride levels with transient polyuria.

**Related Drugs:** A similar interaction may be expected to occur between isoniazid and other fluorinated inhalation anesthetics. There is evidence that isoniazid treatment increased the hepatic microsomal defluorination of isoflurane, methoxyflurane and enflurane. There are no drugs related to isoniazid.

**Mechanism:** Isoniazid may increase the metabolism of enflurane by enzyme induction.

**Detailed Information:** See *EDI*, 2/0.10

Anesthetic

## Ether-Neomycin

**Significance:** 1—highly clinically significant

**Recommendations:** It is important to be prepared to treat the neuromuscular and respiratory depression that is frequently produced by this interaction, particularly if the aminoglycoside is administered intraperitoneally. If neuromuscular blockade and respiratory depression are encountered, the intravenous use of neostigmine (0.2 to 2.5 mg), calcium (1 g), and possibly sodium bicarbonate (dose not reported), either alone or concurrently, may be helpful in reversing the blockade in some but not all patients. The administration of analeptic agents (e.g., doxapram and nikethamide) is of no value. Supportive care and ventilatory assistance should be administered and continued until the neuromuscular blockade has passed. Vital signs should be monitored because secondary circulatory collapse may occur, and volume replacement should be administered as necessary.

**Summary:** Depression of neuromuscular transmission can be produced independently with ether or neomycin. There are data to show that the coadministration of these drugs may enhance respiratory depression or may prolong neuromuscular blockade.

**Related Drugs:** Inhalation anesthetic agents such as cyclopropane, halothane, methoxyflurane, and nitrous oxide have been reported to interact with neomycin. A similar interaction may occur with other inhalation anesthetics and neomycin. Other aminoglycoside antibiotics are known to interact with ether. A similar interaction is expected to occur between ether and the other aminoglycosides, as well as the nonaminoglycoside antibiotics that possess neuromuscular blocking activity.

**Mechanism:** This interaction may be from a synergistic effect of the neuromuscular blocking properties of both agents due to reduced sensitivity of the postjunctional membrane and interference of transmitter release.

**Detailed Information:** See *EDI*, 2/1.00

## Etomidate-Verapamil

**Significance:** 3—minimally clinically significant

**Potential Effects:** Concurrent use of verapamil and etomidate may result in prolonged action of etomidate.

**Recommendations:** The concurrent use of verapamil and etomidate may result in a prolongation of anesthesia and Cheynes-Stokes respirations. Respiratory function should be monitored, and additional ventilatory support may be required.

**Summary:** The coadministration of verapamil may prolong the duration of action of etomidate anesthesia, leading to classic Cheynes-Stokes respirations and necessitating ventilatory assistance.

**Related Drugs:** It is not known whether an interaction would occur between etomidate and other calcium channel blocking agents. There are no drugs related to etomidate.

**Mechanism:** The mechanism of this interaction is not known.

**Detailed Information:** See *EDI*, 2/2.50

## Gallamine-Diazepam

**Significance:** 3—minimally clinically significant

**Potential Effects:** Diazepam may potentiate the neuromuscular blockade of gallamine.

**Recommendations:** The use of these agents together need not be avoided. However, patients should be monitored for an increased neuromuscular blockade when gallamine is given with diazepam.

**Summary:** There are data to show that administration of diazepam increased the magnitude of the neuromuscular blockade of gallamine and caused respiratory depression. However, contrasting data indicate that there is no interaction between these agents.

## Anesthetic

**Related Drugs:** No interaction was shown to occur between diazepam and tubocurarine or pancuronium. Because of conflicting results, it is difficult to determine if an interaction would occur between diazepam and other neuromuscular blocking agents. Diazepam was shown to reduce the neuromuscular blocking activity of the depolarizing agent succinylcholine; however, conflicting data are available. Because of conflicting results, it is not known if an interaction would occur between gallamine and other benzodiazepines.

**Mechanism:** The mechanism of this interaction is unknown. Diazepam may exert a peripheral action involving direct muscle depression and/or limit the release of acetylcholine, prolonging the neuromuscular blockade produced by gallamine.

**Detailed Information:** See *EDI,* 2/3.00

## Halothane-Epinephrine

**Significance:** 1—highly clinically significant

**Potential Effects:** The administration of these agents together may result in ventricular arrhythmias.

**Recommendations:** Avoid the use of these agents together. If IV epinephrine is necessary, the use of nitrous oxide should be considered.

**Summary:** There are data to indicate that administration of epinephrine during halothane anesthesia may lead to serious ventricular arrhythmias.

**Related Drugs:** Norepinephrine has been shown to interact with halothane in a manner similar to epinephrine. A similar interaction is expected to occur with isoproterenol, terbutaline, the other direct-acting sympathomimetics, the indirect-acting sympathomimetics or the mixed-acting sympathomimetics when coadministered with halothane. Chloroform, methoxyflurane, or enflurane when coadministered with epinephrine will increase the incidence of arrhythmias. A similar interaction is expected to occur between epinephrine and other inhalation anesthetics.

**Mechanism:** Although the exact mechanism for this interaction is unknown, the anesthetics' ability to precipitate arrhythmias is enhanced by events that stimulate the release of endogenous catecholamines.

**Detailed Information:** See *EDI,* 2/5.00

## Halothane-Phenytoin

**Significance:** 3—minimally clinically significant

**Recommendations:** Since it is not clear that phenytoin increases the likelihood of halothane-induced toxicity, no additional precautions are warranted. However, if patients receiving phenytoin show signs of hepatitis (fever, elevated transaminase levels, etc.), close monitoring of serum phenytoin concentrations and clinical signs of phenytoin toxicity (e.g., nystagmus, blurring of vision, ataxia) is indicated, and appropriate changes in doses should be made.

**Summary:** There are data to show that phenytoin may increase the likelihood of halothane-induced hepatotoxicity and the hepatic dysfunction may reduce the clearance of phenytoin, resulting in toxicity.

**Related Drugs:** Phenytoin and phenobarbital have been implicated in a patient's fatal fluroxene-induced hepatotoxicity. The hepatotoxicity is usually not seen with the other halogenated anesthetic agents; therefore, a similar interaction is not expected to occur. The other hydantoin anticonvulsants may interact with halothane similar to phenytoin.

**Mechanism:** Hepatotoxicity following halothane anesthesia is expected. Phenytoin metabolism is dependent on the liver microsomal system, and injury to the microsomal system from any source would be expected to inhibit phenytoin metabolism.
**Detailed Information:** See *EDI*, 2/7.00

## Halothane-Rifampin

**Significance:** 2—moderately clinically significant

**Recommendations:** Although a cause and effect relationship was never clearly established, these agents should be used with caution and only when necessary.

**Summary:** There are data to show that coadministration of rifampin and isoniazid may lead to serious hepatotoxicity.

**Related Drugs:** There are no drugs related to rifampin. A similar interaction is not expected to occur between rifampin and other halogenated inhalation anesthetics since hepatotoxicity is usually not observed with these agents.

**Mechanism:** The mechanism is unknown. However, it has been suggested that the interaction is from the combined effects of the two agents on the liver.

**Detailed Information:** See *EDI*, 2/9.00

## Ketamine-Diazepam

**Significance:** 2—moderately clinically significant

**Recommendations:** The clinician should be aware of this interaction, since a patient pretreated with diazepam may need a lower dose of ketamine.

**Summary:** There are data to show that when diazepam and ketamine were coadministered, patients experienced less initial tachycardia and hypertension. Patients also required a significantly lower dose of ketamine.

**Related Drugs:** Documentation is lacking regarding a similar interaction between ketamine and other benzodiazepines. There are no drugs related to ketamine.

**Mechanism:** The mechanism of this interaction is unknown.

**Detailed Information:** See *EDI*, 2/11.00

## Ketamine-Halothane

**Significance:** 2—moderately clinically significant

**Recommendations:** When halothane anesthesia is used, ketamine should be administered with caution. The patient's blood pressure should be carefully monitored, because the hypotension has been severe enough in some reports to necessitate the use of a vasopressor.

**Summary:** There are data to show that during halothane anesthesia, the concurrent use of ketamine caused a rapid increase in arteriolar peripheral resistance and a decrease in cardiac output, stroke volume and blood pressure.

**Related Drugs:** Similar effects were seen when ketamine was used with enflurane. A similar interaction is expected to occur with other halogenated inhalation anesthetics.

**Mechanism:** It is possible that halothane, acting as a sympatholytic, uncovers the direct negative inotropic effects of ketamine, resulting in significant hypotension.

**Detailed Information:** See *EDI*, 2/13.00

## Ketamine-Thyroid

**Significance:** 3—minimally clinically significant

**Recommendations:** Until further clinical studies are done, the concurrent use of these agents need not be avoided. However, if this interaction does occur, propranolol may be useful since it has been shown to control both the heart rate and the increase in blood pressure.

**Summary:** There are data to show that coadministration of thyroid replacement and ketamine resulted in hypertension and tachycardia.

**Related Drugs:** There are no drugs related to ketamine. A similar interaction is expected to occur between ketamine and other thyroid drugs.

**Mechanism:** The mechanism of this interaction is unknown. Ketamine produces hypertension and tachycardia, although less severely. Therefore, it is believed that thyroid replacement is the offender in this interaction.

**Detailed Information:** See *EDI*, 2/15.00

## Methoxyflurane-Secobarbital

**Significance:** 2—moderately clinically significant

**Recommendations:** Methoxyflurane should be avoided in patients who are receiving barbiturates. If the use of methoxyflurane is necessary, the barbiturate should be discontinued well in advance of administering this anesthetic.

**Summary:** There are data to show that coadministration of methoxyflurane and secobarbital will lead to renal insufficiency.

**Related Drugs:** A similar interaction has been documented with pentobarbital and methoxyflurane. A similar interaction between secobarbital and other halogenated anesthetic agents would not be expected. A similar interaction is expected to occur between methoxyflurane and other barbiturates.

**Mechanism:** Barbiturates, which induce hepatic microsomal enzymes, lead to an increased production of toxic metabolites, increasing the incidence of nephrotoxicity.

**Detailed Information:** See *EDI*, 2/17.00

## Methoxyflurane-Tetracycline

**Significance:** 2—moderately clinically significant

**Recommendations:** Until more is known concerning the possible effects of concurrent tetracycline and methoxyflurane administration on renal function, these drugs should not be used together. When alternate therapy is not possible, renal status should be carefully monitored. Concurrent administration of methoxyflurane and other antibiotics known to be nephrotoxic (e.g., aminoglycosides, polymyxin) should be avoided.

**Summary:** There are data to show that the concurrent administration of tetracycline and methoxyflurane may result in severe nephrotoxicity.

**Related Drugs:** Methoxyflurane is expected to interact with the other tetracyclines. Doxycycline may not exhibit a similar toxicity. Methoxyflurane is the only general anesthetic implicated as a causative agent of renal toxicity.

**Mechanism:** The concurrent administration of tetracycline and methoxyflurane may result in additive nephrotoxic effects or create a synergistic basis for the toxicity.

**Detailed Information:** See *EDI*, 2/19.00

Anesthetic

## Metocurine-Phenytoin

**Significance:** 2—moderately clinically significant

**Potential Effects:** Phenytoin may decrease the extent and length of neuromuscular blockade produced by metocurine.

**Recommendations:** Patients receiving phenytoin should be monitored for a decreased response to metocurine when it is administered concurrently. The metocurine dose may need to be increased. Atracurium may be considered as an alternative agent to metocurine.

**Summary:** There are data to show that administration of phenytoin with metocurine may decrease the extent of neuromuscular blockade and higher metocurine plasma concentrations were required to obtain neuromuscular blockade.

**Related Drugs:** A comparable interaction was shown to occur between pancuronium, vecuronium or atracurium with phenytoin; however, all data did not support this. Because of conflicting results, it is difficult to determine if an interaction would occur between phenytoin and other nondepolarizing neuromuscular blocking agents or depolarizing agents. A similar interaction is expected to occur between metocurine and other hydantoin anticonvulsants.

**Mechanism:** Phenytoin may increase anticholinesterase activity, resulting in a higher acetylcholine concentration at the neuromuscular junction.

**Detailed Information:** See *EDI*, 2/20.10

## Nitric Oxide-Alcohol, Ethyl

**Significance:** 2—moderately clinically significant

**Potential Effects:** A lower motor neuron disorder may result when nitric oxide is administered to a patient with chronic ethanol exposure.

**Recommendations:** Caution should be exercised when administering nitric oxide to patients with a history of chronic ethanol exposure.

**Summary:** Nitric oxide may have caused extensive lower motor neuron disorder in a patient with chronic ethanol exposure.

**Related Drugs:** There are no drugs related to nitric oxide, and it is not known if nitric oxide will react with other alcohols or glycols.

**Mechanism:** It is postulated that nitric oxide may mediate excitotoxicity generated by chronic alcohol use, resulting in neuronal disturbances.

**Detailed Information:** See *EDI*, 2/20.50

## Pancuronium-Aminophylline

**Significance:** 2—moderately clinically significant

**Recommendations:** Patients should be monitored during concurrent use of these agents, and the dose of the neuromuscular blocking agent may need to be increased.

**Summary:** There are data to show that the concurrent use of pancuronium and aminophylline causes resistance to the neuromuscular blockade, possibly leading to supraventricular tachycardia.

**Related Drugs:** There is a lack of documentation regarding a similar interaction between pancuronium and other theophylline derivatives, as well as an interaction between theophylline derivatives and other neuromuscular blocking agents.

**Mechanism:** The mechanism of this interaction is unknown.

**Detailed Information:** See *EDI*, 2/21.00

## Pancuronium-Azathioprine

**Significance:** 3—minimally clinically significant

**Recommendations:** Concurrent use or subsequent use of azathioprine following pancuronium administration should be avoided if neuromuscular blockade is desired. If concomitant use is necessary, the dose of pancuronium may need to be increased.

**Summary:** There are data to show that the administration of azathioprine antagonized the neuromuscular blocking action of pancuronium.

**Related Drugs:** There is evidence of azathioprine and gallamine reversing the neuromuscular blockade produced by tubocurarine. A similar interaction is expected to occur with other nondepolarizing neuromuscular blocking agents. The effects of succinylcholine have been shown to be potentiated by azathioprine. Documentation is lacking on whether the other thiopurine antineoplastic agents interact similarly with pancuronium.

**Mechanism:** Azathioprine allows cyclic AMP to accumulate. This prolongs the time of depolarization, causing a generation of repetitive activity, and increases transmitter release.

**Detailed Information:** See *EDI*, 2/23.00

## Pancuronium-Carbamazepine

**Significance:** 3—minimally clinically significant

**Potential Effects:** Carbamazepine decreases the recovery time from pancuronium neuromuscular blockade.

**Recommendations:** Patients receiving carbamazepine should be monitored for a more rapid recovery from neuromuscular blockade when pancuronium is administered. The dose of pancuronium may need to be adjusted.

**Summary:** There are data to show that coadministration of carbamazepine and pancuronium leads to a shorter recovery from neuromuscular blockade.

**Related Drugs:** It is not known if a similar interaction would occur between carbamazepine and other nondepolarizing neuromuscular blocking agents or the depolarizing neuromuscular blocking agents. There are no drugs related to carbamazepine.

**Mechanism:** The mechanism of this interaction is not known.

**Detailed Information:** See *EDI*, 2/24.10

## Pancuronium-Clindamycin

**Significance:** 2—moderately clinically significant

**Recommendations:** These agents should be used concurrently with caution and only if concomitant use is necessary. It is important to be aware of prolonged neuromuscular blockade, and ventilatory assistance should be available if necessary.

**Summary:** There are data to show that clindamycin prolongs the neuromuscular blockade produced by pancuronium.

**Related Drugs:** A similar interaction with clindamycin or lincomycin and two nondepolarizing neuromuscular blocking agents has been documented. A similar interaction may be expected to occur with the other nondepolarizing neuromuscular blocking agents. Succinylcholine has also been reported to be enhanced by clindamycin.

**Mechanism:** There may be an additive or synergistic pharmacologic activity with these agents.

**Detailed Information:** See *EDI*, 2/25.00

## Pancuronium-Cyclosporine

**Significance:** 2—moderately clinically significant

**Potential Effects:** Cyclosporine may prolong the neuromuscular blocking effects of pancuronium.

**Recommendations:** Monitor patients carefully for prolonged neuromuscular blockade when these agents are used concurrently. Atracurium may be an alternative to pancuronium; however, studies are lacking.

**Summary:** There are data to show that coadministration of cyclosporine may prolong the neuromuscular blocking effects of pancuronium, leading to muscle paralysis, increased respiratory distress, blood pressure, heart rate, and respiratory rate.

**Related Drugs:** A similar interaction has been reported between cyclosporine and vecuronium. A similar interaction is expected to occur with other nondepolarizing neuromuscular blocking agents and cyclosporine. Succinylcholine is expected to interact to a lesser extent with cyclosporine. There are no drugs related to cyclosporine.

**Mechanism:** A nonionic surfactant used as a vehicle in cyclosporine may interfere with pancuronium, increasing the concentration at the neuromuscular junction.

**Detailed Information:** See *EDI*, 2/26.50

## Pancuronium-Furosemide

**Significance:** 3—minimally clinically significant

**Potential Effects:** Furosemide may prolong the neuromuscular blockade of pancuronium because of hypokalemia.

**Recommendations:** Avoiding hypokalemia can reduce the potential risks of this interaction in a patient receiving diuretic therapy who will be given pancuronium. The serum potassium level should be determined and corrected if necessary to avoid the possibility of prolonged neuromuscular blockade from a hypokalemic state.

**Summary:** There are data to show that administration of furosemide with pancuronium causes an increase in recovery times.

**Related Drugs:** Theoretically, an enhanced neuromuscular blockade can be predicted to arise from potassium-depleting diuretics and d-tubocurarine. A similar interaction can occur between tubocurarine and other potassium-depleting diuretics and thiazide-related diuretics, as well as with other neuromuscular blocking agents and furosemide.

**Mechanism:** The neuromuscular function is potassium dependent and the disruption of extracellular potassium levels by furosemide could enhance actions of pancuronium.

**Detailed Information:** See *EDI*, 2/26.70

## Pancuronium-Hydrocortisone

**Significance:** 3—minimally clinically significant

**Recommendations:** If the patient is receiving corticosteroids, or if corticosteroids may be used during surgery, the dose of the neuromuscular blocking agent may need to be increased.

**Summary:** There are data to show that following hydrocortisone administration, there was a partial recovery from the neuromuscular blockade produced by pancuronium.

**Related Drugs:** There is evidence to show that prednisone may decrease the neuromuscular blockade. A similar interaction is expected to occur between pancuronium and other corticosteroids or between hydrocortisone and other neuromuscular blocking agents.

**Mechanism:** This interaction may involve competition at the myoneural junction, altered protein binding, or induction of hepatic biotransformation.

**Detailed Information:** See *EDI*, 2/27.00

## Pancuronium-Lithium Carbonate

**Significance:** 3—minimally clinically significant

**Recommendations:** Pancuronium or other neuromuscular blocking agents should be used with caution in patients taking lithium carbonate. Patients should be closely monitored, and ventilatory assistance should be provided as necessary.

**Summary:** There are data to show that lithium carbonate enhanced and prolonged the neuromuscular blockade actions of pancuronium. However, there are conflicting data that did not find similar results.

**Related Drugs:** There are no drugs related to lithium carbonate. There is evidence that lithium and succinylcholine administration has led to prolonged apnea; however, this has been disputed with other data. The effect of lithium on gallamine and tubocurarine is not clear. The neuromuscular blockade of succinylcholine and pancuronium was prolonged by lithium. Because of conflicting results, it is difficult to determine whether an interaction would occur between lithium carbonate and other nondepolarizing neuromuscular blocking agents.

**Mechanism:** Although the mechanism of this interaction is unknown, it has been suggested that it may be caused by the changes in electrolyte balance induced by lithium and the reduction of acetylcholine.

**Detailed Information:** See *EDI*, 2/29.00

## Pancuronium-Nitroglycerin

**Significance:** 3—minimally clinically significant

**Recommendations:** Until further clinical studies are performed in humans, it is important to be aware of the possible prolongation of neuromuscular blockade. If nitroglycerin is to be used, it may be advisable to use a noninteracting neuromuscular blocking agent. Alternatively, neostigmine has been shown to rapidly and completely reverse muscle paralysis, even during the prolongation produced by nitroglycerin.

**Summary:** There are animal data to show that nitroglycerin used prior to pancuronium administration increases the duration and depth of neuromuscular blockade.

**Related Drugs:** The neuromuscular blockade produced by tubocurarine, succinylcholine, and gallamine was not prolonged by nitroglycerin. Due to conflicting reports, it is difficult to determine whether an interaction would occur between nitroglycerin and other nondepolarizing neuromuscular blocking agents, or between pancuronium and other nitrates.

**Mechanism:** The mechanism of this interaction is unknown. However, this interaction is not caused by an altered plasma clearance of pancuronium, circulatory changes, or changes in the acid-base or electrolyte balance.

**Detailed Information:** See *EDI*, 2/31.00

## Pancuronium-Thiotepa (Triethylene Thiophosphoramide)

**Significance:** 3—minimally clinically significant

**Recommendations:** The concurrent use of these agents should be used with caution, and ventilatory assistance should be available.

## Anesthetic

**Summary:** There are data to show that administration of pancuronium followed by thiotepa may lead to rapid and prolonged respiratory depression.

**Related Drugs:** Documentation is lacking of a similar interaction between other neuromuscular blocking agents and other antineoplastic alkylating agents.

**Mechanism:** The mechanism of this interaction is unknown. However, it has been suggested that the presence of myasthenia gravis may be a predisposing and critical factor.

**Detailed Information:** See *EDI*, 2/33.00

### Propofol-Aminophylline

**Significance:** 3—minimally clinically significant

**Potential Effects:** Aminophylline may increase dosage requirements for propofol.

**Recommendations:** Until additional studies are forthcoming, the patient should be monitored and the dose of propofol should be adjusted as necessary for the required effect.

**Summary:** There are data to show that the propofol dosage required for sedation was increased by concomitant aminophylline.

**Related Drugs:** It is not known whether an interaction would occur between propofol and other theophylline derivatives. There are no drugs related to propofol.

**Mechanism:** The mechanism of this interaction is not known.

**Detailed Information:** See *EDI*, 2/34.07

### Propofol-Diazepam

**Significance:** 3—minimally clinically significant

**Potential Effects:** Concurrent use of diazepam and propofol may result in prolonged recovery time.

**Recommendations:** The patient should be monitored for the possibility of prolonged recovery time with concurrent use of propofol and diazepam.

**Summary:** There are data to show that the effects of propofol may be increased with concomitant diazepam and cause prolonged recovery time. However, all data do not support this.

**Related Drugs:** It is not known whether an interaction would occur between propofol and other benzodiazepines. There are no drugs related to propofol.

**Mechanism:** The mechanism of this interaction is not known, although the possibility exists that Cremophor® (a nonionic emulsifying agent in propofol) may be a factor leading to prolonged recovery time.

**Detailed Information:** See *EDI*, 2/34.05

### Succinylcholine-Cimetidine

**Significance:** 2—moderately clinically significant

**Potential Effects:** Cimetidine may prolong the neuromuscular blockade of succinylcholine.

**Recommendations:** Patients receiving cimetidine should be observed for an increased duration of action of succinylcholine. Ventilatory assistance should be provided if necessary. Ranitidine may be an alternative to cimetidine in some cases.

**Summary:** There are data to show that the duration of action of succinylcholine significantly increased with concurrent cimetidine. However, all data do not support this.

**Related Drugs:** There is documentation of a similar interaction with ranitidine and vecuronium. Because the mechanism of the interac-

## Anesthetic

tion is not known, it is not known if a similar interaction would occur between succinylcholine and other $H_2$-receptor antagonists or between cimetidine and other nondepolarizing neuromuscular blocking agents.

**Mechanism:** The mechanism of this interaction is not known.
**Detailed Information:** See *EDI*, 2/34.10

### Succinylcholine-Cyclophosphamide

**Significance:** 2—moderately clinically significant
**Recommendations:** Although the information concerning an interaction between the two drugs is limited, it would be prudent to either determine pseudocholinesterase levels before administering these drugs concurrently in a patient on cyclophosphamide therapy, or avoid the concomitant use of these agents. Alternatively, a neuromuscular blocking agent other than succinylcholine could be used with cyclophosphamide.
**Summary:** There are data to show that cyclophosphamide may potentiate the neuromuscular blockade produced by succinylcholine by inhibiting its metabolism leading to prolonged respiratory depression.
**Related Drugs:** The nondepolarizing neuromuscular blocking agents would not be expected to interact with cyclophosphamide. Other cytotoxic drugs that inhibit pseudocholinesterase would be expected to interact in a similar manner with succinylcholine.
**Mechanism:** Cyclophosphamide decreases pseudocholinesterase activity and this decrease may prolong the neuromuscular blockade produced by succinylcholine.
**Detailed Information:** See *EDI*, 2/35.00

### Succinylcholine-Dexpanthenol

**Significance:** 4—not clinically significant
**Recommendations:** The possibility of an interaction between succinylcholine and dexpanthenol at usual doses appears to be unlikely. Therefore, no additional precautions are necessary when these compounds are used concurrently.
**Summary:** There are data to show that dexpanthenol prolonged the respiratory depression induced by succinylcholine; however, contrasting data are available.
**Related Drugs:** There are no reports of this interaction occurring with the nondepolarizing neuromuscular blocking agents.
**Mechanism:** The excess acetylcholine produced by dexpanthenol may saturate its enzymatic metabolic pathway and then compete with succinylcholine for metabolism.
**Detailed Information:** See *EDI*, 2/37.00

### Succinylcholine-Diethylstilbestrol

**Significance:** 2—moderately clinically significant
**Recommendations:** It may be advisable to measure plasma cholinesterase levels before administration of succinylcholine in patients receiving estrogens or oral contraceptive agents containing estrogens.
**Summary:** There are data to show that the use of succinylcholine with diethylstilbestrol may result in prolonged ventilatory inadequacy secondary to severe depression of plasma cholinesterase.
**Related Drugs:** Oral contraceptive agents containing estrogens can significantly reduce plasma cholinesterase levels. A similar interaction is expected to occur with other estrogens. A similar interaction with diethylstilbestrol would not be expected to occur with the nondepolarizing neuromuscular blocking agents.

**Mechanism:** It has been suggested that estrogens reduce the synthesis or release of cholinesterase in the liver, resulting in a decreased succinylcholine degradation.
**Detailed Information:** See *EDI*, 2/38.10

## Succinylcholine-Echothiophate

**Significance:** 2—moderately clinically significant
**Recommendations:** If a patient is receiving echothiophate, it would be prudent to determine pseudocholinesterase activity before administering succinylcholine. It may be best to decrease the dose of succinylcholine or use a nondepolarizing neuromuscular blocking agent.
**Summary:** There are data to show that the effect of succinylcholine may be prolonged in patients receiving echothiophate ophthalmic preparations, resulting in prolonged neuromuscular blockade and apnea.
**Related Drugs:** A similar interaction may occur between succinylcholine and other ophthalmic cholinesterase inhibitors. It is not known to what extent demecarium and physostigmine would interact with succinylcholine. The nondepolarizing neuromuscular blocking agents would not be expected to interact with echothiophate in a similar manner.
**Mechanism:** Concurrent echothiophate may prevent the metabolism of succinylcholine.
**Detailed Information:** See *EDI*, 2/38.30

## Succinylcholine-Isoflurane

**Significance:** 2—moderately clinically significant
**Potential Effects:** Isoflurane may increase succinylcholine phase II neuromuscular blockade.
**Recommendations:** Patients should be closely observed during concurrent use of these agents because a decreased succinylcholine dose may be necessary.
**Summary:** There are data to show that isoflurane potentiated the neuromuscular blockade produced by succinylcholine leading to tachyphylaxis.
**Related Drugs:** Enflurane and halothane have been shown to have a comparable interaction when administered with succinylcholine. Documentation is lacking for a similar interaction between succinylcholine and other halogenated inhalation anesthetics. Prolonged duration of action was observed for pipecuronium, atracurium and pancuronium when given immediately after enflurane. The effects of atracurium are potentiated by halothane. A similar interaction is expected to occur with the nondepolarizing neuromuscular blocking agents and isoflurane. Enflurane potentiates the neuromuscular blockade of tubocurarine and halothane and decreases the ED50 of tubocurarine and pancuronium.
**Mechanism:** The mechanism of this interaction is not fully known. An increase in muscle blood flow induced by isoflurane may be an explanation. The potentiation of the neuromuscular blocking agents is likely to be caused by decreased acetylcholine at the neuromuscular junction.
**Detailed Information:** See *EDI*, 2/39.00

## Succinylcholine-Lidocaine

**Significance:** 2—moderately clinically significant
**Recommendations:** Patients who receive lidocaine, especially in large intravenous doses concomitantly with succinylcholine, should be observed closely to determine the need for artificial ventilation.

## Anesthetic

**Summary:** There are data to show that lidocaine may prolong and intensify the neuromuscular blocking effect and duration of apnea produced by succinylcholine.

**Related Drugs:** Tubocurarine interacts with lidocaine in a manner similar to succinylcholine. A similar interaction is expected to occur with other nondepolarizing neuromuscular blocking agents. Local anesthetics have been reported to interact similarly with succinylcholine.

**Mechanism:** The mechanism of this interaction has not been fully established. Lidocaine may produce neuromuscular blockade; it displaces succinylcholine from plasma protein and pseudocholinesterase, resulting in greater amounts of succinylcholine. The respiratory depression is probably through a CNS effect.

**Detailed Information:** See *EDI,* 2/41.00

### Succinylcholine-Metoclopramide

**Significance:** 3—minimally clinically significant

**Potential Effects:** Metoclopramide may prolong the neuromuscular blockade of succinylcholine.

**Recommendations:** The dosage of succinylcholine may need to be reduced when coadministered with metoclopramide.

**Summary:** There are data to show that a prolongation of succinylcholine neuromuscular blockade occurred with concurrent metoclopramide.

**Related Drugs:** It is not known whether an interaction would occur between metoclopramide and other nondepolarizing neuromuscular blocking agents. There are no drugs related to metoclopramide.

**Mechanism:** The mechanism of this interaction is unknown. The effect is thought to be related to the prolongation of the neuromuscular blockade induced by succinylcholine.

**Detailed Information:** See *EDI,* 2/46.10

### Succinylcholine-Neostigmine

**Significance:** 2—moderately clinically significant

**Recommendations:** The concurrent use of succinylcholine and an anticholinesterase agent should be avoided during the depolarizing phase of the neuromuscular blockade and should only be used with great caution, if at all, in the desensitizing phase. If concomitant use is necessary, closely monitor the patient and provide ventilatory assistance if necessary.

**Summary:** There are data to show that neostigmine may antagonize or enhance the neuromuscular blocking effect of succinylcholine.

**Related Drugs:** Edrophonium and pyridostigmine prolonged the neuromuscular blockade produced by succinylcholine. A similar interaction is expected to occur between succinylcholine and other anticholinesterases. The nondepolarizing neuromuscular blocking agents would not be expected to interact in a similar manner; however, documentation is lacking.

**Mechanism:** The action of neostigmine effectively increases the concentration of acetylcholine at the neuromuscular junction by decreasing its rate of hydrolysis.

**Detailed Information:** See *EDI,* 2/43.00

### Succinylcholine-Procainamide

**Significance:** 3—minimally clinically significant

**Recommendations:** Patients receiving succinylcholine and procainamide concurrently should be observed for signs of neuromuscular blockade, especially prolonged apnea. Artificial ventilation may be required for a longer time in such patients.

Anesthetic

**Summary:** There are data to show that procainamide may prolong and intensify the neuromuscular blockade produced by succinylcholine.
**Related Drugs:** The same interaction with succinylcholine has been demonstrated with procaine and quinidine. No documentation exists regarding an interaction between procainamide and the nondepolarizing neuromuscular blocking agents.
**Mechanism:** Procainamide may displace succinylcholine from the cholinesterase system or inhibit plasma cholinesterase, leading to a greater concentration of succinylcholine.
**Detailed Information:** See *EDI*, 2/45.00

## Succinylcholine-Promazine

**Significance:** 2—moderately clinically significant
**Recommendations:** Promazine should be used with caution in patients receiving succinylcholine, and ventilatory assistance should be made available. In a study, edrophonium successfully treated the prolonged apnea.
**Summary:** There are data to show that promazine followed by succinylcholine has resulted in total muscle relaxation, prolonged apnea and cyanosis.
**Related Drugs:** A similar interaction is expected to occur with other phenothiazines and succinylcholine. A similar interaction is not expected to occur between promazine and the nondepolarizing neuromuscular blocking agents.
**Mechanism:** The mechanism is not fully known; however, it has been suggested that promazine may lower serum cholinesterase levels, resulting in succinylcholine remaining at the site of action for a prolonged period of time.
**Detailed Information:** See *EDI*, 2/47.00

## Succinylcholine-Thiopental

**Significance:** 2—moderately clinically significant
**Potential Effects:** Concurrent use of these agents in the same IV line may result in anaphylaxis and death.
**Recommendations:** If these agents are to be used together, care should be taken to avoid physical mixing during the administration process.
**Summary:** There are data to show that concurrent use of succinylcholine and thiopental has caused bradycardia, severe bronchospasm, hypotension and cardiac arrest resulting in anaphylaxis and death.
**Related Drugs:** It is not known whether an interaction would occur between thiopental and other neuromuscular blocking agents or between succinylcholine and other barbiturates.
**Mechanism:** The mechanism of this interaction is not known.
**Detailed Information:** See *EDI*, 2/48.10

## Succinylcholine-Trimethaphan

**Significance:** 2—moderately clinically significant
**Recommendations:** Trimethaphan and any neuromuscular blocking agent should be used concurrently with caution. If concomitant use is necessary, ventilatory assistance should be available.
**Summary:** There are data to show that patients on trimethaphan and succinylcholine have exhibited prolonged apnea, indicating an increased neuromuscular blocking effect.
**Related Drugs:** Tubocurarine and trimethaphan may increase the neuromuscular blocking effect of tubocurarine. If trimethaphan causes a neuromuscular blockade, a similar interaction between

## Anesthetic

trimethaphan and other nondepolarizing neuromuscular blocking agents can occur. There are no drugs related to trimethaphan.

**Mechanism:** Trimethaphan can inhibit pseudocholinesterase, which metabolizes succinylcholine.

**Detailed Information:** See *EDI*, 2/49.00

### Thiopental-Morphine

**Significance:** 2—moderately clinically significant

**Recommendations:** Patients should be closely monitored during concurrent use of these agents. If the dose of the narcotic cannot be lowered, it is important to be prepared for ventilatory assistance.

**Summary:** There are data to show that concurrent use of thiopental and morphine may lead to an increased respiratory depression.

**Related Drugs:** Thiopental and meperidine exhibited a similar interaction. A similar interaction may occur with other narcotics and other barbiturate anesthetics.

**Mechanism:** Although the mechanism is not fully known, since each agent produces respiratory depression on its own, an additive synergistic effect may be involved.

**Detailed Information:** See *EDI*, 2/51.00

### Thiopental-Probenecid

**Significance:** 3—minimally clinically significant

**Recommendations:** It is important to be aware of the possibility of prolonged anesthesia after concurrent use of thiopental and probenecid. Probenecid may need to be discontinued prior to the use of thiopental if this effect is not desired.

**Summary:** There are data to show that thiopental anesthesia is prolonged after probenecid administration.

**Related Drugs:** A similar interaction is expected to occur between probenecid and other barbiturate anesthetics. There is no documentation regarding a similar interaction between thiopental and other uricosuric agents.

**Mechanism:** The mechanism of this interaction is unknown.

**Detailed Information:** See *EDI*, 2/53.00

### Thiopental-Reserpine

**Significance:** 2—moderately clinically significant

**Recommendations:** Withdrawal of reserpine prior to surgery is not mandatory; however, it is important to be aware that hypotension and bradycardia may occur. If reserpine is not withdrawn prior to surgery and if hypotension does occur, an exacerbated effect may be noticed since the endogenous catecholamines have already been chronically depleted by reserpine. Therefore, the use of an indirect-acting sympathomimetic agent would be ineffective, and a direct-acting sympathomimetic agent would be required to treat the hypotension.

**Summary:** There are data to show that reserpine may enhance the CNS depression caused by thiopental, resulting in hypotension and bradycardia.

**Related Drugs:** Pentobarbital and thiamylal are reported to interact with reserpine in animals. A similar interaction is expected to occur with other barbiturates and reserpine. All other rauwolfia alkaloids have a potential for interacting with thiopental or other barbiturates.

**Mechanism:** The mechanism for this interaction is unknown. However, reserpine causes a depletion of catecholamines and serotonin in the central and peripheral nervous systems and cardiovascular tissue.

**Detailed Information:** See *EDI*, 2/55.00

## Anesthetic

### Thiopental-Sulfisoxazole
**Significance:** 2—moderately clinically significant

**Recommendations:** When thiopental is used during long-term oral sulfisoxazole therapy, the thiopental dosage may have to be adjusted to provide smaller, more frequent doses in order to compensate for the effect of concomitant sulfisoxazole administration.

**Summary:** There are data to show that sulfisoxazole reduces the amount of thiopental required for anesthesia and shortens the awakening time.

**Related Drugs:** A similar interaction is expected to occur with other ultrashort-acting barbiturate anesthetics. The effect of using longer-acting barbiturates with other sulfonamides is not known.

**Mechanism:** Sulfisoxazole displaces thiopental from plasma protein binding sites, increasing the amount of free thiopental available to exert an anesthetic effect.

**Detailed Information:** See *EDI*, 2/57.00

### Tubocurarine-Gentamicin
**Significance:** 1—highly clinically significant

**Potential Effects:** Concurrent use of these agents may prolong the neuromuscular blockade.

**Recommendations:** Concurrent use should be avoided. Other antibiotics should be considered. Atracurium could possibly be used in place of tubocurarine.

**Summary:** Aminoglycosides have been shown to produce a neuromuscular blockade, prolonging the respiratory depressant and muscle relaxant effects of tubocurarine and other neuromuscular depressant drugs.

**Related Drugs:** All aminoglycosides have been shown experimentally to produce neuromuscular blockade. Potentiation of neuromuscular blocking agents has been reported with all currently available aminoglycosides. The neuromuscular blockade produced by pancuronium, gallamine, vecuronium, succinylcholine and atracurium may be potentiated by these antibiotics.

**Mechanism:** The antibiotics produce neuromuscular blockade by inhibiting acetylcholine release presynaptically and by reducing the sensitivity of the postjunctional membrane.

**Detailed Information:** See *EDI*, 2/61.00

### Tubocurarine-Ketamine
**Significance:** 2—moderately clinically significant

**Recommendations:** These agents should be used concurrently with caution. Patients should be closely monitored throughout anesthesia when ketamine and a neuromuscular blocking agent are used concurrently.

**Summary:** There are data to show that ketamine augments the neuromuscular blocking properties of tubocurarine.

**Related Drugs:** There are no drugs related to ketamine. There are conflicting data concerning the potentiation of ketamine by succinylcholine or pancuronium. Because of this, it is difficult to determine whether an interaction would occur between ketamine and other nondepolarizing neuromuscular blocking agents.

**Mechanism:** Several mechanisms have been suggested. Ketamine may decrease motor end-plate sensitivity, potentiating tubocurarine, or it may interfere with protein binding, making more tubocurarine available.

**Detailed Information:** See *EDI*, 2/65.00

Anesthetic

## Tubocurarine-Morphine

**Significance:** 2—moderately clinically significant

**Recommendations:** If morphine is given to a patient recovering from tubocurarine blockade or to one in whom the blockade has been antagonized recently by neostigmine, ventilation should be monitored and controlled so that the partial pressure of carbon dioxide in the arterial blood does not increase. If it does increase, tubocurarine blockade may reappear or recovery may be delayed. Administration of morphine (5 mg/70 kg) and tubocurarine (9 mg/kg) in small intermittent doses rather than large bolus injections should minimize hypotension.

**Summary:** The administration of morphine augments the neuromuscular blockade produced by tubocurarine. Tubocurarine and morphine both reduce blood pressure and may produce hypotension if used concurrently.

**Related Drugs:** A similar interaction is expected to occur between morphine and other neuromuscular blocking agents. A similar interaction is expected to occur between tubocurarine and other narcotics.

**Mechanism:** Morphine may augment the neuromuscular blockade of tubocurarine and reduce neostigmine's ability to antagonize tubocurarine blockade.

**Detailed Information:** See *EDI*, 2/67.00

## Tubocurarine-Propranolol

**Significance:** 2—moderately clinically significant

**Potential Effects:** The concurrent use of these agents may result in prolonged neuromuscular blockade or hypotension.

**Recommendations:** Patients receiving these agents concurrently should be monitored for prolonged neuromuscular blockade or hypotension. Excessive bradycardia may also occur. If prolonged neuromuscular blockade occurs, neostigmine (1 to 3 mg) with atropine (0.6 to 1.2 mg) may be given.

**Summary:** There are data to show that tubocurarine produced a prolonged neuromuscular blockade in patients receiving propranolol.

**Related Drugs:** The depolarizing neuromuscular blocking agent succinylcholine has been shown to interact with propranolol similar to tubocurarine. The other nondepolarizing neuromuscular blocking agents might also interact with propranolol. Any of the other beta blocking agents may potentially interact with tubocurarine as well.

**Mechanism:** Propranolol depresses post-tetanic repetitive activity and may depress the motor nerve terminal activity of tubocurarine. Propranolol may render the postjunctional membrane insensitive to acetylcholine, as well as enhance the duration of neuromuscular blockade.

**Detailed Information:** See *EDI*, 2/69.00

## Tubocurarine-Quinidine

**Significance:** 2—moderately clinically significant

**Potential Effects:** Concurrent use of these agents may result in additive neuromuscular blockade.

**Recommendations:** Monitor patients closely for prolonged neuromuscular blockade when these agents are used together. Neostigmine (1 to 3 mg IV) with atropine sulfate (0.6 to 1.2 mg IV) may be used to antagonize the action of the tubocurarine. However, this was not effective in one case, and should not be used with succinylcholine.

**Summary:** Quinidine, administered simultaneously with tubocurarine, may cause recurrent neuromuscular effects of tubocurarine, resulting in intensified respiratory depression and apnea.

Anesthetic

**Related Drugs:** Gallamine has been shown to interact with quinidine in animals. A similar interaction is expected to occur with other nondepolarizing neuromuscular blocking agents and quinidine and between tubocurarine and other cinchona alkaloids.

**Mechanism:** The interaction with the neuromuscular blocking agents is caused by an additive pharmacologic effect of quinidine and the neuromuscular blocking agents on skeletal muscle.

**Detailed Information:** See *EDI*, 2/71.00

## Vecuronium-Dantrolene

**Significance:** 3—minimally clinically significant

**Potential Effects:** Dantrolene may prolong the neuromuscular blocking effects of vecuronium.

**Recommendations:** Patients receiving dantrolene prior to vecuronium should be observed for prolonged neuromuscular blockade.

**Summary:** There are data to show that dantrolene administered with vecuronium caused an increase in recovery time from the neuromuscular blockade produced by vecuronium.

**Related Drugs:** A similar interaction is expected to occur between dantrolene and other nondepolarizing neuromuscular blocking agents and the depolarizing neuromuscular blocking agent, succinylcholine. There are no drugs related to dantrolene.

**Mechanism:** The prolonged neuromuscular blockade of vecuronium is related to a dantrolene-induced decrease of transmitter mobilization at the neuromuscular junction.

**Detailed Information:** See *EDI*, 2/72.01

## Vecuronium-Magnesium Sulfate

**Significance:** 2—moderately clinically significant

**Potential Effects:** Vecuronium's action may be potentiated by magnesium sulfate.

**Recommendations:** When these agents are administered together, vecuronium should be carefully titrated to twitch response. Patients should be closely monitored.

**Summary:** There are data to show that magnesium sulfate potentiates the neuromuscular blockade caused by vecuronium.

**Related Drugs:** Pancuronium and atracurium exhibited comparable interactions. A similar interaction may be expected to occur between magnesium sulfate and other nondepolarizing neuromuscular blocking agents. It is not known if a similar interaction would occur with the use of the oral magnesium salts.

**Mechanism:** Increases in plasma magnesium potentiate the activity of nondepolarizing and depolarizing neuromuscular blocking agents, reduce end-plate sensitivity, decrease muscle fiber excitability and suppress peripheral neuromuscular function.

**Detailed Information:** See *EDI*, 2/72.10

## Vecuronium-Piperacillin

**Significance:** 2—moderately clinically significant

**Potential Effects:** Piperacillin may prolong vecuronium's neuromuscular blockade.

**Recommendations:** If vecuronium is used for neuromuscular blockade, the patient should be monitored for a prolonged duration of action of vecuronium if piperacillin is administered. Additional ventilatory support may be required.

**Summary:** Piperacillin may prolong the duration of action of vecuronium.

**Related Drugs:** Vecuronium was prolonged by mezlocillin and azlocillin. It is not known whether an interaction would occur

between vecuronium and the nonacylaminopenicillins or between piperacillin and other nondepolarizing neuromuscular blocking agents.
**Mechanism:** The mechanism of this interaction is not known, but the speculated site of action is prejunctional.
**Detailed Information:** See *EDI*, 2/72.25

## Vecuronium-Testosterone

**Significance:** 3—minimally clinically significant
**Potential Effects:** Testosterone administration may result in resistance to vecuronium.
**Recommendations:** Caution should be used when administering vecuronium to a patient maintained on testosterone.
**Summary:** There are data to show that patients maintained on testosterone will exhibit resistance to the muscle relaxation effects of vecuronium.
**Related Drugs:** A similar resistance has been demonstrated with succinylcholine. An interaction may occur between testosterone and other nondepolarizing neuromuscular blocking agents. It is not known whether an interaction would occur between vecuronium and other androgen derivatives.
**Mechanism:** This interaction involves a combination of factors. The increased volume of distribution may explain the initial resistance. Testosterone may simulate hormones and/or corticosteroids in enhancing neuromuscular transmission and may augment an increased number of acetylcholine receptors from increased skeletal muscle mass.
**Detailed Information:** See *EDI*, 2/72.30

## Vecuronium-Verapamil

**Significance:** 2—moderately clinically significant
**Potential Effects:** Verapamil can prolong the neuromuscular blockade produced by vecuronium.
**Recommendations:** Patients taking verapamil should be administered conservative doses of neuromuscular blocking agents. If reversal of the blockade is not obtained, the use of edrophonium should be considered.
**Summary:** There are data to show that verapamil causes difficulty with the reversal of the neuromuscular blockade caused by vecuronium.
**Related Drugs:** Pancuronium, tubocurarine and succinylcholine have demonstrated similar interactions with the coadministration of verapamil. A similar interaction may occur between verapamil and other nondepolarizing neuromuscular blocking agents. Documentation is lacking regarding an interaction between vecuronium and other calcium channel blockers.
**Mechanism:** Verapamil may reduce the mobilization or release of the transmitter acetylcholine and therefore reduces prejunctional stimulus.
**Detailed Information:** See *EDI*, 2/73.00

# Chapter Three

# Antiarrhythmic Drug Interactions

## Antiarrhythmic

### Amiodarone-Cholestyramine

**Significance:** 3—minimally clinically significant

**Potential Effects:** Cholestyramine may reduce the enterohepatic circulation of amiodarone, leading to an increased elimination of the amiodarone.

**Recommendations:** Cholestyramine may be administered to patients with dose-dependent amiodarone side effects. In other patients, amiodarone levels and effects should be closely monitored. The dose of amiodarone may need to be increased.

**Summary:** There are data to show that amiodarone followed by cholestyramine administration significantly decreases the mean serum level and elimination half-life of amiodarone.

**Related Drugs:** A similar interaction may be expected to occur between amiodarone and other anion exchange resins. There are no drugs related to amiodarone.

**Mechanism:** Cholestyramine significantly reduces the enterohepatic circulation of amiodarone, enhancing its elimination.

**Detailed Information:** See *EDI*, 3/0.01

### Amiodarone-Cyclosporine

**Significance:** 2—moderately clinically significant

**Potential Effects:** The addition of amiodarone to a cyclosporine regimen may result in increased cyclosporine levels and toxicity.

**Recommendations:** Patients should be carefully monitored for changes in cyclosporine levels and clearance with the concurrent use of these agents. The dose of cyclosporine may need to be adjusted to maintain cyclosporine serum levels within the therapeutic range.

**Summary:** Concurrent amiodarone and cyclosporine resulted in decreased cyclosporine clearance, leading to increased levels and potential nephrotoxicity.

**Related Drugs:** There are no drugs related to cyclosporine or amiodarone.

**Mechanism:** Although the mechanism of this interaction is not known, the interaction with cyclosporine may occur in the adipose tissue throughout the body.

**Detailed Information:** See *EDI*, 3/0.02

### Amiodarone-Diltiazem

**Significance:** 2—moderately clinically significant

**Potential Effects:** Use of these agents together may cause a decrease in cardiac function.

**Recommendations:** Patients should be monitored for decreased cardiac function when using these agents together. One or both drugs may need to be discontinued.

**Summary:** There are data to show that coadministration of diltiazem and amiodarone may lead to sinus arrest and severe, low cardiac output with oliguria.

**Related Drugs:** A similar interaction may occur between amiodarone and other calcium channel blockers. There are no drugs related to amiodarone.

**Mechanism:** It has been suggested that the interaction was the result of additive hemodynamic and electrophysiologic effects.

**Detailed Information:** See *EDI*, 3/0.03

### Amiodarone-Lidocaine

**Significance:** 2—moderately clinically significant

**Potential Effects:** Use of these agents together has resulted in adverse cardiac effects.

**Recommendations:** Use these agents together with caution. Monitor the patient's cardiac status.

**Summary:** There are data to show that receiving amiodarone with 2% lidocaine may cause severe sinus bradycardia and sinoatrial arrest.

**Related Drugs:** A similar interaction is expected to occur between amiodarone and tocainide or mexiletine, or the oral antiarrhythmic agents related to lidocaine. There are no drugs related to amiodarone.

**Mechanism:** Lidocaine and amiodarone are known to depress the sinus node; the interaction may be due to an additive effect of the two agents on the sinus node.

**Detailed Information:** See *EDI,* 3/0.05

## Diltiazem-Cisapride

**Significance:** 2—moderately clinically significant

**Potential Effects:** The concurrent administration of cisapride and diltiazem may result in prolongation of the rate corrected QT interval ($QT_c$).

**Recommendations:** The concurrent administration of cisapride and diltiazem should be approached with caution. The manufacturer of cisapride states that an electrocardiogram should be considered prior to the initiation of therapy with cisapride.

**Summary:** The concurrent administration of cisapride and diltiazem may have resulted in prolongation of the $QT_c$ interval in a single case report. When metoclopramide was substituted for cisapride, the patient's $QT_c$ interval was normal ($QT_c$ of 440 msec) within two months.

**Related Drugs:** Although nifedipine plasma concentrations were significantly increased when given with cisapride, no detrimental hypotensive effects occurred. It is not known whether an interaction would occur between cisapride and the other calcium channel blocking agents. However, information concerning a possible interaction between cisapride and bepridil (a calcium channel blocking agent not chemically related to the dihydropyridine or the tetralol calcium channel blocking agents) has been mentioned.

**Mechanism:** It is postulated that diltiazem may inhibit the metabolism of cisapride at the $P450_{3A4}$ isozyme. Cisapride is metabolized at the $P450_{3A4}$ isozyme and elevated levels of cisapride have been shown to result in QT prolongation, torsades de pointes, cardiac arrest, and sudden death.

**Detailed Information:** See *EDI,* 3/0.06

## Diltiazem-Cyclosporine

**Significance:** 1—highly clinically significant

**Potential Effects:** Diltiazem may increase cyclosporine levels, resulting in decreased renal function.

**Recommendations:** Patients should be closely monitored for increased cyclosporine and serum creatinine levels during concurrent therapy with diltiazem. The dose of cyclosporine may need to be adjusted.

**Summary:** Concurrent administration of cyclosporine and diltiazem resulted in increased cyclosporine levels to as high as 1100 ng/ml as well as increased serum creatinine levels.

**Related Drugs:** Concomitant administration of verapamil or nicardipine with cyclosporine also has resulted in significant increases in cyclosporine levels. Several studies have reported that concurrent isradipine had either no effect on cyclosporine kinetics or a beneficial nephroprotective effect. Conversely, one case report documents a threefold increase in trough cyclosporine concentration

## Antiarrhythmic

with concurrent isradipine. Although one study reported a significant increase in plasma cyclosporine levels following a single dose of felodipine, there was an increase in glomerular filtration rate, renal plasma flow, and urinary sodium excretion, suggesting that a single dose of felodipine may have beneficial effects on renal hemodynamics in renal transplant patients. It is difficult to determine whether an interaction would occur between cyclosporine and the other calcium channel blocking agents. There are no drugs related to cyclosporine.

**Mechanism:** It has been suggested that diltiazem interferes with the hepatic metabolism of cyclosporine.

**Detailed Information:** See *EDI*, 3/0.07

## Disopyramide-Alcohol, Ethyl

**Significance:** 3—minimally clinically significant

**Recommendations:** Until further clinical studies are done, the concurrent use of these agents need not be avoided. However, if disopyramide levels increase, the dose of disopyramide may need to be adjusted or the discontinuation of alcohol should be encouraged.

**Summary:** The concurrent use of disopyramide and alcohol has led to a significant reduction in the apparent metabolic clearance of disopyramide.

**Related Drugs:** There are no drugs related to disopyramide.

**Mechanism:** Alcohol may have an inhibitory effect on disopyramide metabolism.

**Detailed Information:** See *EDI*, 3/0.10

## Disopyramide-Atenolol

**Significance:** 3—minimally clinically significant

**Recommendations:** The concurrent use of disopyramide and atenolol need not be avoided. However, since the clearance of disopyramide decreased while the concentration of the metabolite of disopyramide (which has some antiarrhythmic activity) did not change, patients should be monitored for an increased antiarrhythmic effect. During concomitant atenolol therapy the dose of disopyramide may need to be adjusted.

**Summary:** There are data to show that administration of atenolol and disopyramide significantly reduces the clearance of disopyramide, while its other pharmacokinetic parameters remain unchanged.

**Related Drugs:** There are data to show that propranolol does not cause any change in the concentration of disopyramide; however, all data do not support this. Because of conflicting results, it is difficult to determine if an interaction would occur between disopyramide and other beta-blocking agents. There are no drugs related to disopyramide.

**Mechanism:** The effect of atenolol on a small metabolized fraction of disopyramide may account for the change in the elimination of disopyramide. However, a hepatic or renal blood flow cause cannot be excluded.

**Detailed Information:** See *EDI*, 3/0.30

## Disopyramide-Charcoal

**Significance:** 2—moderately clinically significant

**Potential Effects:** Charcoal adsorbs disopyramide, leading to a decrease in disopyramide absorption.

**Recommendations:** Charcoal may be useful in the treatment of disopyramide overdosage. If charcoal is being used for other reasons, the administration of these agents should be separated by as much time as possible.

# Antiarrhythmic

**Summary:** Charcoal significantly decreases the bioavailability and serum concentration of disopyramide.
**Related Drugs:** There are no drugs related to disopyramide.
**Mechanism:** Charcoal adsorbs disopyramide when both drugs are given concurrently.
**Detailed Information:** See *EDI*, 3/0.50

## Disopyramide-Cyclosporine

**Significance:** 3—minimally clinically significant
**Potential Effects:** Cyclosporine may lead to increases in disopyramide levels, leading to pronounced anticholinergic side effects.
**Recommendations:** Monitor the patient for increases in serum creatinine or disopyramide toxicity during concurrent use of these agents.
**Summary:** There are data to show that coadministration of disopyramide and cyclosporine caused serum creatinine levels to increase and potentiate disopyramide-induced anticholinergic side effects.
**Related Drugs:** There are no drugs related to disopyramide or cyclosporine.
**Mechanism:** The exact mechanism of this interaction is unknown, but cyclosporine may have caused nephrotoxicity or a change in the metabolism of disopyramide.
**Detailed Information:** See *EDI*, 3/0.65

## Disopyramide-Erythromycin

**Significance:** 2—moderately clinically significant
**Potential Effects:** Erythromycin may decrease the metabolism of disopyramide, resulting in increased disopyramide levels and possible toxicity.
**Recommendations:** Patients maintained on disopyramide should be closely monitored for changes in cardiac status if erythromycin is added to their drug regimen. The dose of disopyramide may need to be adjusted.
**Summary:** There are data to show that coadministration of disopyramide and erythromycin can increase serum creatinine levels and potentiate cardiac complications, necessitating electrical cardioversion.
**Related Drugs:** A similar interaction may be expected to occur between disopyramide and other macrolide antibiotics. There are no drugs related to disopyramide.
**Mechanism:** It has been suggested that erythromycin interferes with hepatic enzymes used to metabolize disopyramide, causing an increase in the disopyramide level.
**Detailed Information:** See *EDI*, 3/0.67

## Disopyramide-Isosorbide Dinitrate

**Significance:** 2—moderately clinically significant
**Potential Effects:** The occurrence of dry mouth that may be associated with disopyramide therapy because of its anticholinergic side effects may prevent the dissolution of sublingual isosorbide dinitrate tablets, resulting in ineffective therapy.
**Recommendations:** Attempts at increasing salivation (e.g., chewing gum, artificial saliva products) may prove useful in increasing the effectiveness of sublingual isosorbide dinitrate in some patients. If the ineffectiveness of the sublingual isosorbide dinitrate continues, the use of oral, topical, or translingual spray forms of the nitrates, or the substitution of another appropriate antiarrhythmic agent, may need to be considered.

## Antiarrhythmic

**Summary:** There are data to show that disopyramide can cause dry mouth, making the absorption of a sublingual isosorbide dinitrate tablet difficult.
**Related Drugs:** A similar interaction may occur between disopyramide and other sublingual nitrate tablets. There are no drugs related to disopyramide.
**Mechanism:** Dry mouth is a common side effect of disopyramide therapy because of its anticholinergic effects.
**Detailed Information:** See *EDI*, 3/0.70

### Disopyramide-Phenytoin

**Significance:** 2—moderately clinically significant
**Potential Effects:** Phenytoin increases the hepatic metabolism of disopyramide, resulting in decreased disopyramide plasma levels and possibly a decrease in its efficacy. Increased anticholinergic side effects may also occur.
**Recommendations:** Although the metabolite of disopyramide has some antiarrhythmic activity, patients receiving these agents concurrently should be monitored for decreased antiarrhythmic control and increased anticholinergic side effects.
**Summary:** There are data to show that concurrent phenytoin and disopyramide can result in a decrease in the plasma concentration and efficacy of disopyramide.
**Related Drugs:** A similar interaction is expected to occur between disopyramide and other hydantoin anticonvulsants. There are no drugs related to disopyramide.
**Mechanism:** Phenytoin may increase the hepatic metabolism of disopyramide.
**Detailed Information:** See *EDI*, 3/1.00

### Disopyramide-Quinidine

**Significance:** 3—minimally clinically significant
**Recommendations:** The concurrent use of these agents need not be avoided. However, a longer interval between the last dose of disopyramide and the first dose of quinidine may be warranted. Patients on high dose disopyramide therapy should be closely monitored.
**Summary:** There are data to show that the concurrent use of disopyramide and quinidine has led to an increase in disopyramide serum concentration and a decrease in quinidine serum concentration.
**Related Drugs:** There are no drugs related to disopyramide. Documentation is lacking regarding a similar interaction between disopyramide and other cinchona alkaloids.
**Mechanism:** The mechanism of this interaction is unknown.
**Detailed Information:** See *EDI*, 3/3.00

### Disopyramide-Rifampin

**Significance:** 3—minimally clinically significant
**Recommendations:** Although the patients were taking other drugs that could have a role in this interaction, rifampin is still strongly suspected because of its known induction properties. Because the metabolite of disopyramide has some antiarrhythmic activity, the increased rate of metabolism of disopyramide cannot be equated with a shorter duration of response. Therefore, patients should be monitored for a loss of antiarrhythmic effect.
**Summary:** Disopyramide metabolism may be significantly increased with concomitant rifampin. It is not certain if disopyramide will alter the disposition of rifampin.

**Related Drugs:** There are no drugs related to rifampin or disopyramide.
**Mechanism:** Rifampin accelerated disopyramide metabolism by enzyme induction.
**Detailed Information:** See *EDI*, 3/5.00

## Felodipine-Erythromycin

**Significance:** 3—minimally clinically significant
**Potential Effects:** The addition of erythromycin to felodipine may result in elevated plasma felodipine concentrations and increased incidence of adverse events.
**Recommendations:** Patients receiving concurrent therapy should be monitored for an increase in the clinical effects of felodipine. The dosage of felodipine may need to be decreased, or erythromycin may need to be discontinued.
**Summary:** The addition of erythromycin to felodipine may result in elevated plasma felodipine concentrations and increased incidence of adverse events including palpitations, flushing, and lower extremity edema.
**Related Drugs:** *In vitro*, clarithromycin, erythromycin, and rokitamycin did not inhibit the formation of the nifedipine M-1 metabolite when added to nifedipine, although pretreatment with either clarithromycin or erythromycin did inhibit its formation. Only erythromycin inhibited the formation of the nifedipine M-2 metabolite. Erythromycin and roxithromycin appear to be weak inhibitors of nifedipine oxidation. Azithromycin does not produce hepatic cytochrome P450 induction or inactivation as erythromycin estolate does; therefore, an interaction would not be expected to occur between azithromycin and felodipine or nifedipine. An interaction would likely occur between erythromycin and other dihydropyridine calcium channel blocking agents. An interaction may be expected to occur between felodipine and the other macrolide antibiotics.
**Mechanism:** It is hypothesized that erythromycin inhibits the primary metabolic pathway for felodipine. Felodipine is believed to undergo CYP3A4 metabolism both in the gut and the liver, accounting for its low bioavailability.
**Detailed Information:** See *EDI*, 3/5.50

## Felodipine-Itraconazole

**Significance:** 3—minimally clinically significant
**Potential Effects:** Concurrent administration of itraconazole and felodipine resulted in increased levels of felodipine and the development of edema.
**Recommendations:** Concurrent administration of felodipine with itraconazole should be approached with caution. Patients should be observed for increased effects of felodipine. The dosage of felodipine may need to be adjusted or itraconazole may need to be discontinued.
**Summary:** Concurrent administration of itraconazole and felodipine resulted in increased levels of felodipine and the development of edema. Significantly greater effects on both blood pressure and heart rate were also observed.
**Related Drugs:** Concurrent administration of ketoconazole increased the mean AUC and Cmax of nisoldipine and its M9 metabolite; mild headache, orthostatic dysfunction, and moderate dizziness were observed. Plasma levels of nifedipine increased and blood pressure decreased when itraconazole was coadministered; ankle edema has also occurred when itraconazole was given with isradipine. A similar interaction may be expected to occur between

## Antiarrhythmic

itraconazole or ketoconazole and the other calcium channel blockers that are metabolized by the cytochrome $P450_{3A4}$ isoenzyme and between felodipine, isradipine, nifedipine, or nisoldipine and the other azole antifungals that inhibit cytochrome $P450_{3A4}$.

**Mechanism:** Itraconazole may inhibit first-pass and elimination metabolism of felodipine at the cytochrome $P450_{3A4}$ isoenzyme.

**Detailed Information:** See *EDI*, 3/5.60

## Flecainide-Amiodarone

**Significance:** 2—moderately clinically significant

**Recommendations:** Plasma flecainide levels should be closely monitored in patients receiving concurrent flecainide and amiodarone. Because amiodarone has a long half-life, it is important to monitor patients closely for several weeks. When amiodarone is added to flecainide therapy, it may be advisable to decrease the dose of flecainide by one third to one half, and a further dosage reduction may be required.

**Summary:** There are data to show that amiodarone causes an increase in flecainide plasma levels.

**Related Drugs:** Flecainide is unrelated to the Class IB antiarrhythmic agents. There are no drugs related to amiodarone.

**Mechanism:** It was suggested that amiodarone inhibits the hepatic metabolism of flecainide.

**Detailed Information:** See *EDI*, 3/6.01

## Flecainide-Ammonium Chloride

**Significance:** 2—moderately clinically significant

**Potential Effects:** Ammonium chloride, by acidifying the urine, increases flecainide elimination.

**Recommendations:** Patients should be carefully monitored if flecainide and ammonium chloride are used concurrently. The dose of flecainide may need to be increased. Attempts to acidify the urine could be considered as a therapeutic measure in patients with high serum levels of flecainide, but this requires further study.

**Summary:** The renal clearance and urinary elimination of flecainide were increased with decreasing urinary pH caused by ammonium chloride.

**Related Drugs:** A similar interaction may occur between flecainide and other urinary acidifiers. It is not known if a similar interaction would occur between ammonium chloride and the other Class IC antiarrhythmic, encainide.

**Mechanism:** The increased elimination half-life of flecainide may be a result of a change in the degree of ionization of the drug at the adsorption site.

**Detailed Information:** See *EDI*, 3/6.07

## Flecainide-Charcoal

**Significance:** 3—minimally clinically significant

**Potential Effects:** Charcoal adsorbs flecainide, leading to decreased levels.

**Recommendations:** The interaction may be useful in some patients in the case of flecainide intoxication. The administration of charcoal may be useful even after some delay. However, if charcoal is being used for other medical reasons, the administration of these agents should be separated by as much time as possible.

**Summary:** There are data to show that charcoal causes a significant decrease in flecainide plasma levels.

**Related Drugs:** It is not known if a similar interaction would occur with the other Class IC antiarrhythmic agent, encainide. There are no drugs related to charcoal.

## Antiarrhythmic

**Mechanism:** Charcoal adsorbs flecainide when both drugs are given concurrently, reducing the absorption of flecainide in the gastrointestinal tract.
**Detailed Information:** See *EDI*, 3/6.03

## Flecainide-Cimetidine

**Significance:** 2—moderately clinically significant
**Potential Effects:** Cimetidine may increase flecainide levels.
**Recommendations:** Monitor for increased flecainide levels when these agents are used together. The dose of flecainide may need to be decreased.
**Summary:** Cimetidine causes an increase in the peak concentration of flecainide and the amount of flecainide excreted in the urine.
**Related Drugs:** Similar interactions have been documented with cimetidine and encainide or propafenone. A similar interaction may be expected to occur between cimetidine and the other Class IC antiarrhythmic agent, indecainide. The other $H_2$-receptor antagonists would not be expected to interact with flecainide, if the mechanism is caused by flecainide's metabolism by cimetidine.
**Mechanism:** Cimetidine may inhibit the hepatic microsomal enzymes responsible for the metabolism of flecainide.
**Detailed Information:** See *EDI*, 3/6.05

## Flecainide-Isoproterenol

**Significance:** 2—moderately clinically significant
**Potential Effects:** Isoproterenol may decrease the effectiveness of flecainide.
**Recommendations:** Use these agents together with caution. If loss of antiarrhythmic activity occurs, isoproterenol should be discontinued, and the use of a beta-blocking agent may be necessary.
**Summary:** There are data to show that coadministration of flecainide and isoproterenol causes a loss of antiarrhythmic activity of flecainide.
**Related Drugs:** A similar interaction may occur between flecainide and other beta agonist-sympathomimetics. It is not known to what extent the sympathomimetics with both alpha and beta agonist activity would interact with flecainide. Flecainide is unrelated to the Class IB antiarrhythmic agents.
**Mechanism:** Isoproterenol may shorten the refractory period of the accessory pathway through its beta-adrenergic stimulation, resulting in a loss of flecainide's efficacy.
**Detailed Information:** See *EDI*, 3/6.10

## Flecainide-Quinine

**Significance:** 3—minimally clinically significant
**Potential Effects:** The addition of quinine to a flecainide regimen may increase flecainide serum levels.
**Recommendations:** Patients should be monitored if quinine is added to the therapy of a patient maintained on flecainide. The dose of flecainide may need to be adjusted.
**Summary:** Quinine decreased the clearance and increased the half-life of flecainide.
**Related Drugs:** Encainide was shown to similarly interact with quinine. Mexiletine and encainide increased quinidine sulfate serum concentrations, whereas concurrent flecainide and tocainide did not. There is no documentation for an interaction between quinine and other antiarrhythmic agents.

Antiarrhythmic

> **Mechanism:** The inhibition of cytochrome P450 isozymes by quinine is likely to be responsible for the inhibition of flecainide metabolism.
> **Detailed Information:** See *EDI*, 3/6.25

## Flecainide-Sodium Bicarbonate

> **Significance:** 2—moderately clinically significant
> **Potential Effects:** Sodium bicarbonate alkalinizes the urine, resulting in decreased flecainide elimination and possible toxicity.
> **Recommendations:** The patient should be carefully monitored if these agents are used concurrently. The dose of flecainide may need to be decreased.
> **Summary:** The renal clearance and urinary elimination of flecainide were decreased with increasing urinary pH caused by sodium bicarbonate.
> **Related Drugs:** A similar interaction may occur between flecainide and other urinary alkalinizers. It is not known if a similar interaction would occur between sodium bicarbonate and the other Class IC antiarrhythmic, encainide.
> **Mechanism:** A prolonged elimination half-life of flecainide may be the result of a higher degree of renal tubular reabsorption of un-ionized flecainide molecules at an alkaline pH.
> **Detailed Information:** See *EDI*, 3/6.30

## Lidocaine-Cimetidine

> **Significance:** 1—highly clinically significant
> **Potential Effects:** Cimetidine increases lidocaine levels, possibly resulting in lidocaine toxicity.
> **Recommendations:** If these agents are given together, monitor lidocaine levels. The dose of lidocaine may need to be decreased, or ranitidine or possibly famotidine may be used instead of cimetidine.
> **Summary:** There are data to show that the concurrent administration of cimetidine and lidocaine has resulted in increased lidocaine serum concentrations; however, contrasting data are available.
> **Related Drugs:** Ranitidine has shown comparable results when administered with lidocaine. Lidocaine would not be expected to interact with the other $H_2$-receptor antagonists. Mexiletine was shown to react similarly to lidocaine when administered with cimetidine.
> **Mechanism:** Cimetidine may inhibit the microsomal enzymes involved in the metabolism of lidocaine and may induce a reduction in hepatic blood flow, reducing the hepatic clearance of lidocaine.
> **Detailed Information:** See *EDI*, 3/7.00

## Lidocaine-Phenobarbital

> **Significance:** 3—minimally clinically significant
> **Recommendations:** It is recommended that lidocaine plasma levels be monitored to assure that they are in the therapeutic range. However, since induction of metabolism may result in increased levels of pharmacologically active metabolites, the clinical significance of this interaction requires further investigation.
> **Summary:** There are data to show that plasma levels of lidocaine may be decreased during concurrent administration of phenobarbital.
> **Related Drugs:** A similar interaction is expected to occur with other barbiturates and lidocaine. The elimination of tocainide was not influenced by pretreatment with phenobarbital.
> **Mechanism:** The induction of lidocaine metabolism by phenobarbital is most likely responsible for this interaction.
> **Detailed Information:** See *EDI*, 3/9.00

Antiarrhythmic

## Lidocaine-Procainamide

**Significance:** 3—minimally clinically significant

**Recommendations:** Until further clinical studies are performed, the concurrent use of these agents need not be avoided. However, it is important to be aware of a possible interaction, and if CNS symptoms occur, discontinuing lidocaine appears to be beneficial.

**Summary:** There are data to show that the coadministration of procainamide and lidocaine has resulted in restlessness, visual disturbances, and delirium. These symptoms may have been caused by CNS toxicity.

**Related Drugs:** Documentation is lacking regarding a similar interaction between procainamide and tocainide. There are no drugs related to procainamide.

**Mechanism:** The mechanism of this interaction is not fully known; however, the two drugs may have a synergistic effect on the CNS.

**Detailed Information:** See *EDI*, 3/10.10

## Lidocaine-Propranolol

**Significance:** 2—moderately clinically significant

**Recommendations:** Since lidocaine has a narrow therapeutic index, concurrent administration with a beta-blocking agent may require the dosage or infusion rate of lidocaine to be reduced. Lidocaine serum levels should be monitored with appropriate dosage adjustments.

**Summary:** The concurrent administration of propranolol and lidocaine significantly decreased the metabolic clearance of lidocaine.

**Related Drugs:** Pindolol, metoprolol and atenolol did not significantly affect lidocaine metabolism. Nadolol was found to increase lidocaine plasma levels and decrease clearance. Because of conflicting data, it is not known whether the other beta-adrenergic blocking agents would interact with lidocaine. When tocainide and propranolol were administered, severe paranoia and confusion resulted. Tocainide and metoprolol showed no influence on hemodynamic parameters.

**Mechanism:** Propranolol decreases the cardiac output and hepatic blood flow, decreasing the metabolic clearance of lidocaine. Propranolol may also influence the hepatic drug-metabolizing capacity.

**Detailed Information:** See *EDI*, 3/11.00

## Mexiletine-Aluminum Hydroxide, Magnesium Hydroxide

**Significance:** 3—minimally clinically significant

**Potential Effects:** The aluminum hydroxide component may prolong the gastric emptying time, which may prolong the time to reach peak concentration of mexiletine.

**Recommendations:** The concomitant use of these agents need not be avoided since the bioavailability of mexiletine was not altered. However, further studies are necessary.

**Summary:** Administration of an antacid with mexiletine was found to increase mexiletine's peak plasma concentration.

**Related Drugs:** Antacids increased tocainide's area-under-curve and decreased the clearance and maximum plasma concentration. A similar interaction is expected between mexiletine and other antacids; however, only aluminum-containing antacids may interact.

**Mechanism:** The aluminum hydroxide component of the antacid may decrease the gastric emptying rate, prolonging the time to reach peak concentration of mexiletine.

**Detailed Information:** See *EDI*, 3/12.01

## Antiarrhythmic

### Mexiletine-Ammonium Chloride
**Significance:** 3—minimally clinically significant
**Potential Effects:** Ammonium chloride acidifies the urine, which increases the excretion of mexiletine.
**Recommendations:** Monitor mexiletine serum levels and clinical response when these agents are used together.
**Summary:** There are data to show that administration of mexiletine with ammonium chloride acidifies the urine, increasing the excretion of mexiletine.
**Related Drugs:** Other agents that acidify the urine may interact with mexiletine. It is not known if an interaction would occur between ammonium chloride and other antiarrhythmic agents related to mexiletine.
**Mechanism:** As the urine pH decreases, the tubular reabsorption of the ionized mexiletine also decreases, resulting in an increased excretion of unchanged drug.
**Detailed Information:** See *EDI*, 3/12.03

### Mexiletine-Atropine
**Significance:** 3—minimally clinically significant
**Potential Effects:** Atropine decreases the gastric emptying rate, which may lead to a decrease in the rate of mexiletine absorption.
**Recommendations:** The use of these agents concurrently need not be avoided. This interaction may be of significance only when initiating mexiletine therapy.
**Summary:** Administration of atropine reduces the maximum plasma concentration and elimination half-life of mexiletine.
**Related Drugs:** It is not known if a similar interaction would occur between atropine and the other Class IB antiarrhythmic agent, tocainide. A similar interaction may be expected to occur between mexiletine and other anticholinergics.
**Mechanism:** Atropine decreases the rate of mexiletine absorption because of a decrease in the gastric emptying rate.
**Detailed Information:** See *EDI*, 3/12.05

### Mexiletine-Metoclopramide
**Significance:** 3—minimally clinically significant
**Potential Effects:** Metoclopramide increases the gastric emptying rate, which may result in an increase in the absorption of mexiletine.
**Recommendations:** The concomitant use of these agents need not be avoided. However, this interaction may be of some significance when initiating mexiletine therapy.
**Summary:** Metoclopramide increases the gastric emptying rate, resulting in an increased absorption of mexiletine.
**Related Drugs:** It is not known if a similar interaction would occur between metoclopramide and the other Class IB antiarrhythmic agent, tocainide. There are no drugs related to metoclopramide.
**Mechanism:** Metoclopramide may enhance the rate of mexiletine absorption because of an increase in the gastric emptying rate.
**Detailed Information:** See *EDI*, 3/12.07

### Mexiletine-Phenytoin
**Significance:** 3—minimally clinically significant
**Potential Effects:** Phenytoin may decrease plasma levels of mexiletine.
**Recommendations:** Monitor the patient's cardiac status and levels of mexiletine when these agents are used together. The dose of mexiletine may need to be increased.

**Summary:** Phenytoin has been shown to decrease area-under-curve, mean elimination half-life and plasma levels of mexiletine.

**Related Drugs:** Phenytoin has been shown to reduce the bioavailability and increase the clearance of lidocaine. Phenytoin may also interact with tocainide. A similar interaction is expected to occur between mexiletine and other hydantoin anticonvulsants.

**Mechanism:** Phenytoin may induce the hepatic enzymes responsible for the metabolism of mexiletine.

**Detailed Information:** See *EDI*, 3/12.09

## Mexiletine-Rifampin

**Significance:** 3—minimally clinically significant

**Potential Effects:** Rifampin may increase the metabolism of mexiletine.

**Recommendations:** Monitor the patient's cardiac status and mexiletine levels when these agents are used together.

**Summary:** Rifampin has been shown to cause a decrease in the elimination half-life of mexiletine and an increase in its metabolism and nonrenal clearance. There were no pharmacokinetic changes with mexiletine.

**Related Drugs:** Tocainide administered with rifampin has shown altered tocainide pharmacokinetics. Lidocaine may interact similarly with rifampin based on metabolism. There are no drugs related to rifampin.

**Mechanism:** Rifampin induces the hepatic microsomal enzymes responsible for the metabolism of mexiletine.

**Detailed Information:** See *EDI*, 3/12.11

## Mexiletine-Tobacco

**Significance:** 3—minimally clinically significant

**Potential Effects:** Cigarette smoking increases the elimination of mexiletine.

**Recommendations:** Patients stabilized on mexiletine who start or stop smoking should be observed for a change in the therapeutic effects of mexiletine.

**Summary:** There are data to show that cigarette smoking significantly increases the elimination of mexiletine. The effect on the clearance of mexiletine was less marked and the other pharmacokinetic parameters were unaffected.

**Related Drugs:** A similar interaction may be expected to occur with other Class IB antiarrhythmic agents related to mexiletine.

**Mechanism:** Cigarette smoking increases the rate of conjugation of mexiletine with glucuronic acid and induces its aliphatic hydroxylation.

**Detailed Information:** See *EDI*, 3/12.13

## Moricizine-Cimetidine

**Significance:** 3—minimally clinically significant

**Potential Effects:** Cimetidine may decrease the metabolism of moricizine, leading to increased levels.

**Recommendations:** Monitor patients closely during concurrent cimetidine and moricizine administration. The dose of moricizine may need to be decreased.

**Summary:** Cimetidine has been shown to decrease the clearance and to increase the elimination half-life and area-under-curve of moricizine.

**Related Drugs:** Moricizine is not chemically related to the other antiarrhythmic agents. It is not known whether the other $H_2$-receptor antagonists would interact with moricizine.

**Mechanism:** The mechanism of this interaction is not known; however, it has been suggested that cimetidine inhibits the hepatic metabolism of moricizine.
**Detailed Information:** See *EDI,* 3/12.17

## Nifedipine-Cimetidine

**Significance:** 2—moderately clinically significant
**Potential Effects:** Cimetidine inhibits the metabolism of nifedipine, resulting in increased levels and pharmacologic activity.
**Recommendations:** Until further studies are performed, patients should be monitored for increased nifedipine effects during concurrent use of nifedine and cimetidine. Ranitidine, nizatidine, or famotidine may be alternatives to cimetidine.
**Summary:** Cimetidine caused a rise in maximal plasma levels and area-under-curve of nifedipine. Patients also experienced a significant reduction in arterial blood pressure.
**Related Drugs:** Ranitidine was shown to exhibit a similar interaction when administered with nifedipine. Cimetidine caused an increase in the elimination half-life and a reduction in clearance of verapamil.
**Mechanism:** Cimetidine inhibits the hepatic drug metabolizing enzymes by binding to cytochrome P450. It is not known how cimetidine influenced the decreased blood pressure.
**Detailed Information:** See *EDI,* 3/12.20

## Nifedipine-Ethanol

**Significance:** 3—minimally clinically significant
**Potential Effects:** Concurrent nifedipine and ethanol may result in increased nifedipine levels and cardiac effects.
**Recommendations:** Patients maintained on nifedipine should be monitored for potentiation of nifedipine effects if ethanol is given concurrently.
**Summary:** Concurrent nifedipine and ethanol administration resulted in an increase in nifedipine area-under-curve.
**Related Drugs:** Verapamil exhibited a similar interaction when administered with ethanol. Felodipine and ethanol significantly decreased blood pressures. Nifedipine exaggerated the ethanol-induced motor incoordination. A similar interaction is expected between ethanol and other calcium channel blocking agents, if the mechanism involves the inhibition of cytochrome P450 isozymes.
**Mechanism:** Ethanol inhibits nifedipine metabolism, possibly because both agents are metabolized by dehydrogenation.
**Detailed Information:** See *EDI,* 3/12.25

## Nifedipine-Fluoxetine

**Significance:** 3—minimally clinically significant
**Potential Effects:** The concurrent administration of fluoxetine and nifedipine resulted in increased nifedipine effects.
**Recommendations:** If fluoxetine is added to the regimen of a patient maintained on nifedipine, the patient should be monitored for increased nifedipine effects. The dosage of nifedipine may need to be adjusted.
**Summary:** The concurrent administration of fluoxetine and nifedipine resulted in increased nifedipine effects. After being maintained on nifedipine for five years, a patient experienced rapid palpitations, hand tremor, worsening weakness, and upright hypotension 10 days after fluoxetine was added to the regimen. Symptoms gradually improved upon fluoxetine discontinuation.

## Antiarrhythmic

**Related Drugs:** Increased effects of verapamil were noted when fluoxetine was added to the therapy of a patient maintained on verapamil. Based on the postulated mechanism and pharmacologic similarity, a similar interaction would be expected to occur between fluoxetine and the other calcium channel blockers and between nifedipine or verapamil and the other selective serotonin reuptake inhibitors.

**Mechanism:** The mechanism of this interaction is not known. However, it has been postulated that fluoxetine inhibits nifedipine's metabolism. However, nifedipine is metabolized by cytochrome $P450_{3A4}$ isozymes, and the manufacturer of fluoxetine states that fluoxetine's effects on this isozyme are not likely to be clinically significant. An *in vitro* study indicated that fluoxetine's effects may be mediated through a calcium channel-dependent process. The clinical effects of these results are unknown.

**Detailed Information:** See *EDI*, 3/12.27

### Nifedipine-Halothane

**Significance:** 3—minimally clinically significant

**Recommendations:** It is important to be aware of a possible interaction between nifedipine and halothane and to use these agents with caution, especially in patients with decreased left ventricular function.

**Summary:** The concurrent use of nifedipine under halothane anesthesia has led to myocardial depression.

**Related Drugs:** Halothane and verapamil have been shown to have an additive negative inotropic effect. A similar interaction is expected to occur between halothane and other calcium channel blockers. Documentation is lacking regarding an interaction between nifedipine and the other halogenated inhalation anesthetics.

**Mechanism:** Halothane and calcium channel blocking agents have a pronounced independent negative inotropic effects, and an additive effect may explain the mechanism.

**Detailed Information:** See *EDI*, 3/12.30

### Nifedipine-Magnesium Sulfate

**Significance:** 3—minimally clinically significant

**Potential Effects:** Concurrent use of these agents may result in marked hypotension.

**Recommendations:** Concurrent administration of magnesium sulfate and nifedipine should be approached with caution. Blood pressure should be carefully monitored when these agents are used together.

**Summary:** Administration of nifedipine with magnesium sulfate resulted in marked hypotension.

**Related Drugs:** A similar interaction is expected to occur between magnesium sulfate and other calcium-channel blocking agents, if the hypotensive response is related to magnesium sulfate and nifedipine. There are no drugs related to magnesium sulfate.

**Mechanism:** Although the mechanism is not known, the marked hypotension is because of an interaction between magnesium sulfate and nifedipine.

**Detailed Information:** See *EDI*, 3/12.40

### Procainamide-Alcohol, Ethyl

**Significance:** 3—minimally clinically significant

**Recommendations:** Procainamide and N-acetylprocainamide levels should be monitored in patients concurrently ingesting alcohol while on procainamide therapy. The dosage of procainamide may need to be adjusted.

## Antiarrhythmic

**Summary:** The concurrent ingestion of alcohol with procainamide resulted in a significant reduction in procainamide half-life and an increase in the elimination half-life and total clearance.
**Related Drugs:** There are no drugs related to procainamide.
**Mechanism:** Alcohol may affect the acetylation of procainamide.
**Detailed Information:** See *EDI*, 3/13.00

### Procainamide-Amiodarone

**Significance:** 2—moderately clinically significant
**Potential Effects:** Amiodarone may cause an increase in procainamide and NAPA levels.
**Recommendations:** Monitor procainamide and NAPA levels when these agents are used together. The dose of procainamide may need to be decreased by 20% to 50%.
**Summary:** There are data to show that administration of procainamide with amiodarone increases procainamide serum levels, resulting in procainamide toxicity.
**Related Drugs:** There are no drugs related to procainamide or amiodarone.
**Mechanism:** This interaction may be due to a decrease in procainamide tissue binding, releasing procainamide into the serum.
**Detailed Information:** See *EDI*, 3/14.01

### Procainamide-Cimetidine

**Significance:** 2—moderately clinically significant
**Potential Effects:** Cimetidine may cause an increase in procainamide and NAPA levels.
**Recommendations:** Monitor procainamide and NAPA levels when cimetidine is administered concurrently. The dose of procainamide may need to be decreased.
**Summary:** There are data to show that cimetidine increases procainamide serum levels, resulting in procainamide toxicity.
**Related Drugs:** Ranitidine has been shown to cause increases in procainamide serum levels; however, all data do not support this. There are no drugs related to procainamide.
**Mechanism:** It has been suggested that this interaction is a cimetidine-induced reduction in renal blood flow, competing for active tubular secretion.
**Detailed Information:** See *EDI*, 3/14.10

### Procainamide–Para-Aminobenzoic Acid

**Significance:** 3—minimally clinically significant
**Potential Effects:** Administration of PABA to patients receiving procainamide may decrease the NAPA/procainamide serum level ratio. This may lead to an increased antiarrhythmic activity of procainamide.
**Recommendations:** Monitor the NAPA and procainamide levels if these agents are used concomitantly.
**Summary:** There are data to show that coadministration of PABA and procainamide may decrease the NAPA/procainamide serum ratio, leading to an increased antiarrhythmic activity of procainamide.
**Related Drugs:** There are no drugs related to procainamide or PABA.
**Mechanism:** PABA competitively inhibits the acetylation of procainamide, resulting in a decrease in the NAPA/procainamide ratio.
**Detailed Information:** See *EDI*, 3/14.21

## Antiarrhythmic

### Procainamide-Propranolol

**Significance:** 3—minimally clinically significant

**Recommendations:** Until further clinical studies are done, the concurrent use of these agents need not be avoided; however, procainamide and NAPA levels should be routinely monitored.

**Summary:** Propranolol has been shown to decrease the plasma clearance of procainamide and increase the elimination half-life; however, all data do not support this.

**Related Drugs:** Metoprolol and procainamide had no effect on the clearance and elimination half-life of procainamide. Because of conflicting results, it is difficult to determine if an interaction would occur between procainamide and other beta-blocking agents. There are no drugs related to procainamide.

**Mechanism:** The mechanism of the interaction is unknown.

**Detailed Information:** See *EDI*, 3/14.30

### Procainamide-Quinidine

**Significance:** 3—minimally clinically significant

**Potential Effects:** Quinidine may increase the plasma level and half-life of procainamide and its active metabolite.

**Recommendations:** Concurrent use of quinidine and procainamide may be beneficial in certain circumstances. However, high dose procainamide should be used with caution with quinidine. Monitor patients' procainamide and NAPA levels.

**Summary:** The concurrent use of quinidine and procainamide resulted in increased levels of both procainamide and NAPA, an active metabolite.

**Related Drugs:** It is not know if procainamide would interact similarly with quinine. There are no drugs related to procainamide.

**Mechanism:** Quinidine may interfere with the renal elimination of procainamide by interfering with glomerular filtration, proximal tubular secretion, or reabsorption in the distal tubule.

**Detailed Information:** See *EDI*, 3/14.50

### Procainamide-Trimethoprim

**Significance:** 3—minimally clinically significant

**Potential Effects:** Concurrent trimethoprim and procainamide therapy may result in an increase in procainamide and NAPA levels because of competition for excretion of procainamide by trimethoprim.

**Recommendations:** Monitor procainamide and NAPA levels when using procainamide and trimethoprim together.

**Summary:** Trimethoprim decreased the renal clearance of procainamide and of NAPA, an active metabolite of procainamide, and increased serum concentrations were observed.

**Related Drugs:** There are no drugs related to procainamide or trimethoprim.

**Mechanism:** Trimethoprim increases procainamide and NAPA serum concentrations by competing for tubular secretion.

**Detailed Information:** See *EDI*, 3/14.70

### Propafenone-Cyclosporine

**Significance:** 2—moderately clinically significant

**Potential Effects:** Propafenone may inhibit the metabolism of cyclosporine resulting in increased cyclosporine levels.

**Recommendations:** Caution should be used when propafenone therapy is instituted in a patient maintained on cyclosporine. Cyclosporine whole-blood levels should be monitored, and the dose of cyclosporine may need to be reduced.

## Antiarrhythmic

**Summary:** The addition of propafenone to a cyclosporine regimen has been shown to result in an increase in cyclosporine whole blood levels.

**Related Drugs:** It is not known whether an interaction would occur between cyclosporine and other antiarrhythmic agents. There are no drugs related to cyclosporine.

**Mechanism:** Propafenone may inhibit the metabolism of cyclosporine.

**Detailed Information:** See *EDI*, 3/14.80

### Propafenone-Fluoxetine

**Significance:** 2—moderately clinically significant

**Potential Effects:** The concurrent administration of propafenone and fluoxetine may result in increased propafenone serum levels.

**Recommendations:** Caution is advised with the concurrent administration of fluoxetine and propafenone. The patient should be carefully monitored for increased propafenone effects and possible toxicity.

**Summary:** Concomitant administration of propafenone and fluoxetine resulted in increased propafenone serum levels.

**Related Drugs:** An interaction may be expected to occur between propafenone and other selective serotonin reuptake inhibitors known to inhibit the cytochrome $P450_{2D6}$ isozyme (sertraline and paroxetine). It is not known whether an interaction would occur between propafenone and the other selective serotonin reuptake inhibitors (e.g., citalopram, fluvoxamine) or whether an interaction would occur between fluoxetine and the other antiarrhythmic agents.

**Mechanism:** Propafenone undergoes extensive hepatic metabolism and has a low systemic bioavailability following oral administration; therefore, it is likely to interact with inhibitors of the cytochrome $P450_{2D6}$ isozyme such as fluoxetine.

**Detailed Information:** See *EDI*, 3/14.85

### Propafenone-Quinidine

**Significance:** 2—moderately clinically significant

**Potential Effects:** Quinidine may increase propafenone plasma concentration and pharmacologic effects.

**Recommendations:** Patients receiving propafenone should be carefully monitored for cardiac function changes if quinidine is added to therapy. The dose of propafenone may need to be reduced.

**Summary:** Concurrent quinidine and propafenone administration has been shown to increase the propafenone plasma concentration.

**Related Drugs:** Quinine would be expected to interact with propafenone in a similar manner. It is not known whether an interaction would occur between quinidine and other antiarrhythmic agents.

**Mechanism:** Quinidine inhibits the hepatic cytochrome P450 mediated 5-hydroxylation of propafenone, resulting in a decreased clearance of propafenone.

**Detailed Information:** See *EDI*, 3/14.90

### Quinidine-Amiodarone

**Significance:** 1—highly clinically significant

**Potential Effects:** Amiodarone can cause an increase in quinidine levels.

**Recommendations:** Monitor quinidine levels if these agents are used together. The dose of quinidine may need to be decreased.

**Summary:** Amiodarone can cause an increase in quinidine levels, causing atypical ventricular tachycardia and a prolonged QT interval.

Antiarrhythmic

**Related Drugs:** There are no drugs related to amiodarone. It is not known if a similar interaction would occur between amiodarone and quinine.

**Mechanism:** The most likely mechanisms include a decrease in quinidine tissue binding, releasing quinidine into the serum and effectively decreasing the volume of distribution, or decreasing the renal or hepatic clearance of quinidine.

**Detailed Information:** See *EDI,* 3/16.10

## Quinidine-Cimetidine

**Significance:** 2—moderately clinically significant

**Potential Effects:** Cimetidine decreases the clearance of quinidine.

**Recommendations:** Patients taking these agents together should be monitored for signs of quinidine toxicity (e.g., cinchonism, lethargy, tachyarrhythmias, vomiting).

**Summary:** Concurrent administration of cimetidine and quinidine resulted in reduced quinidine clearance, increased half-life, and increased peak plasma concentration.

**Related Drugs:** Quinidine and ranitidine have been shown to cause dizziness, nausea, irregular heart rate, and ventricular bigeminy with ECG changes. However, all data do not support this. It is not known if an interaction would occur between quinidine and other $H_2$-receptor antagonists.

**Mechanism:** An increase in quinidine absorption with concurrent cimetidine may explain the elevated quinidine plasma concentrations.

**Detailed Information:** See *EDI,* 3/17.00

## Quinidine-Diphenoxylate/Atropine

**Significance:** 3—minimally clinically significant

**Potential Effects:** Diphenoxylate/atropine decreases GI motility which may result in a decrease in quinidine levels.

**Recommendations:** Quinidine levels should be monitored and the dosage adjusted as necessary during concomitant administration of diphenoxylate with atropine and quinidine sulfate.

**Summary:** Concurrent administration of quinidine sulfate and diphenoxylate with atropine has been shown to result in a significant decrease in quinidine levels.

**Related Drugs:** A similar interaction between quinidine sulfate and difenoxin/atropine may occur. No documentation is available for an interaction between diphenoxylate and quinine.

**Mechanism:** The ability of diphenoxylate to decrease gastrointestinal motility may affect the absorption of quinidine.

**Detailed Information:** See *EDI,* 3/18.01

## Quinidine-Ketoconazole

**Significance:** 2—moderately clinically significant

**Potential Effects:** Ketoconazole may decrease the clearance of quinidine, resulting in increased levels.

**Recommendations:** Patients maintained on quinidine sulfate should be closely monitored for changes in cardiac status or changes in quinidine serum levels if ketoconazole is added to, or withdrawn from, concurrent quinidine therapy. The dose of quinidine may need to be decreased.

**Summary:** Ketoconazole may decrease the clearance of quinidine, resulting in increased levels and changes in serum creatinine.

**Related Drugs:** Other quinidine salts may interact in a similar manner with ketoconazole. A similar interaction is expected to occur between quinine and ketoconazole.

## Antiarrhythmic

**Mechanism:** The reduction of plasma quinidine concentration is most likely the result of an inhibition of hepatic enzyme activity by ketoconazole.
**Detailed Information:** See *EDI,* 3/18.05

### Quinidine-Metoclopramide

**Significance:** 3—minimally clinically significant
**Potential Effects:** Metoclopramide may decrease the absorption of quinidine, leading to a decrease in quinidine's area-under-curve.
**Recommendations:** Monitor patients for a decrease in quinidine levels during cotherapy with metoclopramide. The dosage of quinidine may need to be increased.
**Summary:** Metoclopramide has been shown to decrease quinidine's area-under-curve and absorption.
**Related Drugs:** It is not known if a similar interaction would occur between metoclopramide and quinine. There are no drugs related to metoclopramide.
**Mechanism:** Metoclopramide may decrease the absorption of quinidine.
**Detailed Information:** See *EDI,* 3/18.10

### Quinidine-Phenobarbital

**Significance:** 2—moderately clinically significant
**Recommendations:** Quinidine plasma levels should be monitored during concurrent use of these agents. If a loss of arrhythmia control is evident, the dose of quinidine may need to be increased. Also, if a patient is stabilized on both agents, the dose of quinidine may have to be decreased upon withdrawal of the barbiturate.
**Summary:** The concurrent administration of quinidine and phenobarbital has been shown to result in a reduction of the elimination half-life of quinidine and the area-under-curve.
**Related Drugs:** Similar changes in quinidine levels after pentobarbital administration have been documented. A similar interaction may occur between quinidine and other barbiturates. The half-life of quinine was reported to be significantly decreased in patients receiving phenobarbital, primidone or phenytoin.
**Mechanism:** Phenobarbital, a known enzyme inducer, may increase the metabolism of quinidine.
**Detailed Information:** See *EDI,* 3/19.00

### Quinidine-Phenytoin

**Significance:** 2—moderately clinically significant
**Recommendations:** Combination therapy of quinidine and phenytoin will probably require an alteration in quinidine dosage to maintain therapeutic quinidine serum levels. Careful monitoring and possible readjustment of quinidine levels will be required when phenytoin therapy is begun or discontinued, as seen in one patient where decreasing the phenytoin dosage resulted in an increased quinidine level.
**Summary:** Quinidine serum levels may be reduced by the concurrent use of phenytoin.
**Related Drugs:** Other hydantoin anticonvulsants may interact with quinidine. The half-life of quinine was found to be significantly decreased in patients receiving phenobarbital, phenytoin, or primidone.
**Mechanism:** Phenytoin, a known enzyme inducer, may increase the metabolism of quinidine.
**Detailed Information:** See *EDI,* 3/21.00

## Antiarrhythmic

### Quinidine-Reserpine

**Significance:** 3—minimally clinically significant

**Recommendations:** To minimize the possible toxic effects resulting from concurrent administration of quinidine and reserpine, treatment with these agents should not be initiated simultaneously. Treatment with reserpine should be initiated first and an interval of at least 24 hours should be allowed before introducing quinidine. When quinidine is added to the regimen of a reserpine-treated patient, the dose should be increased cautiously and cardiac function should be monitored closely.

**Summary:** The antiarrhythmic and cardiodepressant effects of quinidine may be enhanced by the administration of reserpine.

**Related Drugs:** All quinidine salts may have a similar interaction with reserpine. There is no documentation regarding an interaction with quinine. A similar interaction is expected to occur with the other rauwolfia alkaloids.

**Mechanism:** Reserpine depletes myocardial tissue of its catecholamine stores and causes a decrease in the electrical automaticity and excitability of myocardial tissue. This effect may enhance quinidine's direct myocardial tissue depressant activity and could result in quinidine toxicity.

**Detailed Information:** See *EDI*, 3/23.00

### Quinidine-Rifampin

**Significance:** 2—moderately clinically significant

**Recommendations:** When using rifampin concurrently with quinidine, the response to quinidine should be closely monitored and the dose increased if necessary.

**Summary:** The antiarrhythmic effect of quinidine was diminished when rifampin was coadministered with quinidine.

**Related Drugs:** A similar interaction is expected to occur with quinine. There are no drugs related to rifampin.

**Mechanism:** Rifampin, a known enzyme inducer, may increase the metabolism of quinidine.

**Detailed Information:** See *EDI*, 3/25.00

### Quinidine-Sucralfate

**Significance:** 3—minimally clinically significant

**Potential Effects:** Quinidine absorption may be decreased resulting in decreased quinidine levels and effect.

**Recommendations:** Because of the lack of studies, it is not known whether the bioavailability of quinidine can be altered when given concomitantly with sucralfate. Since a potential has been shown for such a reaction, be cautious when using these agents together.

**Summary:** Concomitant quinidine and sucralfate resulted in decreased quinidine levels.

**Related Drugs:** Aluminum hydroxide has been shown to delay the gastrointestinal absorption of quinidine in animals. It is not known whether a similar interaction would occur between quinidine and other aluminum salts.

**Mechanism:** This interaction could occur in humans because of the ability of sucralfate to bind to the quinidine moiety when these two drugs are given simultaneously.

**Detailed Information:** See *EDI*, 3/26.50

### Quinidine-Verapamil

**Significance:** 1—highly clinically significant

**Potential Effects:** Concurrent verapamil and quinidine causes an increase in quinidine levels and possible hypotension.

## Antiarrhythmic

**Recommendations:** Use these agents together with caution. Quinidine levels should be monitored and dosage may have to be decreased. One or both drugs may need to be discontinued.
**Summary:** There are data to show that verapamil causes an increase in quinidine levels, causing hypotension and acute pulmonary edema.
**Related Drugs:** Nifedipine and quinidine resulted in decreased quinidine serum levels. An interaction is expected to occur between quinidine and other calcium channel blockers, but it is difficult to determine if quinidine levels would increase or decrease. Quinidine administered with nifedipine or diltiazem would result in hypotension. No documentation is available regarding an interaction between verapamil quinine.
**Mechanism:** Verapamil inhibits the metabolism of quinidine, which results in increased quinidine levels.
**Detailed Information:** See *EDI,* 3/27.00

### Verapamil-Calcium Gluconate

**Significance:** 2—moderately clinically significant
**Recommendations:** Patients should be monitored for a change in their response to verapamil if calcium is added to, or withdrawn from, their therapy.
**Summary:** There are data to show that coadministration of verapamil and calcium may cause changes in verapamil response.
**Related Drugs:** A similar interaction is expected to occur between calcium gluconate and other calcium channel blockers. The other salts of calcium may be expected to interact similarly with calcium gluconate.
**Mechanism:** This interaction results from an antagonistic effect between the two agents.
**Detailed Information:** See *EDI,* 3/29.00

### Verapamil-Dantrolene

**Significance:** 2—moderately clinically significant
**Potential Effects:** The concurrent use of these agents may result in hyperkalemia and myocardial depression.
**Recommendations:** Monitor for increased potassium levels when the agents are used concurrently. A decreased dose of dantrolene or the use of nifedipine may help circumvent or lessen the magnitude of the interaction.
**Summary:** The concurrent administration of verapamil and dantrolene was shown to result in hyperkalemia and myocardial depression.
**Related Drugs:** Nifedipine exhibits a similar interaction with dantrolene, and in an animal study, nifedipine and dantrolene resulted in hyperkalemia and cardiovascular collapse. A similar interaction is expected to occur between dantrolene and other calcium channel blockers. There are no drugs related to dantrolene.
**Mechanism:** The addition of verapamil may limit the compensatory mechanisms for a dantrolene-induced increases in serum potassium, resulting in a sustained elevation of potassium levels.
**Detailed Information:** See *EDI,* 3/30.01

### Verapamil-Phenobarbital

**Significance:** 3—minimally clinically significant
**Potential Effects:** Phenobarbital may increase the metabolism of verapamil. Also the protein binding of verapamil may be decreased by phenobarbital. These two potential effects may result in an insignificant or no net change in the pharmacologically active unbound concentration of verapamil.

## Antiarrhythmic

**Recommendations:** Although the concurrent administration of phenobarbital and verapamil need not be avoided, patients should be monitored for changes in verapamil serum levels. The dose of verapamil may need to be adjusted.

**Summary:** Phenobarbital has been shown to increase the verapamil free fraction, the total systemic clearance and the rate of elimination of verapamil.

**Related Drugs:** A similar interaction is expected to occur with other calcium channel blockers and phenobarbital and with other barbiturates.

**Mechanism:** Phenobarbital may increase the hepatic metabolism of verapamil.

**Detailed Information:** See *EDI*, 3/30.30

### Verapamil-Propranolol

**Significance:** 2—moderately clinically significant

**Potential Effects:** Concurrent use of verapamil and propranolol may result in serious hypotension, bradycardia, and, rarely, ventricular asystole.

**Recommendations:** Patients undergoing concurrent therapy with verapamil and propranolol should be closely monitored for blood pressure, heart rate and clinical status, especially during the first days of concomitant therapy.

**Summary:** Concurrent use of verapamil and propranolol may result in serious hypotension, decreased cardiac contractility, bradycardia, and ventricular asystole.

**Related Drugs:** Pindolol, metoprolol or atenolol with verapamil has exhibited a similar interaction. There are many documented reports regarding an interaction between other beta-blockers and calcium channel blockers; however, much of the data are conflicting.

**Mechanism:** An additive cardiodepressive response may be seen with concomitant use of these agents, and the concurrent administration of propranolol may block the beta-adrenergic activity originally stimulated by verapamil.

**Detailed Information:** See *EDI*, 3/31.00

### Verapamil-Rifampin

**Significance:** 2—moderately clinically significant

**Potential Effects:** Rifampin induces the hepatic metabolism of oral verapamil, leading to decreased serum levels and efficacy. This effect is significant only with oral verapamil.

**Recommendations:** Patients receiving oral verapamil should be monitored for decreased verapamil levels during concurrent rifampin therapy. If decreased levels or effects of verapamil occur during concomitant rifampin administration, the dose of verapamil may need to be increased.

**Summary:** Rifampin induces the hepatic metabolism of oral verapamil, leading to a decrease in serum levels and efficacy of rifampin.

**Related Drugs:** A similar interaction is expected to occur with other calcium channel blockers and rifampin. There are no drugs related to rifampin.

**Mechanism:** Rifampin decreases the bioavailability of oral verapamil by increasing its first-pass metabolism through the induction of hepatic microsomal enzymes.

**Detailed Information:** See *EDI*, 3/35.00

## Verapamil-Sulfinpyrazone

**Significance:** 3—minimally clinically significant

**Recommendations:** Until further clinical studies are available, the concurrent use of verapamil and sulfinpyrazone need not be avoided. However, if a decreased response to verapamil is noted, the dose of verapamil may need to be increased.

**Summary:** There are data to show that sulfinpyrazone causes an increase in the oral plasma clearance of verapamil.

**Related Drugs:** A similar interaction is expected to occur between sulfinpyrazone and other calcium channel blockers. It is not known if verapamil would interact with probenecid.

**Mechanism:** Sulfinpyrazone decreases the bioavailability of verapamil by increasing its first-pass metabolism.

**Detailed Information:** See *EDI*, 3/37.00

# Chapter Four

# Anticoagulant
Drug Interactions

Anticoagulant

## Acenocoumarol-Cetirizine

**Significance:** 3—minimally clinically significant

**Potential Effects:** The addition of cetirizine to the therapy of a patient maintained on acenocoumarol may result in an increase in international normalized ratio (INR) and anticoagulant activity.

**Recommendations:** Caution is advised when cetirizine is added to or removed from an acenocoumarol regimen. The patient's prothrombin time and INR should be monitored. Cetirizine may need to be discontinued.

**Summary:** The addition of cetirizine to acenocoumarol therapy resulted in an increase in anticoagulant activity and increased the patient's INR values from 1.5 to 14.

**Related Drugs:** A similar interaction would be expected to occur between cetirizine and the other coumarin oral anticoagulants. It is not known whether an interaction would occur between acenocoumarol and the other antihistamines related to cetirizine.

**Mechanism:** It is postulated that cetirizine competitively displaces acenocoumarol from protein binding sites because the carboxylic acid moiety on the cetirizine molecule would enable a strong protein bond. It was also speculated that the patient's renal impairment may have increased cetirizine serum levels, thus further increasing cetirizine's effect on acenocoumarol. These two factors could explain the increased anticoagulant effect noted in the patient.

**Detailed Information:** See *EDI*, 4/0.30

## Acenocoumarol-Ivermectin

**Significance:** 3—minimally clinically significant

**Potential Effects:** The anticoagulant activity of acenocoumarol may be enhanced by the concurrent administration of or exposure to ivermectin.

**Recommendations:** Patients maintained on coumarin anticoagulants should be closely monitored for an increased anticoagulant effect if they are treated with or exposed to ivermectin.

**Summary:** The anticoagulant activity of acenocoumarol was enhanced by concurrent exposure to ivermectin and metidation in a single case report.

**Related Drugs:** A similar interaction may be expected to occur between ivermectin and other coumarin oral anticoagulants. There are no drugs related to ivermectin.

**Mechanism:** Ivermectin may interfere with vitamin K-dependent clotting factors, which are also antagonized by coumarin derivatives. Ivermectin and the insecticide metidation are classified as organophosphates, which may also affect prothrombin time. One study suggests that a two-step reaction may occur, first hypercoagulability and then a period of hypocoagulability.

**Detailed Information:** See *EDI*, 4/0.50

## Dicumarol-Allopurinol

**Significance:** 1—highly clinically significant

**Recommendations:** Patients should be closely monitored for an increased anticoagulant response during concurrent use of dicumarol and allopurinol. If necessary, the dose of the anticoagulant may need to be decreased.

**Summary:** Allopurinol has been documented to significantly prolong dicumarol half-life.

**Related Drugs:** In patients receiving phenprocoumon, bleeding episodes have occurred after allopurinol treatment. Warfarin activity has been shown to increase with allopurinol; however, all data

Anticoagulant

do not support this. Because of conflicting data, it is difficult to determine whether a similar interaction would occur with anisindione and phenindione. There are no drugs related to allopurinol.

**Mechanism:** Allopurinol inhibits the hepatic metabolism of dicumarol, prolonging its half-life.

**Detailed Information:** See *EDI,* 4/1.00

## Dicumarol-Chloramphenicol

**Significance:** 2—moderately clinically significant

**Recommendations:** The concurrent use of dicumarol and chloramphenicol should be avoided. If concomitant use is necessary, frequent monitoring of prothrombin levels is required, and patients should be observed for clinical signs of dicumarol overdosage (e.g., hematuria, melena, bruising).

**Summary:** The anticoagulant activity of dicumarol may be enhanced by the concurrent administration of chloramphenicol. Chloramphenicol has been shown to increase the average dicumarol half-life.

**Related Drugs:** A similar interaction may occur with other coumarin anticoagulants and anisindione or phenindione. There are no drugs related to chloramphenicol.

**Mechanism:** Chloramphenicol may enhance the anticoagulant activity by reducing the availability of vitamin K, and it may interfere with the production of prothrombin.

**Detailed Information:** See *EDI,* 4/3.00

## Dicumarol-Corticotropin

**Significance:** 2—moderately clinically significant

**Recommendations:** Clotting time tests and clinical signs of hemorrhage should be monitored closely during concurrent administration of dicumarol and corticotropin or corticosteroids. The dosage of the anticoagulant may need to be either increased or decreased based on the results of such monitoring.

**Summary:** Corticotropin and corticosteroids have been shown to increase and decrease the hypoprothrombinemic effect of dicumarol and other oral anticoagulants, causing hemorrhagic episodes.

**Related Drugs:** The activity of phenindione is enhanced by corticotropin. Increased sensitivity to warfarin was documented with prednisone administration. Phenprocoumon and anisindione may also interact with corticotropin or corticosteroid. Cortisone and prednisone may interact with dicumarol. A similar interaction is expected to occur with other corticosteroids and dicumarol.

**Mechanism:** Corticosteroids have been shown to increase the coagulability of the blood, and corticotropin and corticosteroids may lower vascular integrity.

**Detailed Information:** See *EDI,* 4/5.00

## Dicumarol-Methylphenidate

**Significance:** 3—minimally clinically significant

**Recommendations:** The concurrent use of these agents need not be avoided. However, it is prudent to be aware of a possible interaction, and prothrombin levels should be frequently monitored.

**Summary:** Methylphenidate has been documented to increase the half-life of dicumarol; however, all data do not support this.

**Related Drugs:** It is difficult to determine whether a similar interaction would occur between methylphenidate and phenprocoumon warfarin, anisindione, phenindione or the other indirect-acting sympathomimetic agents.

## Anticoagulant

**Mechanism:** Methylphenidate may inhibit the hepatic metabolism of dicumarol.
**Detailed Information:** See *EDI*, 4/7.00

## Dicumarol-Oral Contraceptive Agents

**Significance:** 2—moderately clinically significant
**Recommendations:** The evidence is limited, but does indicate that the blood coagulation response of some oral anticoagulant agents may be changed with concurrent oral contraceptive agents. Some adjustment in the anticoagulant dosage may be necessary.
**Summary:** The concurrent administration of oral contraceptive agents and dicumarol has been shown to diminish the anticoagulant response.
**Related Drugs:** Because of conflicting data, it is difficult to determine whether a similar interaction would occur with phenprocoumon, warfarin, anisindione or phenindione.
**Mechanism:** It has been suggested that the estrogenic component of the oral contraceptive agent is responsible for the alterations in blood coagulation.
**Detailed Information:** See *EDI*, 4/9.00

## Dicumarol-Phenytoin

**Significance:** 2—moderately clinically significant
**Recommendations:** If dicumarol, warfarin, or phenprocoumon and phenytoin are coadministered, an increase in phenytoin half-life, serum levels, or side effects should occur within the first four weeks of therapy, particularly when the anticoagulant is added to the drug regimen of a patient previously stabilized on phenytoin. If signs and symptoms of phenytoin toxicity develop (e.g., nystagmus, gait ataxia, poor muscle tone, or lethargy), serum phenytoin levels should be determined and doses of phenytoin reduced to establish therapeutic levels. Similarly, prothrombin times should be monitored closely. Caution should be exercised when establishing anticoagulant doses after discontinuation of phenytoin or carbamazepine because of the possibility of a subsequent increase in anticoagulant effect, which takes approximately three weeks to develop.
**Summary:** Concurrent administration of dicumarol and phenytoin may result in a significant increase in the half-life and serum level of phenytoin. Phenytoin may decrease serum dicumarol levels and decrease its anticoagulant effect.
**Related Drugs:** Warfarin has been documented to cause phenytoin toxicity. Phenytoin has been documented to enhance warfarin's effect. Phenprocoumon has been reported to impair phenytoin metabolism, whereas phenindione had no effect. Phenytoin causes no change in the levels of phenprocoumon. It is difficult to determine whether an interaction would occur with anisindione. A similar interaction is expected to occur with other hydantoin anticonvulsants and dicumarol. Carbamazepine reduces the anticoagulant effect of warfarin.
**Mechanism:** Dicumarol may impair the P-hydroxylation of phenytoin, causing an increase in phenytoin half-life, accumulation, and intoxication. Phenytoin may induce dicumarol metabolism.
**Detailed Information:** See *EDI*, 4/11.00

## Heparin-Aspirin

**Significance:** 1—highly clinically significant
**Recommendations:** Since the combination of low dose heparin and aspirin is effective prophylaxis for postoperative thrombo-

## Anticoagulant

embolism, this combination will continue to be used. Patients should be closely observed for hemorrhagic complications; however, these may not always be predicted by laboratory monitoring of coagulation status. Heparinized patients requiring antipyresis or analgesia should receive acetaminophen rather than aspirin.

**Summary:** The combined use of heparin and aspirin may result in serious bleeding complications. Aspirin also prevents heparin-induced platelet aggregation.

**Related Drugs:** No drugs are related to heparin and there are no reports of heparin interactions with other salicylates.

**Mechanism:** Heparin and aspirin prolong bleeding time, and heparin potentiates aspirin-induced prolongation of bleeding time. Aspirin may decrease platelet aggregation, removing a hemostatic mechanism for protection against heparin-induced bleeding.

**Detailed Information:** See *EDI*, 4/13.00

## Heparin-Carbenicillin

**Significance:** 2—moderately clinically significant

**Potential Effects:** Carbenicillin may prolong bleeding time and may theoretically increase the effects of concurrent heparin. The prolongation of bleeding time may occur only with high doses of carbenicillin.

**Recommendations:** Coagulation must be monitored frequently when these agents are used concurrently.

**Summary:** Carbenicillin and other penicillins have been shown to prolong bleeding time.

**Related Drugs:** Similar effects on bleeding have been reported with penicillin G, ticarcillin, ampicillin, and methicillin. All penicillins may alter platelet function and may interact with heparin. There are no drugs related to heparin. A similar interaction between carbenicillin and dicumarol, warfarin and anisindione may occur.

**Mechanism:** This interaction may be due to the additive pharmacologic activities of heparin and carbenicillin.

**Detailed Information:** See *EDI*, 4/15.00

## Heparin-Dextran

**Significance:** 2—moderately clinically significant

**Recommendations:** Data pertaining to the concurrent use of dextran 40 and heparin suggest baseline studies (thrombin time, activated prothrombin time, or the Lee White clotting time) should be performed before and intermittently during therapy until anticoagulation is achieved. Although sufficient data to formulate a conclusive recommendation for the concomitant use of dextran 70 or 75 and heparin are lacking, the two should only be used in combination when patients can be closely monitored. Limited data suggest dextran 70 or 75 may cause a greater incidence of adverse reactions and have less effect on the sludging of red blood cells than the use of dextran 40; however, a firm recommendation as to the preferred agent cannot be offered.

**Summary:** Use of dextran 70 or dextran 75 in combination with heparin is associated with a significantly higher incidence of bleeding. Dextran 40 has been administered with heparin without untoward effects.

**Related Drugs:** There are no drugs chemically related to either dextran or heparin.

**Mechanism:** Heparin and dextran possess independent and synergistic effects prolonging coagulation time and reducing clot strength.

**Detailed Information:** See *EDI*, 4/17.00

## Anticoagulant

### Heparin-Nitroglycerin
**Significance:** 2—moderately clinically significant
**Potential Effects:** The use of nitroglycerin may decrease the effect of heparin.
**Recommendations:** The effect of heparin should be frequently monitored (e.g., by the use of APTT) when these agents are used together. The dose of one or both agents may need to be adjusted.
**Summary:** There are data to show that the use of nitroglycerin may decrease the effect of heparin. However, one study documented that the propylene glycol vehicle in the nitroglycerin induced heparin resistance; however, all data do not support this.
**Related Drugs:** It is not known if a similar interaction would occur between heparin and other nitrate derivatives. There are no drugs related to heparin.
**Mechanism:** The mechanism of this interaction is not known; however, various theories are documented.
**Detailed Information:** See *EDI*, 4/18.01

### Heparin-Tobacco
**Significance:** 3—minimally clinically significant
**Recommendations:** Based on limited evidence, tobacco smokers may require larger heparin dosages than nonsmokers in order to achieve adequate anticoagulation in the treatment of thromboembolic disease. Further study is needed to determine the clinical significance of this potential interaction.
**Summary:** There are data to show that tobacco smokers may require larger heparin dosages than nonsmokers in order to achieve anticoagulation.
**Related Drugs:** There are no drugs related to heparin.
**Mechanism:** The mechanism of this interaction has not been established.
**Detailed Information:** See *EDI*, 4/18.10

### Phenindione-Haloperidol
**Significance:** 3—minimally clinically significant
**Recommendations:** Until further clinical studies are performed, the concurrent use of these agents need not be avoided. However, it is important to be aware of a possible interaction, and if inadequate anticoagulation occurs a decrease in the haloperidol dose or an increase in the phenindione dose may be necessary.
**Summary:** The concurrent use of phenindione and haloperidol may lead to a reduction in the anticoagulant effect of phenindione.
**Related Drugs:** There is no documentation regarding an interaction between haloperidol and dicumarol, phenprocoumon, warfarin or anisindione. Documentation is lacking regarding an interaction between phenindione and other phenothiazines, thioxanthenes, dihydroindolones or the dibenzoxazepines.
**Mechanism:** The mechanism of this interaction is unknown.
**Detailed Information:** See *EDI*, 4/19.00

### Ticlopidine-Aluminum Hydroxide, Magnesium Hydroxide
**Significance:** 3—minimally clinically significant
**Potential Effects:** Concurrent administration of ticlopidine with aluminum or magnesium hydroxide may result in decreased ticlopidine blood levels.
**Recommendations:** Ticlopidine and antacids should not be administered at the same time.

Anticoagulant

**Summary:** When administered with a combination aluminum-magnesium hydroxide antacid, ticlopidine absorption decreased approximately 20%.

**Related Drugs:** Although documentation is lacking, based on the mechanism of action other antacids could be expected to interact in a similar fashion. There are no drugs related to ticlopidine.

**Mechanism:** The exact mechanism of this interaction is unknown. Both magnesium and aluminum have been shown to form insoluble chelation complexes with drugs. Direct drug adsorption and the formation of poorly soluble salt complexes have also been reported.

**Detailed Information:** See *EDI*, 4/20.00

## Ticlopidine-Cyclosporine

**Significance:** 2—moderately clinically significant

**Potential Effects:** Ticlopidine may decrease whole-blood cyclosporine levels.

**Recommendations:** Caution should be used when ticlopidine is added to a cyclosporine regimen. Cyclosporine whole-blood levels may be reduced to subtherapeutic levels. The dose of cyclosporine may need to be increased or the ticlopidine discontinued.

**Summary:** The addition of ticlopidine to a cyclosporine regimen resulted in decreased cyclosporine whole-blood levels in three patients.

**Related Drugs:** It is unknown whether a similar interaction would occur between cyclosporine and clopidrogel, the other platelet aggregation inhibitor chemically related to ticlopidine. There are no drugs related to cyclosporine.

**Mechanism:** Cyclosporine metabolism may be mediated by the cytochrome $P450_{3A4}$ isozyme. The observed decrease in cyclosporine whole-blood levels may have resulted from ticlopidine-associated induction of the cytochrome $P450_{3A4}$ isozyme, although the exact mechanism is unknown.

**Detailed Information:** See *EDI*, 4/20.50

## Warfarin-Acarbose

**Significance:** 3—minimally clinically significant

**Potential Effects:** The addition of acarbose to a stable warfarin regimen may result in an increased anticoagulant effect.

**Recommendations:** Patients should be carefully monitored for changes in international normalized ratio (INR) or anticoagulant effect when acarbose is added to or removed from the therapy of a patient maintained on warfarin. The dose of warfarin may need to be adjusted.

**Summary:** The addition of acarbose to a stable warfarin regimen resulted in an increased anticoagulant effect and an increase in the patient's INR value to 4.85 after two weeks of acarbose therapy.

**Related Drugs:** It is not known whether an interaction would occur between acarbose and the other coumarin anticoagulant agents. There are no drugs related to acarbose.

**Mechanism:** Since acarbose is not absorbed, it is postulated that this interaction is related to the increased absorption of warfarin, but more studies are needed to determine the precise mechanism of this interaction.

**Detailed Information:** See *EDI*, 4/20.70

## Anticoagulant

### Warfarin-Acetaminophen
**Significance:** 3—minimally clinically significant
**Potential Effects:** Concurrent warfarin and acetaminophen administration may result in a change in hypoprothrombinemic response.
**Recommendations:** Enhancement of warfarin's hypoprothrombinemic effect by acetaminophen appears to be controversial. The use of therapeutic dosages of acetaminophen would thus be preferable to aspirin as an antipyretic or analgesic in the patient requiring oral anticoagulants. However, the use of high doses of acetaminophen may result in an increased prothrombin time. Therefore, the need for monitoring prothrombin time is still necessary for individual patient response to acetaminophen-anticoagulant coadministration.
**Summary:** Concurrent warfarin and acetaminophen administration may result in a change in hypoprothrombinemic response. The risk of this interaction appears to be dose-related, with higher doses of acetaminophen more likely to increase prothrombin time and international normalized ratio values.
**Related Drugs:** High doses of acetaminophen (2600 to 4000 mg/day) have caused significant increases in prothrombin times in patients taking coumarin derivatives, including anisindione, dicumarol, and phenprocoumon. No significant effects on prothrombin times were observed in patients taking phenprocoumon who received two 650 mg doses of acetaminophen administered four hours apart. Phenindione and nicoumalone may also be expected to interact with acetaminophen in a similar manner because they are pharmacologically related to the above agents.
**Mechanism:** The mechanism of this interaction is unknown. More studies are needed, but the mechanism may involve a combination of acetaminophen's effect on prothrombin time and a competitive inhibition of metabolic pathways.
**Detailed Information:** See *EDI,* 4/21.00

### Warfarin-Alcohol, Ethyl
**Significance:** 3—minimally clinically significant
**Recommendations:** No special precautions are necessary when administering warfarin to patients reporting minimal to moderate alcohol consumption as long as routine prothrombin time determinations are regularly obtained. Administration of warfarin to patients who chronically abuse alcohol may require frequent laboratory evaluation to prevent excessive warfarin anticoagulation.
**Summary:** The use of small or moderate amounts of alcohol is unlikely to produce a significant effect on warfarin; however, continuous, heavy alcohol consumption may significantly alter warfarin metabolism and patient response.
**Related Drugs:** Alcohol may be expected to interact with dicumarol, phenprocoumon, anisindione and phenindione.
**Mechanism:** Chronic alcohol abuse may result in exaggerated response to warfarin, possibly secondary to impaired hepatic synthesis of clotting factor precursors or impaired hepatic drug metabolism capacity.
**Detailed Information:** See *EDI,* 4/23.00

### Warfarin-Amiodarone
**Significance:** 1—highly clinically significant
**Potential Effects:** Amiodarone causes an increase in the pharmacologic effect of warfarin.
**Recommendations:** The dosage of warfarin needs to be adjusted based on the prothrombin time when these agents are used together.

## Anticoagulant

**Summary:** The concurrent administration of warfarin and amiodarone has been shown to result in an increase in the hypoprothrombinemic response to warfarin.
**Related Drugs:** Similar results were noted when amiodarone was administered concomitantly with acenocoumarol. A similar interaction may occur between amiodarone and dicumarol, phenprocoumon or anisindione. There are no drugs related to amiodarone.
**Mechanism:** Amiodarone may inhibit the hepatic metabolism of warfarin or an interaction may result from the noncompetitive inhibition of metabolism. Amiodarone may also lower the levels of vitamin K-dependent clotting factors.
**Detailed Information:** See *EDI*, 4/24.10

## Warfarin-Ascorbic Acid

**Significance:** 4—not clinically significant
**Recommendations:** No routine adjustment of warfarin dose needs to be made during concurrent ascorbic acid therapy. However, in patients exhibiting changing (increasing) dosage requirements of warfarin during maintenance anticoagulant therapy, possible concurrent ascorbic acid ingestion should be eliminated as a causative factor.
**Summary:** No significant alteration of warfarin by concurrent ascorbic acid has been demonstrated in controlled clinical studies.
**Related Drugs:** There are no reports demonstrating a similar interaction between ascorbic acid and dicumarol, phenprocoumon, anisindione or phenindione. There are no drugs related to ascorbic acid.
**Mechanism:** The decrease in plasma warfarin concentration during concurrent administration of ascorbic acid may result from diarrhea.
**Detailed Information:** See *EDI*, 4/25.00

## Warfarin-Aspirin

**Significance:** 1—highly clinically significant
**Recommendations:** Concurrent administration of warfarin and salicylate compounds, including aspirin, sodium salicylate, and diflunisal, should be avoided whenever possible. Either acetaminophen or another nonsteroidal anti-inflammatory agent that does not interact with warfarin should be substituted for aspirin according to the indication present. If warfarin and aspirin in moderate to large dosages are administered together, frequent prothrombin time determinations should be performed initially to monitor the transient increase in warfarin effect which is likely to occur.
**Summary:** Concurrent administration of moderate to large doses of aspirin and warfarin may potentiate the anticoagulant action of warfarin and increase the risk of warfarin-induced bleeding.
**Related Drugs:** Dicumarol and phenindione have been shown to not interact with low doses of aspirin. Dicumarol, phenindione, phenprocoumon and anisindione may interact with higher doses of aspirin. Sodium salicylate and diflunisal have been shown to interact with anticoagulants. A similar interaction is expected to occur with other salicylates and warfarin.
**Mechanism:** Aspirin and related compounds will displace warfarin from plasma protein binding sites, increasing an anticoagulant effect and decreasing total plasma warfarin concentrations. Aspirin will directly decrease platelet aggregation and prolong bleeding time, and oral salicylate administration may cause gastrointestinal bleeding.
**Detailed Information:** See *EDI*, 4/27.00

Anticoagulant

## Warfarin-Azathioprine

**Significance:** 2—moderately clinically significant

**Potential Effects:** The addition of azathioprine to the therapy of a patient maintained on warfarin may result in a decrease in the anticoagulant effects of warfarin.

**Recommendations:** The anticoagulant effect of warfarin should be carefully monitored if azathioprine is added to or withdrawn from warfarin therapy.

**Summary:** Concurrent administration of azathioprine in a patient resulted in a decrease in the anticoagulant effects of warfarin.

**Related Drugs:** Mercaptopurine has been reported to have a similar interaction with warfarin. There have been no reports of an interaction between azathioprine and the other coumarin anticoagulants or the indandione derivatives, although because of pharmacologic similarity, an interaction may be expected.

**Mechanism:** Although the exact mechanism is unknown, mercaptopurine might induce the hepatic microsomal enzymes responsible for warfarin metabolism; but a decreased gastrointestinal absorption of warfarin cannot be ruled out. Animal experiments have suggested that synthesis or inactivation of the prothrombin complex may also be involved.

**Detailed Information:** See *EDI*, 4/28.05

## Warfarin-Cefamandole

**Significance:** 2—moderately clinically significant

**Recommendations:** If cefamandole is added to, or withdrawn from, warfarin therapy, the prothrombin time should be monitored. An adjustment of the warfarin dose or the administration of vitamin K may be necessary.

**Summary:** Cefamandole was reported to increase warfarin sensitivity, resulting in increased prothrombin times and possibly severe bleeding.

**Related Drugs:** Coagulation abnormalities have been reported with moxalactam, cefoperazone, cefoxitin, and cefazolin; therefore, cephalosporins would be expected to interact similarly with warfarin. Cefamandole may also interact with dicumarol, phenprocoumon and anisindione.

**Mechanism:** Cefamandole may increase prothrombin time through prothrombin production, suppression of vitamin K-producing bacterial flora, inhibition of warfarin metabolism, and altered ribosomal function.

**Detailed Information:** See *EDI*, 4/28.10

## Warfarin-Chloral Hydrate

**Significance:** 2—moderately clinically significant

**Recommendations:** During initial concurrent administration of warfarin and chloral hydrate, frequent prothrombin time determinations should be made to monitor possible increases in warfarin anticoagulant action. Although temporary warfarin dosage adjustments are not generally necessary, changes in warfarin therapy should be determined on an individual patient basis. For long-term sedative hypnotic therapy, a benzodiazepine is preferable to chloral hydrate (see also Warfarin-Chlordiazepoxide, below).

**Summary:** Concurrent administration of chloral hydrate and warfarin may be associated with a transient increase in warfarin anticoagulant action.

**Related Drugs:** Chloral betaine and triclofos have been shown to produce similar effects on warfarin metabolism. Dicumarol has been shown to interact with chloral hydrate, similar to warfarin. A similar interaction is expected to occur between chloral hydrate and phenprocoumon, anisindione and phenindione.

**Mechanism:** The major metabolite of chloral hydrate displaces warfarin from plasma protein binding sites, increasing the warfarin free fraction in plasma. This elevated free drug concentration is associated with an increased hypoprothrombinemic effect and promotes increased systemic drug clearance.

**Detailed Information:** See *EDI*, 4/29.00

## Warfarin-Chlordiazepoxide

**Significance:** 4—not clinically significant

**Recommendations:** Warfarin therapy during concurrent chlordiazepoxide administration should be monitored in a routine fashion. Therefore, no special precautions are necessary when these drugs are given concurrently.

**Summary:** Concurrent administration of chlordiazepoxide and warfarin produces no clinically significant effect on warfarin.

**Related Drugs:** Benzodiazepines have not demonstrated any interaction with warfarin. The coumarin anticoagulant phenprocoumon has been demonstrated not to interact with nitrazepam. No data describing anisindione and phenindione have been presented. It is not possible to determine whether an interaction would occur with chlordiazepoxide.

**Mechanism:** The benzodiazepines may induce hepatic microsomal enzymes.

**Detailed Information:** See *EDI*, 4/31.00

## Warfarin-Chlorthalidone

**Significance:** 3—minimally clinically significant

**Recommendations:** The concurrent use of warfarin and chlorthalidone may require a higher dose of warfarin. Prothrombin levels should be monitored and the dose of the anticoagulant adjusted as necessary.

**Summary:** The concurrent use of chlorthalidone and warfarin has been shown to reduce the hypoprothrombinemic response.

**Related Drugs:** Documentation is lacking regarding a similar interaction between other thiazide related diuretics and warfarin or between dicumarol, acenocoumarol, anisindione or phenindione and chlorthalidone. A similar interaction is expected to occur with other oral anticoagulants and thiazide related diuretics.

**Mechanism:** The mechanism of this interaction is not known. Chlorthalidone may improve hepatic function and increase clotting factor synthesis. The effects of warfarin may be antagonized by a decrease in plasma, which concentrates circulating clotting factors.

**Detailed Information:** See *EDI*, 4/32.10

## Warfarin-Cholestyramine

**Significance:** 2—moderately clinically significant

**Potential Effects:** Cholestyramine may decrease the anticoagulant action of warfarin. The half-life of warfarin may be decreased and the clearance increased by cholestyramine.

**Recommendations:** Concurrent use of these agents should be avoided. If they must be given together, cholestyramine should be administered three to six hours after the warfarin. Prothrombin times should be carefully monitored during concomitant therapy. Colestipol may be an alternative to cholestyramine.

**Summary:** Concurrent administration of oral cholestyramine and warfarin may result in a significant decrease in the anticoagulant activity of warfarin.

## Anticoagulant

**Related Drugs:** Phenprocoumon showed a similar interaction with warfarin. A similar interaction may be expected to occur between cholestyramine and dicumarol or anisindione. Colestipol has been reported not to interact with phenprocoumon or warfarin. Whether the other coumarin and indandione anticoagulants would also fail to interact with colestipol has not been established.

**Mechanism:** Cholestyramine binds warfarin in a pH dependent fashion, suggesting a direct interaction of the two drugs in the gut.

**Detailed Information:** See *EDI*, 4/33.00

### Warfarin-Cimetidine

**Significance:** 1—highly clinically significant

**Potential Effects:** Cimetidine inhibits the metabolism of warfarin, leading to an increase in the hypoprothrombinemic response of warfarin, resulting in bleeding in some cases.

**Recommendations:** The use of cimetidine should be avoided in patients receiving warfarin. The hypoprothrombinemic response to warfarin should be closely monitored if cimetidine is added to, or withdrawn from, therapy and the warfarin dose adjusted accordingly. Ranitidine should be also be used with caution. Famotidine or nizatidine may be alternatives to cimetidine or ranitidine since they have not been shown to interact.

**Summary:** The concomitant administration of warfarin and cimetidine has been shown to significantly increase plasma warfarin levels and prolong the hypoprothrombinemic response of warfarin.

**Related Drugs:** Phenindione has been shown to react similarly with warfarin; however, phenprocoumon did not show a similar interaction. There is no documentation regarding an interaction with dicumarol or anisindione. Ranitidine did not significantly affect prothrombin time or plasma warfarin concentration; however, all data do not support this. Preliminary studies indicate that warfarin is not affected by the other $H_2$-receptor antagonists.

**Mechanism:** Cimetidine may inhibit the hepatic metabolism of warfarin and may inhibit a specific enantiomer of warfarin.

**Detailed Information:** See *EDI*, 4/35.00

### Warfarin-Cisapride

**Significance:** 2—moderately clinically significant

**Potential Effects:** The addition of cisapride to the therapy of a patient maintained on warfarin may result in hypoprothrombinemia.

**Recommendations:** Patients should be carefully monitored for changes in anticoagulant effect when cisapride is added to or discontinued from the therapy of a patient maintained on warfarin.

**Summary:** The addition of cisapride to the therapy of a patient maintained on warfarin resulted in hypoprothrombinemia, increasing the international normalized ratio values from 2.5 to 10.7.

**Related Drugs:** A similar interaction would be expected to occur between cisapride and the other coumarin anticoagulants provided that the metabolism of these other agents follows a similar metabolic pathway. There are no drugs related to cisapride.

**Mechanism:** A decrease in warfarin metabolism may result from competitive binding with cisapride at active sites on the cytochrome $P450_{3A4}$ isoenzyme, leading to increased warfarin levels and subsequent hypoprothrombinemia.

**Detailed Information:** See *EDI*, 4/36.00

Anticoagulant

## Warfarin-Clofibrate

**Significance:** 1—highly clinically significant

**Recommendations:** Because the concurrent use of clofibrate and warfarin may lead to excessive warfarin-induced anticoagulation and clinically significant hemorrhagic side effects, frequent prothrombin time determinations should be made during concurrent therapy. A reduction in warfarin dosage requirements should be expected, although the magnitude of clofibrate effect will vary among individual patients. Warfarin dosage in patients concurrently receiving clofibrate should be individually titrated using appropriate laboratory evaluation.

**Summary:** Concurrent administration of oral clofibrate and warfarin may enhance warfarin's anticoagulant action.

**Related Drugs:** Phenindione and dicumarol exhibit a similar interaction with warfarin. Phenprocoumon, indandione and anisindione may also interact with clofibrate.

**Mechanism:** Clofibrate displaces warfarin from plasma protein binding sites, competitively and noncompetitively. The enhancement of warfarin's effect in patients may be directly associated with clofibrate's hypolipidemic action.

**Detailed Information:** See *EDI*, 4/37.00

## Warfarin-Cyclosporine

**Significance:** 2—moderately clinically significant

**Potential Effects:** Concurrent use of these agents may result in decreased levels/activity of either agent.

**Recommendations:** Both cyclosporine levels and warfarin activity (prothrombin time) should be monitored during concurrent therapy. The dose of one or both drugs may need to be increased.

**Summary:** There are data to show that the concurrent use of these agents may result in decreased levels and activity of either or both agents.

**Related Drugs:** It is not known if cyclosporine would interact with dicumarol or anisindione.

**Mechanism:** The mechanism of this interaction is not known.

**Detailed Information:** See *EDI*, 4/38.05

## Warfarin-Danshen

**Significance:** 2—moderately clinically significant

**Potential Effects:** The concurrent administration of warfarin and danshen resulted in increased hypoprothrombic effects of warfarin, including bleeding.

**Recommendations:** Concurrent use of warfarin and danshen should be avoided. Patients receiving warfarin therapy should be advised to avoid taking herbal preparations that contain danshen. If concurrent therapy is warranted, patients should be carefully monitored. The dosage of warfarin may need to be adjusted.

**Summary:** Concurrent administration of warfarin and danshen resulted in increased hypoprothrombic effects of warfarin, including bleeding.

**Related Drugs:** A similar interaction would be expected to occur between the other anticoagulants and danshen. There are no agents related to danshen (*Salvia miltiorrhiza*). Common names for danshen include Tan-Shen, Tzu Tan-Ken, Hung Ken, Shu-Wei Ts'ao, Ch'ih Shen, and Pin-Ma Ts'ao.

**Mechanism:** The mechanism is unknown. Danshen may decrease the elimination of warfarin and has been shown to inhibit platelet aggregation *in vitro*.

**Detailed Information:** See *EDI*, 4/38.07

Anticoagulant

## Warfarin-Diazoxide
**Significance:** 3—minimally clinically significant
**Recommendations:** Until further clinical studies are performed, the concurrent use of these agents need not be avoided. However, it is prudent to be aware of a potential interaction and to monitor prothrombin times frequently.
**Summary:** The concurrent administration of warfarin and diazoxide may potentiate the hypoprothrombinemic effect of warfarin.
**Related Drugs:** There are no drugs related to diazoxide. A similar interaction is expected to occur with dicumarol, phenprocoumon, or anisindione and warfarin. An interaction with diazoxide may also occur.
**Mechanism:** Diazoxide can displace warfarin from human albumin.
**Detailed Information:** See *EDI,* 4/38.10

## Warfarin-Diphenhydramine
**Significance:** 4—not clinically significant
**Recommendations:** No specific precautions need be taken during concurrent administration of diphenhydramine and warfarin.
**Summary:** Concurrent administration of oral diphenhydramine and warfarin produces no clinically significant effect on warfarin.
**Related Drugs:** No documentation exists regarding an interaction between diphenhydramine and dicumarol, acenocoumarol, anisindione or phenindione. There is a lack of documentation of this interaction with other antihistamines.
**Mechanism:** Antihistamines have been shown to induce hepatic microsomal enzymes in animal studies.
**Detailed Information:** See *EDI,* 4/39.00

## Warfarin-Disopyramide
**Significance:** 3—minimally clinically significant
**Recommendations:** The pharmacologic activity of warfarin may need to be monitored when disopyramide is added to, or deleted from, therapy.
**Summary:** Disopyramide may enhance the hypoprothrombinemic response to warfarin.
**Related Drugs:** A similar interaction is expected to occur between disopyramide and dicumarol, acenocoumarol, anisindione or phenindione, if the mechanism involves competition for the same metabolic pathways. There are no drugs related to disopyramide.
**Mechanism:** Disopyramide and warfarin may compete for the same hepatic metabolic pathways.
**Detailed Information:** See *EDI,* 4/41.00

## Warfarin-Disulfiram
**Significance:** 1—highly clinically significant
**Recommendations:** The concurrent use of warfarin and disulfiram should be avoided. When these drugs must be administered concurrently, a decrease of usual dosages of warfarin may be necessary. Patient education and careful monitoring of prothrombin activity are recommended.
**Summary:** Concurrent administration of warfarin and disulfiram may result in elevated serum warfarin levels and an enhanced hypoprothrombinemic response.
**Related Drugs:** Disulfiram may interact with dicumarol, acenocoumarol, anisindione or phenindione. No drugs are related to disulfiram.

# Anticoagulant

**Mechanism:** Inhibition of the hepatic enzyme system by disulfiram results in increased warfarin levels and an enhanced hypoprothrombinemic effect.

**Detailed Information:** See *EDI*, 4/43.00

## Warfarin-Dong Quai

**Significance:** 3—minimally clinically significant

**Potential Effects:** Concurrent administration of warfarin and dong quai may result in increased International Normalized Ratio (INR) and increased risk of bleeding.

**Recommendations:** INR values should be carefully monitored if dong quai is added to or discontinued from the regimen of a patient maintained on warfarin. The warfarin dosage may need to be adjusted or the dong quai may need to be discontinued.

**Summary:** The addition of dong quai to the therapy of a patient maintained on a stable warfarin regimen resulted in a significant increase in a patient's INR.

**Related Drugs:** An interaction between dong quai and other coumarin anticoagulants or the indanedione derivatives may occur. No other agents are related to dong quai. Other common names for dong quai include tang-kuei, Dang-gui, and Chinese Angelica.

**Mechanism:** It has been suggested that the dong quai root contains many natural coumarin derivatives and may potentiate the risk of bleeding if combined with anticoagulants.

**Detailed Information:** See *EDI*, 4/43.50

## Warfarin-Erythromycin

**Significance:** 1—highly clinically significant

**Potential Effects:** Erythromycin causes an increase in warfarin's effect on prothrombin time, which may lead to bleeding.

**Recommendations:** Avoid the concurrent use of warfarin and erythromycin. If these agents must be used together, prothrombin times should be carefully monitored.

**Summary:** The concurrent administration of warfarin and erythromycin may increase the hypoprothrombinemic action of warfarin, resulting in bruising and hematuria in some cases. Prothrombin times, which have been shown to significantly increase following the initiation of erythromycin to patients maintained on warfarin, returned to control values when erythromycin was discontinued.

**Related Drugs:** Prolonged prothrombin times have been documented in patients receiving azithromycin concurrently with warfarin and in patients receiving acenocoumarol when erythromycin ethylsuccinate or clarithromycin were added to their regimens. Ponsinomycin had no significant effects on nicoumalone pharmacokinetics. A similar interaction may be expected to occur between erythromycin and the other coumarin anticoagulants and anisindione. Other macrolide antibiotics may also be expected to interact with coumarin anticoagulants.

**Mechanism:** The mechanism is unknown. However, several mechanisms have been postulated, such as antibiotic-induced reduction of vitamin K-producing bacterial flora in the intestine, inhibition of warfarin metabolism, and enhanced responsiveness to warfarin as a result of altered ribosomal function. It has also been suggested that a metabolite of erythromycin inhibits drug metabolism and not erythromycin itself, since erythromycin has been shown to induce microsomal enzymes and promote its own biotransformation into metabolites that form inactive complexes with cytochrome P450.

**Detailed Information:** See *EDI*, 4/45.00

## Anticoagulant

### Warfarin-Ethacrynic Acid
**Significance:** 2—moderately clinically significant
**Recommendations:** Patients stabilized on warfarin should be monitored for prothrombin activity whenever ethacrynic acid is added to, or withdrawn from, the regimen. Furosemide or bumetanide may be suitable alternatives since some studies have reported that warfarin is unaffected by their concurrent use. Since intravenously administered ethacrynic acid has been associated with gastrointestinal bleeding, patients should also be monitored for possible hemorrhage.
**Summary:** Ethacrynic acid has been documented to significantly increase prothrombin time.
**Related Drugs:** Dicumarol, acenocoumarol, anisindione or phenindione may interact with ethacrynic acid. Other loop diuretics have no effect on warfarin.
**Mechanism:** Ethacrynic acid has been shown to displace warfarin from human albumin *in vitro* and enhance warfarin-induced hypoprothrombinemia in rats.
**Detailed Information:** See *EDI*, 4/47.00

### Warfarin-Ethchlorvynol
**Significance:** 2—moderately clinically significant
**Recommendations:** Patients stabilized on dicumarol or warfarin should be monitored for prothrombin activity whenever ethchlorvynol is added to, or withdrawn from, the drug regimen. The substitution of benzodiazepine compounds as an alternative to ethchlorvynol should be considered since benzodiazepines do not significantly affect the activity of oral anticoagulants (see also Warfarin-Chlordiazepoxide, page 79).
**Summary:** Ethchlorvynol may significantly decrease the anticoagulant activity of warfarin when these drugs are administered concurrently.
**Related Drugs:** Dicumarol has been shown to interact with ethchlorvynol. Phenprocoumon, anisindione or phenindione may interact in a similar manner, if the mechanism involves induction of hepatic enzymes by ethchlorvynol.
**Mechanism:** Ethchlorvynol may increase warfarin metabolism by induction of hepatic microsomal enzymes.
**Detailed Information:** See *EDI*, 4/49.00

### Warfarin-Etoposide, Vindesine
**Significance:** 3—minimally clinically significant
**Potential Effects:** Etoposide and/or vindesine may increase the anticoagulant action of warfarin.
**Recommendations:** Monitor prothrombin times when these agents are used together. The dose of warfarin may need to be adjusted.
**Summary:** There are data to show that etoposide and/or vindesine may increase the anticoagulant action of warfarin.
**Related Drugs:** A similar interaction is expected to occur between etoposide and vindesine with dicumarol, acenocoumarol, anisindione or phenindione. Vindesine resembles vincristine in activity; therefore, a similar interaction may occur between these agents and warfarin. A similar interaction is expected to occur with other antineoplastic agents and warfarin.
**Mechanism:** Etoposide may displace warfarin from its binding sites. Etoposide and/or vindesine may competitively inhibit the hepatic enzymes responsible for the metabolism of warfarin.
**Detailed Information:** See *EDI*, 4/50.10

## Anticoagulant

### Warfarin-Etretinate

**Significance:** 2—moderately clinically significant

**Potential Effects:** Warfarin's anticoagulant effect may be decreased.

**Recommendations:** The International Normalized Ratio should be carefully monitored in patients maintained on warfarin when etretinate is added to, or withdrawn from, therapy. The dose of warfarin needs to be adjusted.

**Summary:** The addition of etretinate to the therapy of patients stabilized on warfarin has been shown to result in a decrease in the anticoagulant effect of warfarin.

**Related Drugs:** A similar interaction is expected to occur between warfarin and other retinoic acid derivatives. It is not known whether an interaction would occur between etretinate and acenocoumarol, phenprocoumon, nicoumalone, anisindione or phenindione.

**Mechanism:** Studies in animal models have found that etretinate may cause an induction of hepatic mixed function oxidase system enzymes, increasing the rate of metabolism of warfarin.

**Detailed Information:** See *EDI*, 4/50.60

### Warfarin-Felbamate

**Significance:** 2—moderately clinically significant

**Potential Effects:** An increase in the International Normalized Ratio (INR) may occur with the addition of felbamate to the therapy of a patient maintained on warfarin.

**Recommendations:** Warfarin levels and INR values/prothrombin times should be carefully monitored if felbamate is added to, or withdrawn from, therapy. The dose of warfarin may need to be adjusted.

**Summary:** There are data to show that felbamate increases the INR in patients stabilized on warfarin.

**Related Drugs:** An interaction may occur between felbamate and other coumarin anticoagulant agents. It is not known whether an interaction would occur between felbamate and the indandione anticoagulant agents. An interaction may occur between warfarin and meprobamate (see page 90).

**Mechanism:** Felbamate may inhibit the metabolism of warfarin.

**Detailed Information:** See *EDI*, 4/50.65

### Warfarin-Fluconazole

**Significance:** 2—moderately clinically significant

**Potential Effects:** The anticoagulation effect of warfarin may be potentiated with concurrent fluconazole and may result in bleeding episodes.

**Recommendations:** Patients' prothrombin times and international normalized ratios should be closely monitored during the concomitant use of these agents and when fluconazole is discontinued. The dose of warfarin may need to be adjusted or fluconazole may need to be discontinued. One set of authors recommends a step-wise approach to the reduction of warfarin dosage over the first four days of concurrent therapy by reducing warfarin to 80%, 50%, 43%, and finally 36% of the previous maintenance dosage.

**Summary:** Fluconazole enhances the anticoagulant effects of warfarin and may cause an increase in prothrombin time and possible bleeding episodes.

**Related Drugs:** Ketoconazole and itraconazole have also been shown to potentiate the effects of warfarin and cause bleeding episodes, although the data on ketoconazole are conflicting. Several case reports document the potentiation of warfarin or aceno-

## Anticoagulant

coumarol by concurrent oral miconazole or miconazole oral gel. Prolongation of prothrombin time has also been documented in a patient after fluconazole was added to nicoumalone therapy. A similar interaction would be expected to occur between warfarin and other imidazole antifungal agents and between fluconazole and other coumarin anticoagulants. It is not known whether an interaction would occur with the indanedione derivatives.

**Mechanism:** It is postulated that the mechanism of this interaction involves an inhibition of the cytochrome P450 system. An *in vitro* study has demonstrated that fluconazole inhibits the metabolism of S-warfarin at the cytochrome $P450_{2C9}$ and the metabolism of R-warfarin at the cytochrome $P450_{3A4}$.

**Detailed Information:** See *EDI*, 4/50.70

## Warfarin-Fluoxetine

**Significance:** 3—minimally clinically significant

**Potential Effects:** The addition of fluoxetine to a stable warfarin regimen may result in an increase in the effect of warfarin.

**Recommendations:** Patients maintained on warfarin should be carefully monitored for changes in prothrombin time if fluoxetine is added to, or removed from, therapy. The dose of one or both agents may need to be adjusted.

**Summary:** The addition of fluoxetine may result in an increase in the anticoagulation activity of warfarin.

**Related Drugs:** Paroxetine and sertraline were shown to exhibit a similar interaction with warfarin. The anticoagulant effect of nicoumalone and warfarin may be enhanced by fluvoxamine and paroxetine. It is not known whether an interaction would occur between fluoxetine and dicumarol, acenocoumarol, phenprocoumon, anisindione or phenindione.

**Mechanism:** The mechanism for this interaction in not known, but may involve plasma protein binding.

**Detailed Information:** See *EDI*, 4/50.80

## Warfarin-Ginkgo

**Significance:** 3—minimally clinically significant

**Potential Effects:** The addition of *Ginkgo biloba* to the therapy of a patient maintained on warfarin may result in increased bleeding times and hemorrhagic complications.

**Recommendations:** Caution should be observed if *Ginkgo biloba* is added to the therapy of a patient maintained on warfarin. Patients should be monitored for increased bleeding times and hemorrhagic risk. The dose of warfarin may need to be adjusted.

**Summary:** The addition of *Ginkgo biloba* to the therapy of a patient maintained on warfarin may have resulted in increased bleeding times and an intracerebral hemorrhage.

**Related Drugs:** It is not known whether an interaction would occur between *Ginkgo biloba* and the other coumarin anticoagulant agents.

**Mechanism:** Spontaneous bilateral subdural hematomas have been associated with chronic *Ginkgo biloba* use. Increased bleeding and hemorrhagic complications resulted from the addition of *Ginkgo biloba* to the regimen of a patient maintained on aspirin. It has been suggested that the coadministration of two antiplatelet agents might have contributed to the risk of hemorrhage.

**Detailed Information:** See *EDI*, 4/50.85

## Anticoagulant

### Warfarin-Ginseng
**Significance:** 2—moderately clinically significant

**Potential Effects:** The addition of ginseng to the therapy of a patient maintained on a stable warfarin regimen may result in a significant decline in the international normalized ratio (INR).

**Recommendations:** INR values should be carefully monitored if ginseng is added to or discontinued from the regimen of a patient maintained on warfarin. The warfarin dosage may need to be adjusted or the ginseng may need to be discontinued.

**Summary:** The addition of ginseng to the therapy of a patient maintained on a stable warfarin regimen resulted in a significant decline in the INR from a range of 3.0–4.0 to 1.5.

**Related Drugs:** It is not known whether an interaction would occur between ginseng and the other coumarin or indandione anticoagulants.

**Mechanism:** The mechanism of this interaction is not known.

**Detailed Information:** See *EDI*, 4/50.90

### Warfarin-Glucagon
**Significance:** 1—highly clinically significant

**Recommendations:** It has been suggested that if more than 25mg of glucagon per day is to be given for longer than one to two days, the dosage of warfarin should be reduced and prothrombin time should be monitored closely.

**Summary:** Administration of glucagon was shown to increase the hypoprothrombinemic effect of warfarin.

**Related Drugs:** A similar interaction is expected to occur between glucagon and dicumarol, acenocoumarol, anisindione or phenindione. No drugs are related to glucagon.

**Mechanism:** Glucagon may potentiate the hypoprothrombinemic action of warfarin by acting synergistically to depress hepatic synthesis of vitamin K-sensitive clotting proteins or by increasing the affinity of warfarin.

**Detailed Information:** See *EDI*, 4/51.00

### Warfarin-Glutethimide
**Significance:** 1—highly clinically significant

**Recommendations:** If glutethimide is administered to patients receiving oral anticoagulants, they should be carefully monitored and the dosage of warfarin adjusted as needed, since the enzyme induction by glutethimide can occur from several days to one week after initiation of therapy. Conversely, the withdrawal of glutethimide from the drug regimen could lead to severe bleeding unless the patient is monitored and the anticoagulant dosage adjusted downward as needed. After the discontinuation of glutethimide, it may take up to four weeks for the prothrombin time to return to pretreatment levels. In patients requiring a hypnotic agent, a benzodiazepine can be used as an alternative to glutethimide since these compounds do not significantly affect the prothrombin time achieved with anticoagulants (see also Warfarin-Chlordiazepoxide, page 79).

**Summary:** Glutethimide stimulates the metabolism of warfarin, reducing its anticoagulant effect.

**Related Drugs:** Aminoglutethimide was shown to have a similar interaction with warfarin. A similar interaction is expected to occur between methyprylon and other oral anticoagulants. Glutethimide has been shown to significantly decrease dicumarol plasma levels. Phenprocoumon and anisindione may interact similarly to warfarin.

**Mechanism:** Glutethimide increases the activity of the hepatic microsomal enzymes involved in drug metabolism.

**Detailed Information:** See *EDI*, 4/53.00

## Warfarin-Griseofulvin

**Significance:** 2—moderately clinically significant

**Potential Effects:** Griseofulvin increases the metabolism of warfarin, decreasing the effect on coagulation.

**Recommendations:** If griseofulvin is added to, or withdrawn from, warfarin therapy, the prothrombin time should be monitored and warfarin's dosage may need to be adjusted.

**Summary:** Coadministration of griseofulvin and warfarin has been shown to result in a decreased prothrombin time, requiring an increase in the dose of warfarin. However, data are available indicating that griseofulvin has no effect on warfarin's hypoprothrombinemic response.

**Related Drugs:** A similar interaction may occur between griseofulvin and dicumarol, phenprocoumon, or anisindione. There are no drugs related to griseofulvin.

**Mechanism:** Griseofulvin may induce liver enzymes, increase the rate of metabolic biotransformation or interfere with the absorption of warfarin, decreasing the hypoprothrombinemic effect of warfarin.

**Detailed Information:** See *EDI*, 4/55.00

## Warfarin-Ibuprofen

**Significance:** 2—moderately clinically significant

**Potential Effects:** Although not a significant problem at recommended therapeutic doses, ibuprofen may cause some displacement of warfarin from plasma protein binding sites.

**Recommendations:** No specific adjustments of warfarin's maintenance dosage need to be made during concurrent therapy with ibuprofen. However, prothrombin times should be closely monitored in cases of increasing age or renal impairment if ibuprofen is added to, or withdrawn from, a patient's therapy.

**Summary:** Administration of therapeutic doses of ibuprofen and warfarin should not significantly affect warfarin's anticoagulant action.

**Related Drugs:** Fenoprofen, tolmetin, naproxen and piroxicam have been shown to have a similar interaction with warfarin. Ketoprofen resulted in increasing prothrombin time and gastrointestinal bleeding. Documentation is lacking regarding an interaction between warfarin and meclofenamate. The effects of other NSAIAs appear to be drug-specific. Phenprocoumon has been reported to not interact with ibuprofen. Documentation is lacking regarding an interaction between ibuprofen and dicumarol or anisindione.

**Mechanism:** The mechanism behind this interaction varies depending on the NSAIA.

**Detailed Information:** See *EDI*, 4/57.00

## Warfarin-Ifosfamide

**Significance:** 2—moderately clinically significant

**Potential Effects:** The anticoagulant activity of warfarin may be increased.

**Recommendations:** Patients maintained on warfarin should be closely monitored for changes in anticoagulation activity if ifosfamide is added to, or withdrawn from, therapy. The dose of warfarin may need to be adjusted.

**Summary:** The anticoagulant activity of warfarin may be increased when ifosfamide is added to the therapy of a patient maintained on warfarin.

**Related Drugs:** Cyclophosphamide reduced the anticoagulant effect of warfarin. A similar interaction is expected to occur between ifosfamide and acenocoumarol, dicumarol, phenprocoumon, anisindione or phenindione, if the mechanism involves inhibition of hepatic metabolism.

# Anticoagulant

**Mechanism:** Ifosfamide could displace warfarin from plasma protein binding sites, resulting in an increase in International Normalized Ratio. Ifosfamide may be inhibit the cytochrome P450 mediated metabolism of warfarin.
**Detailed Information:** See *EDI*, 4/58.50

## Warfarin-Indomethacin

**Significance:** 2—moderately clinically significant
**Potential Effects:** Indomethacin can cause gastric ulceration and hemorrhage, and it impairs platelet function. It may also increase the effects of warfarin.
**Recommendations:** Patients receiving these agents concurrently should be monitored closely for changes in prothrombin time as well as for clinical signs of increased anticoagulation.
**Summary:** There are data to show that indomethacin can cause gastric ulceration and hemorrhage, impairing platelet function and prolonging bleeding time. Indomethacin should still be used cautiously in patients receiving oral anticoagulants.
**Related Drugs:** There are many NSAIAs that have interacted with warfarin to some extent. The effects of other NSAIAs on warfarin metabolism and clinical symptoms appear to be drug-specific. A similar interaction is expected to occur between indomethacin and dicumarol or anisindione. Ibuprofen has been shown to have no significant effect on the anticoagulant activity of phenprocoumon.
**Mechanism:** The exact mechanism of the potential interaction between indomethacin and warfarin is unknown but may be related to indomethacin-induced displacement of warfarin from plasma protein binding sites.
**Detailed Information:** See *EDI*, 4/59.00

## Warfarin-Influenza Virus Vaccine

**Significance:** 3—minimally clinically significant
**Potential Effects:** Influenza virus vaccine may increase the anticoagulant effects of warfarin, although several studies reported no interaction between these agents.
**Recommendations:** Patients receiving these agents together should be closely monitored for increases in the anticoagulant effect of warfarin.
**Summary:** The administration of influenza virus vaccine to patients on warfarin therapy may result in an increased prothrombin time; however, all data do not support this.
**Related Drugs:** Documentation is lacking regarding a similar interaction between influenza virus vaccine and dicumarol, phenprocoumon or anisindione. The administration of pneumococcal vaccine did not affect the anticoagulant response.
**Mechanism:** The influenza virus vaccine may affect the metabolism of warfarin and the coagulation pathways.
**Detailed Information:** See *EDI*, 4/61.00

## Warfarin-Isoniazid

**Significance:** 3—minimally clinically significant
**Recommendations:** Until further clinical studies are available, patients should be monitored for an increased anticoagulant action after isoniazid is added to warfarin therapy. The dosage of warfarin may need to be decreased.
**Summary:** Isoniazid causes an increase in the anticoagulant action of warfarin.
**Related Drugs:** There are no drugs related to isoniazid. Dicumarol increased prothrombin time and blood levels after administration of

## Anticoagulant

isoniazid. A similar interaction is expected to occur with phenprocoumon, anisindione or phenindione, if the mechanism of the interaction is related to inhibition of hepatic metabolism by isoniazid.

**Mechanism:** Isoniazid may inhibit the hepatic microsomal enzymes responsible for the metabolism of the anticoagulant.

**Detailed Information:** See *EDI*, 4/63.00

## Warfarin-Lovastatin

**Significance:** 2—moderately clinically significant

**Potential Effects:** Concurrent use of these agents may result in an increase in the hypoprothrombinemic activity of warfarin.

**Recommendations:** The patient should be monitored for changes in prothrombin time if lovastatin is added to or discontinued from therapy of a patient maintained on warfarin. The dose of warfarin may need to be adjusted.

**Summary:** The addition of lovastatin to warfarin therapy resulted in increased prothrombin times and bleeding.

**Related Drugs:** Similar interactions have been reported between fluindione and pravastatin and between acenocoumarol and simvastatin. Conversely, one case reported no interaction between warfarin and simvastatin. An interaction would be expected to occur between warfarin and the other HMG-CoA reductase inhibitors. It is not known whether an interaction would occur between lovastatin and the other oral anticoagulant agents.

**Mechanism:** The mechanism of this interaction is not known, but it has been postulated that lovastatin may inhibit the hepatic hydroxylation of warfarin or that lovastatin, which is highly plasma protein bound, may displace warfarin from its binding site. Either of these possible mechanisms may result in a potentiation of warfarin's hypo-prothrombinemic action.

**Detailed Information:** See *EDI*, 4/64.50

## Warfarin-Magnesium Hydroxide

**Significance:** 4—not clinically significant

**Recommendations:** No special precautions are necessary when antacids containing aluminum or magnesium hydroxide are concurrently administered with warfarin. As a routine practice, however, simultaneous administration of antacids with warfarin should not necessarily be encouraged.

**Summary:** Concurrent administration of warfarin with antacids containing aluminum and/or magnesium hydroxide does not produce any significant effect on warfarin.

**Related Drugs:** The absorption of dicumarol is slightly enhanced by the simultaneous administration of magnesium hydroxide suspension. The effects of aluminum or magnesium hydroxideproducts on phenprocoumon, anisindione or phenindione have not been evaluated.

**Mechanism:** Antacids increase intestinal pH, decreasing the absorption of warfarin.

**Detailed Information:** See *EDI*, 4/65.00

## Warfarin-Meprobamate

**Significance:** 3—minimally clinically significant

**Recommendations:** Since there may be a significant decrease in the prothrombin time only in a rare patient receiving meprobamate and warfarin, it is prudent to routinely check weekly prothrombin times for the first four weeks after initiating meprobamate in warfarin-stabilized patients. The use of another anti-anxiety agent such as a benzodiazepine may be a satisfactory alternative.

## Anticoagulant

**Summary:** Meprobamate has been reported to induce the hepatic microsomal enzymes that metabolize warfarin in animals.

**Related Drugs:** There is a lack of documentation of a similar interaction with the propanediol derivatives, related to meprobamate; however, an interaction may be expected if these agents also induce hepatic enzymes. A similar interaction is expected to occur between meprobamate and dicumarol, acenocoumarol, anisindione or phenindione, if the mechanism involves hepatic microsomal enzyme induction.

**Mechanism:** Meprobamate may accelerate the metabolic inactivation of drugs metabolized hepatic microsomal enzymes.

**Detailed Information:** See *EDI,* 4/69.00

### Warfarin-Methyltestosterone

**Significance:** 1—highly clinically significant

**Recommendations:** It is important to monitor prothrombin times critically in patients receiving these agents concurrently. If methyltestosterone or other C-17-alkylated androgens are administered concomitantly with oral anticoagulants, the anticoagulant dosage may need to be decreased based on changes in prothrombin time.

**Summary:** Concurrent administration of warfarin and methyltestosterone can significantly increase the hypoprothrombinemic actions of warfarin.

**Related Drugs:** Oxymetholone, methandrostenolone, danazol, and stanozolol increase the hypoprothrombinemic action of warfarin, dicumarol, and phenindione. A similar interaction may be expected to occur with phenprocoumon or anisindione. Other C-17-alkylated androgen derivatives may be expected to interact similarly with warfarin.

**Mechanism:** The interaction may be related to an increase in the decay of clotting proteins, a decrease in vitamin K, an increase in warfarin receptor sites, or an alteration in the vitamin K-sensitive clotting factors.

**Detailed Information:** See *EDI,* 4/75.00

### Warfarin-Metronidazole

**Significance:** 2—moderately clinically significant

**Potential Effects:** Concurrent metronidazole may enhance the hypoprothrombinemic effect of warfarin.

**Recommendations:** The racemic mixture is the usual commercially available warfarin. Therefore it can be anticipated that excessive hypoprothrombinemia and bleeding may occur in patients receiving concurrent metronidazole. Appropriate precautions and monitoring of prothrombin levels should be undertaken if these agents are to be used concomitantly, including a decrease in the warfarin dosage if necessary.

**Summary:** In two studies, metronidazole significantly enhanced the hypoprothrombinemic effect of warfarin. The onset of the interaction occurred within four to ten days and appeared as excessive bruising of the legs.

**Related Drugs:** Since the mechanism appears to involve a specific warfarin racemate, it is not known if a similar interaction would occur between metronidazole and the other coumarin anticoagulants and the indandione derivatives. Phenprocoumon is a racemic mixture, as is warfarin, and may be expected to interact similarly. An interaction would be expected to occur between warfarin and the other metronidazole-related antibacterial agents.

## Anticoagulant

**Mechanism:** Studies show that metronidazole inhibits the enzymatic pathway responsible for the ring hydroxylation of S(-) warfarin. This indicates that the S(-) racemate, which is the more potent, is retained in the body whereas the R(+) racemate is unaffected.
**Detailed Information:** See *EDI*, 4/77.00

### Warfarin-Mitotane

**Significance:** 2—moderately clinically significant
**Potential Effects:** Mitotane may increase the metabolism of warfarin, decreasing the anticoagulant effect.
**Recommendations:** Monitor patients' prothrombin time frequently when mitotane is added to, or withdrawn from, warfarin therapy.
**Summary:** Mitotane may increase the metabolism of warfarin, decreasing the anticoagulant effect, necessitating an increase in the warfarin dosage.
**Related Drugs:** A similar interaction is expected to occur between mitotane and dicumarol, phenprocoumon or anisindione. There are no drugs related to mitotane.
**Mechanism:** Mitotane reduces the hypoprothrombinemic effect of warfarin by increasing its metabolism secondary to induction of hepatic microsomal enzymes.
**Detailed Information:** See *EDI*, 4/80.10

### Warfarin-Moricizine

**Significance:** 2—moderately clinically significant
**Potential Effects:** Moricizine may increase the effects of warfarin.
**Recommendations:** Patients maintained on warfarin should be monitored for changes in prothrombin time if moricizine is added to therapy.
**Summary:** The addition of moricizine to the regimen of a patient maintained on warfarin resulted in increased prothrombin time and bleeding.
**Related Drugs:** It is not known whether an interaction would occur between moricizine and acenocoumarol, dicumarol or phenindione. There are no drugs related to moricizine.
**Mechanism:** Moricizine may displace warfarin from plasma protein binding sites.
**Detailed Information:** See *EDI*, 4/80.25

### Warfarin-Nafcillin

**Significance:** 2—moderately clinically significant
**Potential Effects:** Nafcillin may induce warfarin resistance as well as increase the risk of bleeding because of platelet dysfunction.
**Recommendations:** Coagulation should be closely monitored during concurrent use of these agents. The warfarin dosage may need to be adjusted.
**Summary:** There are data to show that nafcillin may induce warfarin resistance and increase the risk of bleeding secondary to platelet dysfunction.
**Related Drugs:** Dicloxacillin sodium, piperacillin, azlocillin and penicillin G have been reported to prolong bleeding time. Amoxicillin and warfarin administration resulted in an embolism. Ticarcillin has been reported to decrease platelet function. Carbenicillin has been reported to decrease platelet function and inhibit fibrinogen conversion. Documentation is lacking regarding an interaction between warfarin and other penicillins and between penicillins and dicumarol, acenocoumarol, phenprocoumon, nicoumalon or anisindione.

Anticoagulant

**Mechanism:** The mechanism by which nafcillin would induce warfarin resistance has not been determined, but may be due to hepatic microsomal enzyme induction.
**Detailed Information:** See *EDI*, 4/80.30

## Warfarin-Nalidixic Acid

**Significance:** 1—highly clinically significant
**Potential Effects:** Nalidixic acid may increase warfarin's anticoagulant effects, possibly by displacing warfarin from plasma albumin.
**Recommendations:** It is important to monitor patients for an increased anticoagulant response when warfarin and nalidixic acid or the fluoroquinolone antibiotics are used concurrently. The dosage of warfarin may need to be decreased.
**Summary:** There are data to show that nalidixic acid may increase warfarin's anticoagulant effects.
**Related Drugs:** Nicoumalone and nalidixic acid were shown to have a similar interaction with warfarin. A similar interaction is expected to occur between nalidixic acid and dicumarol or anisindione. Enoxacin did not affect the hypoprothrombinemic response of warfarin. Norfloxacin has been shown to cause a significant rise in prothrombin time; however, not all data support this. A similar interaction may occur between warfarin and other fluoroquinolones and quinolones.
**Mechanism:** Nalidixic acid has been shown to displace warfarin on plasma albumin *in vitro*.
**Detailed Information:** See *EDI*, 4/81.00

## Warfarin-Neomycin

**Significance:** 3—minimally clinically significant
**Recommendations:** The possibility of a clinically significant enhancement of warfarin activity by the oral aminoglycosides may occur only in certain patients who have a dietary deficiency of vitamin K and are receiving large doses of the aminoglycoside. Nevertheless, monitoring of prothrombin activity is warranted when the two drugs are administered concurrently, as it is whenever any drug is added to, or deleted from, the regimen of a patient receiving an oral anticoagulant.
**Summary:** Concurrent administration of warfarin and oral neomycin may result in a slight increase in the hypoprothrombinemic effect of warfarin.
**Related Drugs:** The other oral aminoglycosides may interact with warfarin. A similar interaction is expected to occur between neomycin and dicumarol, phenprocoumon, anisindione or phenindione.
**Mechanism:** Neomycin may enhance a hypoprothrombinemic response by decreasing vitamin K availability.
**Detailed Information:** See *EDI*, 4/83.00

## Warfarin-Nortriptyline

**Significance:** 4—not clinically significant
**Recommendations:** Avoidance of concurrent administration of these two agents does not appear necessary. However, patients should be monitored for changes in anticoagulant response when antidepressants are added to an oral anticoagulant regimen.
**Summary:** Nortriptyline has been reported not to interfere with warfarin pharmacokinetics.
**Related Drugs:** Hypoprothrombinemic effects were not reported with nortriptyline. No interaction was documented with amitriptyline or nortriptyline with dicumarol or warfarin. Because of conflicting reports, it is difficult to determine whether an interaction would

## Anticoagulant

occur between phenprocoumon, anisindione or phenindione with nortriptyline, or between warfarin and the other tricyclic antidepressants or tetracyclic antidepressants.

**Mechanism:** Nortriptyline may inhibit the metabolism of dicumarol. The tricyclic antidepressants may slow gastrointestinal motility. It has been shown that warfarin is not affected by nortriptyline.

**Detailed Information:** See *EDI*, 4/85.00

### Warfarin-Omeprazole

**Significance:** 3—minimally clinically significant

**Potential Effects:** The anticoagulant effect of warfarin may be increased.

**Recommendations:** The concurrent administration of omeprazole and warfarin may result in an increase in the hypoprothrombinemic effect of warfarin. Patients receiving warfarin should be closely monitored if omeprazole is added to, or withdrawn from, therapy.

**Summary:** There are data to show that administration of omeprazole may increase the anticoagulation effect of warfarin.

**Related Drugs:** A similar interaction is expected to occur between omeprazole and dicumarol or anisindione. There are no drugs related to omeprazole.

**Mechanism:** Omeprazole inhibits metabolism through inhibition of the cytochrome P450 isoenzymes, and the increase in warfarin may be due to inhibition, affecting the elimination of warfarin.

**Detailed Information:** See *EDI*, 4/86.10

### Warfarin-Phenobarbital

**Significance:** 1—highly clinically significant

**Recommendations:** If possible, it is best to avoid the concurrent use of warfarin and phenobarbital. If phenobarbital therapy is initiated in a patient stabilized on a particular dosage of warfarin, it is likely that an increase in the dosage of warfarin will be required. If phenobarbital is discontinued, the therapy should be monitored closely and the need for reducing the anticoagulant dosage must be carefully considered.

**Summary:** The anticoagulant effect of warfarin can be decreased by the administration of phenobarbital, and it may be necessary to increase the warfarin dose.

**Related Drugs:** Amobarbital, aprobarbital, barbital, butabarbital, pentobarbital, and secobarbital interact with coumarin anticoagulants. Other barbiturates may act similarly to phenobarbital. Reports indicate that warfarin or dicumarol may need dosage adjustments when administered with phenobarital. Phenprocoumon is also influenced. Caution is indicated with anisindione and phenindione because of a similar metabolic fate.

**Mechanisms:** Phenobarbital increases the hepatic microsomal enzymes responsible for metabolizing warfarin, resulting in a decreased anticoagulant response.

**Detailed Information:** See *EDI*, 4/87.00

### Warfarin-Phenylbutazone

**Significance:** 1—highly clinically significant

**Recommendations:** Concurrent warfarin and phenylbutazone therapy threatens all patients with the potential for serious hemorrhage and should be avoided. If the combination must be used, close observation for bleeding is mandatory, and alternatives to phenylbutazone should be administered whenever possible. These alternatives (e.g., acetaminophen, other non-steroidal anti-inflammatory agents) are discussed in other monographs. Exces-

Anticoagulant

sive hypoprothrombinemia can be treated with phytonadione (vitamin K, 5 to 10 mg) given subcutaneously or orally and by discontinuing the anticoagulant until prothrombin levels return to the proper range. Larger doses of vitamin K do not hasten response and will make the patient resistant to subsequent warfarin therapy. Evidence of hemorrhage requires immediate return of prothrombin levels to normal ranges, attention to blood volume restoration, and other medical and surgical treatments as indicated. If hemorrhage is severe, fresh frozen plasma may be given to supply clotting factors.

**Summary:** Phenylbutazone enhances the hypoprothrombinemic effect of warfarin and can cause serious bleeding episodes.

**Related Drugs:** Phenprocoumon has been reported to interact with phenylbutazone or its analogs. Phenindione has shown a similar interaction with phenylbutazone. A similar interaction is expected to occur between dicumarol or anisindione and phenylbutazone. Oxyphenbutazone interacts with dicumarol and acenocoumarol.

**Mechanism:** Phenylbutazone increases the plasma concentration of unbound warfarin, inhibits the metabolism of warfarin and may cause gastric ulceration and decrease platelet aggregation.

**Detailed Information:** See *EDI*, 4/89.00

## Warfarin-Phytonadione

**Significance:** 1—highly clinically significant

**Potential Effects:** Phytonadione antagonizes the anticoagulant effect of warfarin.

**Recommendations:** It is prudent to monitor the International Normalized Ratio of patients stabilized on warfarin when large quantities of tube feedings are instituted or stopped. Excessive or fluctuating intake of foods containing vitamin K, such as green leafy vegetables, should be avoided in patients stabilized on warfarin.

**Summary:** Although it is the preparation of choice to treat hypopothrombinemia caused by warfarin, excessive intake of phytonadione (vitamin $K_1$), particularly from foods such as green leafy vegetables, should be avoided in patients stabilized on oral anticoagulants.

**Related Drugs:** Drugs with vitamin K activity include menadione (vitamin $K_3$) and menadione sodium diphosphate. Vitamin K is also found in green leafy vegetables and in oral nutritional supplements, which, if taken in large amounts, may affect warfarin response. Ingestion of excessive amounts of foods with relatively low (avocado) or high (green tea) vitamin K content has caused warfarin antagonism.

**Mechanism:** Coumarin anticoagulants inhibit vitamin K-dependent hepatic synthesis of clotting factors II, VII, IX, and X. Warfarin may inhibit cyclic regeneration of vitamin $K_1$ from its inactive epoxide, which is formed during the synthesis of these clotting factors. Since the amount of available vitamin K influences the rate of clotting factor synthesis, excessive vitamin K intake may reverse or impair the anticoagulant effect of warfarin.

**Detailed Information:** See *EDI*, 4/91.00

## Warfarin-Propafenone

**Significance:** 2—moderately clinically significant

**Potential Effects:** Concurrent propafenone may result in an enhanced warfarin anticoagulant effect.

**Recommendations:** The addition or removal of propafenone from the therapy of a patient maintained on warfarin should be approached with caution. The prothrombin time should be monitored for changes and the warfarin dose may need to be adjusted.

## Anticoagulant

**Summary:** Concurrent propafenone and warfarin has been shown to result in an enhanced warfarin anticoagulant effect.

**Related Drugs:** Propafenone potentiated the anticoagulant effect of fluindione. A similar interaction may occur between propafenone and acenocoumarol, phenprocoumon, nicoumalone, anisindione and phenindione. It is not known if an interaction would occur between warfarin and other Class IC antiarrhythmics.

**Mechanism:** Both drugs are metabolized by the hepatic cytochrome P450 system, and the interaction reflects the higher binding affinity of propafenone for cytochrome P450.

**Detailed Information:** See *EDI,* 4/92.50

## Warfarin-Propoxyphene

**Significance:** 2—moderately clinically significant

**Recommendations:** Patients' prothrombin times should be monitored closely during concurrent use of these agents. The dose of warfarin may need to be decreased, the propoxyphene may need to be discontinued, or the use of a noninteracting analgesic may be considered.

**Summary:** The concurrent use of warfarin and propoxyphene may lead to decreased prothrombin levels and bleeding episodes.

**Related Drugs:** A similar interaction is expected to occur between warfarin and other narcotic analgesics and between propoxyphene and dicumarol, phenprocoumon, anisindione or phenindione.

**Mechanism:** Propoxyphene, which is metabolized by the same hepatic microsomal enzymes that hydroxylate warfarin, may compete for metabolism.

**Detailed Information:** See *EDI,* 4/93.00

## Warfarin-Propranolol

**Significance:** 2—moderately clinically significant

**Potential Effects:** Propranolol may increase warfarin serum levels, which may lead to an increase in anticoagulation.

**Recommendations:** Although propranolol may increase serum warfarin concentrations, the clinical significance of this potential interaction has not been established. However, patients should be monitored for increased effects of warfarin, and prothrombin time should be monitored routinely. Acebutolol might be considered as a possible alternative therapy to propranolol in patients maintained on anticoagulation therapy.

**Summary:** There are data to show that propranolol may increase warfarin serum levels, leading to an increase in anticoagulation.

**Related Drugs:** Neither atenolol nor metoprolol altered the effects of warfarin. Acebutolol did not result in a change in prothrombin time. Esmolol did not affect warfarin plasma levels. It is difficult to determine if an interaction would occur between warfarin and other beta-blocking agents. Phenprocoumon with metoprolol increased plasma phenprocoumon levels. It is difficult to determine whether an interaction would occur between propranolol and dicumarol or anisindione.

**Mechanism:** Beta-blocking agents may increase serum warfarin concentrations by inhibiting the hepatic metabolism of warfarin.

**Detailed Information:** See *EDI,* 4/94.10

## Warfarin-Quinidine

**Significance:** 2—moderately clinically significant

**Recommendations:** Concurrent administration of warfarin and quinidine is not recommended, but if necessary there should be frequent monitoring of prothrombin times as well as monitoring for

## Anticoagulant

clinical symptoms of warfarin overdose. Use of an alternative antiarrhythmic agent that does not interact with the anticoagulant may be preferable to the use of quinidine.

**Summary:** Concurrent administration of quinidine and warfarin may result in enhanced hypoprothrombinemic activity. Quinidine can inhibit the production of vitamin K-dependent clotting factors.

**Related Drugs:** Quinine may exert a hypoprothrombinemic effect. Dicumarol and phenindione have been reported to enhance hypoprothrombinemic activity; however, dicumarol has been reported to decrease the anticoagulant effect. A similar interaction is expected to occur between quinidine and phenprocoumon or anisindione.

**Mechanism:** The additive effect shown by quinidine may be related to the depressant effect on the vitamin K-dependent clotting factors. The decreased anticoagulant effects may be due to the enhanced production of prothrombin and other coagulation factors.

**Detailed Information:** See *EDI*, 4/95.00

### Warfarin-Rifampin

**Significance:** 1—highly clinically significant

**Potential Effects:** Rifampin induces the metabolism of warfarin, decreasing warfarin's pharmacologic effects.

**Recommendations:** Monitor patients' prothrombin times when rifampin is added to, or withdrawn from, cotherapy with warfarin.

**Summary:** The administration of rifampin has been shown to result in a decreased warfarin pharmacologic effect.

**Related Drugs:** A similar interaction may occur between rifampin and dicumarol or anisindione. There are no drugs related to rifampin.

**Mechanism:** Rifampin, a known inducer of hepatic microsomal enzymes, increases the hepatic metabolism of warfarin.

**Detailed Information:** See *EDI*, 4/97.00

### Warfarin-Spironolactone

**Significance:** 3—minimally clinically significant

**Recommendations:** The clinical significance of long-term cotherapy has not been determined. If a reduction in the hypopro-thrombinemic effect should occur with long-term administration, suitable dosage adjustments of warfarin may be indicated.

**Summary:** The concurrent administration of spironolactone has been shown to decrease the hypoprothrombinemic effect of warfarin.

**Related Drugs:** An interaction may occur between spironolactone and dicumarol, phenprocoumon, anisindione or phenindione. A similar interaction is expected between other potassium sparing diuretics and warfarin.

**Mechanism:** Spironolactone-induced diuresis may concentrate the blood clotting factors as a result of plasma water loss, leading to a reduced anticoagulant effect.

**Detailed Information:** See *EDI*, 4/99.00

### Warfarin-Sucralfate

**Significance:** 3—minimally clinically significant

**Potential Effects:** Sucralfate may possibly decrease the action of warfarin.

**Recommendations:** Monitor the patient's prothrombin time when these agents are used together.

**Summary:** There are data to show that administration of sucralfate may possibly decrease the action of warfarin.

## Anticoagulant

**Related Drugs:** There are no drugs related to sucralfate. No documentation exists concerning whether a similar interaction would occur between sucralfate and dicumarol, phenprocoumon or anisindione.
**Mechanism:** The mechanism of this potential interaction is unknown.
**Detailed Information:** See *EDI*, 4/101.00

## Warfarin-Sulfamethoxazole

**Significance:** 1—highly clinically significant
**Potential Effects:** Sulfamethoxazole may be expected to enhance warfarin's anticoagulant effect.
**Recommendations:** Patients receiving sulfamethoxazole, either alone or as cotrimoxazole, and warfarin would be expected to display enhanced anticoagulant effects. Appropriate precautions should be taken to prevent excessive hypoprothrombinemia and bleeding.
**Summary:** Concurrent administration of sulfamethoxazole and trimethoprim, as cotrimoxazole, has augmented the hypoprothrombinemic effect of warfarin, significantly increasing warfarin levels.
**Related Drugs:** Sulfisoxazole and sulfamethazole have been shown to increase the hypoprothrombinemic activity of warfarin. A similar interaction is expected to occur between warfarin and other sulfonamides. Phenindione has been shown to not interact with cotrimoxazole. No documentation demonstrates that dicumarol, phenprocoumon or anisindione interacts similarly with sulfonamides. Proguanil was shown to potentiate the effect of warfarin. Trimethoprim would also be expected to interact with warfarin.
**Mechanism:** Several mechanisms have been proposed. Sulfonamides may displace plasma protein bound warfarin, the antibiotics may reduce vitamin K synthesis or the sulfonamides may inhibit warfarin metabolism.
**Detailed Information:** See *EDI*, 4/103.00

## Warfarin-Sulfinpyrazone

**Significance:** 1—highly clinically significant
**Potential Effects:** Sulfinpyrazone decreases the metabolism of warfarin, thereby increasing warfarin's pharmacologic effect.
**Recommendations:** The use of these agents together should be avoided. If they are given together, the prothrombin time should be monitored and the dose of warfarin decreased as necessary.
**Summary:** Concomitant sulfinpyrazone and warfarin therapy significantly potentiates the hypoprothrombinemic effect of warfarin.
**Related Drugs:** Sulfinpyrazone has been shown to not interact with phenprocoumon. It is not known if an interaction would occur between sulfinpyrazone and dicumarol or anisindione, or between warfarin and probenecid.
**Mechanism:** Sulfinpyrazone inhibits certain metabolic pathways, decreases the clearance of warfarin, displaces warfarin from plasma proteins and has been shown to displace phenprocoumon.
**Detailed Information:** See *EDI*, 4/105.00

## Warfarin-Tamoxifen

**Significance:** 2—moderately clinically significant
**Potential Effects:** Tamoxifen may increase the hypoprothrombinemic effects of warfarin. The antitumor activity of tamoxifen may also be reduced as a result of cotherapy.
**Recommendations:** Patients maintained on warfarin should have prothrombin times closely monitored if tamoxifen is added to, or withdrawn from, cotherapy. The dose of warfarin may need to be adjusted.

**Summary:** Tamoxifen may increase the hypoprothrombinemic effects of warfarin.
**Related Drugs:** A similar interaction may occur between tamoxifen and dicumarol or anisindione.
**Mechanism:** Tamoxifen and warfarin are metabolized by hepatic microsomal enzyme systems. Tamoxifen may increase the pharmacological activity of warfarin by competitive enzyme inhibition.
**Detailed Information:** See *EDI,* 4/107.00

## Warfarin-Terbinafine

**Significance:** 2—moderately clinically significant
**Potential Effects:** The addition of terbinafine to or discontinuation from the therapy of a patient maintained on warfarin may result in changes in international normalized ratio (INR) and anticoagulant effect.
**Recommendations:** The addition of terbinafine to, or the discontinuation from, the therapy of a patient maintained on warfarin should be approached with caution. The patient should be carefully monitored for changes in INR and anticoagulant effect, which may take several weeks to develop. The dose of warfarin may need to be adjusted.
**Summary:** The addition of oral terbinafine to the therapy of a patient maintained on warfarin resulted in decreased warfarin anticoagulant effect, although another study in 16 subjects showed no interaction.
**Related Drugs:** It is not known whether an interaction would occur between terbinafine and the other coumarin anticoagulants. It is not known whether a similar interaction would occur with warfarin and butenafine, a benzylamine derivative with a mode of action similar to the allylamine antifungal agent terbinafine.
**Mechanism:** The mechanism may involve enzyme induction, but documentation is lacking.
**Detailed Information:** See *EDI,* 4/108.50

## Warfarin-Tetracycline

**Significance:** 3—minimally clinically significant
**Recommendations:** The possibility of enhanced warfarin activity caused by tetracycline or its analogs appears to be slight when dietary intake of vitamin K is maintained at adequate levels and antibiotic clearance is normal. Nevertheless, close monitoring of prothrombin activity is warranted when the two drugs are administered concurrently or when one or the other is deleted from the regimen.
**Summary:** A broad spectrum antibiotic such as tetracycline can potentiate the hypoprothrombinemic effect of warfarin.
**Related Drugs:** Various tetracycline analogs may interact in a similar manner. Doxycycline has been implicated as the cause of an increased hypothrombinemic effect of warfarin. Dicumarol, phenprocoumon, anisindione or phenindione may interact similarly.
**Mechanism:** This interaction has often been considered to be inhibition of bacterial synthesis of vitamin K, resulting in an increased hypoprothrombinemic effect.
**Detailed Information:** See *EDI,* 4/109.00

## Warfarin-Thyroid

**Significance:** 1—highly clinically significant

**Recommendations:** Initiation of thyroid replacement therapy in patients stabilized on warfarin carries a significant risk of excessive prothrombin response and hemorrhage. Conversely, warfarin therapy should be started in small doses in hyperthyroid patients, and any change of thyroid status in patients already receiving warfarin may necessitate a change in the warfarin dosage requirement. A decrease in the dosage of warfarin required for anticoagulation usually becomes necessary within one to four weeks after starting therapy with thyroid compounds. Since hyperthyroidism may increase patient sensitivity to warfarin, individuals undergoing unexplained changes in warfarin requirements should have an evaluation of thyroid function. Patients' prothrombin times should be closely monitored while they are on antithyroid therapy, since a dosage increase or discontinuation of the antithyroid drug may necessitate an increase or a decrease, respectively, of the warfarin dosage.

**Summary:** Thyroid compounds increase the hypoprothrombinemic effect of warfarin and other anticoagulants.

**Related Drugs:** Levothyroxine has exhibited a similar interaction. Dicumarol and phenindione have been shown to interact with thyroid derivatives. A similar interaction is expected to occur with phenprocoumon and anisindione. All thyroid compounds are expected to interact with the anticoagulants.

**Mechanism:** Hyperthyroidism may reduce serum albumin and there may be an enhanced degradation of vitamin K-dependent factors.

**Detailed Information:** See *EDI*, 4/111.00

## Warfarin-Tobacco

**Significance:** 4—not clinically significant

**Recommendations:** Although there is a theoretical basis for an interaction between warfarin and tobacco, the limited evidence to date suggests that no special precautions are necessary when warfarin is administered to tobacco smokers. Further clinical studies designed specifically to evaluate this interaction are necessary.

**Summary:** There is no evidence that tobacco smokers require different maintenance doses of warfarin than nonsmokers.

**Related Drugs:** There is no documentation regarding an interaction between tobacco smoking and dicumarol, phenprocoumon or anisindione.

**Mechanism:** An increased maintenance dosage requirement in smokers could theoretically result from induction of warfarin metabolism.

**Detailed Information:** See *EDI*, 4/112.10

## Warfarin-Tolterodine

**Significance:** 2—moderately clinically significant

**Potential Effects:** The addition of tolterodine to the therapy of a patient maintained on warfarin may result in an increase in the International Normalized Ratio (INR).

**Recommendations:** Careful monitoring of INR values should be conducted on patients maintained on warfarin if tolterodine is added to, or discontinued from, concurrent therapy. The warfarin dosage may need to be adjusted.

**Summary:** The addition of tolterodine to the therapy of two patients maintained on warfarin resulted in an increase in the patients' INR.

**Related Drugs:** It is not known whether an interaction would occur between warfarin and the other anticholinergics or between tolterodine and the other coumarin anticoagulant agents.

**Mechanism:** Tolterodine is extensively metabolized by the cytochrome $P450_{2D6}$ isoenzyme; the alternative pathway for poor metabolizers lacking this isoenzyme is dealkylation by the cytochrome $P450_{3A4}$ isoenzyme. Warfarin is metabolized by several isoenzymes. An interaction between tolterodine and warfarin involving the cytochrome P450 isoenzyme system seems more likely in poor metabolizers of tolterodine, because the 3A4 isoenzyme is the only common metabolic pathway. A competing interaction is possible because both agents act as substrates for enzymes rather than inhibitors or inducers.
**Detailed Information:** See *EDI*, 4/112.20

## Warfarin-Trastuzumab

**Significance:** 2—moderately clinically significant
**Potential Effects:** The addition of trastuzumab to the therapy of a patient maintained on warfarin resulted in an increase in hypoprothrombinemic events and International Normalized Ratio (INR) values.
**Recommendations:** Careful monitoring of INR values, prothrombin time, and clinical status should be conducted on patients maintained on warfarin if therapy with trastuzumab is instituted. The warfarin dosage may need to be adjusted and other clinical measures may need to be instituted.
**Summary:** The addition of trastuzumab to the therapy of two patients maintained on long-term stable warfarin regimens resulted in an increase in hypoprothrombinemic events and INR values.
**Related Drugs:** It is not known whether an interaction would occur between warfarin and other monoclonal antibodies. If the mechanism involves displacement of warfarin from albumin binding sites, then an interaction might be expected to occur between trastuzumab and the other coumarin anticoagulant agents.
**Mechanism:** Trastuzumab might displace warfarin from albumin binding sites; however, it is not clear why the increased plasma warfarin takes a long time to manifest a clinical effect. Other mechanisms may be involved.
**Detailed Information:** See *EDI*, 4/112.25

## Warfarin-Trazodone

**Significance:** 3—minimally clinically significant
**Potential Effects:** Concomitant administration of trazodone with warfarin may result in decreased pharmacologic effects of the warfarin.
**Recommendations:** Patients receiving warfarin should be closely monitored when trazodone is added to, or withdrawn from, their therapy. A report recommends monitoring prothrombin and partial thromboplastin times three times a week, when trazodone is initiated, until the drug's effects are optimal. The dosage of warfarin may need to be adjusted.
**Summary:** There are data to show that concomitant administration of trazodone with warfarin may result in decreased warfarin effects.
**Related Drugs:** It is not known if a similar interaction would occur between trazodone and dicumarol or anisindione. Trazodone is unrelated to tricyclic, tetracyclic, or other available antidepressant agents.
**Mechanism:** The mechanism of this interaction is not known.
**Detailed Information:** See *EDI*, 4/112.30

Anticoagulant

## Warfarin-Troglitazone

**Significance:** 3—minimally clinically significant

**Potential Effects:** The addition of troglitazone to the therapy of a patient maintained on warfarin may result in an increased international normalized ratio (INR) and the possible need for warfarin dosage adjustment.

**Recommendations:** Patients should be closely monitored for increased INR and warfarin anticoagulant effects when troglitazone is added to or removed from the therapy of a patient maintained on warfarin. The dose of warfarin may need to be adjusted.

**Summary:** The addition of troglitazone to the therapy of a patient maintained on warfarin resulted in an increased INR and necessitated warfarin dosage adjustment.

**Related Drugs:** It is not known whether an interaction would occur between troglitazone and the other coumarin anticoagulant or the indanedione anticoagulant agents. There are no drugs related to troglitazone.

**Mechanism:** The mechanism is thought to be due to either inhibition of the cytochrome P450 enzyme system (which would result in decreased warfarin metabolism) or displacement of warfarin from plasma protein binding sites. Either of these suggested pathways would result in increased warfarin serum levels and subsequent effects.

**Detailed Information:** See *EDI*, 4/112.60

## Warfarin-Vitamin E

**Significance:** 2—moderately clinically significant

**Recommendations:** Until further clinical studies are reported, the concurrent use of these agents need not be avoided. However, it is prudent to monitor patients during concomitant administration, and a lower dose of warfarin may be necessary. It should be noted that the vitamin E effect can be overcome by either stopping the vitamin E or administering vitamin K.

**Summary:** The concurrent use of vitamin E may enhance the hypoprothrombinemic effect of warfarin.

**Related Drugs:** A similar interaction is expected to occur between vitamin E and phenprocoumon, anisindione or phenindione. No drugs are related to vitamin E.

**Mechanism:** The mechanism is unknown. Vitamin E may interfere with the oxidation of the reduced form of vitamin K.

**Detailed Information:** See *EDI*, 4/113.00

# Chapter Five

# Anticonvulsant Drug Interactions

Anticonvulsant

## Carbamazepine-Charcoal

**Significance:** 1—highly clinically significant

**Recommendations:** It has been recommended that activated charcoal be administered as soon as possible after an acute carbamazepine overdose. Also, activated charcoal may significantly increase the elimination of carbamazepine if given in multiple doses thereafter. If charcoal is not used for carbamazepine overdose, it may be advisable to separate the administration of these agents by as much time as possible.

**Summary:** Charcoal significantly reduces carbamazepine absorption and increases elimination.

**Related Drugs:** There are no drugs related to carbamazepine or charcoal.

**Mechanism:** Charcoal adsorbs carbamazepine and prevents its absorption and may prevent enterohepatic recycling of carbamazepine, increasing its elimination.

**Detailed Information:** See *EDI*, 5/1.00

## Carbamazepine-Cimetidine

**Significance:** 2—moderately clinically significant

**Potential Effects:** Cimetidine may increase carbamazepine levels. Monitor carbamazepine levels if cimetidine is added to, or withdrawn from, therapy.

**Recommendations:** Ranitidine may be used as an alternative to cimetidine.

**Summary:** Cimetidine has been shown to decrease the clearance of carbamazepine, resulting in increased carbamazepine plasma concentrations; however, all data do not support this.

**Related Drugs:** Ranitidine was documented to not change the carbamazepine area-under-curve or elimination half-life. There are no drugs related to carbamazepine.

**Mechanism:** Cimetidine inhibits the hepatic metabolism of carbamazepine and the autoinduction of carbamazepine.

**Detailed Information:** See *EDI*, 5/3.00

## Carbamazepine-Danazol

**Significance:** 2—moderately clinically significant

**Potential Effects:** Danazol may inhibit the metabolism of carbamazepine, leading to increased carbamazepine levels and carbamazepine toxicity in some cases.

**Recommendations:** Although plasma carbamazepine levels were increased above the therapeutic range by danazol, toxicity did not occur in all patients. Therefore, the patient's clinical condition and carbamazepine serum levels should be monitored. The dosage of carbamazepine may need to be decreased or danazol may need to be discontinued.

**Summary:** Danazol may increase carbamazepine levels and toxicity.

**Related Drugs:** A similar interaction may be expected to occur between carbamazepine and other androgen derivatives. There are no drugs related to carbamazepine.

**Mechanism:** Danazol causes an inhibition of carbamazepine metabolism and a reduction in the clearance of carbamazepine.

**Detailed Information:** See *EDI*, 5/4.01

## Carbamazepine-Desipramine

**Significance:** 3—minimally clinically significant

**Recommendations:** Although concurrent use of these agents need not be avoided, if desipramine is added to, or withdrawn from, carbamazepine therapy, serum carbamazepine concentrations

## Anticonvulsant

should be monitored. Additionally, the patient should be monitored for signs of carbamazepine toxicity or lack of efficacy.

**Summary:** Desipramine has been shown to cause an acute episode of nausea, vomiting, visual illusions, slurred speech, and ataxia in a patient taking carbamazepine.

**Related Drugs:** A similar interaction is expected to occur between carbamazepine and other tricyclic antidepressants or the tetracyclic antidepressants. Nomifensine may be expected to interact with carbamazepine. There are no drugs related to carbamazepine.

**Mechanism:** Desipramine and carbamazepine may compete for hydroxylation by the hepatic microsomal enzyme system, increasing the carbamazepine concentration.

**Detailed Information:** See *EDI*, 5/4.10

## Carbamazepine-Erythromycin

**Significance:** 1—highly clinically significant

**Potential Effects:** Erythromycin will cause an increase in carbamazepine levels, resulting in carbamazepine toxicity (e.g., nausea, nystagmus, ataxia).

**Recommendations:** Use of the agents together should be avoided. If they must be given together, patients should be monitored for increased carbamazepine levels and side effects. A decreased carbamazepine dose may be necessary.

**Summary:** The concurrent administration of erythromycin and carbamazepine has resulted in significant increases in plasma concentrations of carbamazepine.

**Related Drugs:** Administration of carbamazepine and troleandomycin has resulted in a similar interaction. Clarithromycin has been documented to double carbamazepine's concentration and dose ratio. There are no drugs related to carbamazepine.

**Mechanism:** Erythromycin may inhibit the hepatic metabolism of carbamazepine through competitive binding to cytochrome P450.

**Detailed Information:** See *EDI*, 5/5.00

## Carbamazepine-Felbamate

**Significance:** 2—moderately clinically significant

**Potential Effects:** Coadministration of carbamazepine and felbamate results in decreases in both the concentration of carbamazepine plasma levels and clearance of felbamate, in addition to an increase in carbamazepine epoxide plasma levels, thus possibly leading to an increase in carbamazepine epoxide concentrations.

**Recommendations:** Patients should be carefully monitored for changes in seizure potential with initial concomitant use of these agents. The concurrent use of these agents may be purposeful and the dose of one or both agents may need to be adjusted.

**Summary:** There are data to show that coadministration of carbamazepine and felbamate results in decreases in the concentration of carbamazepine plasma levels and clearance of felbamate, in addition to an increase in carbamazepine epoxide plasma levels and concentrations.

**Related Drugs:** There are no related drugs to carbamazepine. It is not known whether meprobamate would interact similarly with carbamazepine.

**Mechanism:** The interaction between carbamazepine and felbamate occurs via an alteration in the metabolic pathway. Felbamate has been shown to induce isozymes responsible for the conversion of carbamazepine to the epoxide. Carbamazepine also causes an increase in the clearance of felbamate.

**Detailed Information:** See *EDI*, 5/5.50

## Anticonvulsant

### Carbamazepine-Hydrochlorothiazide
**Significance:** 3—minimally clinically significant
**Potential Effects:** Concurrent use of these agents may result in hyponatremia as a result of a synergistic effect of both agents.
**Recommendations:** Patients should be monitored for hyponatremia when carbamazepine and hydrochlorothiazide are administered concurrently. One or both drugs may need to be discontinued. Also, if a patient's serum sodium levels are adequate during concurrent therapy, the levels should be monitored if the carbamazepine dose is increased.
**Summary:** Hyponatremia has been documented to occur when carbamazepine and hydrochlorothiazide are coadministered.
**Related Drugs:** Furosemide was shown to exhibit a similar interaction with carbamazepine. A similar interaction may occur between carbamazepine and other thiazide diuretics, the thiazide-related diuretics, and other loop diuretics. There are no drugs related to carbamazepine.
**Mechanism:** It is possible that a synergistic effect occurs between the two agents, causing hyponatremia.
**Detailed Information:** See *EDI*, 5/6.10

### Carbamazepine-Isoniazid
**Significance:** 2—moderately clinically significant
**Recommendations:** It is important to monitor carbamazepine levels during concurrent use of these agents. It may be necessary to reduce the dose of carbamazepine if toxic symptoms appear since this has been shown to reverse toxicity.
**Summary:** Concurrent administration of carbamazepine and isoniazid may lead to neurologic changes secondary to elevated carbamazepine levels.
**Related Drugs:** There are no drugs related to carbamazepine or isoniazid.
**Mechanism:** Isoniazid inhibits the hepatic metabolism of carbamazepine. Isoniazid-induced hepatotoxicity has been attributed to a reactive intermediate that results in cell death, and carbamazepine may potentiate this.
**Detailed Information:** See *EDI*, 5/7.00

### Carbamazepine-Isotretinoin
**Significance:** 3—minimally clinically significant
**Potential Effects:** Isotretinoin may cause a decrease in carbamazepine levels, resulting in loss of seizure control.
**Recommendations:** Patients maintained on carbamazepine should be closely monitored for decreases in carbamazepine levels or seizure control if isotretinoin is added to therapy. The dose of carbamazepine may need to be adjusted.
**Summary:** Isotretinoin may cause a decrease in carbamazepine and carbamazepime epoxide (CPZ-E, the active metabolite) levels, resulting in loss of seizure control.
**Related Drugs:** There are no drugs related to carbamazepine or isotretinoin.
**Mechanism:** It is suggested that isotretinoin alters the bioavailability or clearance or both of carbamazepine and CPZ-E.
**Detailed Information:** See *EDI*, 5/8.05

### Carbamazepine-Ketoconazole
**Significance:** 3—minimally clinically significant
**Potential Effects:** The concurrent administration of carbamazepine and an imidazole antifungal may result in elevated levels of carbamazepine or in decreased levels of the antifungal agent.

Anticonvulsant

**Recommendations:** Patients receiving concurrent therapy with carbamazepine and an imidazole antifungal should be monitored for increased levels of carbamazepine and possible decreased effectiveness of the imidazole antifungal.

**Summary:** The concurrent administration of carbamazepine and ketoconazole resulted in increased levels of carbamazepine. Carbamazepine levels increased by 25% and 28% by days 7 and 10, respectively, of concurrent therapy with ketoconazole. There were no significant effects on the levels of the active metabolite of carbamazepine. No signs or symptoms of carbamazepine toxicity were noted and there was no change in seizure frequency.

**Related Drugs:** It is not known whether an interaction would occur between carbamazepine and the other imidazole antifungal agents. There are no drugs related to carbamazepine.

**Mechanism:** It has been postulated that ketoconazole inhibited the metabolism of carbamazepine and that the extent of the effects seen on carbamazepine levels may have been limited by once daily ketoconazole administration.

**Detailed Information:** See *EDI*, 5/8.07

## Carbamazepine-Methylphenidate

**Significance:** 3—minimally clinically significant

**Potential Effects:** The concurrent administration of methylphenidate and carbamazepine may result in decreased methylphenidate serum levels and efficacy.

**Recommendations:** Methylphenidate serum levels and efficacy should be monitored if carbamazepine is added to or withdrawn from therapy. The dose of methylphenidate may need to be adjusted.

**Summary:** Coadministration of methylphenidate and carbamazepine resulted in decreased methylphenidate serum levels and efficacy in two patients.

**Related Drugs:** An interaction may occur between carbamazepine and other indirect-acting sympathomimetics due to similarities in metabolism. There are no drugs related to carbamazepine.

**Mechanism:** The interaction may involve the induction of hepatic cytochrome P450 metabolism of methylphenidate by carbamazepine. This may appear more prominently in children due to their accelerated hepatic metabolism compared to that of adults.

**Detailed Information:** See *EDI*, 5/8.09

## Carbamazepine-Metoclopramide

**Significance:** 3—minimally clinically significant

**Recommendations:** Patients receiving carbamazepine and metoclopramide concurrently should be monitored for signs and symptoms of neurotoxicity, and carbamazepine levels should be measured. One or both drugs may need to be discontinued, as this reduces the neurotoxic symptoms.

**Summary:** There are data to show that the administration of metoclopramide has led to carbamazepine-induced neurotoxicity.

**Related Drugs:** There are no drugs related to carbamazepine or metoclopramide.

**Mechanism:** The mechanism of this interaction is unknown.

**Detailed Information:** See *EDI*, 5/8.10

## Carbamazepine-Metronidazole

**Significance:** 2—moderately clinically significant

**Potential Effects:** Concurrent carbamazepine and metronidazole may result in increased carbamazepine serum levels and signs of carbamazepine toxicity.

## Anticonvulsant

**Recommendations:** Patients on carbamazepine who begin therapy with metronidazole should be carefully monitored for increased carbamazepine levels and signs of toxicity.

**Summary:** In a case report, the concurrent use of carbamazepine and metronidazole resulted in increased levels of carbamazepine and symptoms of carbamazepine toxicity.

**Related Drugs:** There are no drugs related to carbamazepine. Although documentation is lacking, a similar interaction would be expected to occur between carbamazepine and anti-infective agents related to metronidazole based on the postulated mechanism and pharmacological and structural similarity.

**Mechanism:** It is postulated that the interaction is a result of selective inhibition of the aromatic hydroxylation of carbamazepine by metronidazole.

**Detailed Information:** See *EDI*, 5/8.25

## Carbamazepine-Niacinamide

**Significance:** 3—minimally clinically significant

**Recommendations:** Carbamazepine plasma levels should be monitored in patients receiving concurrent niacinamide, especially when niacinamide is added to, or withdrawn from, therapy or the dose is changed. The dose of carbamazepine may need to be decreased. It is not known if a smaller dose of niacinamide (e.g., the amount that may be found in a multivitamin preparation) would interact with carbamazepine.

**Summary:** The administration of niacinamide decreased the clearance and increased the plasma levels of carbamazepine.

**Related Drugs:** There are no drugs related to carbamazepine. Niacin (nicotinic acid) may be expected to interact similarly with carbamazepine.

**Mechanism:** Niacinamide may inhibit the hepatic metabolism of carbamazepine. The decrease in carbamazepine clearance correlated highly with increasing niacinamide doses.

**Detailed Information:** See *EDI*, 5/8.30

## Carbamazepine-Oral Contraceptive Agents

**Significance:** 3—minimally clinically significant

**Potential Effects:** Carbamazepine may induce the metabolism of ethinylestradiol, leading to decreased levels.

**Recommendations:** The concomitant use of oral contraceptives and carbamazepine need not be avoided. However, the potential for reduced efficacy of the oral contraceptive should be a consideration in patients receiving both drugs.

**Summary:** There are data to show that carbamazepine causes oral contraceptive failure; however, it is unclear if other factors such as patient compliance are responsible. The potential for reduced efficacy of oral contraceptives should be considered.

**Related Drugs:** There are no drugs related to carbamazepine.

**Mechanism:** The cytochrome P450 metabolism of ethinylestradiol may be induced by administration of carbamazepine.

**Detailed Information:** See *EDI*, 5/8.50

## Carbamazepine-Phenobarbital

**Significance:** 3—minimally clinically significant

**Recommendations:** Carefully monitor patients receiving both phenobarbital and carbamazepine to assure that adequate therapeutic carbamazepine concentrations are maintained. The possibility of shortened carbamazepine half-life should be taken into consideration when establishing dosage frequency to prevent large fluctu-

## Anticonvulsant

ations in plasma concentration. One report suggests giving carbamazepine three times a day—morning, evening, and bedtime—to keep carbamazepine plasma levels fairly constant during the day and to counteract subtherapeutic levels in the morning.

**Summary:** Phenobarbital has been shown to decrease serum carbamazepine half-life and plasma concentration levels when given in combination; however, all data do not support this.

**Related Drugs:** Carbamazepine has been reported to lower serum concentrations of primidone. Other barbiturates may interact in a manner similar to phenobarbital. There are no drugs related to carbamazepine.

**Mechanism:** Phenobarbital is thought to induce the metabolism of carbamazepine to its epoxide metabolite.

**Detailed Information:** See *EDI,* 5/9.00

### Carbamazepine-Propoxyphene

**Significance:** 2—moderately clinically significant

**Potential Effects:** Propoxyphene may increase carbamazepine levels.

**Recommendations:** The use of these agents together should be avoided. Monitor for increased carbamazepine levels and toxicity. Propoxyphene may need to be discontinued.

**Summary:** Propoxyphene has been documented to increase carbamazepine levels.

**Related Drugs:** A similar interaction may occur between carbamazepine and other narcotic analgesics. There are no drugs related to carbamazepine.

**Mechanism:** Propoxyphene may inhibit the hepatic metabolism of carbamazepine, resulting in increased carbamazepine levels.

**Detailed Information:** See *EDI,* 5/11.00

### Carbamazepine-Terfenadine

**Significance:** 3—minimally clinically significant

**Potential Effects:** Terfenadine administration may result in increased levels of free carbamazepine and toxicity.

**Recommendations:** Patients receiving terfenadine and carbamazepine should be closely monitored for increased serum levels of free carbamazepine and signs of carbamazepine toxicity.

**Summary:** The addition of terfenadine to carbamazepine therapy has resulted in increased carbamazepine adverse effects and toxicity.

**Related Drugs:** A similar interaction may occur between carbamazepine and other $H_1$-receptor antagonists. An interaction would be expected to occur between terfenadine and other tricyclic antidepressant agents. A recent study has shown that terfenadine has no effect on phenytoin (see also Phenytoin-Carbamazepine, page 115).

**Mechanism:** Terfenadine may displace carbamazepine from plasma proteins, leading to an increase in the toxicities associated with carbamazepine.

**Detailed Information:** See *EDI,* 5/12.05

### Carbamazepine-Ticlopidine

**Significance:** 2—moderately clinically significant

**Potential Effects:** The concurrent administration of ticlopidine with carbamazepine may result in increased carbamazepine serum levels and toxic effects.

**Recommendations:** Serum carbamazepine levels should be monitored when ticlopidine is added to or discontinued from concurrent therapy. The dosage of carbamazepine may need to be adjusted.

**Summary:** Concurrent administration of ticlopidine and carbamazepine may result in increased carbamazepine serum levels and toxic effects including dizziness, ataxia, and a decreased level of consciousness.

## Anticonvulsant

**Related Drugs:** An interaction between carbamazepine and clopidogrel (a thienopyridine derivative similar to ticlopidine), which inhibits cytochrome $P450_{2C9}$ seems possible, although no documentation exists. There are no drugs related to carbamazepine.

**Mechanism:** It has been postulated that ticlopidine may inhibit the cytochrome $P450_{3A4}$ isoenzyme, the major metabolic pathway of carbamazepine.

**Detailed Information:** See *EDI*, 5/12.07

### Carbamazepine-Trazodone

**Significance:** 3—minimally clinically significant

**Potential Effects:** The concurrent administration of carbamazepine and trazodone resulted in decreased levels of trazodone and increased levels of carbamazepine.

**Recommendations:** Patients receiving concurrent therapy with carbamazepine and trazodone should be monitored for elevated levels of carbamazepine and possible carbamazepine toxicity, as well as decreased effectiveness of trazodone. The dosage of one or both agents may need to be adjusted at the initiation of concurrent therapy. If concurrent therapy is discontinued, the dosage of the remaining agent may need to be adjusted.

**Summary:** Concurrent administration of carbamazepine and trazodone may result in decreased levels of trazodone and increased levels of carbamazepine.

**Related Drugs:** A similar interaction would be expected to occur between trazodone and oxcarbazepine. Trazodone is a triazolopyridine derivative antidepressant that is chemically unrelated to tricyclic, tetracyclic, or other available antidepressant agents.

**Mechanism:** Carbamazepine may induce the metabolism of trazodone and its active metabolite, *m*-CPP. Trazodone may inhibit the metabolism of carbamazepine by the cytochrome $P450_{3A4}$ isoenzyme.

**Detailed Information:** See *EDI*, 5/12.08

### Carbamazepine-Verapamil

**Significance:** 2—moderately clinically significant

**Potential Effects:** Verapamil may cause an increase in carbamazepine levels, resulting in increased side effects.

**Recommendations:** Monitor the patient for increased carbamazepine levels and side effects when these agents are used together.

**Summary:** There are data to show that verapamil causes an increase in carbamazepine levels, resulting in increased side effects and neurotoxicity.

**Related Drugs:** Diltiazem exhibited a similar interaction with carbamazepine. Nifedipine did not interact with carbamazepine and its levels were unaffected. Felodipine plasma levels were shown to decrease. It is not known whether an interaction would occur between carbamazepine and other calcium channel blocking agents. There are no drugs related to carbamazepine.

**Mechanism:** It was suggested that verapamil and diltiazem may inhibit the hepatic metabolism of carbamazepine.

**Detailed Information:** See *EDI*, 5/12.10

### Clonazepam-Carbamazepine

**Significance:** 3—minimally clinically significant

**Potential Effects:** Carbamazepine may decrease clonazepam levels when used concurrently.

**Recommendations:** Monitor clonazepam levels when carbamazepine is added to, or withdrawn from, clonazepam

# Anticonvulsant

**Summary:** Concurrent carbamazepine reduced plasma clonazepam concentrations, making seizure control difficult since these agents may have an additive anticonvulsant action.

**Related Drugs:** Carbamazepine was shown to decrease alprazolam serum levels. A similar interaction is expected to occur with other benzodiazepines that are metabolized by phase I reactions and carbamazepine, if the mechanism involves induction of hepatic enzymes. There are no drugs related to carbamazepine.

**Mechanism:** Carbamazepine is known to induce hepatic enzymes, which is thought to be the mechanism responsible for the reduced clonazepam levels.

**Detailed Information:** See *EDI*, 5/13.00

## Clonazepam-Primidone

**Significance:** 4—not clinically significant

**Recommendations:** The clinical significance of this interaction is difficult to assess. Clonazepam has exhibited therapeutic effects over a wide range of plasma concentrations, and the possible change in primidone levels may offset any decreased levels of clonazepam.

**Summary:** Reports concerning an interaction between primidone and clonazepam are contradictory.

**Related Drugs:** Nitrazepam has been reported to decrease the primidone serum concentration. Clorazepate given with primidone resulted in personality changes. A similar interaction is expected to occur with other benzodiazepines and primidone and other barbiturates with clonazepam.

**Mechanism:** Phenobarbital, a known inducer of microsomal enzymes, can cause an increased clearance of drugs that undergo hepatic elimination.

**Detailed Information:** See *EDI*, 5/15.00

## Ethosuximide-Carbamazepine

**Significance:** 3—minimally clinically significant

**Potential Effects:** The concurrent use of these agents may result in decreased ethosuximide serum levels.

**Recommendations:** Patients should be monitored for decreased ethosuximide levels during concurrent therapy with carbamazepine. The dose of ethosuximide may need to be increased.

**Summary:** There are data to show that the concurrent use of these agents may result in decreased ethosuximide serum levels.

**Related Drugs:** A similar interaction is expected to occur between carbamazepine and other succinimide anticonvulsants. There are no drugs related to carbamazepine.

**Mechanism:** Carbamazepine increased the clearance and reduced the levels of ethosuximide by inducing the hepatic microsomal enzymes.

**Detailed Information:** See *EDI*, 5/16.01

## Ethosuximide-Isoniazid

**Significance:** 3—minimally clinically significant

**Recommendations:** If gastrointestinal symptoms and psychotic behavior occur during concurrent use of these agents, ethosuximide plasma levels should be monitored. The dose of ethosuximide may need to be decreased.

**Summary:** There are data to show that the admintration of isoniazid and ethosuximide may induce gastrointestinal symptoms and psychotic behavior.

Anticonvulsant

**Related Drugs:** An interaction may occur between isoniazid and other succinimides. There are no drugs related to isoniazid.
**Mechanism:** Isoniazid inhibits the metabolism of ethosuximide.
**Detailed Information:** See *EDI,* 5/16.03

## Ethosuximide-Valproic Acid

**Significance:** 3—minimally clinically significant
**Recommendations:** Concomitant use of ethosuximide and valproic acid need not be avoided; however, if valproic acid is added to, or withdrawn from, therapy, the serum ethosuximide concentration should be monitored and the patient observed for signs of toxicity or lack of efficacy.
**Summary:** Valproic acid and ethosuximide have been shown to increase, decrease, or have no effect on serum ethosuximide concentrations, toxicity, or efficacy.
**Related Drugs:** Similar interactions may occur between valproic acid and other succinimide anticonvulsants. There are no drugs related to valproic acid; however, sodium valproate and divalproex sodium would be expected to interact in the same manner as valproic acid. Valproic acid has been reported to increase levels of trimethadione. There is no documentation regarding an interaction between valproic acid and paramethadione.
**Mechanism:** Valproic acid may inhibit the hepatic metabolism of ethosuximide. The inhibition of metabolism may be dependent upon serum valproic acid concentrations or the administration of other agents that compete for metabolism.
**Detailed Information:** See *EDI,* 5/16.10

## Lamotrigine-Acetaminophen

**Significance:** 3—minimally clinically significant
**Potential Effects:** Acetaminophen may result in an increase in lamotrigine clearance.
**Recommendations:** When acetaminophen and lamotrigine are given concurrently (particularly when multiple doses of acetaminophen are necessary), patients should be monitored for a possible decrease of lamotrigine clinical effects. Although further studies are needed, the dose of lamotrigine may need to be increased.
**Summary:** Concurrent acetaminophen and lamotrigine may result in an increase in lamotrigine clearance and a decreased clinical effect, a study suggested.
**Related Drugs:** There are no drugs related to lamotrigine or acetaminophen.
**Mechanism:** It was suggested that acetaminophen facilitated lamotrigine removal through an unknown mechanism which may involve acetaminophen-mediated activation of a glucuronyl transferase.
**Detailed Information:** See *EDI,* 5/16.30

## Lamotrigine-Rifampin

**Significance:** 3—minimally clinically significant
**Potential Effects:** Concurrent administration of rifampin and lamotrigine may result in decreased half-life and area-under-curve of lamotrigine.
**Recommendations:** Patients receiving concurrent therapy with lamotrigine and rifampin should be monitored for possible decreased effects of lamotrigine. The dosage of lamotrigine may need to be adjusted.
**Summary:** Concomitant administration of rifampin and lamotrigine may result in decreased half-life and AUC of lamotrigine.
**Related Drugs:** A similar interaction may occur between the other rifamycins and lamotrigine. There are no drugs related to lamotrigine.

## Anticonvulsant

**Mechanism:** Pretreatment with rifampin may reduce lamotrigine half-life and increase clearance/bioavailability due to induction of the hepatic enzymes that cause glucuronidation.
**Detailed Information:** See *EDI*, 5/16.40

## Lamotrigine-Sodium Valproate

**Significance:** 3—minimally clinically significant
**Potential Effects:** Concurrent lamotrigine and sodium valproate may result in a decrease in clearance of lamotrigine.
**Recommendations:** Patients receiving lamotrigine should be monitored for changes in levels and possible toxicity if sodium valproate is added to, or withdrawn from, therapy. The dosage of lamotrigine may need to be adjusted.
**Summary:** Concurrent sodium valproate and lamotrigine resulted in a decreased clearance of lamotrigine.
**Related Drugs:** Valproic acid and divalproex sodium would be expected to interact similarly with lamotrigine. There are no drugs related to lamotrigine.
**Mechanism:** The reduced clearance of lamotrigine by sodium valproate is as a result of impaired glucuronide formation in the liver.
**Detailed Information:** See *EDI*, 5/16.50

## Phenobarbital-Valproic Acid

**Significance:** 2—moderately clinically significant
**Potential Effects:** The concomitant administration of these agents may result in increased phenobarbital serum levels and toxicity and/or decreased valproic acid serum levels.
**Recommendations:** Patients receiving these agents concurrently should be monitored for increased phenobarbital serum levels and/or decreased valproic acid serum levels. The dose of one or both agents may need to be adjusted.
**Summary:** The concurrent administration of phenobarbital and valproic acid has been shown to result in increased phenobarbital serum concentrations, and studies have shown decreased serum valproic acid concentrations.
**Related Drugs:** Valproic acid and primidone have shown significant increases in primidone concentrations; however, contrasting data exist. Mephobarbital decreased the serum level and dose ratio of valproic acid. It is difficult to determine if an interaction would occur between valproic acid and other barbiturates. Sodium valproate has been shown to increase phenobarbital levels. Divalproex sodium would be expected to interact similarly.
**Mechanism:** Valproic acid may inhibit the hepatic metabolism of phenobarbital. Phenobarbital may induce the hepatic metabolism of valproic acid.
**Detailed Information:** See *EDI*, 5/17.00

## Phenytoin-Acetazolamide

**Significance:** 4—not clinically significant
**Recommendations:** The concurrent use of these agents need not be avoided. However, special attention to the early detection of osteomalacia should be given to patients receiving this combination of agents.
**Summary:** Use of phenytoin and acetazolamide may accelerate the osteomalacia induced by anticonvulsant therapy.
**Related Drugs:** An interaction between acetazolamide and other hydantoin anticonvulsants has not been documented. No reports are available regarding an interaction between hydantoins and other carbonic anhydrase inhibitors.

## Anticonvulsant

**Mechanism:** Acetazolamide enhances urinary calcium excretion and urinary phosphate excretion, causing systemic acidosis, which retards the dihydroxycholecalciferol.
**Detailed Information:** See *EDI*, 5/19.00

## Phenytoin-Alcohol, Ethyl

**Significance:** 2—moderately clinically significant
**Recommendations:** If phenytoin is administered to patients who ingest alcohol chronically, the serum phenytoin level should be monitored to assure that they are in the therapeutic range. Conversely, in alcoholic patients whose phenytoin dose has been titrated to therapeutic levels, a decrease in serum phenytoin levels may occur when alcohol is discontinued, necessitating an increase in the phenytoin dose.
**Summary:** Long-term alcohol ingestion may increase the metabolism and clearance of phenytoin. However, it has been shown that long-term alcohol ingestion can inhibit phenytoin metabolism, decreasing serum phenytoin levels.
**Related Drugs:** The other hydantoin derivatives may interact with alcohol in a similar manner.
**Mechanism:** Increased phenytoin clearance during alcohol withdrawal results from an increased metabolic rate, secondary to enzyme induction by alcohol.
**Detailed Information:** See *EDI*, 5/21.00

## Phenytoin-Allopurinol

**Significance:** 2—moderately clinically significant
**Recommendations:** Close patient attention is necessary during the concurrent administration of phenytoin and allopurinol. If phenytoin toxicity appears, the dosage may need to be adjusted downward.
**Summary:** Concurrent allopurinol administration has resulted in an increase in phenytoin serum concentration.
**Related Drugs:** A similar interaction is expected to occur between allopurinol and other hydantoin anticonvulsants. There are no drugs related to allopurinol.
**Mechanism:** Allopurinol inhibits the oxidative metabolism of phenytoin in the liver, resulting in an increased serum concentration.
**Detailed Information:** See *EDI*, 5/23.00

## Phenytoin-Aluminum Hydroxide, Magnesium Trisilicate

**Significance:** 3—minimally clinically significant
**Recommendations:** There is no need to routinely avoid concurrent use of these agents. However, if loss of seizure control occurs, the administration of phenytoin and the antacid should be separated by as much time as possible and the dose of phenytoin modified as required.
**Summary:** A combination antacid containing aluminum hydroxide and magnesium trisilicate was shown to reduce phenytoin serum concentrations; however, data have shown no alterations in phenytoin absorption.
**Related Drugs:** It is not possible to determine if antacids will interact with phenytoin. Documentation is lacking regarding an interaction with other hydantoin anticonvulsants and a magnesium trisilicate-aluminum hydroxide combination antacid.
**Mechanism:** The aluminum hydroxide and magnesium trisilicate may adsorb phenytoin, reducing phenytoin absorption.
**Detailed Information:** See *EDI*, 5/24.10

Anticonvulsant

## Phenytoin-Amiodarone

**Significance:** 2—moderately clinically significant

**Potential Effects:** Amiodarone may cause an increase in phenytoin levels.

**Recommendations:** Monitor phenytoin levels when these agents are used together; the dose of phenytoin may need to be decreased.

**Summary:** Amiodarone increased phenytoin serum concentrations and was associated with ataxia, nystagmus, clouding of vision, and bilateral leg weakness.

**Related Drugs:** A similar interaction may occur between amiodarone and other hydantoin anticonvulsants. There are no drugs related to amiodarone.

**Mechanism:** The hepatic metabolism of phenytoin may be inhibited by amiodarone, and amiodarone may displace phenytoin from serum and tissue protein binding sites.

**Detailed Information:** See *EDI*, 5/24.30

## Phenytoin-Aspirin

**Significance:** 4—not clinically significant

**Recommendations:** Although the patient's phenytoin levels (free and total) should be monitored closely during concurrent salicylate therapy, these agents need not be avoided.

**Summary:** Several studies have indicated that aspirin and other salicylates may cause a transient increase in phenytoin plasma levels.

**Related Drugs:** A similar interaction is expected to occur between other hydantoin anticonvulsants and other salicylates.

**Mechanism:** Salicylates have been shown to displace phenytoin from plasma protein binding sites; however, the metabolic clearance of phenytoin may increase, resulting in a lower total phenytoin plasma level.

**Detailed Information:** See *EDI*, 5/25.00

## Phenytoin-Carbamazepine

**Significance:** 3—minimally clinically significant

**Potential Effects:** The concurrent use of these agents may result in increased or decreased phenytoin levels or decreased carbamazepine levels.

**Recommendations:** Serum concentrations of both agents should be monitored during concomitant therapy. Seizure control and serum levels should be monitored if either agent is added to, or withdrawn from, therapy.

**Summary:** Conflicting results have occurred when phenytoin and carbamazepine were administered concurrently. The use of these agents may result in increased or decreased phenytoin levels or decreased carbamazepine levels.

**Related Drugs:** A similar interaction is expected to occur between carbamazepine and other hydantoin anticonvulsants; however, it is not known which agent will be affected or if the levels will increase or decrease. There are no drugs related to carbamazepine.

**Mechanism:** Carbamazepine induces the hepatic metabolism of phenytoin, causing a decrease in serum levels, and inhibits the hepatic metabolism of phenytoin, causing an increase in serum levels. The decreased carbamazepine levels may occur by induction of hepatic metabolism, and phenytoin may increase the drug's biotransformation.

**Detailed Information:** See *EDI*, 5/27.00

Anticonvulsant

## Phenytoin-Carmustine, Methotrexate, Vinblastine
**Significance:** 2—moderately clinically significant
**Potential Effects:** The serum levels of phenytoin may be decreased. This may lead to loss of seizure control.
**Recommendations:** Monitor phenytoin levels when these agents are used together. The dosage of phenytoin may need to be adjusted.
**Summary:** There are data to show that administration of phenytoin and carmustine may lead to a high incidence of partial seizures.
**Related Drugs:** Use of vinblastine, bleomycin and cisplatin necessitated a doubling in phenytoin dosage. It is not known if a similar interaction would occur with ethotoin or mephenytoin.
**Mechanism:** Decreased gastrointestinal absorption of phenytoin may be the cause of this interaction, secondary to the antineoplastic agents.
**Detailed Information:** See *EDI*, 5/29.00

## Phenytoin-Charcoal
**Significance:** 2—moderately clinically significant
**Potential Effects:** Charcoal may decrease the adsorption of phenytoin. This effect may be used to treat acute phenytoin overdose.
**Recommendations:** Multiple activated charcoal doses (30G in 26% sorbitol) may be given for acute phenytoin toxicity. Administer charcoal as far apart from phenytoin administration as possible. The patient should be monitored for changes in phenytoin levels.
**Summary:** There are data to show that administration of charcoal significantly decreases the absorption of phenytoin.
**Related Drugs:** Ethotoin and mephenytoin may also interact with charcoal.
**Mechanism:** Charcoal adsorbs phenytoin, limiting its absorption.
**Detailed Information:** See *EDI*, 5/31.00

## Phenytoin-Chloramphenicol
**Significance:** 2—moderately clinically significant
**Recommendations:** In view of the increases in serum phenytoin concentration that have been observed after a single dose of chloramphenicol, it is recommended that frequent phenytoin levels be obtained after the initiation of chloramphenicol therapy, and that careful observation of the patient for signs and symptoms of phenytoin toxicity (e.g., ataxia, nystagmus) be undertaken with subsequent proper phenytoin dosage adjustments if needed. With regard to potential chloramphenicol toxicity, it has been recommended that a dosage of chloramphenicol no greater than 75 mg/kg/day be considered in patients receiving phenytoin concomitantly.
**Summary:** It has been shown that chloramphenicol has a direct inhibitory effect on the metabolism of phenytoin, decreasing the metabolic clearance and increasing the serum concentration of phenytoin; however, there are conflicting data.
**Related Drugs:** A similar interaction is expected to occur between other hydantoin anticonvulsants and chloramphenicol. There are no drugs related to chloramphenicol.
**Mechanism:** Concurrent administration of chloramphenicol may inhibit phenytoin metabolism, causing elevated serum levels. Competition for hepatic enzyme binding sites may explain the inhibition of chloramphenicol metabolism.
**Detailed Information:** See *EDI*, 5/33.00

Anticonvulsant

## Phenytoin-Chlorpheniramine

**Significance:** 2—moderately clinically significant

**Recommendations:** Although this interaction is based on isolated case reports, it is necessary to monitor phenytoin levels during concurrent use of these agents. If toxicity does occur, the dose of phenytoin may need to be decreased, or chlorpheniramine may need to be discontinued.

**Summary:** Phenytoin toxicity has been reported after the concurrent administration of chlorpheniramine.

**Related Drugs:** A similar interaction is expected to occur between phenytoin and other antihistamines. An interaction between chlorpheniramine and other hydantoin anticonvulsants may be expected.

**Mechanism:** Chlorpheniramine may inhibit the liver microsomal enzymes responsible for phenytoin metabolism.

**Detailed Information:** See *EDI*, 5/35.00

## Phenytoin-Chlorpromazine

**Significance:** 3—minimally clinically significant

**Potential Effects:** The concomitant administration of these agents may result in an increase or decrease in phenytoin serum levels. This interaction is subject to individual variability.

**Recommendations:** Patients receiving phenytoin should be monitored for increases or decreases in their phenytoin levels when chlorpromazine is added to, or withdrawn from, their therapy. Also, epileptic patients should be monitored closely for a possible increase in seizure frequency.

**Summary:** There are data to show the concomitant administration of these agents may result in an increase or decrease in phenytoin serum levels, indicating that this interaction is subject to individual variability.

**Related Drugs:** Prochlorperazine and thioridazine have been reported to increase phenytoin levels, but inconsistent data are available. Mesoridazine has been shown to decrease phenytoin concentrations. Phenytoin decreased clozapine plasma concentrations. It is difficult to determine if an interaction would occur between phenytoin and the phenothiazines, the thioxanthenes, the dihydroindolones or the dibenzoxazepines. Documentation is lacking regarding an interaction between chlorpromazine and other hydantoin anticonvulsants.

**Mechanism:** Chlorpromazine, other phenothiazines, and phenytoin probably compete for the limited metabolic capacity of the microsomal hydroxylation enzymes in the liver.

**Detailed Information:** See *EDI*, 5/37.00

## Phenytoin-Cimetidine

**Significance:** 1—highly clinically significant

**Potential Effects:** Cimetidine inhibits the metabolism of phenytoin, leading to increased phenytoin serum levels and toxicity.

**Recommendations:** If these agents are used concomitantly, patients should be monitored for increased phenytoin serum levels and toxicity. Famotidine may be an alternative to cimetidine.

**Summary:** There are data to show that coadministration of these agents causes increased phenytoin levels and phenytoin toxicity.

**Related Drugs:** A similar interaction is expected to occur between cimetidine and other hydantoin anticonvulsants. Ranitidine exhibited a similar interaction; however, ranitidine has also been reported not to interact with phenytoin. The clearance of phenytoin was not affected by famotidine. It cannot be determined if an interaction would be expected to occur between other $H_2$-receptor antagonists and phenytoin.

**Mechanism:** Cimetidine inhibits hepatic microsomal enzymes and impairs the metabolism of phenytoin, resulting in increased serum phenytoin levels.

**Detailed Information:** See *EDI*, 5/39.00

## Phenytoin-Ciprofloxacin

**Significance:** 2—moderately clinically significant

**Potential Effects:** Ciprofloxacin may decrease phenytoin levels and/or increase seizure frequency.

**Recommendations:** Patients maintained on phenytoin should be carefully monitored for changes in plasma phenytoin levels or seizure frequency if ciprofloxacin is added to or discontinued from therapy. The dose of phenytoin may need to be adjusted.

**Summary:** The addition of ciprofloxacin to the therapy of several patients maintained on phenytoin resulted in decreased phenytoin serum levels and an increased frequency of seizures. In conflicting reports, ciprofloxacin may have caused an increase in phenytoin levels or no effect at all.

**Related Drugs:** Although there is no documentation for an interaction between ciprofloxacin and the other hydantoin anticonvulsants, or between phenytoin and the other quinolone antibiotics, an interaction could occur.

**Mechanism:** The reduction in phenytoin serum concentration may be due to ciprofloxacin's induction of phenytoin metabolism; however, the timing of the decrease in phenytoin concentrations is not consistent with enzyme induction and ciprofloxacin is usually an inhibitor rather than an inducer of cytochrome P450. A disruption in the enterohepatic circulation of phenytoin by ciprofloxacin and a ciprofloxacin-induced shift in the volume of distribution of phenytoin have also been proposed. Ciprofloxacin may increase the renal excretion of phenytoin by inhibiting its tubular reabsorption.

**Detailed Information:** See *EDI*, 5/40.50

## Phenytoin-Clarithromycin

**Significance:** 2—moderately clinically significant

**Potential Effects:** The concomitant use of phenytoin and clarithromycin may result in elevated phenytoin plasma levels.

**Recommendations:** Patients maintained on phenytoin should be closely monitored for increased phenytoin levels and phenytoin toxicity if clarithromycin is added to therapy. The dose of phenytoin may need to be adjusted.

**Summary:** Concurrent therapy with phenytoin and clarithromycin may result in elevated phenytoin plasma levels.

**Related Drugs:** Single-dose phenytoin clearance appears to be unaffected by erythromycin; however, occasional, large interindividual changes in phenytoin clearance have occurred when it was given with erythromycin. A similar interaction is possible between phenytoin and other macrolide antibiotics that inhibit cytochrome $P450_{3A4}$ (dirithromycin, josamycin, spiramycin, and troleandomycin) but is not likely to occur with azithromycin, which does not affect cytochrome P450. An interaction may be expected to occur between clarithromycin and other hydantoin anticonvulsants.

**Mechanism:** Clarithromycin and phenytoin are metabolized by cytochrome $P450_{3A4}$. Clarithromycin also inhibits cytochrome $P450_{3A4}$. Elevated phenytoin levels may be caused by clarithromycin inhibiting phenytoin metabolism.

**Detailed Information:** See *EDI*, 5/39.30

## Anticonvulsant

### Phenytoin-Cyclosporine
**Significance:** 2—moderately clinically significant
**Potential Effects:** Phenytoin may decrease the concentration of cyclosporine, which may lead to graft rejection.
**Recommendations:** Monitor cyclosporine levels when phenytoin is added to therapy. An increase in the cyclosporine dose may be necessary.
**Summary:** The administration of phenytoin has resulted in a reduction in the cyclosporine maximum concentration and area-under-curve and an increase in total body clearance. Decreased cyclosporine levels could lead to graft rejection.
**Related Drugs:** A similar interaction is expected to occur between cyclosporine and other hydantoin anticonvulsants. There are no drugs related to cyclosporine.
**Mechanism:** It is possible that phenytoin induces the hepatic metabolism of cyclosporine.
**Detailed Information:** See *EDI*, 5/41.00

### Phenytoin-Dexamethasone
**Significance:** 2—moderately clinically significant
**Recommendations:** If the dexamethasone suppression test is used in patients who have been receiving phenytoin long term, the test should be interpreted with caution and a higher dose of dexamethasone may be necessary. Patients receiving both drugs concurrently should be observed for possible diminution of the therapeutic effect of dexamethasone or other corticosteroids and/or signs and symptoms of phenytoin toxicity (e.g., nystagmus, gait ataxia, poor muscle tone, or lethargy). These effects may require an increase in corticosteroid dosage, a decrease in phenytoin dose, or both, to establish therapeutic levels.
**Summary:** Phenytoin impairs the response to dexamethasone and may result in a decrease in the therapeutic response to dexamethasone. Administration of dexamethasone may result in a significant increase in the half-life and serum level of phenytoin.
**Related Drugs:** Phenytoin has been reported to increase the metabolism of hydrocortisone, methylprednisolone, prednisolone, and prednisone. A similar interaction is expected to occur with other corticosteroids and phenytoin. Primidone has increased the metabolism of dexamethasone and reduced its clinical effectiveness. A similar interaction is expected to occur with other hydantoin anticonvulsants and other anticonvulsants that cause enzyme induction.
**Mechanism:** Phenytoin affects corticosteroid metabolism by stimulating hepatic enzymes responsible for corticosteroid metabolism, and phenytoin and dexamethasone may compete for the metabolic capacity of these enzymes.
**Detailed Information:** See *EDI*, 5/43.00

### Phenytoin-Diazepam
**Significance:** 3—minimally clinically significant
**Potential Effects:** Diazepam may increase or decrease phenytoin levels.
**Recommendations:** Monitor phenytoin levels when these agents are used together. Phenytoin dosage may need to be adjusted.
**Summary:** There are conflicting reports regarding the effect of diazepam on phenytoin serum concentrations. Diazepam may increase or decrease phenytoin levels.
**Related Drugs:** Phenytoin serum levels have been shown to be increased during administration of chlordiazepoxide, clonazepam, and nitrazepam. Phenytoin levels have been shown to be decreased with chlordiazepoxide and clonazepam. Other benzo-

## Anticonvulsant

diazepines have not been reported to alter phenytoin levels. It is difficult to determine whether an interaction would occur between diazepam and other hydantoin anticonvulsants.

**Mechanism:** Possible mechanisms include a benzodiazepine microsomal enzyme induction or inhibition of phenytoin metabolism. The apparent volume of distribution of phenytoin may also be affected by benzodiazepines.

**Detailed Information:** See *EDI*, 5/45.00

### Phenytoin-Diazoxide

**Significance:** 2—moderately clinically significant

**Recommendations:** Phenytoin plasma levels should be monitored, and an increased phenytoin dosage may be necessary if loss of seizure control occurs. Also, when diazoxide is discontinued, phenytoin dosage may need to be decreased to avoid toxicity.

**Summary:** Phenytoin serum levels may be decreased to subtherapeutic levels by concurrent oral diazoxide.

**Related Drugs:** A similar interaction may occur between diazoxide and other hydantoin anticonvulsants. There are no drugs related to diazoxide.

**Mechanism:** Diazoxide may increase the hepatic metabolism of phenytoin and increase its clearance. Displacement from plasma protein binding sites may also play a role. The reduced effects of diazoxide may be the result of induction of diazoxide's metabolism by phenytoin.

**Detailed Information:** See *EDI*, 5/47.00

### Phenytoin-Disulfiram

**Significance:** 1—highly clinically significant

**Recommendations:** If a patient must be treated with both drugs, a baseline phenytoin level should be drawn before disulfiram is added to the regimen. The levels should be measured again in two to four days, and once or twice weekly until a new steady-state is established. In most cases, the plateau will be reached two to three weeks after the last dosage adjustment. The patient should also be monitored clinically for signs of phenytoin toxicity (e.g., ataxia, nystagmus) since symptom severity and height of serum level usually are parallel. Both parameters may be used as guides for adjusting the phenytoin dose if necessary. In most cases, decreasing the phenytoin dose will be sufficient to avoid toxicity, but some patients may require withdrawal of the disulfiram.

**Summary:** Addition of disulfiram to a stable phenytoin regimen will result in decreased phenytoin metabolism and increased phenytoin levels that may lead to toxicity.

**Related Drugs:** A similar interaction is expected to occur with the other hydantoin anticonvulsants and disulfiram.

**Mechanism:** Increased phenytoin levels result from disulfiram inhibition of the major route of metabolism of phenytoin.

**Detailed Information:** See *EDI*, 5/49.00

### Phenytoin-Dopamine

**Significance:** 1—highly clinically significant

**Recommendations:** Although this precaution is based on one report, phenytoin should be used with the greatest care, or not at all, in patients receiving dopamine to support blood pressure. If hypotension occurs, discontinue phenytoin.

**Summary:** The administration of dopamine and phenytoin has been shown to produce a dramatic hypotension effect, possibly causing death.

**Related Drugs:** There is no documentation concerning the interaction of dopamine with other hydantoin anticonvulsants. No reports are available regarding an interaction between phenytoin and other agents used to treat shock; therefore, it cannot be determined if an interaction exists between other anticonvulsants and other sympathomimetics.

**Mechanism:** The hypotensive effect may be due to dopamine preventing the uptake at storage sites and increasing the synthesis of norepinephrine while phenytoin exerts a greater myocardial depressant effect secondary to catecholamine depletion.

**Detailed Information:** See *EDI*, 5/51.00

## Phenytoin-Ethosuximide

**Significance:** 3—minimally clinically significant

**Recommendations:** Patients receiving phenytoin should be closely monitored for increased serum phenytoin concentrations or signs of toxicity (e.g., ataxia, nystagmus) when ethosuximide is coadministered. Patients stabilized on both drugs should also be monitored for subtherapeutic phenytoin levels if ethosuximide is discontinued.

**Summary:** Increased serum phenytoin concentrations with concurrent administration of ethosuximide have been reported; however, reports that no interaction occurs with these agents are documented.

**Related Drugs:** Increased serum phenytoin concentrations have been seen with concurrent methsuximide. A similar interaction is expected to occur between ethosuximide and other hydantoin anticonvulsants and between phenytoin and phensuximide.

**Mechanism:** Ethosuximide induced inhibition of phenytoin metabolism is a suggested mechanism for this interaction.

**Detailed Information:** See *EDI*, 5/53.00

## Phenytoin-Felbamate

**Significance:** 2—moderately clinically significant

**Potential Effects:** Coadministration of felbamate and phenytoin will cause an increase in phenytoin levels and a decrease in felbamate clearance, resulting in phenytoin adverse effects.

**Recommendations:** As felbamate is added to existing phenytoin therapy, it may be necessary to reduce the dosage of phenytoin (20-33%) in order to control plasma phenytoin concentrations and symptoms of toxicity. Additional reductions of the concomitant phenytoin dosage may also be necessary to minimize side effects and toxicity. Patient serum phenytoin levels and changes in seizure control should be monitored during all phases of therapy.

**Summary:** Coadministration of phenytoin and felbamate resulted in an increase in plasma phenytoin concentrations and a decrease in felbamate clearance.

**Related Drugs:** It is not known whether meprobamate would interact similarly with phenytoin. A similar interaction may occur between felbamate and other hydantoin anticonvulsant agents.

**Mechanism:** Felbamate may act as a competitive inhibitor of phenytoin metabolism.

**Detailed Information:** See *EDI*, 5/54.50

## Phenytoin-Fluconazole

**Significance:** 1—highly clinically significant

**Potential Effects:** Fluconazole may decrease the metabolism of phenytoin, leading to increased phenytoin levels and toxicity.

**Recommendations:** Patients maintained on phenytoin should be closely monitored for increased serum phenytoin levels and

## Anticonvulsant

phenytoin toxicity if fluconazole is added to, or withdrawn from, therapy. The dose of phenytoin may need to be adjusted.

**Summary:** The addition of fluconazole to a phenytoin regimen resulted in an increase in serum phenytoin concentration.

**Related Drugs:** Miconazole has been shown to increase serum phenytoin concentrations. A similar interaction is expected to occur between phenytoin and other imidazole systemic antifungal agents and between fluconazole and other hydantoin anticonvulsants.

**Mechanism:** Fluconazole may inhibit the hepatic metabolism of phenytoin by interfering with fungal demethylation.

**Detailed Information:** See *EDI*, 5/54.10

## Phenytoin-Fluoxetine

**Significance:** 2—moderately clinically significant

**Potential Effects:** The addition of fluoxetine to phenytoin therapy may cause an increase in phenytoin levels and resultant phenytoin toxicity.

**Recommendations:** Patients receiving concurrent fluoxetine and phenytoin should be monitored for increased phenytoin levels and an increase in phenytoin toxic effects (e.g., nystagmus, gait ataxia, poor muscle tone, lethargy). If phenytoin toxicity occurs, both fluoxetine and phenytoin doses may need to be reduced until toxic signs and symptoms subside.

**Summary:** Fluoxetine has been shown to increase phenytoin levels, leading to signs and symptoms of phenytoin intoxication.

**Related Drugs:** An interaction may occur between fluoxetine and other hydantoin anticonvulsants and between phenytoin and other serotonin-selective reuptake inhibitors. Paroxetine may interact with phenytoin.

**Mechanism:** This interaction may involve the inhibition of the hepatic metabolism of phenytoin by fluoxetine and cause an enhancement of serotonergic neurotransmission, leading to enhanced anticonvulsant effects.

**Detailed Information:** See *EDI*, 5/54.20

## Phenytoin-Folic Acid

**Significance:** 2—moderately clinically significant

**Potential Effects:** Folic acid administration (5 mg or more per day) to patients stabilized on phenytoin may increase the incidence of seizures. Long-term phenytoin administration may precipitate signs of folic acid deficiency.

**Recommendations:** If signs of folic acid deficiency are observed in patients receiving phenytoin, folic acid (0.1 to 1 mg/day) may be added to therapy. Larger doses of folic acid are not more effective and may cause a loss in seizure control.

**Summary:** Folic acid administration has been associated with increased seizure frequency and lowered serum phenytoin concentrations. Long-term administration of phenytoin may cause low serum folate concentrations and may precipitate folic acid deficiency.

**Related Drugs:** The other hydantoin anticonvulsants may also interact with folic acid in a similar manner. There are no drugs related to folic acid.

**Mechanism:** Phenytoin-induced increases in hepatic metabolizing enzymes may cause a greater demand for folate, and phenytoin may inhibit folate conversion. Folic acid may enhance the parahydroxylation of phenytoin, and higher doses of folate may result in a competitive effect on phenytoin binding sites.

**Detailed Information:** See *EDI*, 5/55.00

# Anticonvulsant

## Phenytoin-Hormonal Contraceptive Agents

**Significance:** 3—minimally clinically significant

**Potential Effects:** Concurrent use of phenytoin and levonorgestrel-containing hormonal contraceptives may result in decreased plasma concentration of levonorgestrel, decreased levonorgestrel area-under-curve, and, in some cases, loss of contraceptive effect resulting in pregnancy.

**Recommendations:** Patients maintained on phenytoin and hormonal contraceptives should be carefully monitored for decreased contraceptive efficacy. Another method of contraception should be considered. Also, patients should be monitored for loss of seizure control since an increased phenytoin dose may be necessary.

**Summary:** Concurrent use of phenytoin and hormonal contraceptive agents may result in breakthrough bleeding, spotting, decreased hormonal contraceptive AUC and serum concentration, and, in some cases, loss of contraceptive effect resulting in pregnancy.

**Related Drugs:** A similar interaction may occur between hormonal contraceptive agents and other hydantoin derivatives. Besides taking phenytoin, some patients were receiving phenobarbital, primidone, or carbamazepine. Menopausal symptoms and depressed estradiol and estrone levels occurred when a patient received concomitant phenytoin and conjugated estrogens. A similar interaction may also occur between phenytoin and other estrogens.

**Mechanism:** Phenytoin and other anticonvulsants may cause contraceptive failure because they induce hepatic microsomal enzymes, thereby increasing the rate of metabolism of oral contraceptives. Loss of seizure control may result from changes in fluid retention induced by oral contraceptives. Contraceptive agents may also affect plasma protein binding of phenytoin or inhibit its metabolism; however, one study found no effect on phenytoin binding. Other studies have postulated that treatment with phenytoin enhances levonorgestrel metabolism and clearance and that, because phenytoin induces sex hormone binding globulin, less biologically active free levonorgestrel is available in the bloodstream. Phenytoin induces the $CYP_{3A4}$ isoenzyme, which is responsible for 6β-hydroxylation of certain progestins.

**Detailed Information:** See *EDI*, 5/69.00

## Phenytoin-Ibuprofen

**Significance:** 2—moderately clinically significant

**Potential Effects:** Ibuprofen may cause an increase in phenytoin levels.

**Recommendations:** If these agents are used together, phenytoin levels should be monitored. If increased levels occur, ibuprofen should be discontinued or the dosage of phenytoin decreased.

**Summary:** The concomitant administration of phenytoin and ibuprofen may increase phenytoin plasma levels, resulting in phenytoin toxicity.

**Related Drugs:** Phenylbutazone and oxyphenbutazone have been reported to interact with phenytoin (see also Phenytoin-Phenylbutazone, page 127). Other NSAIAs may increase phenytoin plasma levels. A similar interaction is expected to occur between ibuprofen and other hydantoin anticonvulsants.

**Mechanism:** Ibuprofen may inhibit the hepatic microsomal enzymes responsible for phenytoin metabolism.

**Detailed Information:** See *EDI*, 5/57.00

Anticonvulsant

## Phenytoin-Imipramine

**Significance:** 3—minimally clinically significant

**Potential Effects:** Imipramine may cause an increase in phenytoin levels, leading to toxicity. Phenytoin may also cause a decrease in desipramine levels.

**Recommendations:** Phenytoin levels and signs of toxicity (e.g., nystagmus, gait ataxia, lethargy) should be monitored during cotherapy with imipramine. Since the tricyclics may cause an increase in seizures, the phenytoin dosage may need to be increased. In addition, tricyclic antidepressant levels should be monitored for decreases during concurrent phenytoin therapy.

**Summary:** Imipramine has been reported to cause an increase in phenytoin levels and phenytoin toxicity.

**Related Drugs:** The action of other antidepressants on phenytoin levels is varied and conflicting; therefore, it is difficult to determine whether an interaction would occur between phenytoin and the other tricyclic antidepressants and the tetracyclic antidepressants. Amitriptyline, amoxapine, desipramine, imipramine, nortriptyline, and protriptyline have been reported to cause seizures in patients. A similar interaction is expected to occur between imipramine and other hydantoin anticonvulsants.

**Mechanism:** Imipramine may inhibit the metabolism of phenytoin, which results in increased levels.

**Detailed Information:** See *EDI*, 5/59.00

## Phenytoin-Influenza Virus Vaccine

**Significance:** 3—minimally clinically significant

**Potential Effects:** Influenza Virus Vaccine has been shown to increase, decrease, and have no serum phenytoin levels.

**Recommendations:** Plasma phenytoin levels should be monitored and adjusted if necessary following influenza virus vaccination.

**Summary:** The administration of influenza virus vaccine was shown to decrease, increase, and have no effect on phenytoin plasma levels.

**Related Drugs:** It is not known if an interaction would occur between influenza virus vaccine and other hydantoin anticonvulsants.

**Mechanism:** The influenza virus vaccine is thought to enhance the metabolism of phenytoin. Phenytoin levels may be increased secondary to a decrease in metabolism caused by the influenza virus vaccine.

**Detailed Information:** See *EDI*, 5/60.10

## Phenytoin-Isoniazid

**Significance:** 2—moderately clinically significant

**Recommendations:** Patients receiving phenytoin and isoniazid concurrently should have periodic determinations of serum phenytoin concentrations and should be observed closely for signs and symptoms of toxicity (e.g., ataxia, nystagmus). Patients known to be slow acetylators of isoniazid should have the phenytoin dosage reduced when isoniazid is added to the regimen. If phenytoin toxicity occurs, phenytoin should be discontinued or the dosage reduced until toxic signs and symptoms subside. Phenytoin may then be reinstituted and the dosage adjusted until therapeutic concentrations are obtained.

**Summary:** Isoniazid increases the serum phenytoin concentration, which can result in an increased incidence of phenytoin toxicity.

**Related Drugs:** Isoniazid may interact with other hydantoin anticonvulsants. Aminosalicylic acid and cycloserine have been shown to interact with phenytoin.

**Mechanism:** Studies have shown that isoniazid blocks the para-hydroxylation of phenytoin and conjugation of the principal metabolite.

**Detailed Information:** See *EDI*, 5/61.00

## Anticonvulsant

### Phenytoin-Levodopa
**Significance:** 3—minimally clinically significant
**Recommendations:** If the concurrent use of levodopa and phenytoin is necessary, a higher dose of levodopa may be required.
**Summary:** The therapeutic effects of levodopa were inhibited by the concurrent use of phenytoin, and Parkinson patients showed a worsening of symptoms and a reduction of dyskinesias.
**Related Drugs:** There are no drugs related to levodopa. A similar interaction may occur between levodopa and other hydantoins; however, documentation is lacking.
**Mechanism:** The mechanism of this interaction is unknown.
**Detailed Information:** See *EDI*, 5/63.00

### Phenytoin-Levothyroxine
**Significance:** 3—minimally clinically significant
**Recommendations:** Since patients may remain euthyroid during concurrent administration of phenytoin and levothyroxine, concomitant use need not be avoided. However, patients should be frequently observed for signs of hypothyroidism. The dose of levothyroxine may need to be increased, since an increase in dose was shown to improve the symptoms of hypothyroidism.
**Summary:** Data have shown that patients on levothyroxine may develop clinical hypothyroidism after initiation of phenytoin therapy; however, patients remained euthyroid.
**Related Drugs:** A similar interaction may occur between phenytoin and other thyroid preparations and between levothyroxine and other hydantoin anticonvulsants.
**Mechanism:** Phenytoin may displace thyroid hormones or it may increase the rate of clearance and catabolism of thyroid hormones.
**Detailed Information:** See *EDI*, 5/64.10

### Phenytoin-Methoxsalen
**Significance:** 2—moderately clinically significant
**Potential Effects:** Phenytoin may decrease the serum levels of methoxsalen.
**Recommendations:** The use of methoxsalen (PUVA therapy) in patients receiving phenytoin may result in treatment failure. However, if phenytoin is discontinued or the dose decreased, methoxsalen serum levels may increase, resulting in serious erythema or blistering reactions. It is not known if adjusting the dose of methoxsalen would be beneficial.
**Summary:** A patient maintained on phenytoin received PUVA treatment and no beneficial effect was observed. Phenytoin was discontinued, and PUVA therapy had to be stopped secondary to intense PUVA erythema with blisters.
**Related Drugs:** A similar interaction may occur between methoxsalen and other hydantoin anticonvulsants and between phenytoin and trioxsalen.
**Mechanism:** Phenytoin may induce the hepatic microsomal enzymes responsible for the metabolism of methoxsalen. There may be a decreased gastrointestinal absorption or altered plasma protein binding of methoxsalen by phenytoin.
**Detailed Information:** See *EDI*, 5/64.21

### Phenytoin-Methylphenidate
**Significance:** 3—minimally clinically significant
**Recommendations:** Serum concentrations of phenytoin should be monitored and the dose altered to bring the anticonvulsant level into the therapeutic range.

## Anticonvulsant

**Summary:** Methylphenidate raises serum phenytoin concentration and may cause symptoms of phenytoin toxicity in children; these effects were not seen in adults.
**Related Drugs:** Primidone has been reported to interact with methylphenidate in a similar manner. A similar interaction is expected to occur with other hydantoin anticonvulsants and methylphenidate.
**Mechanism:** Methylphenidate is a competitive inhibitor of the hepatic metabolism of phenytoin.
**Detailed Information:** See *EDI*, 5/65.00

## Phenytoin-Metronidazole

**Significance:** 3—minimally clinically significant
**Potential Effects:** Concomitant metronidazole therapy may cause an increase in phenytoin levels.
**Recommendations:** Although these agents may be used together, patients' phenytoin levels should be monitored.
**Summary:** Metronidazole has been shown to significantly prolong phenytoin's half-life and reduce its clearance; however, in another study, there was no change in the elimination of phenytoin.
**Related Drugs:** A similar interaction may occur between metronidazole and other hydantoin anticonvulsants. There are no drugs related to metronidazole.
**Mechanism:** Metronidazole may impair the oxidative metabolism of phenytoin.
**Detailed Information:** See *EDI*, 5/66.01

## Phenytoin-Nifedipine

**Significance:** 2—moderately clinically significant
**Potential Effects:** Nifedipine may cause an increase in phenytoin levels, leading to phenytoin toxicity.
**Recommendations:** Monitor phenytoin levels if nifedipine is added to, or withdrawn from, therapy.
**Summary:** Nifedipine has been shown to induce signs of phenytoin toxicity revealing nystagmus, dysarthria and cerebellar ataxia.
**Related Drugs:** A similar interaction may occur between phenytoin and other calcium channel blockers and between nifedipine and other hydantoin anticonvulsants.
**Mechanism:** Nifedipine may displace phenytoin from plasma proteins or inhibit the parahydroxylation of phenytoin, resulting in increased phenytoin levels.
**Detailed Information:** See *EDI*, 5/66.30

## Phenytoin-Nitrofurantoin

**Significance:** 3—minimally clinically significant
**Recommendations:** These agents need not be avoided. However, patients should be monitored for an increase in seizure frequency. If loss of seizure control occurs, the dose of phenytoin may need to be increased or nitrofurantoin may have to be discontinued.
**Summary:** Phenytoin has been shown to reduce plasma phenytoin levels after the initiation of nitrofurantoin.
**Related Drugs:** A similar interaction is expected to occur between nitrofurantoin and other hydantoin anticonvulsants. There is a lack of documentation concerning an interaction between phenytoin and furazolidone, and it is not possible to predict whether a similar interaction could occur.
**Mechanism:** Impaired phenytoin absorption and increased phenytoin metabolism by nitrofurantoin may be responsible.
**Detailed Information:** See *EDI*, 5/67.00

## Anticonvulsant

### Phenytoin-Omeprazole

**Significance:** 2—moderately clinically significant

**Potential Effects:** Omeprazole may increase the phenytoin area-under-curve.

**Recommendations:** Caution should be used if omeprazole is added to, or withdrawn from, cotherapy with phenytoin. Phenytoin levels should be monitored, and the dose of phenytoin may need to be adjusted.

**Summary:** Omeprazole increased the area-under-curve of phenytoin when compared to subjects on phenytoin alone; however, it has been found that omeprazole will not significantly affect the steady-state plasma levels.

**Related Drugs:** A similar interaction is expected to occur between omeprazole and other hydantoin anticonvulsants. There are no drugs related to omeprazole.

**Mechanism:** This interaction may result from a decreased elimination or an increased absorption of phenytoin. Omeprazole may inhibit hepatic cytochrome P450 monooxygenase.

**Detailed Information:** See *EDI*, 5/68.10

### Phenytoin-Phenobarbital

**Significance:** 3—minimally clinically significant

**Recommendations:** Concurrent phenytoin and phenobarbital therapy need not be avoided when indicated. However, the unpredictable clinical outcome of the drug interaction requires that the serum phenytoin concentrations be determined when initiating concurrent therapy, and that phenytoin and phenobarbital concentrations be determined periodically thereafter until the serum drug levels are stabilized. A determination of serum phenytoin and phenobarbital concentrations after three or four weeks of therapy may serve as a good indicator of the quality of the therapeutic regimen. Serum drug concentrations should be determined at the first sign of phenytoin or phenobarbital toxicity. If toxicity occurs, phenytoin or phenobarbital should be discontinued or the dosage should be reduced until toxic signs and symptoms disappear. Then the drug can be reinstituted or the dosages can be adjusted until therapeutic concentrations are attained.

**Summary:** Phenobarbital may increase, decrease, or cause no change in serum phenytoin concentrations. Other evidence indicates that phenobarbital levels may be increased with concomitant phenytoin.

**Related Drugs:** Primidone has been shown to interact like phenobarbital with phenytoin (see also Primidone-Phenytoin, page 131). A similar interaction is expected to occur with phenobarbital and other hydantoin anticonvulsants. There is no information regarding possible interactions of other barbiturates with phenytoin.

**Mechanism:** Phenobarbital induces hepatic microsomal enzyme activity, increasing the rate of metabolism of phenytoin and decreasing its half life. The two drugs may compete for the hepatic microsomal enzyme system.

**Detailed Information:** See *EDI*, 5/71.00

### Phenytoin-Phenylbutazone

**Significance:** 2—moderately clinically significant

**Recommendations:** If phenylbutazone, oxyphenbutazone, or sulfinpyrazone and phenytoin are coadministered, an increase in phenytoin half-life, serum levels, or side effects may occur within the first four weeks of therapy, particularly when phenylbutazone, oxyphenbutazone, or sulfinpyrazone is added to the drug regimen of a patient previously stabilized on phenytoin. If signs and symptoms of phenytoin toxicity develop (e.g., nystagmus, gait ataxia, poor muscle tone, or lethargy), serum phenytoin levels should be determined and doses of phenytoin reduced to establish therapeutic levels.

**Summary:** Concurrent administration of phenytoin and phenylbutazone may result in a significant increase in the half-life, free fraction, and serum level of phenytoin in some patients.

**Related Drugs:** Oxyphenbutazone, phenylbutazone, and sulfinpyrazone have been reported to interact with phenytoin in a similar manner. A similar interaction is expected to occur with phenylbutazone, oxyphenbutazone, or sulfinpyrazone and other hydantoin anticonvulsants.

**Mechanism:** This interaction may be due to the competition for the limited metabolic capacity of hydroxylation enzymes, impaired p-hydroxylation, or phenytoin displacement from its protein binding sites.

**Detailed Information:** See *EDI*, 5/73.00

## Phenytoin-Pyridoxine

**Significance:** 2—moderately clinically significant

**Recommendations:** Because not all patients appear to be affected by concurrent pyridoxine and phenytoin, these agents need not be avoided. However, the possibility of an interaction does exist, and patients should be monitored for decreased phenytoin levels or loss of seizure control during concurrent administration.

**Summary:** Pyridoxine has been shown to cause a marked reduction in phenytoin serum levels.

**Related Drugs:** A similar interaction is expected to occur between pyridoxine and other hydantoin anticonvulsants, if the mechanism involves induction of hepatic enzymes by pyridoxine. There are no drugs related to pyridoxine.

**Mechanism:** Pyridoxine may increase the liver enzyme activity responsible for phenytoin metabolism.

**Detailed Information:** See *EDI*, 5/75.00

## Phenytoin-Rifampin

**Significance:** 2—moderately clinically significant

**Recommendations:** Patients stabilized on phenytoin should be closely monitored for decreased serum phenytoin concentrations or signs of seizure activity when rifampin is coadministered. Conversely, discontinuation of rifampin in a patient stabilized on phenytoin may necessitate a reduction in the phenytoin dose.

**Summary:** Rifampin has been shown to decrease serum phenytoin concentrations.

**Related Drugs:** A similar interaction is expected to occur between rifampin and other hydantoin anticonvulsants. There are no drugs related to rifampin.

**Mechanism:** Rifampin appears to increase the rate of metabolism of phenytoin, decreasing its half-life and serum concentration.

**Detailed Information:** See *EDI*, 5/76.10

## Phenytoin-Sucralfate

**Significance:** 2—moderately clinically significant

**Potential Effects:** Phenytoin levels may be decreased, which may lead to a loss of seizure control.

**Recommendations:** Monitor phenytoin levels. Phenytoin dosage may need to be increased.

**Summary:** Sulcralfate was shown to reduce phenytoin's area-under-curve and absorption, risking loss of seizure control.

## Phenytoin-Sulfamethizole

**Significance:** 2—moderately clinically significant

**Recommendations:** If sulfamethizole and phenytoin are coadministered, an increase in phenytoin half-life, serum levels, or side effects should occur within the first four weeks of therapy, particularly when the sulfonamide is added to the drug regimen of a patient previously stabilized on phenytoin. If signs and symptoms of phenytoin toxicity develop (e.g., nystagmus, gait ataxia, poor muscle tone, or lethargy), serum phenytoin levels should be determined and doses of phenytoin reduced to establish therapeutic levels.

**Summary:** Sulfamethizole may cause a significant increase in the half-life and serum level of phenytoin.

**Related Drugs:** Sulfadiazine and sulfamethoxazole, alone and in combination with trimethoprim, have been reported to impair phenytoin metabolism and increase its half-life. Sulfisoxazole does not impair phenytoin metabolism; however, it has been reported to displace phenytoin. It is difficult to predict possible interactions with other sulfonamides and phenytoin. A similar interaction is expected to occur with other hydantoin anticonvulsants and other anticonvulsants metabolized by hepatic microsomal hydroxylation.

**Mechanism:** Sulfamethizole and phenytoin may compete for the limited metabolic capacity of enzymes. Phenytoin's p-hydroxylation is impaired. Sulfisoxazole displaces phenytoin from its protein binding sites.

**Detailed Information:** See *EDI*, 5/77.00

## Phenytoin-Ticlopidine

**Significance:** 2—moderately clinically significant

**Potential Effects:** The addition of ticlopidine to phenytoin therapy may result in increased phenytoin serum levels and toxicity.

**Recommendations:** The patient should be carefully monitored for changes in phenytoin serum levels and toxicity if ticlopidine is added to or seizures if it is removed from a phenytoin regimen.

**Summary:** Increased phenytoin serum levels and toxicity resulted when ticlopidine was added to phenytoin therapy.

**Related Drugs:** Although documentation is lacking regarding an interaction between ticlopidine and the other hydantoin anticonvulsant agents, an interaction may be expected to occur. There are no drugs related to ticlopidine.

**Mechanism:** It is postulated that this interaction involves ticlopidine's effect on the cytochrome $P450_{2C19}$ isozyme system.

**Detailed Information:** See *EDI*, 5/78.05

## Phenytoin-Trazodone

**Significance:** 3—minimally clinically significant

**Potential Effects:** Trazodone may increase phenytoin levels.

**Recommendations:** Phenytoin levels should be monitored when trazodone is added to, or withdrawn from, therapy.

**Summary:** The administration of trazodone has been shown to increase phenytoin levels.

## Anticonvulsant

**Related Drugs:** Documentation is lacking regarding an interaction between trazodone and other hydantoin anticonvulsants. There are no drugs related to trazodone.
**Mechanism:** The mechanism of this interaction is unknown.
**Detailed Information:** See *EDI*, 5/78.10

### Phenytoin-Trimethoprim

**Significance:** 2—moderately clinically significant
**Recommendations:** Patients should be monitored for increased phenytoin plasma levels since a lower dosage of phenytoin may be necessary during concurrent use of these agents.
**Summary:** Trimethoprim has been shown to cause an increased phenytoin elimination half-life and a reduced metabolic clearance rate.
**Related Drugs:** There are no drugs related to trimethoprim. A similar interaction may occur between trimethoprim and other hydantoin anticonvulsants.
**Mechanism:** Trimethoprim may inhibit the hepatic metabolism of phenytoin.
**Detailed Information:** See *EDI*, 5/79.00

### Phenytoin-Valproic Acid

**Significance:** 2—moderately clinically significant
**Recommendations:** Surveillance of the patient requiring both phenytoin and valproic acid for seizure control should not be limited solely to the serum concentration of total phenytoin, because measurements may grossly underestimate the concentration of free (active) drug. Dosage adjustments should be determined by clinical signs of over- or underdose. Phenytoin serum levels should be determined before valproic acid is administered. After valproic acid is given, a change in serum concentration of phenytoin is used to determine any phenytoin dose adjustments that might be necessary. The measurement of free (active) phenytoin levels should provide a better therapeutic guide than total serum concentrations. The serum concentration of free phenytoin should be determined by ultrafiltration methods or by using saliva samples.
**Summary:** Valproic acid will decrease phenytoin concentrations and increase the percentage of free phenytoin.
**Related Drugs:** A similar interaction is expected to occur with valproic acid and other hydantoin anticonvulsants. There are no drugs related to valproic acid; however, sodium valproate and divalproex sodium would be expected to interact in a similar manner.
**Mechanism:** This interaction will depend on the combination of the displacement of phenytoin from plasma protein binding sites and its reduction in clearance.
**Detailed Information:** See *EDI*, 5/81.00

### Primidone-Acetazolamide

**Significance:** 3—minimally clinically significant
**Recommendations:** Patients receiving these agents concomitantly should be monitored for decreases in primidone and/or phenobarbital serum concentrations or lack of seizure control.
**Summary:** Concurrent administration of primidone and acetazolamide has been reported to decrease or delay the absorption of primidone.
**Related Drugs:** No documentation exists regarding an interaction between acetazolamide and other barbiturates. No reports exist of barbiturates interacting with other carbonic anhydrase inhibitors.
**Mechanism:** Acetazolamide may decrease the gastrointestinal absorption of primidone.
**Detailed Information:** See *EDI*, 5/83.00

## Anticonvulsant

### Primidone-Phenytoin

**Significance:** 2—moderately clinically significant

**Recommendations:** Because these agents are often administered together successfully, their concurrent use need not be avoided. However, patients taking phenytoin and primidone concurrently should be monitored to assure effective anticonvulsant control. Additionally, they may have to be monitored for possible phenobarbital toxicity.

**Summary:** Concomitant phenytoin therapy increases the plasma concentrations of phenobarbital, and primidone may increase phenytoin clearance.

**Related Drugs:** Ethosuximide had no effect on primidone levels, but primidone caused a slight increase in ethosuximide levels. Methsuximide increased primidone and phenobarbital levels. Phenobarbital has been shown to interact with phenytoin (see also Phenytoin-Phenobarbital, page 127). An interaction may be expected between primidone and the other hydantoin anticonvulsants.

**Mechanism:** Phenytoin may induce the microsomal enzymes responsible for the oxidation of primidone to phenobarbital, or phenytoin may inhibit phenobarbital metabolism or excretion.

**Detailed Information:** See *EDI,* 5/85.00

### Sodium Valproate-Cimetidine

**Significance:** 3—minimally clinically significant

**Recommendations:** These agents may be given together; however, valproic acid levels should be monitored. The dose of sodium valproate may need to be decreased.

**Summary:** Administration of cimetidine has been shown to increase the serum levels of valproic acid.

**Related Drugs:** Ranitidine did not affect any pharmacokinetic parameters of sodium valproate. Valproic acid and divalproex sodium would be expected to interact similarly with cimetidine.

**Mechanism:** Cimetidine may inhibit the hepatic metabolism of sodium valproate.

**Detailed Information:** See *EDI,* 5/86.01

### Sodium Valproate-Naproxen

**Significance:** 3—minimally clinically significant

**Recommendations:** Patients receiving these agents concurrently should be monitored for valproic acid toxicity. Although the change in free fraction could theoretically alter the relationship between total drug level and clinical response, in practice the magnitude of the interaction does not appear to be sufficiently marked to have clinical relevance for the interpretation of serum drug levels.

**Summary:** Naproxen was shown to displace valproic acid, increasing the clearance of total drug, but leaving free valproic acid levels unchanged.

**Related Drugs:** A similar interaction is expected to occur between valproic acid and other NSAIAs. Valproic acid and divalproex sodium would be expected to interact similarly with naproxen.

**Mechanism:** Naproxen appears to exert a displacing effect on valproic acid, increasing the clearance of total drug, but leaving the clearance of free drug unchanged.

**Detailed Information:** See *EDI,* 5/86.10

Anticonvulsant

## Valproic Acid-Aluminum Hydroxide, Magnesium Hydroxide

**Significance:** 3—minimally clinically significant

**Recommendations:** Whether this interaction is clinically significant with steady-state valproic acid therapy or with smaller amounts of antacids is not known. Since antacids are often recommended to relieve gastrointestinal symptoms common to valproic acid administration (indigestion, nausea and vomiting, cramps, diarrhea, etc.), it is important to monitor patients closely for signs of valproic acid toxicity when antacids are used concurrently.

**Summary:** Aluminum hydroxide-magnesium hydroxide antacid preparations have been shown to significantly increase area-under-curve and steady-state serum levels of valproic acid.

**Related Drugs:** No drugs are related to valproic acid; however, sodium valproate and divalproex sodium may be expected to interact similarly.

**Mechanism:** The aluminum/magnesium hydroxide antacid may increase the bioavailability of valproic acid.

**Detailed Information:** See *EDI,* 5/87.00

## Valproic Acid-Amitriptyline

**Significance:** 3—minimally clinically significant

**Potential Effects:** Concurrent administration of valproic acid or its derivatives with a tricyclic antidepressant may result in alterations in the pharmacokinetics of either agent.

**Recommendations:** Monitor for changes in valproic acid levels and tricyclic antidepressant levels when these agents are used together.

**Summary:** Concurrent administration of valproic acid or its derivatives with a tricyclic antidepressant may result in alterations in the pharmacokinetics of either agent. The clinical significance of this interaction was not determined.

**Related Drugs:** A similar interaction may occur between valproic acid, divalproex, and valproate with the other tricyclic antidepressants.

**Mechanism:** The volume of distribution of valproic acid may increase as a result of drug displacement from plasma proteins and/or an enhancement in tissue binding. However, displacement is unlikely since amitriptyline and valproic acid bind predominantly to different classes of plasma proteins. Therefore, an increase in tissue binding of valproic acid by amitriptyline appears more probable. The exact mechanism resulting in increased levels of tricyclic antidepressants is unknown, although it is postulated to involve inhibition of the hydroxylation of the tricyclic agent.

**Detailed Information:** See *EDI,* 5/88.10

## Valproic Acid-Aspirin

**Significance:** 2—moderately clinically significant

**Potential Effects:** Aspirin may increase valproic acid half-life, resulting in increased levels of valproic acid and toxicity.

**Recommendations:** Patients receiving valproic acid should be closely monitored for toxicity if aspirin is added. Especially during a period of febrile illness. Another analgesic/antipyretic may be used as an alternative to aspirin (e.g., acetaminophen).

**Summary:** Administration of aspirin has been shown to increase valproic acid half-life resulting in increased levels of valproic acid and toxicity.

**Related Drugs:** A similar interaction is expected to occur between valproic acid and other salicylates. There are no drugs related to valproic acid; however, sodium valproate and divalproex sodium would be expected to interact similarly.

# Anticonvulsant

**Mechanism:** Salicylic acid may compete for active transport sites in the renal tubules or liver. Aspirin may displace valproic acid from plasma proteins and may increase glucuronide excretion, inhibiting the conjugation of valproic acid.
**Detailed Information:** See *EDI*, 5/89.00

## Valproic Acid-Carbamazepine

**Significance:** 2—moderately clinically significant
**Recommendations:** Serum valproic acid determinations may be helpful in assessing the need of changing the valproic acid dosage when carbamazepine is added to, or withdrawn from, valproate therapy. There is not enough documentation to substantiate a need to reduce carbamazepine dosage in the presence of valproic acid.
**Summary:** Concurrent use of carbamazepine and valproic acid results in a decrease in serum valproic acid concentrations. Valproic acid may cause an increase in serum carbamazepine concentrations.
**Related Drugs:** There are no drugs related to valproic acid; however, sodium valproate and divalproex sodium would be expected to interact similarly.
**Mechanism:** Carbamazepine is thought to induce hepatic microsomal enzymes, enhancing the metabolism of valproic acid.
**Detailed Information:** See *EDI*, 5/91.00

## Valproic Acid-Chlorpromazine

**Significance:** 3—minimally clinically significant
**Potential Effects:** Chlorpromazine may cause an increase in valproic acid levels.
**Recommendations:** Valproic acid levels should be monitored if these agents are used together. The dose of valproic acid may need to be decreased or haloperidol used instead of chlorpromazine.
**Summary:** Administration of chlorpromazine was shown to significantly increase the serum levels of valproic acid.
**Related Drugs:** A similar interaction may occur between valproic acid and other phenothiazines. Haloperidol has been shown to not affect the pharmacokinetic parameters of valproic acid. It is difficult to determine if an interaction would occur between valproic acid and the thioxanthenes, the dihydroindolones and the dibenzoxazepines. There are no drugs related to valproic acid; however, sodium valproate and divalproex sodium would be expected to interact similarly with chlorpromazine.
**Mechanism:** Chlorpromazine may inhibit the hepatic metabolism of valproic acid.
**Detailed Information:** See *EDI*, 5/92.10

## Valproic Acid-Clonazepam

**Significance:** 3—minimally clinically significant
**Recommendations:** The incidence of this interaction is expected to be low. Nevertheless, it should be considered a possibility when these agents are used together. If drowsiness occurs, reduction of the clonazepam dosage may be required.
**Summary:** Concurrent administration of clonazepam and valproic acid does not appear to cause any alterations in plasma concentrations of either drug; however, some patients have experienced drowsiness.
**Related Drugs:** Nitrazepam and valproic acid have been reported to cause drowsiness. Valproic acid may increase the free diazepam serum concentration and inhibit diazepam metabolism. A similar

## Anticonvulsant

interaction is expected to occur between valproic acid and other benzodiazepines. No drugs are related to valproic acid; however, sodium valproate and divalproex sodium would be expected to interact similarly.

**Mechanism:** Drowsiness may be the result of an increase in benzodiazepine serum levels.

**Detailed Information:** See *EDI*, 5/93.00

### Valproic Acid-Erythromycin

**Significance:** 2—moderately clinically significant

**Potential Effects:** The addition of erythromycin to a valproic acid regimen may result in increased valproate levels and toxicity.

**Recommendations:** Caution should be used in patients maintained on valproic acid if the addition of erythromycin to therapy is contemplated. Possibly an alternative choice of antibiotic therapy should be made.

**Summary:** Concomitant valproic acid and erythromycin has been shown to result in increased valproic acid serum levels.

**Related Drugs:** A similar interaction may be expected to occur between valproic acid and other macrolide antibiotics. There are no drugs related to valproic acid; however, sodium valproate and divalproex sodium would be expected to interact similarly.

**Mechanism:** Erythromycin may inhibit the metabolism of valproate by competitive inhibition of hepatic microsomal enzymes.

**Detailed Information:** See *EDI*, 5/88.50

### Valproic Acid-Felbamate

**Significance:** 2—moderately clinically significant

**Potential Effects:** The addition of felbamate to valproic acid results in increased valproic acid plasma drug concentrations.

**Recommendations:** Patients should be closely monitored for changes in valproic acid serum levels and signs of toxicity with concurrent use of these agents. The dose of one or both agents may need to be adjusted. Initial adverse effects may be minimized by slowly increasing the felbamate dosage or reducing the initial valproic acid dosage during rapid felbamate titration.

**Summary:** The coadministration of felbamate and valproic acid results in increased steady-state valproate concentrations.

**Related Drugs:** There are no drugs related to valproic acid. It is not known whether meprobamate would interact similarly with valproic acid. Sodium valproate and divalproex sodium would be expected to interact similarly.

**Mechanism:** Valproic acid may cause elevations in felbamate concentration through enzyme inhibition.

**Detailed Information:** See *EDI*, 5/94.50

### Valproic Acid-Fluoxetine

**Significance:** 3—minimally clinically significant

**Potential Effects:** Serum valproic acid levels may be increased by concurrent fluoxetine.

**Recommendations:** Patients in whom fluoxetine is added to or discontinued from a valproic acid regimen should be monitored for possible changes in valproic acid serum levels.

**Summary:** In a single case report, increased serum valproic acid levels resulted when fluoxetine was added.

**Related Drugs:** Paroxetine has been reported not to interact with valproic acid. No documentation exists regarding an interaction between valproic acid and the other selective serotonin reuptake inhibitors.

Anticonvulsant

**Mechanism:** It was postulated that fluoxetine may increase valproic acid levels by decreasing the hepatic metabolism of valproic acid.
**Detailed Information:** See *EDI*, 5/94.70

## Valproic Acid-Isoniazid

**Significance:** 3—minimally clinically significant
**Potential Effects:** Concurrent use of these agents may result in hepatic and CNS toxicity.
**Recommendations:** Patients receiving valproic acid and isoniazid concurrently should be monitored for increased liver enzymes and increased central nervous system effects such as vomiting and drowsiness. Valproic acid may need to be discontinued.
**Summary:** The concurrent use of these agents has been shown to result in hepatic and CNS toxicity.
**Related Drugs:** There are no drugs related to isoniazid or valproic acid; however, sodium valproate and divalproex sodium would be expected to interact similarly.
**Mechanism:** Isoniazid may inhibit the metabolism of valproic acid, or valproic acid may increase the risk of isoniazid-induced toxicity.
**Detailed Information:** See *EDI*, 5/95.00

## Valproic Acid-Methylphenidate

**Significance:** 3—minimally clinically significant
**Potential Effects:** Concomitant administration of methylphenidate and valproic acid may increase valproic acid adverse effects and the risk of central nervous system toxicities including dyskinesia, bruxism, fidgeting hands, and agitation.
**Recommendations:** Patients should be carefully monitored for increased valproic acid adverse effects if methylphenidate therapy is instituted or the dosage is increased. The dose of methylphenidate may need to be adjusted.
**Summary:** Concurrent administration of methylphenidate increased valproic acid adverse effects and the risk of CNS toxicities including dyskinesia, bruxism, fidgeting hands, and agitation. One study revealed a large inter-patient variability in response, ranging from valproic acid levels decreasing, increasing, or remaining unchanged.
**Related Drugs:** An interaction may occur between methylphenidate and valproic acid derivatives due to similar effects on dopamine and a similar metabolic pathway. It is not known whether an interaction would occur between valproic acid and the other indirect-acting sympathomimetics.
**Mechanism:** The postulated mechanisms for this interaction include increased dopamine availability and competitive inhibition of methylphenidate metabolism mediated by cytochrome $P450_{2D6}$. Methylphenidate and valproic acid may exert additive or synergistic pharmacologic activity by increasing the availability of dopamine, since valproic acid decreases the ability of methylphenidate to be eliminated, resulting in increased dopamine.
**Detailed Information:** See *EDI*, 5/100.00

# Chapter Six

# Antidepressant Drug Interactions

# Antidepressant

## Amitriptyline-Chlordiazepoxide

**Significance:** 3—minimally clinically significant

**Potential Effects:** Concurrent use of these agents may result in impairment of motor function and enhanced anticholinergic effects.

**Recommendations:** Although a significant interaction is rare, concurrent use of these agents may result in enhanced central nervous system depression. Concurrent use of these agents has not proved to be superior to the tricyclic antidepressant alone. Monitor serum levels of the tricyclic antidepressant.

**Summary:** The concurrent administration of amitriptyline and chlordiazepoxide may cause impairment of motor function, and chlordiazepoxide may enhance the anticholinergic action of the tricyclic antidepressant.

**Related Drugs:** Diazepam has been shown to interact with amitriptyline; however, the data are conflicting. Triazolam and tricyclic antidepressants resulted in increased sedation. Alprazolam decreased the clearance of imipramine. Clonazepam has been shown to decrease desipramine serum levels. It is difficult to determine if an interaction would occur with other tricyclic antidepressants and the other benzodiazepines or with the administration of chlordiazepoxide and the other tricyclic antidepressants or the tetracyclic antidepressants.

**Mechanism:** Amitriptyline and other tricyclic antidepressants may enhance the sedation produced by chlordiazepoxide.

**Detailed Information:** See *EDI*, 6/1.00

## Amitriptyline-Disulfiram

**Significance:** 3—minimally clinically significant

**Potential Effects:** Central nervous system changes (organic brain syndrome) may occur if these agents are used together.

**Recommendations:** Discontinue one or both agents if signs or symptoms of acute organic brain syndrome develop (e.g., impaired consciousness, orientation or memory; hallucinations; illusions).

**Summary:** Amitriptyline has been shown to exhibit signs of organic brain syndrome when added to disulfiram therapy.

**Related Drugs:** Disulfiram has been shown to increase imipramine area-under-curve and elimination half-life and increase desipramine area-under-curve. A similar interaction is expected to occur between disulfiram and other tricyclic antidepressants or the tetracyclic antidepressants. There are no drugs related to disulfiram.

**Mechanism:** Disulfiram and amitriptyline administration may lead to elevated levels of monoamines and dopamine, resulting in organic brain syndromes and psychoses.

**Detailed Information:** See *EDI*, 6/3.00

## Amitriptyline-Fluconazole

**Significance:** 2—moderately clinically significant

**Potential Effects:** The addition of fluconazole to the therapy of a patient maintained on amitriptyline may result in increased amitriptyline serum levels and associated toxicity.

**Recommendations:** Tricyclic antidepressant serum levels should be carefully monitored when fluconazole or other systemic triazole or imidazole antifungal agents are added to or discontinued from concurrent therapy. The dose of the antidepressant may need to be adjusted.

**Summary:** Concurrent amitriptyline and fluconazole administration resulted in increased amitriptyline levels to as high as 1,464 ng/ml (therapeutic range: 150–250 ng/ml) and amitriptyline toxicity.

## Antidepressant

**Related Drugs:** An interaction may be expected to occur between fluconazole and the other tricyclic antidepressants or between amitriptyline and the other imidazole antifungal agents or triazole antifungal agents. If the interaction occurs by the postulated mechanism, then clomipramine and desipramine would not be expected to interact with fluconazole to the same extent.

**Mechanism:** The mechanism of this interaction is not known, but it has been suggested that fluconazole and ketoconazole, both known inhibitors of cytochrome $P450_{3A4}$, may interfere with the demethylation of tricyclic antidepressants whose metabolism is mediated by this isoenzyme. It has also been suggested that ketoconazole, which is relatively specific for inhibition of the cytochrome $P450_{3A4}$ isoenzyme, does not significantly affect desipramine metabolism, which is mediated primarily by the cytochrome $P450_{2D6}$ isoenzyme. Also, because the metabolism of clomipramine occurs primarily through cytochrome $P450_{2D6}$, it is possible that clomipramine, like desipramine, may be less likely to interact with fluconazole.

**Detailed Information:** See *EDI*, 6/4.01

## Bupropion-Amantadine

**Significance:** 3—minimally clinically significant

**Potential Effects:** The addition of amantadine to a concurrent bupropion regimen may cause neurotoxicity.

**Recommendations:** Concurrent administration of bupropion and amantadine should be used with caution. Patients receiving concurrent therapy should be monitored for neurotoxicity.

**Summary:** The addition of amantadine to a concurrent bupropion regimen may have caused neurotoxicity, including symptoms of restlessness, agitation, gross motor tremors, ataxia, gait disturbance, dizziness, and vertigo.

**Related Drugs:** A similar interaction would be expected between bupropion and rimantadine. There are no drugs related to bupropion.

**Mechanism:** Bupropion is a specific inhibitor of neuronal norepinephrine reuptake and a weak inhibitor of dopamine reuptake. Amantadine is an N-methyl-D-aspartate antagonist and a dopamine agonist. The increase of dopamine caused by both bupropion and amantadine may have caused the neurotoxicity.

**Detailed Information:** See *EDI*, 6/4.02

## Bupropion-Carbamazepine

**Significance:** 3—minimally clinically significant

**Potential Effects:** Concurrent carbamazepine administration may lead to decreased bupropion serum levels and possible decreased pharmacologic effects.

**Recommendations:** Patients should be carefully monitored for signs of central nervous system toxicity and seizures with concurrent administration of these agents.

**Summary:** Concurrent carbamazepine and bupropion administration may lead to decreased bupropion serum levels and possible decreased pharmacologic effects. Carbamazepine may decrease bupropion peak plasma concentration and area-under-curve (AUC) values by as much as 87%.

**Related Drugs:** Bupropion is an antidepressant agent chemically unrelated to the other antidepressant agents; there are no drugs related to carbamazepine. Although unrelated to carbamazepine, valproic acid did not affect the bupropion AUC or peak serum concentration, but it did decrease the time to peak serum concentration. Its sodium salt, sodium valproate, and divalproex sodium would be expected to interact similarly.

**Mechanism:** It is postulated that the mechanism of this interaction involves the induction by carbamazepine of cytochrome $P450_{3A4}$-mediated hydroxylation of bupropion.
**Detailed Information:** See *EDI*, 6/4.03

## Buspirone-Erythromycin

**Significance:** 3—minimally clinically significant
**Potential Effects:** Concurrent administration of buspirone and erythromycin may result in elevated levels of buspirone and a slight increase in buspirone-related adverse effects.
**Recommendations:** Although the pharmacodynamic changes in a single dose study were small, it would be prudent to reduce the dosage of buspirone during concomitant administration of erythromycin. Buspirone may exhibit nonlinear pharmacokinetics, thus elevations of buspirone during concomitant administration of erythromycin with multiple doses of buspirone may be more dramatic.
**Summary:** Concurrent administration of buspirone and erythromycin resulted in elevated levels of buspirone and a slight increase in buspirone-related adverse effects. There were interindividual differences in the extent of the interaction.
**Related Drugs:** Because it is believed that azithromycin does not produce hepatic cytochrome P450 induction or inactivation as erythromycin estolate does, an interaction between buspirone and azithromycin is not likely. Although documentation is lacking, an interaction would be expected to occur between buspirone and the other macrolide antibiotics. Buspirone is an antianxiety agent that is not chemically or pharmacologically related to the benzodiazepines, barbiturates, or other sedative/anxiolytic agents.
**Mechanism:** Buspirone undergoes extensive first-pass metabolism. It is postulated that erythromycin inhibits the metabolism of buspirone at the cytochrome $P450_{3A4}$ isoenzyme.
**Detailed Information:** See *EDI*, 6/4.04

## Buspirone-Fluoxetine

**Significance:** 3—minimally clinically significant
**Potential Effects:** Fluoxetine may decrease the effects of buspirone. Buspirone may augment the effects of fluoxetine.
**Recommendations:** The concomitant use of buspirone and fluoxetine may be desirable for the treatment of obsessive-compulsive disorder (OCD) or in refractory depression in some patients. However, this combination may decrease the efficacy of buspirone in other conditions.
**Summary:** The addition of fluoxetine to buspirone therapy may decrease the anxiolytic action of buspirone or may result in adverse effects. The addition of buspirone to fluoxetine therapy in OCD patients may result in augmentation of the effect of fluoxetine.
**Related Drugs:** A similar effect between buspirone and the other selective serotonin reuptake inhibitors would be expected to occur. Based on the postulated mechanisms, similar effects may result with concurrent buspirone and agents such as venlafaxine or nefazodone that inhibit serotonin reuptake as a part of their mechanism of action. There are no drugs related to buspirone.
**Mechanism:** The mechanism of this interaction is not known. It has been postulated that efficacy of buspirone in the treatment of OCD is due to its high affinity for the 5-HT1a receptor. The potentiation of fluoxetine by buspirone may cause an effective increase in the amount of synaptic 5-HT. Fluoxetine may impair the oxidative metabolism of buspirone, which may result in increased plasma levels of buspirone.
**Detailed Information:** See *EDI*, 6/4.05

Antidepressant

## Desipramine-Quinidine
**Significance:** 3—minimally clinically significant
**Potential Effects:** Concurrent quinidine administration may result in a decrease in desipramine clearance.
**Recommendations:** The interaction between desipramine and quinidine does not occur in all patients, and it appears to be dependent on the metabolic state of the patient. The clinical effects of this interaction have not been clearly established; therefore, patients taking both medications concurrently should be monitored for changes in clinical efficacy and in serum levels early in the course of therapy.
**Summary:** Concurrent quinidine and desipramine may result in decreased desipramine clearance.
**Related Drugs:** Nortriptyline and quinidine produced a decrease in nortriptyline metabolism and an increase in the excretion of unchanged nortriptyline. Imipramine oral clearance was decreased when administered concurrently with quinidine sulfate. A similar interaction is expected to occur between quinidine and other tricyclic antidepressant agents.
**Mechanism:** Inhibition of cytochrome $P450_{DB1}$ metabolism by quinidine is responsible for this interaction.
**Detailed Information:** See *EDI*, 6/4.06

## Desipramine-Thioridazine
**Significance:** 2—moderately clinically significant
**Potential Effects:** Thioridazine may inhibit the metabolism of desipramine, resulting in increased levels and toxicity.
**Recommendations:** Monitor the desipramine level closely during concurrent thioridazine therapy. One or both agents may need to be discontinued or the doses decreased.
**Summary:** Concomitant use if thioridazine and desipramine has resulted in increased desipramine levels.
**Related Drugs:** Imipramine and chlorpromazine may result in increased serum levels of either drug. Perphenazine, haloperidol, and thiothixene have been shown to inhibit metabolism of imipramine, and nortriptyline and desipramine have been shown to elevate butaperazine. Fluphenazine has been shown to increase imipramine and desipramine levels. Nortriptyline caused increases in chlorpromazine levels.
**Mechanism:** This interaction involves an inhibition of desipramine metabolism by thioridazine.
**Detailed Information:** See *EDI*, 6/4.07

## Donepezil-Paroxetine
**Significance:** 2—moderately clinically significant
**Potential Effects:** The addition of donepezil to a regimen including paroxetine may result in gastrointestinal and neurologic side effects.
**Recommendations:** The addition of donepezil to patients maintained on paroxetine should be performed with careful monitoring in the early days of concurrent therapy. Initiation of donepezil therapy at a lower dose with titration upward based on tolerability and absence of adverse effects would be prudent in these patients.
**Summary:** The addition of donepezil to a regimen including paroxetine has resulted in gastrointestinal and neurologic side effects including severe diarrhea, flatulence, insomnia, agitation, confusion, and aggression.
**Related Drugs:** It is not known whether an interaction would occur between donepezil and other selective serotonin reuptake inhibitors. There are no drugs related to donepezil.

**Mechanism:** The metabolism of donepezil by cytochrome $P450_{2D6}$ isozymes in the liver may have been impaired by paroxetine, which is a potent inhibitor *in vitro* of cytochrome $P450_{2D6}$. Also, patients affected may have had lower than average cytochrome $P450_{3A4}$ activity, either from genetic causes or secondary to other medications, and this, in combination with paroxetine-induced $P450_{2D6}$ inhibition, caused the effects.

**Detailed Information:** See *EDI*, 6/4.08

## Doxepin-Cholestyramine

**Significance:** 2—moderately clinically significant

**Potential Effects:** Concurrent administration of doxepin and cholestyramine may result in decreased serum doxepin levels and an increase in the manifestation of depressive symptoms.

**Recommendations:** Careful monitoring of antidepressant blood levels and effectiveness should be made in patients receiving concurrent doxepin and cholestyramine.

**Summary:** A patient maintained on doxepin was administered concurrent cholestyramine, and the serum levels of doxepin and n-desmethyldoxepin, an active metabolite, decreased.

**Related Drugs:** *In vitro* studies found that amitriptyline, desipramine, imipramine and nortriptyline were significantly adsorbed to cholestyramine in gastric fluid. There are no *in vivo* reports of an interaction between cholestyramine and other tricyclic antidepressants; however, an interaction may be expected to occur. An interaction between tricyclic antidepressants and colestipol may also be expected to occur.

**Mechanism:** *In vitro*, doxepin has been reported to be 80–83% bound to cholestyramine. One *in vitro* study demonstrated that doxepin adsorption onto cholestyramine decreased with increasing pH of the simulated gastric fluid and with increasing ethanol, suggesting that the true binding effect *in vivo* may be variable.

**Detailed Information:** See *EDI*, 6/4.10

## Doxepin-Propoxyphene

**Significance:** 3—minimally clinically significant

**Recommendations:** Further studies are necessary to confirm the interaction; however, patients should be monitored for increased central nervous system side effects. The dose of doxepin may have to be decreased or propoxyphene may need to be discontinued.

**Summary:** The concurrent use of propoxyphene and doxepin has been shown to result in increased doxepin levels.

**Related Drugs:** A similar interaction is expected to occur between propoxyphene and other tricyclic antidepressants or maprotiline. No documentation exists regarding a similar interaction between doxepin and other narcotic analgesics.

**Mechanism:** Propoxyphene may inhibit the hepatic metabolism of doxepin.

**Detailed Information:** See *EDI*, 6/5.00

## Fluoxetine-Aspirin

**Significance:** 3—minimally clinically significant

**Potential Effects:** The addition of aspirin following the discontinuation of fluoxetine therapy may result in a display of fluoxetine adverse effects.

**Recommendations:** The use of concurrent aspirin and fluoxetine should be approached with caution and the patient should be monitored for signs of fluoxetine adverse reactions. It is recommended that fluoxetine be discontinued for longer than 48 hours after the resolution of an allergic reaction before switching to another drug.

## Antidepressant

**Summary:** The addition of aspirin following fluoxetine discontinuation because of hives resulted in a reappearance of hives.

**Related Drugs:** Sudden precordial chest pain occurred in a patient with coronary artery disease maintained on propranolol and aspirin two days after sertraline therapy was instituted and after another subsequent dose. Serotonin has a vasodilatory effect on healthy human arteries, but causes vasoconstriction in endothelium damaged by coronary artery disease. It was postulated that serotonin-induced coronary spasms might be a result of excess activation of serotonin receptors. It is not known whether an interaction would occur between fluoxetine and the other salicylates or between aspirin and other selective serotonin reuptake inhibitors.

**Mechanism:** A pharmacodynamic interaction may have occurred between aspirin and fluoxetine in which aspirin may have sensitized the patient to develop hives during the declining fluoxetine plasma levels after its discontinuation; however, similarities in the appearance and distribution of hives with fluoxetine and then with aspirin suggest a pharmacokinetic interaction. Aspirin acetylates serum albumin, which alters the binding of other drugs to this protein. Salicylic acid is strongly bound to serum albumin and can displace other drugs from their protein binding sites. Fluoxetine is approximately 94.5% bound to human serum proteins *in vitro*.

**Detailed Information:** See *EDI*, 6/5.20

## Fluoxetine-Ayahuasca

**Significance:** 2—moderately clinically significant

**Potential Effects:** The consumption of ayahuasca by a patient maintained on fluoxetine resulted in tremors, sweating, shivering, and confusion lasting several hours.

**Recommendations:** Patients maintained on fluoxetine or other serotonin-reuptake inhibitors should be warned of the potential for serious adverse effects if ayahuasca is used concurrently.

**Summary:** Consumption of ayahuasca by a patient maintained on fluoxetine resulted in tremors, sweating, shivering, confusion, nausea, and vomiting lasting several hours.

**Related Drugs:** Ayahuasca is a psychoactive beverage that has been used for centuries in South America and has had increased interest in North America and Europe in recent years. Also known as *hoasca, daime, yage, caapi, natema,* and other names, it contains harmala alkaloids (including harmine and harmaline) which are derived from the vine *Banisteriopsis caapi*, one of the major plant components from which ayahuasca is brewed. Another plant component, the leaves of *Psychotria viridis*, contains N,N-dimethyltryptamine (DMT). An interaction may occur between ayahuasca and other selective serotonin reuptake inhibitors. An interaction between ayahuasca and the newer antidepressants that inhibit both serotonin and norepinephrine uptake, such as venlafaxine or nefazodone, may also be possible.

**Mechanism:** Ayahuasca exerts its psychoactive properties in part from harmala alkaloids infused from *B. caapi* that block the enzymatic activity of monoamine oxidase. DMT, from the leaves of *P. virdis*, is a potent and short-acting psychedelic agent when smoked or injected; however, it is not active orally due to its rapid oxidation by monoamine oxidase A. The doses of harmine and harmaline administered in ayahuasca tea (1-3 mg/kg) are essentially devoid of psychedelic activity, while higher doses (3-5 mg/kg) achieved with administration of pure harmine or harmaline may cause tremors, nystagmus, vomiting, and diarrhea.

**Detailed Information:** See *EDI*, 6/5.30

## Antidepressant

### Fluoxetine-Clarithromycin

**Significance:** 3—minimally clinically significant

**Potential Effects:** The addition of clarithromycin to fluoxetine therapy may have resulted in delirium.

**Recommendations:** Patients receiving fluoxetine therapy who begin treatment with clarithromycin should be monitored for mental status changes and other signs of fluoxetine toxicity. Alternative antibiotic therapy may need to be instituted, or the dose of fluoxetine may need to be adjusted.

**Summary:** The addition of clarithromycin to fluoxetine therapy may have resulted in confusion, agitation, delusions, and hallucinations.

**Related Drugs:** Concomitant administration of erythromycin and sertraline has resulted in symptoms of nervousness, irritability, paresthesias, tremor, decreased concentration, and confusion. A similar interaction would be expected to occur between fluoxetine and the other macrolide antibiotic agents, as well as between clarithromycin and the other selective-serotonin reuptake inhibitors (fluvoxamine, paroxetine, and sertraline) or venlafaxine and nefazodone, non-selective serotonin reuptake inhibitors. Because azithromycin does not produce either hepatic cytochrome P450 inactivation via cytochrome-metabolite complex formation or induction, it would not be expected to interact with fluoxetine

**Mechanism:** Clarithromycin may have inhibited the metabolism of fluoxetine at the cytochrome P450 site, resulting in accumulation of fluoxetine. The macrolide antibiotics clarithromycin, troleandomycin, and erythromycin potently inhibit the isoenzyme $CYP_{3A4}$.

**Detailed Information:** See *EDI*, 6/5.50

### Fluoxetine-Cyclosporine

**Significance:** 3—minimally clinically significant

**Potential Effects:** The addition of fluoxetine to a cyclosporine regimen may result in increased cyclosporine levels and toxicity.

**Recommendations:** Cyclosporine blood levels should be carefully monitored when fluoxetine is initiated or discontinued in patients maintained on cyclosporine. The dosage of one or both agents may need to be adjusted.

**Summary:** The addition of fluoxetine to a cyclosporine regimen may result in increased cyclosporine levels and toxicity. However, conflicting data are available.

**Related Drugs:** A similar interaction would be expected to occur between cyclosporine and the other selective serotonin reuptake inhibitors or the other nonselective serotonin reuptake inhibitor, venlafaxine. There are no drugs related to cyclosporine.

**Mechanism:** It has been suggested that because cyclosporine is primarily metabolized by the hepatic cytochrome $P450_{3A3/4}$ isoenzyme, drugs that inhibit this isoenzyme may be the most likely to reduce the clearance of cyclosporine and thus produce increases in whole blood levels of cyclosporine. It has also been postulated that inhibition of the cytochrome $P450_{2D6}$ isoenzyme may play a role in the interaction of cyclosporine and fluoxetine.

**Detailed Information:** See *EDI*, 6/5.70

### Fluoxetine-Cyproheptadine

**Significance:** 2—moderately clinically significant

**Potential Effects:** The therapeutic effects of fluoxetine may be reversed by the addition of cyproheptadine.

**Recommendations:** The addition of cyproheptadine to a fluoxetine regimen may result in a decreased effect of fluoxetine. The cyproheptadine may have to be discontinued.

## Antidepressant

**Summary:** The therapeutic effects of fluoxetine may be reversed by the addition of cyproheptadine. However, conflicting data are available.

**Related Drugs:** Paroxetine has interacted with cyproheptadine in a similar fashion. It is not known whether a similar interaction would occur between cyproheptadine and the other selective or nonselective serotonin reuptake inhibitors. It is not known whether a similar interaction would occur between fluoxetine and the other antihistamines.

**Mechanism:** Fluoxetine's increase of the deficient serotonin activity in bulimia nervosa results in its antibulimic efficacy. Cyproheptadine blocks both serotonergic and histaminic function and is effective in reversing sexual dysfunction resulting from antidepressant use. It is postulated that the effects of fluoxetine, a serotonin agonist, are canceled by cyproheptadine, a serotonin antagonist.

**Detailed Information:** See *EDI*, 6/6.03

### Fluoxetine-Marijuana

**Significance:** 2—moderately clinically significant

**Potential Effects:** Concurrent use of fluoxetine and marijuana may result in severe mania.

**Recommendations:** Patients maintained on fluoxetine therapy should be cautioned against the concomitant use of marijuana.

**Summary:** Marijuana usage by a patient on a fluoxetine regimen resulted in severe mania.

**Related Drugs:** There are no drugs related to fluoxetine. A similar interaction may occur between fluoxetine and dronabinol.

**Mechanism:** Marijuana could potentiate the action of fluoxetine at central serotonergic neurons.

**Detailed Information:** See *EDI*, 6/6.05

### Fluoxetine-Tranylcypromine

**Significance:** 1—highly clinically significant

**Potential Effects:** Concurrent fluoxetine and tranylcypromine may result in severe toxic and possibly fatal reactions.

**Recommendations:** The concurrent use of these agents should be avoided. It is recommended that a patient currently maintained on a monoamine oxidase inhibitor have the drug withdrawn for at least 14 days prior to initiating therapy with fluoxetine. A patient currently maintained on fluoxetine should have the drug withdrawn for at least five weeks prior to starting therapy with a monoamine oxidase inhibitor. This five-week period is necessary because of the long half-life (7.6 days) of fluoxetine and its active metabolite, norfluoxetine.

**Summary:** The administration of tranylcypromine within one to ten days after discontinuation of fluoxetine resulted in adverse effects and death in several patients.

**Related Drugs:** Phenelzine has produced adverse reactions when combined with or administered shortly after the discontinuation of fluoxetine. Patients being treated with phenelzine or tranylcypromine concurrently with sertraline have also experienced adverse reactions. There is a report of three fatal overdoses of concurrent moclobemide and citalopram. Selegiline has also been reported to interact with fluoxetine. Venlafaxine has interacted similarly with isocarboxazid and phenelzine. Other selective serotonin reuptake inhibitors may be expected to interact with tranylcypromine, and other monoamine oxidase inhibitors may be expected to interact with the selective serotonin reuptake inhibitors.

**Mechanism:** The exact mechanism is not known. It has been suggested that the combined pharmacologic effects of tranylcypromine, which prevents the breakdown of serotonin in the central nervous system (CNS), and fluoxetine, which prevents the

reuptake of serotonin into presynaptic neurons, may result in increased serotonin levels in the CNS.
**Detailed Information:** See *EDI*, 6/6.07

## Fluoxetine-Tryptophan
**Significance:** 3—minimally clinically significant
**Potential Effects:** Concurrent use of these agents may result in decreased efficacy of fluoxetine. This may result from stimulation of the serotonergic system by a combination of the two agents.
**Recommendations:** Patients receiving fluoxetine should be monitored for decreased efficacy of fluoxetine when tryptophan is added to their therapy. The tryptophan may need to be discontinued since this has been shown to resolve the adverse effects.
**Summary:** Administration of tryptophan may decrease the efficacy of fluoxetine.
**Related Drugs:** There are no drugs related to tryptophan or fluoxetine.
**Mechanism:** A stimulation of the serotonergic system by the two agents may be the cause of this interaction.
**Detailed Information:** See *EDI*, 6/6.10

## Fluvoxamine-Melatonin
**Significance:** 3—minimally clinically significant
**Potential Effects:** The concurrent use of melatonin and fluvoxamine may result in elevated plasma concentrations of melatonin.
**Recommendations:** The patient should be monitored for increased effects of melatonin when melatonin and fluvoxamine are used concomitantly.
**Summary:** Concurrent use of melatonin and fluvoxamine resulted in elevated plasma concentrations of melatonin.
**Related Drugs:** Concomitant use of sertraline, melatonin, and a high-protein diet resulted in visual acuity loss, dyschromatopsia, and altered light adaptation. Visual acuity and color vision improved after discontinuing the high-protein diet and melatonin. It is not known if melatonin would interact with other selective serotonin reuptake inhibitors. There are no drugs related to melatonin.
**Mechanism:** Fluvoxamine inhibits metabolic reactions mediated by cytochrome $P450_{1A2}$, $P450_{2C19}$, and $P450_{3A3/4}$. Elevated levels of melatonin following coadministration of melatonin with fluvoxamine may result from the inhibition of hepatic metabolism of melatonin. Further studies are required to isolate which isoenzyme(s) is/are involved. The combination of sertraline, melatonin, and a high-protein diet may have resulted in an imbalance of melatonin and dopamine in the retina, resulting in toxic optic neuropathy.
**Detailed Information:** See *EDI*, 6/6.20

## Fluvoxamine-Tacrine
**Significance:** 2—moderately clinically significant
**Potential Effects:** The concurrent administration of tacrine and fluvoxamine resulted in increased levels of tacrine and an increase in tacrine-induced side effects.
**Recommendations:** Patients receiving concurrent tacrine and fluvoxamine should be monitored for possible increased effects and side effects of tacrine. The dosage of tacrine may need to be adjusted or one or both agents may need to be discontinued.
**Summary:** The concurrent administration of tacrine and fluvoxamine resulted in increased levels of tacrine and an increase in tacrine-induced side effects. There was an eightfold increase in tacrine area-under-curve and an 88% decrease in nonrenal tacrine clearance with concurrent fluvoxamine administration.

## Antidepressant

**Related Drugs:** Although documentation is lacking, if the proposed mechanism is correct an interaction between tacrine and the other selective serotonin reuptake inhibitors would be expected to occur, but with less severity than that observed with fluvoxamine.

**Mechanism:** It has been postulated that fluvoxamine inhibits the metabolism of tacrine at the $P450_{1A2}$ isozyme. Tacrine has been shown to be metabolized at the cytochrome $P450_{1A2}$ isozyme. *In vitro* studies in human liver microsomes and an *in vivo* study indicated that fluvoxamine is a potent inhibitor of cytochrome $P450_{1A2}$.

**Detailed Information:** See *EDI*, 6/5.15

## Imipramine-Aspirin

**Significance:** 3—minimally clinically significant

**Potential Effects:** The addition of aspirin to an imipramine regimen resulted in increased imipramine serum levels and adverse effects.

**Recommendations:** In patients who are maintained on a regimen of imipramine, it may be prudent to consider alternatives to aspirin for occasional use. In addition, patients who report an increase in severity or number of adverse effects while taking imipramine should be questioned concerning occasional aspirin use. If patients require routine low-dose aspirin for beneficial cardiac effects, consideration may be given to increased monitoring of the imipramine regimen and a possible dosage adjustment, although further research is needed.

**Summary:** The addition of aspirin to an imipramine regimen resulted in increased imipramine serum levels and imipramine-related adverse effects.

**Related Drugs:** An interaction may occur between aspirin and other tricyclic antidepressants, and between imipramine and other salicylates, although there is no documentation.

**Mechanism:** Because imipramine is highly bound to plasma proteins, competition by aspirin for protein binding sites may increase the amount of unbound imipramine, resulting in a greater proportion of adverse effects. Exact mechanisms are unknown.

**Detailed Information:** See *EDI*, 6/6.70

## Imipramine-Bupropion

**Significance:** 3—minimally clinically significant

**Potential Effects:** Concurrent administration of bupropion and imipramine may result in decreased imipramine and desipramine clearance and increased imipramine and desipramine levels.

**Recommendations:** Until further studies are performed, patients should be monitored for increased imipramine and desipramine levels and effects during concurrent use of imipramine and bupropion. Other tricyclic antidepressants may also interact in the same way and should be monitored accordingly.

**Summary:** Concurrent administration of bupropion and imipramine resulted in decreased imipramine and desipramine clearance (by 57% and 82%, respectively) and increased imipramine and desipramine levels.

**Related Drugs:** A similar interaction may be expected to occur between bupropion and the other tricyclic antidepressants. There are no agents related to bupropion.

**Mechanism:** Imipramine is converted to desipramine by demethylation via cytochrome P450 isoenzymes 1A2, 2C19, and 3A4. Desipramine and imipramine are also hydroxylated by the 2D6 isoenzyme to 2-hydroxymetabolites. It is possible that bupropion may inhibit the 2D6 isoenzyme and increase levels of both parent and metabolite compounds. It has been postulated that the metabolism of bupropion to hydroxybupropion is mediated by the cytochrome $P450_{3A4}$ isoenzyme which could result in competitive inhibition of imipramine metabolism.

**Detailed Information:** See *EDI*, 6/7.50

Antidepressant

## Imipramine-Cimetidine

**Significance:** 2—moderately clinically significant

**Potential Effects:** Cimetidine may cause an increase in imipramine levels, leading to increased side effects.

**Recommendations:** If cimetidine and imipramine are taken together, a decreased dose of imipramine may be necessary. If cimetidine is withdrawn from cotherapy, an increased dose of imipramine may be required. Ranitidine may be used instead of cimetidine.

**Summary:** Cimetidine may decrease the clearance of imipramine, resulting in increased serum concentrations and consequent anticholinergic adverse effects.

**Related Drugs:** Cimetidine has been shown to decrease nortriptyline steady-state serum concentration and increase amitriptyline plasma levels, desipramine plasma levels and doxepin's area-under-curve; however, all data do not support these interactions. A similar interaction is expected to occur between cimetidine and other tricyclic antidepressants. Ranitidine has been shown to not alter imipramine, amitriptyline and doxepin's pharmacokinetics. A similar interaction is not expected to occur between imipramine and the other $H_2$-receptor antagonists, if the mechanism involves hepatic inhibition.

**Mechanism:** It has been postulated that cimetidine suppresses the conversion of imipramine to desipramine by inhibition of the hepatic metabolism of imipramine.

**Detailed Information:** See *EDI,* 6/9.00

## Imipramine-Epinephrine

**Significance:** 2—moderately clinically significant

**Recommendations:** The concurrent use of epinephrine or other direct-acting sympathomimetic amines and tricyclic antidepressants should be avoided. When concurrent therapy is necessary, the initial dose of the sympathomimetic should be lowered, and the patient should be carefully monitored for adverse cardiovascular effects.

**Summary:** Epinephrine and other direct-acting sympathomimetic amines have shown enhanced cardiovascular effects in those taking imipramine or other tricyclic antidepressants.

**Related Drugs:** Norepinephrine, phenylephrine, dopamine, and methoxamine have been shown to interact with tricyclic antidepressants. Maprotiline has been shown to reduce tyramine sensitivity. Protriptyline, amitriptyline, and desipramine have been reported to interact with direct-acting sympathomimetics. A similar interaction is expected to occur with other tricyclic antidepressants and imipramine.

**Mechanism:** There is an enhanced cardiovascular effect because tricyclic antidepressants block the reuptake of norepinephrine, increasing concentrations at receptor sites.

**Detailed Information:** See *EDI,* 6/11.00

## Imipramine-Ethinyl Estradiol

**Significance:** 3—minimally clinically significant

**Recommendations:** A patient receiving concurrent ethinyl estradiol and imipramine therapy should be observed for lack of effect or enhanced toxicities of imipramine. Should such effects occur, the dose of one of the agents should be adjusted accordingly. One report suggested reducing the dosage of imipramine by approximately one third when the patient is also taking oral contraceptive agents.

**Summary:** Patients taking ethinyl estradiol have been reported to be relatively unresponsive to therapy with imipramine.

**Related Drugs:** Similar reactions have been reported in patients taking conjugated estrogens and imipramine or doxepin. There are no

## Antidepressant

reports with other tricyclic antidepressants or maprotiline. Ethinyl estradiol has been shown to increase elimination half-life, and volume of distribution, and reduce clearance of imipramine. A similar interaction is expected to occur with other estrogenic substances and imipramine.

**Mechanism:** This interaction may be dose related and dependent on baseline hormonal balance. Imipramine may inhibit oral contraceptive metabolism and enhance the effect of the estrogens.

**Detailed Information:** See *EDI*, 6/13.00

### Imipramine-Levodopa

**Significance:** 3—minimally clinically significant

**Recommendations:** Because tricyclic antidepressants have been used successfully and uneventfully for depression in patients with Parkinson's disease, the concurrent use of these agents need not be avoided. However, it is advisable to be aware of a possibility of decreased levodopa levels since a dosage adjustment may be necessary.

**Summary:** There are data to show that imipramine causes a reduction in the absorption of levodopa.

**Related Drugs:** A similar interaction is expected to occur between levodopa and other tricyclic antidepressants or tetracyclic antidepressants.

**Mechanism:** Imipramine may slow gastric emptying time, allowing more time for levodopa to be metabolized and reducing the amount of levodopa available for absorption.

**Detailed Information:** See *EDI*, 6/15.00

### Imipramine-Liothyronine

**Significance:** 3—minimally clinically significant

**Recommendations:** Since a patient's thyroid function can affect the response to tricyclic antidepressant agents, patients who fail to respond to such drugs should be examined for hypothyroidism. The addition of liothyronine (25 µg/day) to tricyclic antidepressant therapy may be considered in selected patients who do not respond to tricyclic antidepressants alone.

**Summary:** Liothyronine may enhance and accelerate the onset of the antidepressant effects in euthyroid patients.

**Related Drugs:** Liothyronine has been shown to potentiate the effect of protriptyline and amitriptyline. A similar interaction is expected to occur with other tricyclic antidepressants and tetracyclic antidepressants. A similar interaction is expected to occur with other thyroid preparations.

**Mechanism:** The mechanism may involve the thyroid enhancement of antidepressant receptor sensitivity.

**Detailed Information:** See *EDI*, 6/17.00

### Imipramine-Lithium Carbonate

**Significance:** 3—minimally clinically significant

**Potential Effects:** Lithium may potentiate the antidepressant effects of imipramine.

**Recommendations:** Patients maintained on imipramine should be monitored carefully if cotherapy with lithium is instituted. Lithium levels should be monitored, and the dosage of one or both agents may need to be adjusted.

**Summary:** Concurrent use of imipramine and lithium carbonate may result in increased antidepressant effects.

**Related Drugs:** A similar interaction is expected to occur with other tricyclic antidepressants and lithium carbonate.

## Antidepressant

**Mechanism:** There may be a synergistic effect or a potentiation of the pharmacologic activity of imipramine by lithium. The potentiation of the tricyclic may be due to lithium's enhancement of the serotonin metabolite.
**Detailed Information:** See *EDI*, 6/18.10

## Imipramine-Methyltestosterone

**Significance:** 3—minimally clinically significant
**Recommendations:** If paranoid reactions occur during concomitant use of imipramine and methyltestosterone, one or both drugs may have to be discontinued.
**Summary:** There are data to show that the concurrent use of methyltestosterone and imipramine may cause paranoid reactions.
**Related Drugs:** A similar interaction is expected to occur between the other tricyclic antidepressants, the tetracyclic antidepressants, and other androgen derivatives.
**Mechanism:** The mechanism of this interaction is unknown.
**Detailed Information:** See *EDI*, 6/19.00

## Imipramine-Nitroglycerin

**Significance:** 2—moderately clinically significant
**Potential Effects:** The occurrence of dry mouth that may be associated with imipramine therapy because of its anticholinergic side effects may prevent the dissolution of sublingual nitroglycerin tablets, resulting in ineffective therapy.
**Recommendations:** Attempts at increasing salivation (e.g., chewing gum, artificial saliva products) may prove useful in increasing the effectiveness of sublingual nitroglycerin in some patients. If the ineffectiveness of the sublingual nitroglycerin continues, use of the oral, topical, or translingual spray forms of the nitrates or discontinuation of the tricyclic antidepressant may need to be considered.
**Summary:** There are data to show that imipramine can cause a lack of dissolution of nitroglycerin, secondary to the dry mouth caused by imipramine.
**Related Drugs:** A similar interaction may occur between sublingual nitroglycerin and other tricyclic antidepressant agents and between imipramine and other nitrates available as a sublingual tablet.
**Mechanism:** Dry mouth is a common side effect of imipramine therapy because of its anticholinergic effects, making dissolution of the sublingual nitroglycerin difficult.
**Detailed Information:** See *EDI*, 6/20.10

## Imipramine-Reserpine

**Significance:** 3—minimally clinically significant
**Recommendations:** These agents should be used concurrently to induce an antidepressant response only in the most recalcitrant patients. Experience with this combination is limited to a few patients, and the risk of adverse effects may outweigh potential therapeutic gains. Also, since reserpine may itself cause depression, this fact should be considered before concurrent administration with imipramine.
**Summary:** Reserpine used in combination with tricyclic antidepressants has been shown to cause hypotension, flushing, diarrhea, and manic reactions.
**Related Drugs:** The other tricyclic antidepressants and tetracyclic antidepressants may react similarly. A similar interaction is expected to occur between imipramine and other rauwolfia alkaloids.
**Mechanism:** When reserpine is added to imipramine therapy, there is a release of norepinephrine into the synapse where imipramine inhibits its reuptake.
**Detailed Information:** See *EDI*, 6/21.00

Antidepressant

## Imipramine-Tobacco

**Significance:** 3—minimally clinically significant

**Potential Effects:** Tobacco smoking may increase the metabolism of imipramine, leading to decreased levels.

**Recommendations:** Although no specific adjustments in the imipramine dose need be made in smokers, these patients should be monitored for a decreased response to imipramine.

**Summary:** There are data to show that tobacco smoking may increase the metabolism of imipramine, leading to decreased levels and response.

**Related Drugs:** Smoking has been associated with lower plasma amitriptyline and/or nortriptyline levels. Because of conflicting results, it is difficult to determine whether an interaction would occur with tobacco smoking and other tricyclic antidepressants or tetracyclic antidepressants.

**Mechanism:** The interaction between tobacco and imipramine may result from an increased metabolism of imipramine by tobacco.

**Detailed Information:** See *EDI*, 6/22.10

## Imipramine-Tranylcypromine

**Significance:** 2—moderately clinically significant

**Potential Effects:** Concurrent use of these agents may result in hyperpyrexia, excitability, muscular rigidity, fluctuations in blood pressure, convulsions, grand mal seizures, and coma.

**Recommendations:** Concurrent use of these agents should be avoided. Chlorpromazine has been shown to be useful in treating the effects of this interaction.

**Summary:** Severe toxic and fatal reactions have been reported when tricyclic antidepressants have been given with a MAOI. However, other studies have described beneficial and uneventful concurrent use. Adverse effects may include hyperpyrexia, excitability, muscular rigidity, fluctuations in blood pressure, convulsions, grand mal seizures, and coma.

**Related Drugs:** Doxepin, nortriptyline, and protriptyline may interact with MAOIs. Isocarboxazid and amitriptyline have been shown to adversely interact. Tranylcypromine and clomipramine have been shown to cause fatal disseminated intravascular coagulation. Moclobemide with imipramine and clomipramine have been shown to cause serotonin syndrome. A similar interaction may occur with other tricyclic antidepressants. Cyclobenzaprine may react with the MAOIs. Other MAOIs may interact with imipramine.

**Mechanism:** The MAOIs may enhance the effect of the tricyclic antidepressants through inhibition of microsomal enzymes, or the tricyclic antidepressants may sensitize adrenergic receptors to amines which accumulate extraneuronally.

**Detailed Information:** See *EDI*, 6/23.00

## Mirtazapine-Levodopa

**Significance:** 3—minimally clinically significant

**Potential Effects:** The addition of mirtazapine to a levodopa regimen resulted in development of psychosis.

**Recommendations:** Patients maintained on levodopa therapy should be carefully monitored for changes in their mental status if mirtazapine is added to their regimen.

**Summary:** The addition of mirtazapine to a levodopa regimen resulted in development of psychosis. On day 24 of concurrent mirtazapine and levodopa therapy, the patient complained of sleeplessness, vivid dreams, and a dysphoric mood. Two days later she attempted to commit suicide. There was a complete recovery from all psychotic symptoms within 10 days of discontinuation of mirtazapine therapy.

Antidepressant

**Related Drugs:** Mirtazapine has a tetracyclic structure that is unrelated to the selective serotonin reuptake inhibitors, tricyclics, or monoamine oxidase inhibitors. There are no drugs related to levodopa.

**Mechanism:** It has been concluded that the psychosis experienced by a patient was dopamine-induced and triggered by mirtazapine. Mirtazapine acts as an alpha$_2$-receptor antagonist. Studies suggest the inhibition of dopamine release by presynaptic alpha$_2$-receptors. This would allow mirtazapine to cause an increase in central dopamine levels.

**Detailed Information:** See *EDI*, 6/23.50

## Mirtazapine-Sertraline

**Significance:** 3—minimally clinically significant

**Potential Effects:** The addition of mirtazapine to the therapy of a patient maintained on sertraline may result in hypomania in a patient with major affective disorder.

**Recommendations:** In patients maintained on a regimen including sertraline, the addition of mirtazapine should be approached with caution. It may be prudent to monitor the patient for symptoms of mania or hypomania following the start of combination therapy with these two drugs.

**Summary:** The addition of mirtazapine to a sertraline regimen was associated with hypomania in a patient with major depressive disorder.

**Related Drugs:** It is not known whether an interaction would occur between mirtazapine and other selective serotonin reuptake inhibitors. There are no drugs related to mirtazapine.

**Mechanism:** The mechanism of this interaction is not known. Mirtazapine has minimal inhibitory effects *in vitro* on cytochrome P450 1A2, 3A4, and 2D6 isoenzymes. Mirtazapine alone has been reported to induce mania in a small percentage of patients. It is not clear what role sertraline played in the onset of hypomanic symptoms.

**Detailed Information:** See *EDI*, 6/23.70

## Nortriptyline-Charcoal

**Significance:** 3—minimally clinically significant

**Recommendations:** Activated charcoal may be effective in an acute tricyclic antidepressant overdose, and it may even be useful several hours after the overdose since nortriptyline delays gastric emptying. However, if charcoal is not used for nortriptyline overdose, the administration of these agents should be separated by as much time as possible.

**Summary:** There are data to show that activated charcoal significantly reduces the absorption of nortriptyline.

**Related Drugs:** Activated charcoal has been shown to greatly accelerate the elimination of amitriptyline. Other tricyclic and tetracyclic antidepressants may be adsorbed by charcoal. There are no drugs related to charcoal.

**Mechanism:** Nortriptyline delays gastric emptying, and activated charcoal limits its absorption.

**Detailed Information:** See *EDI*, 6/24.10

## Nortriptyline-Fluoxetine

**Significance:** 2—moderately clinically significant

**Potential Effects:** Fluoxetine may inhibit the metabolism of nortriptyline, resulting in increased levels and toxicity.

**Recommendations:** Patients receiving concurrent fluoxetine and nortriptyline or carbamazepine should be monitored for increased levels of nortriptyline or carbamazepine and toxicity. The dosage of nortriptyline or carbamazepine may need to be decreased.

**Summary:** The administration of fluoxetine may inhibit the metabolism of nortriptyline, resulting in increased levels.

**Related Drugs:** Data concerning the coadministration of the tricyclic antidepressant drugs and fluoxetine have been well documented; however, much of the data are conflicting.

**Mechanism:** Fluoxetine may inhibit the hepatic metabolism of notriptyline, which may result in elevated plasma levels of nortriptyline.

**Detailed Information:** See *EDI*, 6/24.30

## Nortriptyline-Marijuana

**Significance:** 2—moderately clinically significant

**Potential Effects:** The use of marijuana cigarettes while receiving concurrent nortriptyline may result in tachycardia, delirium, and transient cognitive changes.

**Recommendations:** It was suggested that patients receiving tricyclic antidepressants should be informed of the potential risks of an interaction with marijuana.

**Summary:** The use of marijuana cigarettes while receiving concurrent nortriptyline resulted in tachycardia, delirium, and transient cognitive changes in a 16-year-old male and a 21-year-old female.

**Related Drugs:** Another report documents a similar interaction of marijuana and desipramine. A similar interaction may be expected to occur between marijuana and other tricyclic antidepressants. It is not known whether an interaction would occur between nortriptyline and dronabinol, although an interaction would be expected based on the postulated mechanism.

**Mechanism:** The concurrent use of tricyclic antidepressants may slow the metabolism of tetrahydrocannabinol (THC), thereby increasing levels of THC in the central nervous system. Marijuana, generally in larger doses than were used by these patients, is known to cause symptoms of delirium and tachycardia similar to the ones reported. More data are needed to determine the exact mechanism of this interaction.

**Detailed Information:** See *EDI*, 6/24.50

## Nortriptyline-Phenobarbital

**Significance:** 3—minimally clinically significant

**Recommendations:** Although the clinical data are limited, they are sufficient to indicate that phenobarbital will decrease serum nortriptyline levels in patients receiving these drugs concurrently. Because the change in therapeutic effect caused by decreased serum nortriptyline levels is not known, the clinical significance of this drug interaction is difficult to assess. If patients are unresponsive to nortriptyline therapy, concurrent barbiturate therapy should be considered as a possible underlying cause. If additional drugs must be used, the benzodiazepines may be useful in treating anxiety symptoms since they do not affect the metabolism of the tricyclic drugs. Flurazepam, a benzodiazepine, apparently does not affect the metabolism of tricyclic antidepressants; therefore, it maybe an alternative to barbiturate cotherapy.

**Summary:** Limited data indicate that phenobarbital may decrease the serum concentrations of nortriptyline.

**Related Drugs:** Amobarbital, pentobarbital, and secobarbital have been suggested to interact similarly with nortriptyline. Desipramine and phenobarbital, and protriptyline and amobarbital undergo a similar interaction. A similar interaction may occur between all other barbiturates, other tricyclic antidepressants, and the tetracyclic antidepressants.

Antidepressant

**Mechanism:** Barbiturates can stimulate the metabolism of the tricyclic antidepressants.

**Detailed Information:** See *EDI*, 6/25.00

## Nortriptyline-Rifampin

**Significance:** 3—minimally clinically significant

**Potential Effects:** Concurrent rifampin may induce the metabolism of nortriptyline, resulting in decreased nortriptyline levels.

**Recommendations:** Nortriptyline serum levels should be closely monitored with the addition or discontinuation of rifampin from concurrent therapy. The dose of nortriptyline may need to be adjusted.

**Summary:** Nortriptyline serum levels increased following rifampin discontinuation from concurrent nortriptyline therapy.

**Related Drugs:** Similar interactions between other tricyclic antidepressants and rifampin may be expected to occur. If the interaction occurs based on the proposed mechanism, one would be expected to occur between nortriptyline and rifabutin, which is structurally and pharmacologically related to rifampin.

**Mechanism:** It is postulated that rifampin, which is known to induce cytochrome P450 enzymatic activity, induces the metabolism of nortriptyline, which undergoes oxidation through this system.

**Detailed Information:** See *EDI*, 6/26.05

## Nortriptyline-Terbinafine

**Significance:** 2—moderately clinically significant

**Potential Effects:** The addition of terbinafine to the therapy of a patient maintained on nortriptyline may result in increased nortriptyline serum levels and nortriptyline toxicity.

**Recommendations:** The addition of terbinafine to the therapy of a patient maintained on nortriptyline should be approached with caution. The patient should be carefully monitored for increased nortriptyline serum levels and toxicity. The dose of nortriptyline may need to be adjusted.

**Summary:** The addition of terbinafine to the therapy of a patient maintained on nortriptyline resulted in increased nortriptyline levels and nortriptyline toxicity. After discontinuation of terbinafine and normalization of nortriptyline levels, the patient was rechallenged with terbinafine with the same adverse effects.

**Related Drugs:** It is not known whether an interaction would occur between terbinafine and the other tricyclic antidepressants. It is not known whether a similar interaction would be expected to occur with nortriptyline and butenafine, a benzylamine derivative with a mode of action similar to the allylamine antifungal agent terbinafine.

**Mechanism:** It has been postulated that the increased nortriptyline concentration was due to a pharmacokinetic interaction because there were no increases in the concentrations of gamma-glutamyl transferase, aspartate aminotransferase, or alanine aminotransferase.

**Detailed Information:** See *EDI*, 6/26.08

## Pargyline-Methyldopa

**Significance:** 3—minimally clinically significant

**Recommendations:** Until further clinical studies are performed, the concurrent use of these agents need not be avoided. However, it is prudent to be aware of a possible interaction, and if adverse central nervous system effects develop, it may be advisable to discontinue one or both drugs.

**Summary:** The concomitant administration of pargyline and methyldopa may result in hallucinations and prolonged nervous system excitement.

**Related Drugs:** A similar interaction may occur between methyldopa and other monoamine oxidase inhibitors. There are no drugs related to methyldopa.

**Mechanism:** A combination may be mediated by increased levels of free cerebral catecholamines released from binding sites.

**Detailed Information:** See *EDI*, 6/26.10

## Paroxetine-Cimetidine

**Significance:** 3—minimally clinically significant

**Potential Effects:** Serum paroxetine levels may be increased by concurrent cimetidine administration.

**Recommendations:** The dose of paroxetine may need to be adjusted when cimetidine is added to or removed from concurrent therapy.

**Summary:** Studies have shown increased serum paroxetine levels may result with cimetidine administration.

**Related Drugs:** Based on the postulated mechanism, an interaction may be expected to occur between cimetidine and the other serotonin-selective reuptake inhibitors, although documentation is lacking. It cannot be determined whether an interaction would be expected to occur between paroxetine and the other $H_2$ receptor antagonists.

**Mechanism:** It is postulated that cimetidine may increase paroxetine levels by inhibiting the hepatic metabolism of paroxetine.

**Detailed Information:** See *EDI*, 6/26.22

## Paroxetine-Dextromethorphan

**Significance:** 2—moderately clinically significant

**Potential Effects:** The addition of dextromethorphan to paroxetine may produce serotonin syndrome.

**Recommendations:** The use of dextromethorphan in patients receiving paroxetine or other agents that inhibit the reuptake of serotonin should be avoided if possible.

**Summary:** The addition of dextromethorphan to a drug regimen that included paroxetine resulted in serotonin syndrome (mental status changes, restlessness, hypertension, tremor, and myoclonus).

**Related Drugs:** Fluoxetine has interacted similarly with dextromethorphan and pentazocine; however, in one study, pretreatment with fluoxetine prior to dental surgery had no significant effect on pentazocine analgesia, but significantly attenuated morphine-produced analgesia and shortened morphine's duration of action. When fluvoxamine was added to maintenance methadone therapy, two patients experienced approximately a 20% increase in the methadone plasma level/dose ratio and the remaining three patients had from a 40% to a 100% increase in this ratio. A serotonin-like syndrome has occurred when tramadol was added to a regimen including sertraline. It is likely that a similar effect would occur between dextromethorphan and sertraline and between paroxetine and the narcotic agents related to dextromethorphan. It is also likely that similar effects would occur when dextromethorphan is combined with agents such as nefazodone and venlafaxine that inhibit serotonin reuptake as a part of their mechanism of action.

**Mechanism:** Dextromethorphan inhibits the reuptake of serotonin at the synapse. The addition of dextromethorphan to a selective serotonin reuptake inhibitor regimen may result in additively or synergistically increased serotonin levels and serotonin syndrome. Con-

# Antidepressant

comitant pseudoephedrine and ischemic disease may contribute to the adverse event. The 5-HT$_2$ receptors in the brain are responsible for the hallucinogenic effects of lysergic acid diethylamide (LSD), and the synergistic action of fluoxetine and dextromethorphan on serotonin levels may lead to the hallucinations. Because paroxetine is a potent inhibitor of cytochrome P450$_{2D6}$ in *in vitro* studies and has a tenfold greater affinity for this enzyme than does dextromethorphan, it is postulated that the interaction may result from a reduction in the clearance of dextromethorphan and a subsequent increase in dextromethorphan plasma levels.

**Detailed Information:** See *EDI,* 6/26.24

## Paroxetine-Hypericum

**Significance:** 3—minimally clinically significant

**Potential Effects:** The addition of paroxetine to the therapy of a patient receiving hypericum (St. John's Wort) may result in nausea, weakness, and extreme fatigue.

**Recommendations:** Patients taking hypericum should discontinue this medication for a 14-day washout period prior to instituting therapy with a selective serotonin reuptake inhibitor (SSRI). Patients receiving an SSRI should discontinue this medication prior to instituting hypericum. The length of the washout period may vary depending on the SSRI that the patient was receiving, but prudence dictates at least a 14-day washout period.

**Summary:** The addition of paroxetine to the therapy of a patient receiving hypericum resulted in nausea, weakness, and extreme fatigue. The patient reported that she had stopped taking paroxetine 10 days before starting hypericum. The evening after starting hypericum the patient took a single 20 mg dose of paroxetine. At noon the following day she was able to be awakened but was incoherent, groggy, and almost unable to get out of bed. She did not take any additional paroxetine, and when seen the following day she was back to her baseline status.

**Related Drugs:** There is no documentation regarding an interaction between hypericum and the other SSRIs, although an interaction might be expected to occur based on the proposed mechanism.

**Mechanism:** Standardized hypericum extract inhibited serotonin, dopamine, and norepinephrine synaptosomal uptake with about equal affinity and was found to be a weak inhibitor of monoamine oxidase (MAO)-A and MAO-B activity. Concomitant administration of MAO inhibitors and SSRIs should be avoided (see Fluoxetine-Tranylcypromine, page 144) because of the possibility of a "serotonin syndrome." *In vitro* measurements of the activity of hypericum for MAO-A and MAO-B receptors have indicated that the concentration of hypericum extract required is unlikely to be attained in humans.

**Detailed Information:** See *EDI,* 6/26.25

## Paroxetine-Interferon Alpha

**Significance:** 3—minimally clinically significant

**Potential Effects:** A patient maintained on a regimen of paroxetine and trazodone experienced a recurrence of depressive symptoms following the addition of interferon.

**Recommendations:** In patients with depression who require therapy with interferon alpha, the activity of selective serotonin reuptake inhibitors might be impaired; the use of alternative antidepressant agents should be considered. For patients who are already maintained on a selective serotonin reuptake inhibitor for depression, a relapse in depressive symptoms after the introduction of an interferon product may indicate the need to switch to alternative antidepressant therapy.

## Antidepressant

**Summary:** A patient maintained on a regimen of paroxetine and trazodone experienced a recurrence of depressive symptoms following the addition of interferon.

**Related Drugs:** An interaction may occur between the other selective serotonin reuptake inhibitors and interferon alpha, and between paroxetine and other interferon preparations.

**Mechanism:** Interferon alpha might impair the body's production of serotonin by inducing enzymes that degrade tryptophan, a precursor in serotonin synthesis. Dietary tryptophan depletion can reverse the antidepressant effect of selective serotonin reuptake inhibitors.

**Detailed Information:** See *EDI*, 6/26.26

### Paroxetine-Zolpidem

**Significance:** 3—minimally clinically significant

**Potential Effects:** Concurrent paroxetine and zolpidem may result in delirium.

**Recommendations:** The concurrent use of these agents should be approached with caution. The use of an alternative medication for zolpidem may be considered in those patients receiving paroxetine.

**Summary:** The concomitant administration of zolpidem and paroxetine may have induced delirium in a patient taking paroxetine after receiving her first dose of zolpidem. The delirium resolved spontaneously without treatment within four hours.

**Related Drugs:** It is not known whether an interaction would occur between zolpidem and the other selective serotonin reuptake inhibitors (SSRIs). It is possible that a similar interaction may occur between zolpidem and the SSRIs that are highly protein bound, fluoxetine and sertraline.

**Mechanism:** It has been proposed that since both paroxetine and zolpidem are highly protein bound, this interaction may occur through competition for binding sites. Both of these agents are known to only infrequently cause hallucinations without the presence of other drugs. Further studies are needed.

**Detailed Information:** See *EDI*, 6/26.27

### Phenelzine-Buspirone

**Significance:** 3—minimally clinically significant

**Potential Effects:** Concurrent administration of buspirone and a monoamine oxidase inhibitor (MAOI) may result in blood pressure elevation.

**Recommendations:** Concurrent therapy with a MAOI and buspirone is not recommended. However, if these agents are administered together, the patient's blood pressure should be carefully monitored.

**Summary:** There are data to show that the concurrent administration of buspirone and a MAOI may result in blood pressure elevation.

**Related Drugs:** Tranylcypromine was shown to exhibit a similar interaction. A similar interaction is expected to occur between buspirone and other MAOIs. Furazolidone and procarbazine may interact similarly with buspirone.

**Mechanism:** The affinity of buspirone for serotonin receptors may explain the observed change in blood pressure.

**Detailed Information:** See *EDI*, 6/26.30

### Phenelzine-Clonazepam

**Significance:** 3—minimally clinically significant

**Potential Effects:** Concurrent use of these agents may result in a tyramine-type reaction.

## Antidepressant

**Recommendations:** The concomitant use of phenelzine and clonazepam should be approached with caution. The patient should be monitored for signs of a tyramine-type reaction (e.g., headache, flushing, hypertension). The dose of one or both agents may need to be decreased, or one may need to he discontinued.

**Summary:** Concurrent administration of phenelzine and clonazepam resulted in a tyramine-type reaction.

**Related Drugs:** A similar interaction is expected to occur between clonazepam and other MAOIs, and between clonazepam and furazolidone, procarbazine, or selegiline. An interaction may occur between phenelzine and other benzodiazepines.

**Mechanism:** Clonazepam and other benzodiazepines may elevate serotonin levels.

**Detailed Information:** See *EDI*, 6/26.31

### Phenelzine-Ginseng

**Significance:** 3—minimally clinically significant

**Potential Effects:** The addition of ginseng to the therapy of a patient maintained on phenelzine may result in unexpected toxic effects.

**Recommendations:** Patients should be carefully monitored for changes in efficacy and toxic effects if ginseng is added to or removed from the therapy of a patient maintained on phenelzine.

**Summary:** Adding ginseng to the therapies of patients maintained on phenelzine resulted in unexpected toxic effects including irritability, insomnia, headaches, tremulousness, and visual hallucinations.

**Related Drugs:** A similar interaction could occur between ginseng and the other monoamine oxidase inhibitors. There are no agents related to ginseng. There are several different species of the genus *Panax* that include ginseng in their names. These include Korean ginseng, Sanchi ginseng, American ginseng, Chikusetsu ginseng, Himalayan ginseng, and Dwarf ginseng. Another species is called Zhuzishen.

**Mechanism:** Ginsenosides (saponin glycosides in ginseng) inhibit cyclic adenosine monophosphate phosphodiesterase (cAMP) and the effects of various ginsenosides on cortical steroid secretion and cAMP activity appear to be parallel. These effects may account partly for their psychoactive effects.

**Detailed Information:** See *EDI*, 6/26.50

### Phenelzine-Levodopa

**Significance:** 1—highly clinically significant

**Recommendations:** Levodopa and monoamine oxidase inhibitors should not be administered concurrently. If an antidepressant must be used in a patient receiving levodopa, a tricyclic antidepressant should be considered. If a monoamine oxidase inhibitor must be used concurrently with levodopa, a carbidopa-levodopa combination product should be considered instead of levodopa alone. The effects of monoamine oxidase inhibition usually last two weeks after the drug is discontinued; therefore, levodopa should not be given until at least four weeks after the monoamine oxidase inhibitor is discontinued.

**Summary:** Levodopa has been documented to cause a significant rise in blood pressure as well as flushing and palpitations when used in combination with phenelzine.

**Related Drugs:** Isocarboxazid, pargyline and tranylcypromine have been shown to exhibit a similar interaction. This interaction would be expected to occur with agents that possess MAOI activity. There are no drugs related to levodopa.

Antidepressant

**Mechanism:** The concurrent administration of carbidopa, a peripheral decarboxylase inhibitor, with levodopa may suppress the hypertensive reaction caused by monoamine oxidase inhibitors.
**Detailed Information:** See *EDI*, 6/27.00

## Phenelzine-Sulfisoxazole

**Significance:** 3—minimally clinically significant
**Recommendations:** If an increased incidence of adverse effects occurs following concurrent administration of these agents, one or both drugs may need to be discontinued. In a case report, symptoms subsided upon discontinuation of sulfisoxazole.
**Summary:** There are data to show that coadministration of these agents may cause an increased incidence of adverse effects.
**Related Drugs:** A similar interaction is expected to occur between sulfisoxazole and other MAOIs or between phenelzine and other sulfonamides.
**Mechanism:** The concurrent use of these agents may saturate the acetylation mechanism, resulting in higher plasma levels and increased side effects.
**Detailed Information:** See *EDI*, 6/28.10

## Pimozide-Sulfamethoxazole, Trimethoprim

**Significance:** 3—minimally clinically significant
**Potential Effects:** Combination sulfamethoxazole-trimethoprim may alter a patient's response to pimozide.
**Recommendations:** Patients receiving these agents together should be closely monitored for changes in their response to pimozide.
**Summary:** There are data to show that administration of sulfamethoxazole-trimethoprim may alter a patient's response to pimozide.
**Related Drugs:** It is not known if a similar interaction would occur between pimozide and other sulfonamides. There are no drugs related to pimozide.
**Mechanism:** This interaction may have occurred at pimozide's receptor site.
**Detailed Information:** See *EDI*, 6/28.30

## S-Adenosylmethionine-Clomipramine

**Significance:** 3—minimally clinically signifiicant
**Potential Effects:** Concomitant use of S-adenosylmethionine and clomipramine may result in serotonin syndrome.
**Recommendations:** Concurrent use of S-adenosylmethionine and clomipramine should be approached with caution. Patients should be monitored for signs of serotonin syndrome. One or both of these agents may need to be discontinued.
**Summary:** Concomitant use of intramuscular S-adenosylmethionine and oral clomipramine resulted in serotonin syndrome. Initial effects of anxiety, agitation, and confusion progressed to more severe symptoms, including rigidity, stupor, tachycardia, tachypnea, profuse diaphoresis, myoclonus, generalized tremors, hyperreflexia, and hyperpyrexia.
**Related Drugs:** Interactions between S-adenosylmethionine and other tricyclic antidepressants have not been reported. No other known agents are related to S-adenosylmethionine. Other common names for S-adenosylmethionine are SAMe, SAM, ADE-SD4, and ademetionine.
**Mechanism:** It has been suggested that the interaction was caused by synergistic action between S-adenosylmethionine and clomipramine.
**Detailed Information:** See *EDI*, 6/28.33

## Sertraline-Rifampin

**Significance:** 3—minimally clinically significant

**Potential Effects:** The addition of rifampin to the therapy of a patient maintained on sertraline may result in a decrease in antidepressant efficacy and symptoms suggestive of selective serotonin reuptake inhibitor (SSRI) withdrawal syndrome.

**Recommendations:** If rifampin is added to, or discontinued from, the therapy of a patient who is maintained on a stable regimen of sertraline, the patient should be carefully monitored for changes in sertraline levels and clinical effect. The dose of sertraline may need to be adjusted.

**Summary:** Adding rifampin to the therapy of a patient maintained on sertraline resulted in a decrease in sertraline blood levels and antidepressant efficacy and symptoms suggestive of SSRI withdrawal syndrome.

**Related Drugs:** It is not known whether an interaction would occur between rifampin and the other selective serotonin reuptake inhibitors or between sertraline and the other rifamycins.

**Mechanism:** It has been postulated that the induction of cytochrome $P450_{3A4}$ isozymes by rifampin led to the decreased sertraline serum levels.

**Detailed Information:** See *EDI*, 6/28.40

## Tranylcypromine-Atracurium

**Significance:** 3—minimally clinically significant

**Potential Effects:** Concurrent use of these agents may result in hypertension.

**Recommendations:** Patients should be monitored for hypotension during co-therapy with these agents. If necessary, phentolamine may be useful in reversing the hypertension.

**Summary:** There are data to show that administration of tranylcypromine when patients are induced with atracurium may result in hypertension.

**Related Drugs:** It is difficult to determine if a similar interaction would occur between atracurium and other MAOIs or between tranylcypromine and other nondepolarizing neuromuscular blocking agents.

**Mechanism:** The mechanism of this interaction is not known.

**Detailed Information:** See *EDI*, 6/28.50

## Tranylcypromine-Phenylpropanolamine

**Significance:** 1—highly clinically significant

**Recommendations:** Patients receiving monoamine oxidase inhibitors should be instructed to avoid indirect-acting sympathomimetic agents, foods containing tyramine, and nonprescription items with the potential to interact (e.g., cough and cold preparations). Symptoms such as headache, gastrointestinal upset, fever, and visual disturbances should be pointed out as indicators of hypertension caused by such combinations. Marked elevation of blood pressure under these circumstances may be treated by alpha-adrenergic blocking agents like phentolamine (5 mg intramuscularly or intravenously).

**Summary:** Indirect acting sympathomimetic amines may cause an abrupt elevation of blood pressure when administered with tranylcypromine or other MAOIs, resulting in hypertensive crisis.

**Related Drugs:** Other MAOIs have been reported to interact with other indirect-acting sympathomimetics. Pseudoephedrine may interact similarly. Mixed acting sympathomimetics have been shown to interact with monoamine oxidase inhibitors. Procarbazine and

## Antidepressant

dopamine administered with indirect and mixed acting sympathomimetics may cause hypertensive reactions. Furazolidone has been shown to interact with indirect acting sympathomimetics (see also Furazolidone-Amphetamine, page 191).

**Mechanism:** The stimulation of norepinephrine released by the indirect-acting adrenergic agents results in an increase of neurotransmitters. The enhancement results from an inhibition of the hepatic microsomal enzymes.

**Detailed Information:** See *EDI*, 6/29.00

### Tranylcypromine-Propranolol

**Significance:** 4—not clinically significant

**Recommendations:** One study suggests that monamine oxidase inhibitors should be discontinued at least two weeks before the institution of propranolol therapy, but this is a theoretical consideration only and no clinical interaction has been documented. Therefore, this combination need not be avoided at this time.

**Summary:** The concomitant administration of tranylcypromine and propranolol does not result in an increase in pressor activity or tachycardia.

**Related Drugs:** Documentation is lacking regarding an interaction between other MAOIs and other beta-blocking agents and with furazolidone and procarbazine.

**Mechanism:** The mechanism of this interaction is unknown.

**Detailed Information:** See *EDI*, 6/31.00

### Tranylcypromine-Tryptophan

**Significance:** 3—minimally clinically significant

**Potential Effects:** Use of these agents together may cause sudden changes in mental status.

**Recommendations:** Use these agents together with caution. Monitor patients for mental status changes. Tryptophan may need to be discontinued.

**Summary:** There are data to show that coadministration of these agents may cause sudden changes in mental status, exhibiting symptoms such as hyperreflexia, ankle clonus, nystagmus, incoordination, tremor, myoclonic jerks, and nausea.

**Related Drugs:** Phenelzine was shown to have a similar interaction. A similar interaction may occur between tryptophan and other MAOIs. There are no drugs related to tryptophan.

**Mechanism:** This interaction may result from a stimulation of the serotonergic system by the combination of the two agents.

**Detailed Information:** See *EDI*, 6/33.00

### Trazodone-Fluoxetine

**Significance:** 3—minimally clinically significant

**Potential Effects:** Fluoxetine may decrease the metabolism of trazodone, resulting in increased levels.

**Recommendations:** Monitor patients for increased trazodone levels and side effects when fluoxetine is added to trazodone therapy.

**Summary:** There are data to show that the ratio of trazodone plasma level to dose increases when fluoxetine is added to therapy, decreasing trazodone levels.

**Related Drugs:** There are no drugs related to fluoxetine or trazodone.

**Mechanism:** Fluoxetine may decrease the hepatic metabolism of trazodone, resulting in an increase in plasma levels and adverse reactions.

**Detailed Information:** See *EDI*, 6/35.00

## Trazodone-Ginkgo

**Significance:** 3—minimally clinically significant

**Potential Effects:** Concurrent trazodone and *Ginkgo biloba* administration may result in an increase in trazodone effects and possible adverse events.

**Recommendations:** Concurrent trazodone and *Ginkgo biloba* administration should be approached with caution. The patient should be monitored for signs of trazodone toxicity and adverse events. The dose of trazodone may need to be reduced or *Ginkgo biloba* administration may need to be discontinued.

**Summary:** Concurrent trazodone and *Ginkgo biloba* administration resulted in coma in a patient diagnosed with Alzheimer's disease. The patient awoke immediately after flumazenil was injected.

**Related Drugs:** Trazodone is chemically and pharmacologically unrelated to the tricyclic and tetracyclic antidepressant agents. *Ginkgo biloba* L. is the world's oldest living tree species and is also commonly known as maidenhair tree, kew tree, fossil tree, or ginkgo.

**Mechanism:** It has been postulated that the increase of the GABAergic activity from the gingko flavonoid's effect and mCPP production from trazodone metabolism could potentially lead to excess GABA activity. It was also postulated that a blockade by flumazenil of flavonoid direct effects may have resulted in a decrease in GABAergic activity, leading to reversal of the coma.

**Detailed Information:** See *EDI*, 6/35.50

## Venlafaxine-Cimetidine

**Significance:** 3—minimally clinically significant

**Potential Effects:** Concurrent use of venlafaxine and cimetidine may result in an inhibition of venlafaxine first-pass metabolism.

**Recommendations:** The concomitant use of these agents may result in a more pronounced interaction in the elderly and in patients with hepatic impairment or pre-existing hypertension. Therefore, caution is advised with such patients, and dosage adjustments may be necessary.

**Summary:** Cimetidine may inhibit the first-pass metabolism of venlafaxine.

**Related Drugs:** It is not known whether an interaction would occur between venlafaxine and other $H_2$-receptor antagonists. There are no drugs related to venlafaxine.

**Mechanism:** Cimetidine may inhibit venlafaxine metabolism to its active metabolite, increase the plasma concentrations of venlafaxine and lower the concentrations of the active metabolite.

**Detailed Information:** See *EDI*, 6/37.00

# Chapter Seven

# Antihypertensive Drug Interactions

Antihypertensive

### Bethanidine-Mazindol

**Significance:** 2—moderately clinically significant

**Recommendations:** The concomitant use of these agents may need to be avoided. If concurrent use is required, blood pressure should be monitored frequently.

**Summary:** A report has shown that mazindol reversed the antihypertensive effect of bethanidine and caused a loss of bethanidine-induced side effects.

**Related Drugs:** Other antihypertensives related to bethanidine may interact with mazindol. Other anorexiants that possess indirect-acting sympathomimetic activity may interact with bethanidine (see Guanethidine-Dextroamphetamine, page 170). Phenylpropanolamine has been shown to antagonize the antihypertensive effects of bethanidine.

**Mechanism:** Anorexiants with indirect-acting sympathomimetic activity may compete with bethanidine for uptake or displace bethanidine from adrenergic neurons.

**Detailed Information:** See *EDI,* 7/1.00

### Captopril-Allopurinol

**Significance:** 3—minimally clinically significant

**Recommendations:** Until further clinical studies are done, the concurrent use of these agents need not be avoided. However, these drugs should be prescribed with caution, especially in patients with chronic renal failure. One or both drugs may need to be discontinued.

**Summary:** The coadministration of allopurinol and captopril have been shown to result in Stevens-Johnson syndrome, pyrexia, arthralgia, and myalgia.

**Related Drugs:** There are no drugs related to captopril or allopurinol.

**Mechanism:** Allopurinol and captopril have been associated with skin eruptions of the erythema multiforme type and, in some cases, have led to toxic epidermal necrolysis and Stevens-Johnson syndrome.

**Detailed Information:** See *EDI,* 7/2.10

### Captopril-Aluminum Hydroxide, Magnesium Carbonate, Magnesium Hydroxide

**Significance:** 3—minimally clinically significant

**Potential Effects:** The antacid combination may decrease the bioavailability of captopril.

**Recommendations:** If these agents are used together, their administration should be separated by as much time as possible.

**Summary:** There are data to show that coadministration of these agents will cause a decrease in captopril concentration and in the bioavailability of captopril.

**Related Drugs:** A similar interaction may occur between captopril and other antacids because of pharmacologic similarity. It is not known if a similar interaction would occur between the antacid combinations and other ACE inhibitors.

**Mechanism:** A transient rise in gastric pH caused by the antacid preparation may have increased the ionization of captopril, decreasing membrane penetration.

**Detailed Information:** See *EDI,* 7/2.30

## Antihypertensive

### Captopril-Aspirin

**Significance:** 2—moderately clinically significant

**Recommendations:** Patients should be closely monitored for blood pressure changes during concurrent use of these agents. If blood pressure control decreases, discontinuation of the aspirin may be necessary.

**Summary:** Coadministration of captopril and aspirin showed a decreased antihypertensive effect after a single dose of captopril.

**Related Drugs:** There are no drugs related to captopril. A similar interaction is expected to occur between captopril and other salicylates.

**Mechanism:** Aspirin may interfere with the release of vasodilating prostaglandins enhanced by long-term captopril therapy.

**Detailed Information:** See *EDI*, 7/3.00

### Captopril-Chlorpromazine

**Significance:** 3—minimally clinically significant

**Potential Effects:** Concurrent use of these agents may result in hypotension.

**Recommendations:** If these agents are used together, blood pressure should be closely monitored. One or both agents may need to be discontinued.

**Summary:** Data have shown that the coadministration of these agents may cause hypotension.

**Related Drugs:** An interaction may occur between chlorpromazine and other ACE inhibitors and between captopril and other phenothiazines, thioxanthenes, butyrophenones, dihydroindolones, and dibenzoxazepines.

**Mechanism:** A synergistic effect may have occurred when chlorpromazine and captopril were used concurrently.

**Detailed Information:** See *EDI*, 7/4.10

### Captopril-Furosemide

**Significance:** 2—moderately clinically significant

**Potential Effects:** Furosemide may induce severe postural hypotension in patients receiving captopril.

**Recommendations:** The hypotension is transient. If it occurs, place the patient in a supine position and, if needed, start an IV with normal saline.

**Summary:** There are data to show that coadministration of these agents may induce severe postural hypotension; however, this hypotensive response is transient.

**Related Drugs:** Enalapril and furosemide have been shown to potentiate renal problems; however, conflicting data are available. A similar interaction is expected to occur between captopril and other loop diuretics, thiazide diuretics, mercurial diuretics, and thiazide-related diuretics.

**Mechanism:** Furosemide, as well as other diuretics that cause sodium and water loss, may exaggerate the hypotensive state.

**Detailed Information:** See *EDI*, 7/5.00

### Captopril-Indomethacin

**Significance:** 2—moderately clinically significant

**Potential Effects:** Indomethacin may decrease or abolish the antihypertensive effect of captopril.

**Recommendations:** Blood pressure should be monitored if indomethacin is added to, or withdrawn from, captopril therapy. Indomethacin may need to be discontinued.

## Antihypertensive

**Summary:** There are data to show that coadministration of indomethacin and captopril has led to a decreased or a total invalidation of the antihypertensive effect of captopril.
**Related Drugs:** Enalapril was not affected by indomethacin or sulindac; however, conflicting data are available. A similar interaction is expected to occur between captopril and other NSAIAs. An interaction may also be expected to occur between indomethacin and other ACE inhibitors.
**Mechanism:** Indomethacin, which inhibits endogenous prostaglandin synthesis, may interfere with the release of vasodilating prostaglandins.
**Detailed Information:** See *EDI*, 7/7.00

### Captopril-Naloxone

**Significance:** 3—minimally clinically significant
**Potential Effects:** Naloxone may decrease the hypotensive effect of captopril.
**Recommendations:** Monitor the patient's blood pressure if these agents are used together.
**Summary:** There are data to show that coadministration of these agents may lead to a decrease in the hypotensive effect of captopril.
**Related Drugs:** A similar interaction may occur between captopril and naltrexone.
**Mechanism:** Administration of the opiate antagonist naloxone with captopril would prevent a decrease in baroreflex sensitivity, attenuating the hypotensive response to the captopril.
**Detailed Information:** See *EDI*, 7/8.10

### Captopril-Potassium Chloride

**Significance:** 3—minimally clinically significant
**Potential Effects:** The concurrent use of these agents may cause an increase in potassium levels.
**Recommendations:** Monitor potassium levels when using these agents together. The dose of either agent may need to be reversed or discontinued.
**Summary:** There are data to show that coadministration of these agents may increase serum potassium; however, no clinical signs or symptoms associated with hyperkalemia were present. There are data indicating that coadministration of these agents caused no change in serum potassium.
**Related Drugs:** The other ACE inhibitors would also be expected to interact with potassium chloride. Captopril may also be expected to interact with other potassium salts.
**Mechanism:** Concurrent administration of captopril and a potassium supplement may result in an additive pharmacologic effect, increasing serum potassium concentrations.
**Detailed Information:** See *EDI*, 7/8.30

### Captopril-Probenecid

**Significance:** 3—minimally clinically significant
**Recommendations:** Because it is not clear whether a moderate increase in captopril levels will have any significant effect on the antihypertensive action of captopril, the concurrent use of these agents need not be avoided. However, it is prudent to monitor the patient's blood pressure regularly, and a decrease in the dose of captopril may be necessary.

## Antihypertensive

**Summary:** There are data to show that probenecid reduces the total body clearance and renal clearance of captopril, increasing captopril levels.
**Related Drugs:** There are no drugs related to captopril. A similar interaction is expected to occur between captopril and sulfinpyrazone.
**Mechanism:** Probenecid may interfere with tubular secretion of drugs and this may interfere with captopril excretion.
**Detailed Information:** See *EDI*, 7/9.00

## Clonidine-Cyclosporine

**Significance:** 2–moderately clinically significant
**Potential Effects:** Concurrent administration of clonidine and cyclosporine may result in elevated levels of cyclosporine. Clonidine may help prevent cyclosporine-induced renal toxicity.
**Recommendations:** Cyclosporine levels should be monitored in patients maintained on cyclosporine in whom clonidine is initiated or discontinued. Dosage adjustments of cyclosporine may be necessary or clonidine may need to be discontinued.
**Summary:** Concurrent administration of clonidine and cyclosporine resulted in elevated levels of cyclosporine from 300–927 µg/L (therapeutic range: 150–300 µg/L) within five days, despite a reduction in cyclosporine dosage. Following the discontinuation of clonidine, cyclosporine levels decreased rapidly to below 200 µg/L within two days. In other studies, bone marrow transplant patients and renal allograft recipients also had elevated levels of cyclosporine, but mean serum creatinine levels were significantly lower than in patients who did not receive clonidine.
**Related Drugs:** There are no agents related to cyclosporine or clonidine.
**Mechanism:** It is postulated that clonidine inhibits the metabolism of cyclosporine by the cytochrome P450 enzyme system. It is also postulated that clonidine's beneficial effects on kidney function may be the result of a combination of clonidine's inhibition of renin release, reduction in the responsiveness of the kidneys to vasopressin, and reduction of preglomerular vasoconstriction.
**Detailed Information:** See *EDI*, 7/9.80

## Clonidine-Mirtazapine

**Significance:** 2—moderately clinically significant
**Potential Effects:** The addition of mirtazapine to the therapy of a patient on a hypertension regimen that included clonidine resulted in hypertensive urgency.
**Recommendations:** The concurrent use of mirtazapine and clonidine should be approached with caution. Patients receiving concurrent therapy should be monitored for lack of efficacy of both agents. One or both agents may need to be discontinued.
**Summary:** The addition of mirtazapine to a hypertension regimen that included clonidine resulted in hypertensive urgency.
**Related Drugs:** A similar interaction would be expected between mirtazapine and other alpha-agonists (guanabenz, guanfacine, lofexidine, methyldopa, and methyldopate). An interaction might also be expected to occur between clonidine and maprotiline, a tetracyclic antidepressant agent structurally related to mirtazapine.
**Mechanism:** Clonidine is an $alpha_2$ agonist that suppresses the release of norepinephrine, thereby lowering blood pressure. Mirtazapine increases noradrenaline by blocking inhibitory $alpha_2$ receptors, antagonizing the antihypertensive effects of clonidine.
**Detailed Information:** See *EDI*, 7/9.90

Antihypertensive

## Clonidine-Naloxone
**Significance:** 3—minimally clinically significant
**Potential Effects:** Patients taking clonidine who are given naloxone may have a diminished antihypertensive effect.
**Recommendations:** If a loss of antihypertensive control occurs, naloxone may need to be discontinued or another antihypertensive chosen.
**Summary:** Several studies have shown that the concurrent administration of clonidine and naloxone decreases the antihypertensive effect of clonidine; however, there are conflicting data available.
**Related Drugs:** Naltrexone has been shown to inhibit the hypotension and bradycardia produced by clonidine. There are no drugs related to clonidine.
**Mechanism:** This interaction may result from the similarities that may exist between central alpha adrenergic receptors and opiate receptors.
**Detailed Information:** See *EDI*, 7/10.10

## Clonidine-Propranolol
**Significance:** 1—highly clinically significant
**Potential Effects:** Abrupt discontinuation of clonidine from cotherapy with propranolol results in severe hypertension and tachycardia.
**Recommendations:** Propranolol should be discontinued well in advance of clonidine withdrawal. Labetalol may be substituted for propranolol, or it may be used to reverse the resulting hypertension after clonidine withdrawal.
**Summary:** The rapid discontinuation of clonidine from combined therapy with propranolol may produce severe symptoms of sympathetic activity, rapid blood pressure elevations and a paradoxic hypertension.
**Related Drugs:** Timolol and metoprolol have been documented to exhibit a similar interaction. It is not known if other beta cardioselective beta blocking agents would interact similarly. Other noncardioselective beta-blocking agents may interact similarly to propranolol.
**Mechanism:** Propranolol neutralizes the vasodilatory effect of beta$_2$-adrenergic receptors. When clonidine is stopped, neurotransmitters are released and manifest vasoconstriction.
**Detailed Information:** See *EDI*, 7/11.00

## Clonidine-Rifampin
**Significance:** 4—not clinically significant
**Recommendations:** Rifampin has not been shown to alter the elimination of clonidine, and no special precautions need to be taken when these two agents are used concomitantly.
**Summary:** The results of a study involving six normal volunteers indicates that no change occurred in the elimination kinetics of clonidine during rifampin administration.
**Related Drugs:** There are no drugs related to rifampin or clonidine.
**Mechanism:** Clonidine is biotransformed by the liver and eliminated unchanged by the kidney. Rifampin does not appear to induce the metabolism of clonidine.
**Detailed Information:** See *EDI*, 7/13.00

## Antihypertensive

### Enalapril-Azathioprine

**Significance:** 3—minimally clinically significant

**Potential Effects:** Concurrent use of azathioprine and an ACE inhibitor may result in hematological changes such as anemia, neutropenia, or granulocytopenia.

**Recommendations:** Patients receiving concurrent azathioprine and an ACE inhibitor should be closely monitored for hematological changes.

**Summary:** Concurrent use of azathioprine and enalapril resulted in significantly reduced hematocrit and hemoglobin.

**Related Drugs:** Captopril has been reported to reduce white blood cell counts when combined with azathioprine. Based on the postulated mechanism and pharmacologic similarity, an interaction would be expected to occur between azathioprine and the other ACE inhibitors and between enalapril and the other nitrosourea alkylating agents, although documentation is lacking.

**Mechanism:** The exact mechanism of this interaction is unknown. The impairment of hematopoiesis by azathioprine may have made any inherent ability of ACE inhibitors to trigger anemia, possibly through decreased or low erythropoietin or hemolysis, clinically significant.

**Detailed Information:** See *EDI,* 7/14.00

### Enalapril-Rifampin

**Significance:** 3—minimally clinically significant

**Potential Effects:** Rifampin may increase the clearance of enalapril leading to hypertensive control.

**Recommendations:** Patients maintained on enalapril should be closely monitored for changes in blood pressure if rifampin cotherapy is instituted. The rifampin may need to be discontinued or the enalapril dose may need to be adjusted.

**Summary:** Concurrent administration of enalapril and rifampin may result in a decrease in the effects of enalapril.

**Related Drugs:** It is not known whether an interaction would occur between rifampin and other ACE inhibitors. There are no drugs related to rifampin.

**Mechanism:** Rifampin may enhance the renal clearance of enalaprilat.

**Detailed Information:** See *EDI,* 7/14.50

### Guanethidine-Alcohol, Ethyl

**Significance:** 2—moderately clinically significant

**Recommendations:** Patients prescribed guanethidine should be informed of the following: (1) concurrent alcohol ingestion may increase the incidence of guanethidine-induced orthostatic hypotension, dizziness, and syncope, thus alcohol intake should be limited, if possible; (2) these adverse reactions are most likely to occur during hot weather or while standing for long periods, rising rapidly from a sitting or prone position, or exercising; (3) if such symptoms occur, one should lie, sit, or squat immediately.

**Summary:** Alcohol may enhance the orthostatic hypotension and syncope caused by guanethidine.

**Related Drugs:** Other drugs pharmacologically related to guanethidine may interact with alcohol.

**Mechanism:** Alcohol may inhibit the ability of a patient taking guanethidine to respond to orthostatic changes.

**Detailed Information:** See *EDI,* 7/15.00

## Guanethidine-Chlorpromazine

**Significance:** 1—highly clinically significant

**Recommendations:** Because this interaction is clinically significant, patients should not receive chlorpromazine and guanethidine concomitantly, if possible. If concurrent administration is required, patients should be closely monitored for a reversal of the hypotensive effect of guanethidine. The dose of guanethidine may have to be increased to maintain the hypotensive effect. Antihypertensive drugs, such as methyldopa, which do not interact with chlorpromazine may be considered as alternatives to guanethidine. Also, molindone, which does not appear to alter the antihypertensive effect of guanethidine, may be a suitable alternative to chlorpromazine.

**Summary:** Chlorpromazine may reverse the antihypertensive effects of guanethidine.

**Related Drugs:** Chlorpromazine may interact with guanethidine to a greater degree than other phenothiazines, thioxanthenes, and dibenzoxazepines. Administration of haloperidol and thiothixene has been shown to cause a significant increase in blood pressure. Molindone does not alter the antihypertensive effects of guanethidine. Bethanidine, debrisoquin, and guanadrel may be expected to interact with chlorpromazine.

**Mechanism:** Guanethidine exerts its antihypertensive effects by competing with norepinephrine. Chlorpromazine apparently blocks the transport of guanethidine into the neuron.

**Detailed Information:** See *EDI*, 7/17.00

## Guanethidine-Desipramine

**Significance:** 1—highly clinically significant

**Recommendations:** The concurrent administration of guanethidine and desipramine or other tricyclic antidepressants should be avoided. If cotherapy is selected, the patient should be closely monitored for one to two weeks, with the expectation that the guanethidine dose may have to be increased. High doses (300 mg) of guanethidine have been successful in overcoming the antidepressant antagonism. Antihypertensive agents such as prazosin, atenolol, or other beta blockers may be considered as guanethidine substitutes since they do not interact with desipramine. The antidepressant doxepin (in doses less than 150 mg daily) may be substituted for desipramine. However, doxepin in this dosage rarely produces an adequate antidepressant effect.

**Summary:** The antihypertensive effect of guanethidine has been shown to be antagonized within three to seven days of initiating desipramine therapy.

**Related Drugs:** Amitriptyline, imipramine, protriptyline, nortriptyline, and doxepin have been shown to inhibit the antihypertensive effects of guanethidine. Cyclobenzaprine may antagonize the antihypertensive effect of guanethidine. Bethanidine and debrisoquin have shown a loss of antihypertensive effect when administered with tricyclic antidepressants. An interaction may occur between desipramine and guanadrel.

**Mechanism:** Desipramine antagonizes guanethidine's antihypertensive and neuronal blocking effects, and this is dependent upon the concentration of guanethidine.

**Detailed Information:** See *EDI*, 7/19.00

Antihypertensive

## Guanethidine-Dextroamphetamine

**Significance:** 2—moderately clinically significant

**Recommendations:** The reversal of guanethidine's effect by dextroamphetamine, and its resultant effect on blood pressure, suggests that the two drugs should not be administered concurrently. If dextroamphetamine and antihypertensive therapy are indicated for the treatment of a given patient, clonidine, methyldopa, or a beta blocking agent whose effect has not been reported to be antagonized by dextroamphetamine should be considered. In addition, since the effect of guanethidine on blood pressure is known to last for several days after discontinuation, the effects of amphetamines on blood pressure must be monitored even after guanethidine discontinuation because these patients may quickly revert to pretreatment levels of blood pressure. One should also note that this prolonged antihypertensive effect of guanethidine may also enhance the effect of alternative forms of blood pressure control, even after drug therapy has been altered.

**Summary:** The concurrent use of guanethidine and dextroamphetamine may result in a decrease in the antihypertensive effect of guanethidine.

**Related Drugs:** Bethanidine, debrisoquin, and guanadrel have shown to decrease antihypertensive effects. Methamphetamine, ephedrine, methylphenidate, and mephentermine have shown a similar effect. Phenylpropanolamine has antagonized the effects of bethanidine. The interaction of other direct and mixed acting sympathomimetics with guanethidine are discussed in another monograph (see Guanethidine-Phenylephrine, page 171).

**Mechanism:** The antihypertensive effect of guanethidine is the result of its ability to block the release of norepinephrine.

**Detailed Information:** See *EDI*, 7/21.00

## Guanethidine-Hydrochlorothiazide

**Significance:** 2—moderately clinically significant

**Recommendations:** The addition of hydrochlorothiazide to long-term guanethidine therapy may result in the need to reduce the dose of guanethidine. The thiazide diuretic will enhance the antihypertensive effect of guanethidine. Patients should be informed of the possible occurrence of dizziness or syncope from the enhanced antihypertensive effect of the combination therapy.

**Summary:** Concurrent hydrochlorothiazide and guanethidine therapy reduces sodium and water retention and increases blood volume, necessitating a decrease in guanethidine.

**Related Drugs:** Other diuretics that possess antihypertensive properties may be expected to undergo a similar interaction with guanethidine. Bethanidine, debrisoquin, and guanadrel may be expected to interact with hydrochlorothiazide.

**Mechanism:** The thiazides appear to cause fluid and sodium depletion, and long-term use of guanethidine results in a progressive resistance to its antihypertensive effect because of increasing sodium retention and edema formation.

**Detailed Information:** See *EDI*, 7/23.00

## Guanethidine-Minoxidil

**Significance:** 2—moderately clinically significant

**Recommendations:** It is recommended that guanethidine be discontinued at least one week before initiation of minoxidil, if possible. If not possible, it is suggested that minoxidil therapy be started in a hospital setting and that the patient remain in the hospital until the severe orthostatic effects dissipate or until the patient learns how to avoid activities that produce these effects.

## Antihypertensive

**Summary:** The coadministration of guanethidine and minoxidil may result in profound orthostatic hypotension.

**Related Drugs:** Bethanidine, debrisoquin, and guanadrel may be expected to produce a similar hypotensive episode with minoxidil. There are no drugs related to minoxidil.

**Mechanism:** Guanethidine is known to cause orthostatic hypotension, and minoxidil may accentuate this effect.

**Detailed Information:** See *EDI*, 7/25.00

### Guanethidine-Phenelzine

**Significance:** 2—moderately clinically significant

**Recommendations:** To avoid any risk in compromise of blood pressure control, MAO inhibitors should not be added to any antihypertensive regimen including guanethidine. Careful monitoring of blood pressure is required if this combination cannot be avoided.

**Summary:** Addition of a MAOI to guanethidine may result in a compromise in the antihypertensive effectiveness of guanethidine.

**Related Drugs:** Other MAOIs may be expected to interact similarly with guanethidine. Bethanidine, debrisoquin, and guanadrel may interact in the same manner.

**Mechanism:** MAOIs antagonize guanethidine's hypotensive effect by interfering with catecholamine depletion.

**Detailed Information:** See *EDI*, 7/27.00

### Guanethidine-Phenylephrine

**Significance:** 2—moderately clinically significant

**Recommendations:** A compromise in blood pressure control may occur when direct or mixed-acting sympathomimetic agents are used by patients who are receiving or have recently received guanethidine. The concurrent use of these agents should be avoided.

**Summary:** Direct and mixed acting sympathomimetics may antagonize the hypotensive effects of patients pretreated with guanethidine, resulting in hypertension.

**Related Drugs:** Bethanidine, debrisoquin, and guanadrel may show potential to interact in the same manner. Other sympathomimetics may show an effect similar to phenylephrine's. Interactions between indirect-acting sympathomimetics and guanethidine are discussed in another monograph (see Guanethidine-Dextroamphetamine, page 170).

**Mechanism:** Guanethidine blocks the release of norepinephrine, causing a supersensitivity, and this may be related to guanethidine indirectly interfering with neuron amine uptake and/or a sensitizing action of the drug.

**Detailed Information:** See *EDI*, 7/29.00

### Guanfacine-Bupropion

**Significance:** 3—minimally clinically significant

**Potential Effects:** The addition of guanfacine to a bupropion regimen may result in seizures.

**Recommendations:** Patients maintained on bupropion therapy should be closely monitored for changes in seizure activity if guanfacine is added to their regimen. Until more documentation is available, alternate therapy should be considered.

**Summary:** The addition of guanfacine to a bupropion regimen may have resulted in a grand mal seizure. All medications were discontinued and the patient remained seizure-free 10 months later. A subsequent neurological workup was negative.

Antihypertensive

**Related Drugs:** It is not known whether an interaction would occur between bupropion and the other centrally acting antiadrenergic agents. Bupropion is an antidepressant agent chemically unrelated to the other antidepressant agents.

**Mechanism:** The mechanism of this interaction is not known. Bupropion has been associated with an increased rate of seizures (0.4%) at doses up to 450 mg per day, and the risk of seizures with bupropion administration increases almost tenfold with dosages between 450 mg and 600 mg per day. Adding guanfacine to the therapy of a patient maintained on bupropion may decrease the seizure threshold, increase bupropion levels, or result in an increased incidence of seizures.

**Detailed Information:** See *EDI*, 7/30.03

## Guanfacine-Phenobarbital

**Significance:** 3—minimally clinically significant

**Potential Effects:** Phenobarbital induces the metabolism of guanfacine leading to decreased blood pressure control.

**Recommendations:** Monitor blood pressure closely if phenobarbital is added to, or discontinued from, a guanfacine regimen. The guanfacine dose may need to be adjusted.

**Summary:** The antihypertensive effect of guanfacine may be decreased by the addition of phenobarbital.

**Related Drugs:** A similar interaction is expected to occur between guanfacine and other barbiturates. There are no drugs related to guanfacine.

**Mechanism:** Enzyme induction of guanfacine metabolism by phenobarbital may be the cause of this interaction.

**Detailed Information:** See *EDI*, 7/30.05

## Hydralazine-Indomethacin

**Significance:** 3—minimally clinically significant

**Potential Effects:** The hypotensive effect of hydralazine may be blocked or decreased by indomethacin.

**Recommendations:** Monitor the patient's blood pressure when using these agents together.

**Summary:** There are data to show that administration of indomethacin may block or decrease the hypotensive effect of hydralazine; however, conflicting data are available.

**Related Drugs:** Diclofenac was shown to diminish the antihypertensive effect of hydralazine. It is not known if a similar interaction would occur between hydralazine and other NSAIAs. There are no drugs related to hydralazine.

**Mechanism:** Indomethacin, by inhibiting prostaglandin synthesis, may attenuate the hypotensive response to hydralazine.

**Detailed Information:** See *EDI*, 7/30.10

## Losartan-Rifampin

**Significance:** 2—moderately clinically significant

**Potential Effects:** The concurrent administration of rifampin and losartan may result in decreased losartan levels and clinical effects.

**Recommendations:** Patients receiving concurrent therapy with rifampin and losartan should be monitored for decreased losartan levels and clinical effects.

**Summary:** The concurrent administration of rifampin and losartan resulted in decreased losartan serum concentrations. Although clinical effects were not measured in the study, this interaction is likely to be clinically significant, resulting in loss of blood pressure control, because of the magnitude of the changes observed in the serum levels of losartan and E3174 (an active metabolite of losartan with greater potency than the parent drug).

## Antihypertensive

**Related Drugs:** It is not known whether an interaction would occur between rifampin and the other angiotensin II receptor antagonists. If the other rifamycins are also inducers of cytochrome $P450_{3A4}$, then a similar interaction would be expected to occur with these agents and losartan, although documentation is lacking.

**Mechanism:** Approximately 14% of an oral dose of losartan is converted to E3174. Cytochrome $P450_{3A4}$ is involved in the oxidation of losartan to E3174. Rifampin has been shown to be a potent inducer of E3174. Changes in E3174 levels are likely to be more meaningful than changes in losartan levels. It was therefore postulated that rifampin was a potent inducer of the elimination of both losartan and E3174.

**Detailed Information:** See *EDI*, 7/30.50

## Methyldopa-Amitriptyline

**Significance:** 3—minimally clinically significant

**Recommendations:** Based on the information available, it would seem that an interaction between methyldopa and amitriptyline is unlikely to occur in most patients; however, it is prudent to monitor blood pressure if tricyclic antidepressants are added to methyldopa therapy. An interaction between clonidine and desipramine is more firmly established and appears to occur regularly, although it can be overcome by increasing the dose of clonidine. Patients who receive tricyclic antidepressants in combination with clonidine should have their blood pressure closely monitored during the first several days of combined therapy. Alternatively, the tetracyclic antidepressant maprotiline may be substituted for the tricyclic antidepressant if clonidine therapy is chosen.

**Summary:** Loss of blood pressure control occurred when amitriptyline was added to a methyldopa regimen.

**Related Drugs:** Methyldopa was reported not to interact with desipramine. Clonidine has been reported to interact with tricyclic antidepressants. Imipramine has been reported to antagonize the antihypertensive effects of clonidine. Guanabenz may interact similarly with other tricyclic antidepressants. Mianserin was shown to have no interaction with the antihypertensive action of clonidine or methyldopa.

**Mechanism:** Methyldopa and clonidine depend on central alpha-adrenergic stimulation, and the tricyclic antidepressants could directly antagonize their effect.

**Detailed Information:** See *EDI*, 7/31.00

## Methyldopa-Ferrous Sulfate

**Significance:** 2—moderately clinically significant

**Potential Effects:** Concurrent use of these agents may decrease the hypertensive effects of methyldopa.

**Recommendations:** Patients should be monitored closely if ferrous sulfate is added to, or withdrawn from, concomitant therapy with methyldopa. The dose of methyldopa may need to be adjusted.

**Summary:** Ferrous sulfate may decrease the absorption of methyldopa, decreasing its hypertensive effects.

**Related Drugs:** Ferrous gluconate has been shown to decrease excretion and absorption of methyldopa. Ferrous fumarate would be expected to interact in a similar manner. There are no drugs related to methyldopa.

**Mechanism:** The decrease in excretion of methyldopa is due to a reduction in methyldopa absorption and an increase in methyldopa sulfation, and the decrease in absorption may result from chelation of methyldopa.

**Detailed Information:** See *EDI*, 7/32.50

## Methyldopa-Haloperidol

**Significance:** 3—minimally clinically significant

**Recommendations:** Reports suggest that the concurrent use of these agents can lead to abnormal central nervous system symptoms. Although the incidence may be low, it is important to be aware of this possible interaction. Should central nervous system symptoms occur, discontinuation of haloperidol should resolve the reaction.

**Summary:** Data have shown that dementia has occurred after haloperidol was added to an existing methyldopa regimen.

**Related Drugs:** A similar interaction is expected to occur with the phenothiazines, thioxanthenes, dihydroindolones and dibenzoxazepines. There are no drugs related to methyldopa.

**Mechanism:** This interaction results from an additive inhibition of dopamine in the central nervous system.

**Detailed Information:** See *EDI*, 7/33.00

## Methyldopa-Levodopa

**Significance:** 3—minimally clinically significant

**Recommendations:** Although several reports indicate that concurrent use of levodopa and methyldopa may produce a beneficial effect on the symptoms of parkinsonism without increasing the risk of adverse drug reactions, the possibility that this combination influences the therapeutic response to levodopa in certain patients should be considered. The occurrence of side effects such as vomiting and drowsiness induced by either drug may require a dose reduction or discontinuation of methyldopa.

**Summary:** Coadministration of levodopa and methyldopa can result in increased therapeutic effectiveness of either drug or adverse effects, depending on dose of either drug used.

**Related Drugs:** There are no drugs related to levodopa or methyldopa.

**Mechanism:** This interaction may be due to additive or synergistic hypotensive effects.

**Detailed Information:** See *EDI*, 7/35.00

## Methyldopa-Norepinephrine

**Significance:** 2—moderately clinically significant

**Recommendations:** It is important to be aware of a possible interaction between methyldopa and norepinephrine or other sympathomimetics (direct, indirect, and mixed acting), which may lead to hypertension. Phentolamine or another alpha-adrenergic blocking agent may be useful if hypertension does occur. It may also be necessary to discontinue the sympathomimetic amine. The norepinephrine dose should initially be reduced when used concurrently with methyldopa, and one study suggests beginning with one-tenth the usual dose.

**Summary:** The pressor effect of norepinephrine was found to increase and to be prolonged with the concurrent administration of methyldopa. A possible hypertensive episode may result.

**Related Drugs:** Other direct-acting sympathomimetics may interact similarly with methyldopa. The pressor effect of tyramine was found to be increased when coadministered with methyldopa. Phenylpropanolamine was reported to cause a severe hypertensive reaction. A similar interaction is expected to occur between methyldopa and other mixed and indirect-acting sympathomimetics.

**Mechanism:** There may be an additive effect between the false transmitter and normal transmitter at the same alpha receptor sites, or methyldopa's metabolites may facilitate the access to alpha-adrenergic receptor sites.

**Detailed Information:** See *EDI*, 7/37.00

Antihypertensive

## Methyldopa-Phenobarbital
**Significance:** 4—not clinically significant

**Recommendations:** The clinical significance of the potential interaction between methyldopa and phenobarbital has not been substantiated. Therefore, it appears that no dosage adjustments or additional precautions are necessary when these two agents are administered concurrently.

**Summary:** Barbiturate therapy could result in lowered methyldopa blood levels.

**Related Drugs:** Other barbiturates may act in a similar manner with phenobarbital. There are no drugs related to methyldopa.

**Mechanism:** Phenobarbital may increase methyldopa metabolism, resulting in decreased serum methyldopa levels.

**Detailed Information:** See *EDI*, 7/39.00

## Methyldopa-Phenoxybenzamine
**Significance:** 3—minimally clinically significant

**Potential Effects:** Use of these agents together may cause urinary incontinence, especially in patients who undergo a bilateral lumbar sympathectomy.

**Recommendations:** If urinary incontinence occurs, phenoxybenzamine may need to be discontinued.

**Summary:** There are data to show that coadministration of these agents may cause urinary incontinence.

**Related Drugs:** A similar interaction is expected to occur with the other nonspecific alpha-adrenergic blocking agents. Phentolamine may produce a similar interaction with methyldopa. There are no drugs related to methyldopa.

**Mechanism:** Methyldopa and phenoxybenzamine may decrease alpha-adrenergic stimulation of the bladder, increasing cholinergic activity and leading to the relaxation of the trigone and contraction of the detrusor.

**Detailed Information:** See *EDI*, 7/40.10

## Methyldopa-Propranolol
**Significance:** 2—moderately clinically significant

**Recommendations:** These interactions are potentially serious. It would seem prudent to consider the possibility of this interaction in patients taking methyldopa and beta-adrenergic blocking agents, especially when a drug or clinical situation may cause an increased release of the neurotransmitter.

**Summary:** There are data to show that coadministration of methyldopa and propranolol leads to increased blood pressure.

**Related Drugs:** Other nonselective beta blocking agents may interact in a similar manner with methyldopa.

**Mechanism:** Beta-blocking agents, when administered concurrently, would block the beta receptor activity, allowing the alpha receptor activity to occur unopposed, resulting in hypertension.

**Detailed Information:** See *EDI*, 7/41.00

## Nitroprusside-Captopril
**Significance:** 3—minimally clinically significant

**Recommendations:** Patients who are receiving captopril for control of hypertension and who require nitroprusside for acute lowering of blood pressure should be closely monitored to prevent extreme hypotension.

**Summary:** The concurrent administration of captopril with nitroprusside can reduce the dosage requirement for nitroprusside while maintaining adequate hypotensive control.

## Antihypertensive

**Related Drugs:** A similar interaction may occur between nitroprusside and other ACE inhibitors. There are no drugs related to nitroprusside.
**Mechanism:** The concurrent use of these two drugs can diminish the body's compensatory mechanism to nitroprusside-induced hypotension and reduce the dose of nitroprusside required.
**Detailed Information:** See *EDI*, 7/42.10

### Prazosin-Indomethacin

**Significance:** 2—moderately clinically significant
**Recommendations:** Patients' blood pressure should be closely monitored during concurrent use of these agents. An increased prazosin dose may be necessary.
**Summary:** The concurrent use of prazosin and indomethacin may reduce the hypotensive effect of prazosin.
**Related Drugs:** There are no drugs related to prazosin. A similar interaction is expected to occur with other NSAIAs and prazosin, if the mechanism involves prostaglandin inhibition.
**Mechanism:** Indomethacin prevents the rise in plasma renin activity that is seen following the administration of prazosin.
**Detailed Information:** See *EDI*, 7/43.00

### Prazosin-Propranolol

**Significance:** 2—moderately clinically significant
**Recommendations:** Patients should be advised of the increased risk involved with the first dose of prazosin, especially when it is added to a beta-blocking agent. Initiation of prazosin treatment with a dose of 0.5 mg or less has been suggested.
**Summary:** The concurrent use of prazosin and propranolol may enhance the acute postural hypotensive reaction.
**Related Drugs:** Prazosin and alprenolol exhibited a similar interaction. A similar interaction is expected to occur between prazosin and other beta-blocking agents. There are no drugs related to prazosin.
**Mechanism:** The compensatory responses of the heart, after the first dose of prazosin, is blocked by the beta-blockade produced by propranolol.
**Detailed Information:** See *EDI*, 7/45.00

### Prazosin-Verapamil

**Significance:** 3—minimally clinically significant
**Recommendations:** Patients should be monitored for a rapid decrease in blood pressure if the agents are used concurrently. A decreased prazosin dose may be necessary.
**Summary:** The concurrent administration of verapamil and prazosin have been shown to decrease systolic and diastolic blood pressures.
**Related Drugs:** Prazosin and nifedipine resulted in an acute hypotensive response; however, conflicting data are available. A similar interaction may occur between prazosin and other calcium channel blockers. There are no drugs related to prazosin.
**Mechanism:** This greater hypotensive activity may be due in part to a pharmacokinetic interaction that enhances the bioavailability of prazosin. A pharmacodynamic interaction at the level of vascular smooth muscle or compensatory cardiac activity may also play a role.
**Detailed Information:** See *EDI*, 7/46.10

## Antihypertensive

### Reserpine-Ephedrine
**Significance:** 2—moderately clinically significant

**Recommendations:** Patients receiving reserpine who are not responsive to therapeutic doses of ephedrine should be switched to a direct acting sympathomimetic agent such as norepinephrine or phenylephrine. The direct acting adrenergic agents will bypass the vesicle depletion action of reserpine and initiate the desired hypertensive action. Should norepinephrine be used, the added reuptake action of this agent will partially restore normal catecholamine activity. Smaller doses of direct acting sympathomimetics may be sufficient since the vasculature in reserpine treated patients is often more sensitive to these drugs.

**Summary:** The indirect sympathomimetic action of ephedrine may be antagonized as a result of depletion of norepinephrine from adrenergic vesicles by reserpine.

**Related Drugs:** Amphetamine, methylphenidate, tyramine, and phenylpropanolamine may interact with reserpine. Other rauwolfia alkaloids may interact with ephedrine.

**Mechanism:** When reserpine is given before ephedrine, it may antagonize the indirect action of ephedrine, resulting in a decreased cardiovascular response to this sympathomimetic.

**Detailed Information:** See *EDI,* 7/47.00

### Reserpine-Halothane
**Significance:** 3—minimally clinically significant

**Recommendations:** Clinical evidence indicates that long-term reserpine therapy is not a contraindication to anesthesia and surgery. However, patients on reserpine therapy should be observed for any unexpected hypotensive episodes during administration of halothane, particularly when there is associated blood loss, excessive speed of induction of anesthesia, surgical manipulation, position change, or excessive amount of anesthetic agents used. If reserpine is not withdrawn before surgery and if hypotension does occur, an exacerbated effect may be noticed since the endogenous catecholamines have already been chronically depleted by reserpine. Therefore, the use of an indirect-acting sympathomimetic agent would be ineffective, and a direct-acting sympathomimetic agent would be required to treat the hypotension.

**Summary:** Several studies have suggested that administration of halothane in patients receiving reserpine may be tolerated without increased risk of hypotension; however, conflicting data are available.

**Related Drugs:** Other anesthetic agents may interact similarly with reserpine. Other rauwolfia alkaloids may interact with halothane and other general anesthetics.

**Mechanism:** Halothane adds to the catecholamine depleting action of reserpine, causing enhanced depressant effects on the heart and resulting in decreased cardiac output and hypotension.

**Detailed Information:** See *EDI,* 7/49.00

### Sodium Nitroprusside-Esmolol
**Significance:** 3—minimally clinically significant

**Potential Effects:** Esmolol may potentiate sodium nitroprusside hypotension.

**Recommendations:** Monitor patients for excessive hypotension during concurrent use of these agents.

**Summary:** The hypotensive action of sodium nitroprusside is potentiated when esmolol is given concurrently.

**Related Drugs:** No documentation exists regarding an interaction between sodium nitroprusside and other cardioselective beta-blocking agents or the noncardioselective beta-blocking agents. There are no drugs related to sodium nitroprusside.

**Mechanism:** The activation of the renin-angiotensin system and the production of angiotensin II is thought to be the cause of resistance to the effects of sodium nitroprusside.

**Detailed Information:** See *EDI*, 7/51.00

## Spironolactone-Cholestyramine

**Significance:** 2—moderately clinically significant

**Potential Effects:** Concurrent spironolactone and cholestyramine may result in metabolic acidosis and hyperkalemia.

**Recommendations:** Concurrent cholestyramine and spironolactone should be approached with caution. Patients receiving concurrent therapy should be monitored for potential acidosis and hyperkalemia. Either cholestyramine or spironolactone may need to be discontinued.

**Summary:** Concurrent spironolactone and cholestyramine may have resulted in metabolic acidosis and hyperkalemia in patients with pre-existing hepatic dysfunction.

**Related Drugs:** Although documentation is lacking, based on the proposed mechanism a similar reaction would be expected to occur between spironolactone and the other anion exchange resin and between cholestyramine and the other potassium sparing diuretics.

**Mechanism:** Bicarbonate has been shown to bind to cholestyramine, an anionic exchange resin. It is postulated that cholestyramine may have exchanged chloride for bicarbonate and concurrent spironolactone may have prevented the kidneys from adequately acidifying the urine and correcting the excess chloride and loss of bicarbonate.

**Detailed Information:** See *EDI*, 7/52.00

# Chapter Eight

# Anti-infective Drug Interactions

Anti-infective

### Acyclovir-Probenecid

**Significance:** 3—minimally clinically significant

**Recommendations:** Until further information concerning this interaction is available, the clinical significance is difficult to assess. However, when acyclovir is used parenterally with probenecid, the resulting reduced elimination of acyclovir should be considered and any necessary dosage adjustments made.

**Summary:** The administration of probenecid caused a decrease in the elimination rate of acyclovir.

**Related Drugs:** A similar interaction may occur between acyclovir and sulfinpyrazone. There are no drugs related to acyclovir.

**Mechanism:** Acyclovir is eliminated by urinary excretion, by glomerular filtration and tubular secretion. Probenecid blocks the tubular secretion of acyclovir.

**Detailed Information:** See *EDI,* 8/1.00

### Ampicillin-Allopurinol

**Significance:** 3—minimally clinically significant

**Recommendations:** The concurrent use of these agents need not be avoided; however, one or both drugs may have to be discontinued if a rash develops.

**Summary:** The concurrent use of allopurinol and ampicillin may result in an increased incidence of drug-induced skin rash.

**Related Drugs:** Similar results were reported in patients receiving both allopurinol and amoxicillin. A similar interaction may occur between bacampicillin and hetacillin. There are no drugs related to allopurinol.

**Mechanism:** It is not known if the increased rash incidence is the result of a drug-drug interaction or an ampicillin-hyperuricemia interaction.

**Detailed Information:** See *EDI,* 8/3.00

### Ampicillin-Khat

**Significance:** 3—minimally clinically significant

**Potential Effects:** The concurrent use of ampicillin and khat chewing may result in decreased bioavailability of ampicillin.

**Recommendations:** The dosing of ampicillin and khat chewing should be separated by two hours. Patients chewing khat and taking ampicillin concurrently should be monitored for decreased ampicillin bioavailability and/or efficacy.

**Summary:** Concurrent use of ampicillin and khat chewing resulted in decreased bioavailability of ampicillin.

**Related Drugs:** A similar interaction has been reported with amoxicillin and might be expected between khat and other orally administered penicillins. There are no agents related to khat. Other common names for khat include qut, kat, chaat, Kus es Salahin, Tchaad, Tschut, Tohat, Tohai, and Gat.

**Mechanism:** Ampicillin may combine with tannins, one of the alkaloids found in khat leaves, to form an insoluble and poorly absorbed complex. It has also been suggested that the tannins from the khat leaf interfere with the gastrointestinal absorption process.

**Detailed Information:** See *EDI,* 8/4.00

### Ampicillin-Oral Contraceptive Agents

**Significance:** 2—moderately clinically significant

**Potential Effects:** Ampicillin may decrease the effect of the oral contraceptive agents.

## Anti-infective

**Recommendations:** The concomitant use of oral contraceptive agents and ampicillin need not be avoided. However, the potential for reduced efficacy of the oral contraceptive should be a consideration in patients receiving both drugs.

**Summary:** Ampicillin may cause a loss of contraceptive protection.

**Related Drugs:** Oral contraceptive failures have been further reported for amoxicillin, penicillin G, and oxacillin. A similar interaction is expected to occur with other penicillins.

**Mechanism:** Antibiotics destroy gut flora and prevent steroid reabsorption, resulting in lower than normal concentrations.

**Detailed Information:** See *EDI*, 8/5.00

### Bacampicillin–N-Acetylcysteine

**Significance:** 3—minimally clinically significant

**Potential Effects:** Bacampicillin may decrease the absorption of N-acetylcysteine (NAC), resulting in decreased levels.

**Recommendations:** Patients being administered oral NAC should be monitored for decreased plasma levels of NAC if bacampicillin is added to the regimen, and the dosage should be adjusted as necessary. Erythromycin has been shown not to interact significantly with NAC.

**Summary:** Administration of bacampicillin resulted in a decrease in the NAC peak concentration.

**Related Drugs:** A similar interaction may occur between NAC and other penicillins. There are no drugs related to NAC.

**Mechanism:** Absorption of bacampicillin is dose-dependent. A capacity-limited transport system exists in the intestine for the aminopenicillins and NAC may be expected to utilize the same transport system.

**Detailed Information:** See *EDI*, 8/6.50

### Cefoperazone-Alcohol, Ethyl

**Significance:** 2—moderately clinically significant

**Potential Effects:** A disulfiram-like reaction may occur when alcohol is ingested while a patient is receiving cefoperazone.

**Recommendations:** Patients receiving cefoperazone or other cephalosporins with a methyltetrazolethiol side chain should avoid ingesting products containing alcohol.

**Summary:** A disulfiram-like reaction including symptoms like flushing, tachycardia, bronchospasm, sweating, nausea, and vomiting may occur in patients ingesting alcohol and receiving cefoperazone.

**Related Drugs:** Moxalactam, cefamandole and cefotetan have exhibited this reaction. Cefoperazone, cefonicid and ceforanide may exhibit an interaction with alcohol. An interaction would not be expected to occur between alcohol and other cephalosporins that do not have the methyltetrazolethiol side chain.

**Mechanism:** Disulfiram-like reactions are caused when there is interference with acetaldehyde dehydrogenase activity and acetaldehyde subsequently accumulates.

**Detailed Information:** See *EDI*, 8/7.00

### Cefotaxime-Cimetidine

**Significance:** 3—minimally clinically significant

**Potential Effects:** Concurrent bolus administration of cimetidine and cefotaxime has been reported to result in tachycardia.

**Recommendations:** If a bolus of cimetidine is given with cefotaxime, the patient should be monitored for tachycardia. The use of continuous infusion of cimetidine may circumvent the tachycardia.

## Anti-infective

**Summary:** There are data to show that coadministration of cimetidine and cefotaxime results in tachycardia.

**Related Drugs:** It is not known if a similar interaction would occur between cimetidine and other cephalosporins or between cefotaxime and other $H_2$-receptor antagonists.

**Mechanism:** The mechanism of this interaction is not known.

**Detailed Information:** See *EDI*, 8/8.10

### Cephaloridine-Furosemide

**Significance:** 2—moderately clinically significant

**Recommendations:** Concurrent use of furosemide and cephaloridine should be avoided in patients with even mild pre-existing renal disease or impaired renal function, the elderly, and those receiving other nephrotoxic drugs. Use of a less nephrotoxic cephalosporin may be preferable if this combination is required, and renal function should be monitored regularly.

**Summary:** Cephaloridine nephrotoxicity may be enhanced by concurrent furosemide administration, but reports are complicated.

**Related Drugs:** Cephacetrile and cephalothin have exhibited a similar interaction. There is no documentation regarding a similar interaction with bumetanide. No other reports have appeared involving an interaction between cephaloridine and the thiazide diuretics or the thiazide-related diuretics.

**Mechanism:** An additive stimulation of renin release by both agents may lead to acute renal failure. Furosemide inhibits water reabsorption, leading to a higher concentration of cephaloridine. Natriuresis may lead to higher concentrations of cephaloridine.

**Detailed Information:** See *EDI*, 8/9.00

### Cephalothin-Colistimethate

**Significance:** 2—moderately clinically significant

**Recommendations:** Renal function should be closely monitored if these drugs are used together or sequentially. It has been recommended that the colistimethate dosage be determined according to kidney function rather than body weight.

**Summary:** Concurrent use of cephalothin and colistimethate have been associated with an increased risk of nephrotoxicity.

**Related Drugs:** Other cephalosporins may interact in a similar manner with colistimethate or other polypeptide antibiotics.

**Mechanism:** Cephalothin may interfere with the renal excretion of colistimethate.

**Detailed Information:** See *EDI*, 8/11.00

### Cephalothin-Probenecid

**Significance:** 2—moderately clinically significant

**Potential Effects:** Administration of probenecid and a cephalosporin may result in higher and prolonged serum cephalosporin concentrations with a resultant increase in potential nephrotoxicity.

**Recommendations:** Concurrent use of a cephalosporin and probenecid may increase and prolong the serum levels of the cephalosporin. Since cephalosporins are thought to be potentially nephrotoxic, these elevated serum levels can increase this effect. Therefore, the dosage may need to be decreased. In certain situations this interaction may prove useful to allow for a decrease in dosing frequency of the cephalosporin.

**Summary:** Ample documentation shows that concurrent administration of probenecid and a cephalosporin results in higher and prolonged serum cephalosporin concentrations, as shown with cephalothin.

## Anti-infective

**Related Drugs:** Increased serum levels of cefazolin, cephacetrile, cephaloglycin, cephalexin, cephradine, cefoxitin, cefadroxil, cefamandole, ceftizoxime, cefuroxime, cefprozil, cefonicid, cefaclor, cefotaxime, and cefmetazole have occurred when given with probenecid; it has not affected the elimination of moxalactam or cefonaride, or the half-life and AUC of ceftazidime. Conversely, concurrent probenecid use caused an increase in the systemic clearance and a subsequent decrease in terminal half-life of ceftriaxone. Cefoperazone, which is extensively excreted in the bile, would not be expected to interact with probenecid. Other cephalosporins may be expected to interact with probenecid in a manner similar to cephalothin.

**Mechanism:** Probenecid may compete with cephalothin for active renal secretion by the proximal tubule and may also restrict its volume of distribution. The unusual interaction of ceftriaxone and probenecid may occur because high doses of probenecid may compete with ceftriaxone for plasma protein binding sites and also decrease biliary secretion of ceftriaxone. Competition for binding sites has been noted with concurrent administration of probenecid and methotrexate, rifampin, and indomethacin. This is significant since ceftriaxone has been shown to possess dose-dependency in its rate of systemic clearance.

**Detailed Information:** See *EDI*, 8/13.00

## Chloramphenicol-Acetaminophen

**Significance:** 3—minimally clinically significant

**Potential Effects:** Acetaminophen may increase the clearance of chloramphenicol. In the presence of malnutrition, the net effect may be a decrease in chloramphenicol.

**Recommendations:** Because of conflicting results, it is not possible to recommend avoiding the concurrent administration of acetaminophen and chloramphenicol. However, it is prudent to be aware of a possible interaction between these agents. Patients should be closely monitored since a dosage adjustment of either agent may be necessary.

**Summary:** Acetaminophen may increase the clearance of chloramphenicol; however, there are conflicting data available.

**Related Drugs:** There are no drugs related to chloramphenicol or acetaminophen.

**Mechanism:** Acetaminophen and chloramphenicol may compete for metabolism, resulting in a decreased clearance of chloramphenicol. The increased clearance of chloramphenicol may be a result of increased glucuronidation of chloramphenicol.

**Detailed Information:** See *EDI*, 8/14.10

## Chloramphenicol-Cyclosporine

**Significance:** 3—minimally clinically significant

**Potential Effects:** The addition of chloramphenicol to the therapy of a patient maintained on cyclosporine may result in increased cyclosporine serum levels.

**Recommendations:** Cyclosporine concentrations should be carefully monitored if chloramphenicol is added to or discontinued from concurrent therapy.

**Summary:** The addition of chloramphenicol to the therapeutic regimen of two patients maintained on cyclosporine resulted increased cyclosporine serum levels.

**Related Drugs:** There are no drugs related to cyclosporine or chloramphenicol.

Anti-infective

**Mechanism:** The mechanism of this interaction is not known. It has been postulated that chloramphenicol may inhibit enzymes that mediate cyclosporine metabolism.
**Detailed Information:** See *EDI*, 8/14.70

### Chloramphenicol-Phenobarbital

**Significance:** 3—minimally clinically significant
**Recommendations:** It will be necessary to carefully monitor patients who receive these agents concomitantly. Chloramphenicol dosage may need to be significantly increased within a few days of initiating combined therapy. The possible rise in phenobarbital concentrations may cause sedation or other toxic symptoms, thereby necessitating a decreased phenobarbital dosage.
**Summary:** Concurrent administration of these agents has resulted in decreased chloramphenicol serum concentrations in infants and children.
**Related Drugs:** A similar interaction is expected to occur between chloramphenicol and other barbiturates.
**Mechanism:** Chloramphenicol may inhibit phenobarbital metabolism.
**Detailed Information:** See *EDI*, 8/15.00

### Chloramphenicol-Rifampin

**Significance:** 2—moderately clinically significant
**Recommendations:** Since there is a risk that serum concentrations of chloramphenicol will be reduced to subtherapeutic levels when rifampin is administered concomitantly, it appears prudent to monitor these concentrations when rifampin is added to chloramphenicol therapy, and consideration may be given to increasing the dose of chloramphenicol.
**Summary:** This interaction may lead to a decrease in the effectiveness of chloramphenicol.
**Related Drugs:** There are no drugs related to chloramphenicol or rifampin.
**Mechanism:** Rifampin can increase the rate of glucuronide, and chloramphenicol is metabolized by glucuronide conjugation.
**Detailed Information:** See *EDI*, 8/16.01

### Chloroquine-Cimetidine

**Significance:** 3—minimally clinically significant
**Potential Effects:** Cimetidine may inhibit the metabolism of chloroquine, resulting in increased levels.
**Recommendations:** Concurrent use of these agents should be done with caution. Ranitidine, or possibly famotidine, may be an alternative to cimetidine.
**Summary:** There are data to show that administration of cimetidine may inhibit the metabolism of chloroquine, resulting in increased levels.
**Related Drugs:** Ranitidine did not significantly alter chloroquine pharmacokinetics. An interaction may occur between cimetidine and other aminoquinolines.
**Mechanism:** Cimetidine may inhibit the hepatic mixed-function oxidases responsible for chloroquine's metabolism.
**Detailed Information:** See *EDI*, 8/16.03

### Chloroquine-Cyclosporine

**Significance:** 2—moderately clinically significant
**Potential Effects:** Concurrent administration of cyclosporine and chloroquine may result in an increase in cyclosporine levels and serum creatinine.

## Anti-infective

**Recommendations:** Cyclosporine levels and serum creatinine should be monitored in patients receiving cyclosporine when chloroquine is initiated or discontinued. The dose of cyclosporine may need to be significantly lowered.

**Summary:** In two case reports, concurrent administration of cyclosporine and chloroquine resulted in an increase in cyclosporine levels and serum creatinine.

**Related Drugs:** It is not known if there is an interaction between chloroquine and tacrolimus. Although documentation is lacking, based on the proposed mechanism a similar interaction would be expected to occur between cyclosporine and hydroxychloroquine or primaquine.

**Mechanism:** One set of authors proposed that chloroquine may have increased cyclosporine levels by interfering with cyclosporine metabolism either by direct action at the cytochrome P450 site or by decreasing enzyme release from lysosomes.

**Detailed Information:** See *EDI*, 8/16.07

## Chloroquine-Kaolin

**Significance:** 3—minimally clinically significant

**Recommendations:** Simultaneous administration of these agents should be avoided. It may be best to separate the administration of these drugs by at least four hours to reduce the possibility of an interaction. The dose of chloroquine may need to be increased.

**Summary:** There are data to show that administration of kaolin can result in a decrease in the chloroquine area-under-curve and in chloroquine plasma level and absorption.

**Related Drugs:** It is not known if a similar interaction would occur between kaolin and other aminoquinolines. There are no drugs related to kaolin; however, it is possible that other aluminum salts may interact similarly with chloroquine.

**Mechanism:** The gastrointestinal absorption of chloroquine may decrease because of the adsorption of chloroquine onto the surface of kaolin.

**Detailed Information:** See *EDI*, 8/16.10

## Chloroquine-Levothyroxine

**Significance:** 3—minimally clinically significant

**Potential Effects:** The addition of chloroquine to a stable levothyroxine regimen may result in an increase in the thyroid stimulating hormone (TSH) concentration.

**Recommendations:** TSH levels should be monitored if chloroquine is added to or discontinued from the therapy of a patient maintained on levothyroxine. The dose of levothyroxine may need to be adjusted.

**Summary:** The addition of chloroquine to a stable levothyroxine regimen may have resulted in an increase in the TSH, which returned to normal one week after discontinuation of the chloroquine. Upon rechallenge, TSH levels increased from 3.2 to 26 mU/L and, after two months, reached 54.7 mU/L. Free tri-iodothyronine concentrations also increased. Four weeks after completing therapy, levels of TSH and free tri-iodothyronine returned to normal ranges.

**Related Drugs:** It is not known whether a similar interaction would occur between chloroquine and dextrothyroxine or between levothyroxine and hydroxychloroquine or primaquine.

**Mechanism:** The mechanism of this interaction is not known. However, it is postulated that chloroquine increases the catabolism of thyroid hormones by enzymatic induction.

**Detailed Information:** See *EDI*, 8/16.20

## Anti-infective

### Ciprofloxacin-Aluminum Hydroxide, Magnesium Hydroxide

**Significance:** 2—moderately clinically significant

**Potential Effects:** Concurrent use of ciprofloxacin and aluminum hydroxide/magnesium hydroxide may result in decreased absorption of ciprofloxacin, leading to a decrease in serum levels.

**Recommendations:** Patients receiving these agents concomitantly should be monitored for decreased ciprofloxacin levels and/or efficacy. The dose of ciprofloxacin may need to be increased or an alternative antacid may need to be considered.

**Summary:** The concurrent administration of ciprofloxacin and a combination antacid containing aluminum hydroxide and magnesium hydroxide resulted in a decrease in plasma ciprofloxacin levels by as much as 94%.

**Related Drugs:** Calcium carbonate antacid has shown both no effect and a decrease in ciprofloxacin area-under-curve and bioavailability. Dairy products also may cause a significant decrease in ciprofloxacin bioavailability. A similar interaction was noted with lomefloxacin and aluminum/magnesium hydroxide. Single doses of bismuth subsalicylate did not significantly alter ciprofloxacin absorption. Because of conflicting results, it is difficult to determine if an interaction would occur between ciprofloxacin and the other antacids; however, a similar interaction may be expected to occur with those antacids that contain aluminum or magnesium ions. A decrease of 73% in serum ofloxacin levels has been seen with aluminum hydroxide/magnesium hydroxide use, and the antacid combination has reportedly decreased the antibiotic efficacy of norfloxacin. Enoxacin bioavailability was decreased by 49–73% when magnesium/aluminum hydroxide was given 0.5–2 hours prior to administration of the antibiotic. The bioavailability of enoxacin was not affected when the antacid was given eight hours before or two hours after enoxacin administration. A similar interaction has been described with pefloxacin. The concurrent administration of levofloxacin and aluminum hydroxide, rufloxacin and magnesium/aluminum hydroxides, and fleroxacin with calcium-rich foods have all demonstrated similar interactions. Since the fluoroquinolones have been modified chemically to a great extent compared to the other quinolones, cinoxacin and nalidixic acid, it is difficult to determine if an interaction would occur with these two agents.

**Mechanism:** Reduced levels of ciprofloxacin may result from reduced gastrointestinal absorption probably related to the formation of inactive chelate complexes between ciprofloxacin and the aluminum and magnesium ions. In one report, supplementation of agar media for testing quinolone sensitivities with magnesium sulfate results in the production of smaller inhibition zone diameters as compared to agar that has not been supplemented with magnesium sulfate. Fewer effects or no effects were noted with agar supplemented with zinc sulfate or calcium nitrate.

**Detailed Information:** See *EDI*, 8/16.30

### Ciprofloxacin-Cyclosporine

**Significance:** 2—moderately clinically significant

**Potential Effects:** Ciprofloxacin may increase cyclosporine levels, resulting in nephrotoxicity.

**Recommendations:** Patients maintained on cyclosporine should be monitored for increased cyclosporine levels and for signs of nephrotoxicity when ciprofloxacin is added to therapy.

**Summary:** There are data to show that administration of ciprofloxacin may increase cyclosporine levels resulting in nephrotoxicity.

## Anti-infective

**Related Drugs:** Norfloxacin was shown to exhibit a similar interaction. It is not known if an interaction would occur between cyclosporine and other quinolone antibacterials. There are no drugs related to cyclosporine.

**Mechanism:** There may be a synergistic nephrotoxicity between ciprofloxacin and cyclosporine.

**Detailed Information:** See *EDI*, 8/16.45

## Ciprofloxacin-Ferrous Sulfate

**Significance:** 2—moderately clinically significant

**Potential Effects:** Ferrous sulfate has been shown to decrease ciprofloxacin peak concentrations and area under curve.

**Recommendations:** The concurrent use of ciprofloxacin and ferrous sulfate should be avoided. This is prudent since decreased ciprofloxacin absorption occurs even with separation of administration of these agents.

**Summary:** Concurrent ciprofloxacin and ferrous sulfate resulted in a decrease in the ciprofloxacin peak serum concentration.

**Related Drugs:** Multiple vitamin and/or mineral preparations have shown similar changes in ciprofloxacin concentrations. Ferrous sulfate and zinc sulfate have been shown to reduce excretion of norfloxacin. A similar interaction may occur between the ferrous salts and other fluoroquinolone anti-infective agents. It is difficult to determine if an interaction would occur with cinoxacin or nalidixic acid.

**Mechanism:** A ciprofloxacin-$Fe^{+3}$ complex formation has been demonstrated *in vitro* in pH conditions similar to the small bowel.

**Detailed Information:** See *EDI*, 8/16.48

## Ciprofloxacin-Nutritional Supplements

**Significance:** 3—minimally clinically significant

**Potential Effects:** Concurrent administration of ciprofloxacin and nutritional supplement products may result in changes in ciprofloxacin pharmacokinetics.

**Recommendations:** Further studies are needed to determine the potential for clinical significance of this interaction. Until that time, it is recommended that patients receiving concurrent therapy with fluoroquinolones and nutritional supplements be closely monitored for efficacy of their anti-infective therapy.

**Summary:** Studies of ciprofloxacin administered concurrently with three different nutritional supplements have documented varying effects of these products on ciprofloxacin pharmacokinetics. Conflicting results have been seen with ciprofloxacin and Osmolite®, with one study reporting a reduction of 26% in the maximum concentration ($C_{max}$) and of 33% in the area-under-curve (AUC) of the antibiotic. The second study did not report any significant reduction in absorption of ciprofloxacin. Results with Pulmocare® have also shown significant decreases in $C_{max}$ and AUC. When ciprofloxacin was administered in conjunction with Resource®, no significant differences were noted in either $C_{max}$ or time to $C_{max}$ ($T_{max}$); however, the AUC for ciprofloxacin was reduced by 25%. The combination of ciprofloxacin and Ensure revealed significant lowering of the $C_{max}$ by 53% and lengthening of the $T_{max}$. The AUC for ciprofloxacin was substantially reduced, with a resultant 72% reduction in the bioavailability of the antibiotic.

**Related Drugs:** Ofloxacin has also been studied when used in combination with Ensure®. The nutritional product's coadministration resulted in a decrease in the $C_{max}$ of 64% and lengthened the $T_{max}$ of ofloxacin. The AUC for ofloxacin was also increased, resulting in

Anti-infective

an 88% reduction in ofloxacin's bioavailability. Similar interactions may occur between other enteral nutritional supplements and these or other fluoroquinolones. Since the fluoroquinolones have been modified chemically to a great extent compared to the other quinolones, cinoxacin and nalidixic acid, it is difficult to determine if an interaction would also occur with these agents.

**Mechanism:** Many nutritional supplements contain divalent cations that may be involved in a chelation reaction with ciprofloxacin. This type of interaction has been reported in the past with concurrent administration of ciprofloxacin with antacids, sucralfate, and ferrous sulfate.

**Detailed Information:** See *EDI,* 8/16.49

## Cyclosporine-Amphotericin B

**Significance:** 2—moderately clinically significant

**Potential Effects:** Concurrent use of these agents may result in nephrotoxicity.

**Recommendations:** Monitor serum creatinine levels carefully. The dose of cyclosporine may need to be decreased or an alternative therapy used.

**Summary:** There are data to show that concurrent use of these agents may result in nephrotoxicity. There are data available indicating that amphotericin B increases cyclosporine concentrations.

**Related Drugs:** There are no drugs related to cyclosporine or amphotericin B.

**Mechanism:** Cyclosporine alone is potentially nephrotoxic, and the addition of amphotericin B may increase cyclosporine concentrations and the occurrence of nephrotoxicity.

**Detailed Information:** See *EDI,* 8/2.50

## Dapsone-Rifampin

**Significance:** 3—minimally clinically significant

**Potential Effects:** Rifampin may induce the metabolism of dapsone, leading to decreased levels.

**Recommendations:** If rifampin is used on a regular basis with dapsone, the patient should be monitored for decreased dapsone efficacy or levels. The dosage of dapsone may need to be increased.

**Summary:** There are data to show that coadministration of rifampin may induce the metabolism of dapsone, leading to decreased levels.

**Related Drugs:** There are no drugs related to dapsone or rifampin.

**Mechanism:** Rifampin may induce the hepatic microsomal enzymes responsible for the metabolism of dapsone.

**Detailed Information:** See *EDI,* 8/16.50

## Dapsone-Trimethoprim

**Significance:** 3—minimally clinically significant

**Potential Effects:** Concurrent use of these agents may result in increased serum levels of both drugs.

**Recommendations:** The concurrent administration of dapsone and trimethoprim results in increased serum concentration of both drugs. This may result in an increased cure rate for AIDS-associated *Pneumocystis carinii* pneumonia. Patients receiving this therapy should be observed for a greater risk of developing methemoglobinemia.

**Summary:** Concurrent administration of dapsone and trimethoprim resulted in an increase in the serum concentration of both agents.

**Related Drugs:** There are no drugs related to either dapsone or trimethoprim.

Anti-infective

**Mechanism:** A competitive inhibition may occur between dapsone and/or monoacetyldapsone and trimethoprim for renal secretion.
**Detailed Information:** See *EDI,* 8/16.70

## Doxycycline-Carbamazepine
**Significance:** 2—moderately clinically significant
**Recommendations:** To maintain adequate serum levels of doxycycline, the antibiotic should be given every 12 hours to patients on long-term therapy with carbamazepine, or another noninteracting tetracycline product may be used.
**Summary:** The administration of doxycycline to patients receiving carbamazepine therapy will result in a reduction of antimicrobial effectiveness.
**Related Drugs:** For tetracycline, methacycline, oxytetracycline, demeclocycline, and chlortetracycline, half-lives and quantity excreted have not been shown to be affected by carbamazepine. There is a lack of data concerning whether this interaction occurs with minocycline.
**Mechanism:** Carbamazepine is known to induce liver enzymes and possibly accelerate the metabolism of doxycycline.
**Detailed Information:** See *EDI,* 8/17.00

## Doxycycline-Phenobarbital
**Significance:** 2—moderately clinically significant
**Recommendations:** A higher dosage of doxycycline or a normal dosage of a noninteracting tetracycline derivative should be used during concurrent administration with phenobarbital.
**Summary:** Doxycycline serum levels, half-life, and urinary excretion may be reduced by concurrent administration of phenobarbital.
**Related Drugs:** Amobarbital and pentobarbital have been reported to decrease the half-life of doxycycline, and other barbiturates may be expected to interact similarly. A similar interaction is expected to occur with minocycline.
**Mechanism:** Phenobarbital induces hepatic microsomal enzymes, resulting in enhanced doxycycline elimination.
**Detailed Information:** See *EDI,* 8/19.00

## Doxycycline-Phenytoin
**Significance:** 2—moderately clinically significant
**Recommendations:** The clinical response to doxycycline in patients receiving concurrent anticonvulsants should be monitored closely. It has been suggested that doxycycline's daily dose be doubled.
**Summary:** The concurrent use of doxycycline and phenytoin may result in a decreased half-life of doxycycline, lower serum levels and an inadequate antibacterial effect.
**Related Drugs:** Other tetracycline derivatives were shown to be unaffected by these anticonvulsants. A similar interaction is expected to occur with minocycline and with the other hydantoin anticonvulsants.
**Mechanism:** The decrease in half-life of doxycycline has been attributed to the induction of microsomal enzymes by phenytoin.
**Detailed Information:** See *EDI,* 8/21.00

## Erythromycin-Cimetidine
**Significance:** 3—minimally clinically significant
**Potential Effects:** Concurrent erythromycin and cimetidine may result in increased erythromycin levels with possible erythromycin-induced reversible hearing loss.

## Anti-infective

**Recommendations:** Patients receiving concurrent cimetidine and erythromycin (especially high dose erythromycin) in the presence of renal insufficiency should be monitored for hearing loss.

**Summary:** Concurrent erythromycin and cimetidine resulted in increased erythromycin levels and one report of erythromycin-induced deafness.

**Related Drugs:** Although documentation is lacking, based on the postulated mechanism and pharmacologic and structural similarity a similar interaction would be expected to occur between cimetidine and the other macrolide antibiotics (except azithromycin) and between erythromycin and the other $H_2$ receptor antagonists.

**Mechanism:** It is thought that cimetidine may have increased erythromycin levels by inhibiting the metabolism of erythromycin at the cytochrome P450 site or by increasing erythromycin absorption from the gastrointestinal tract.

**Detailed Information:** See *EDI*, 8/21.50

## Erythromycin-Cyclosporine

**Significance:** 1—highly clinically significant

**Potential Effects:** Erythromycin causes an increase in cyclosporine levels, which can lead to nephrotoxicity and neurotoxicity.

**Recommendations:** Concurrent used of these agents should be avoided. Monitor cyclosporine levels and renal function if these agents must be used together.

**Summary:** There are data to show that erythromycin causes an increase in cyclosporine levels, and this interaction may lead to nephrotoxicity and neurotoxicity.

**Related Drugs:** A similar interaction may occur between cyclosporine and other macrolide antibiotics. There are no drugs related to cyclosporine.

**Mechanism:** Erythromycin may inhibit the hepatic metabolism of cyclosporine.

**Detailed Information:** See *EDI*, 8/22.01

## Erythromycin-Ergotamine

**Significance:** 2—moderately clinically significant

**Potential Effects:** The concurrent use of these agents may result in the development of the clinical signs of ergotism.

**Recommendations:** If clinical signs of ergotism develop during concurrent administration of these agents, one or both drugs may need to be discontinued and the patient treated symptomatically. It has been shown that nitroprusside reduces the duration of vasospasm.

**Summary:** The concurrent administration of erythromycin and ergotamine may result in the development of the clinical signs of ergotism as evidenced by peripheral vasospasm, dysesthesia, and renal ischemia. This effect occurred with small doses of ergotamine (1.2–2 mg). Concurrent erythromycin and ergotamine may also result in lower extremity ischemia.

**Related Drugs:** Concurrent use of ergotamine and troleandomycin has been reported to cause peripheral vasospasm. A similar interaction occurred between ergotamine and oleandomycin. Dihydroergotamine, administered concurrently with erythromycin, troleandomycin, or ponsinomycin has shown similar results. The concurrent administration of erythromycin and bromocriptine resulted in a 268% increase in bromocriptine area-under-curve and a 4.6-fold increase in bromocriptine maximum concentration. An interaction between erythromycin and the other ergot alkaloids may be expected to occur.

## Anti-infective

**Mechanism:** The mechanism is unknown. Erythromycin may interfere with the hepatic metabolism of ergotamine. It has been shown in animal models that the cytochrome $P450_{3A1}$ isozyme induced by macrolides is similar to the metabolite-cytochrome P450 complex formed by macrolides that impairs the metabolism of dihydroergotamine.
**Detailed Information:** See *EDI,* 8/22.03

### Erythromycin-Terfenadine

**Significance:** 1—highly clinically significant
**Potential Effects:** Concurrent use of these agents may result in increased terfenadine levels with cardiotoxicity.
**Recommendations:** The concurrent use of these agents is contraindicated according to the manufacturer's package insert for terfenadine. Loratadine or cetirizine may be alternatives to terfenadine; azithromycin may be an alternative to erythromycin.
**Summary:** Concurrent erythromycin and terfenadine may result in increased terfenadine levels and possible cardiotoxicity, studies have shown.
**Related Drugs:** There have been reports of serious cardiac events with concomitant troleandomycin and terfenadine. Similar cardiac events have been reported with concomitant terfenadine and josamycin. Clarithromycin may interact with terfenadine in a manner similar to erythromycin, but azithromycin does not interact with terfenadine. Though erythromycin caused a significant increase in loratidine concentration, there were no statistically significant changes in any electrocardiogram parameter, including $QT_c$ interval. Although documentation is lacking, based on the proposed mechanism and structural and pharmacologic similarity a similar interaction would be expected to occur between terfenadine or astemizole and other macrolide antibiotics.
**Mechanism:** It is postulated that erythromycin and clarithromycin inhibit the cytochrome P450 metabolism of terfenadine and astemizole, thus allowing an increase in plasma levels. The cardiac changes produced by elevated levels of terfenadine and astemizole may be due to the ability of terfenadine and astemizole to inhibit the delayed rectifier potassium channel.
**Detailed Information:** See *EDI,* 8/22.07

### Ethambutol-Aluminum Hydroxide

**Significance:** 3—minimally clinically significant
**Recommendations:** The results of a study do not indicate that the concomitant administration of aluminum hydroxide and ethambutol should be avoided. Should a patient receiving these agents exhibit a reduced antitubercular effectiveness, the possibility of this interaction should be considered.
**Summary:** Aluminum hydroxide may delay or reduce the absorption of ethambutol.
**Related Drugs:** Other antacids containing aluminum salts may delay the absorption of ethambutol.
**Mechanism:** Aluminum hydroxide is thought to reduce ethambutol absorption by delaying gastric emptying.
**Detailed Information:** See *EDI,* 8/22.10

### Furazolidone-Amphetamine

**Significance:** 1—highly clinically significant
**Recommendations:** Tyramine containing foods, amphetamines, other indirect acting sympathomimetic agents, and mixed acting sympathomimetics are contraindicated in patients receiving furazolidone.
**Summary:** Furazolidone has a progressive and generalized monoamine oxidase inhibition, and concurrent administration of amphetamine could result in a hypertensive crisis.

**Related Drugs:** Tyramine has been reported to interact with furazolidone. Other sympathomimetics may have the potential for interacting with furazolidone. Other monoamine oxidase inhibitors have been shown to interact with indirect-acting sympathomimetics (see also Tranylcypromine-Phenylpropanolamine, page 159). Procarbazine may be expected to interact similarly.

**Mechanism:** Inhibition of monoamine oxidase by furazolidone causes a supersensitivity to amphetamine because of an increased amount of norepinephrine released.

**Detailed Information:** See *EDI*, 8/23.00

## Gentamicin-Carbenicillin

**Significance:** 1—highly clinically significant

**Recommendations:** To prevent *in vitro* inactivation, the antibiotics should not be mixed in infusion fluids. There apparently is no contraindication for using these agents together in patients with normal renal function. For patients with renal failure, the dosage of the aminoglycoside and the penicillin must be adjusted for renal impairment and the serum levels of both agents should be monitored. Concurrent use of neomycin and orally administered penicillins should be avoided.

**Summary:** Concurrent gentamicin and carbenicillin are more effective against certain susceptible organisms than either drug alone; however, gentamicin can be significantly diminished if mixed with carbenicillin *in vitro*.

**Related Drugs:** Carbenicillin and ticarcillin have been reported to cause the *in vitro* inactivation of sisomicin, netilmicin, tobramycin, amikacin and gentamicin. Ampicillin and penicillin G decrease gentamicin activity when mixed *in vitro*.

**Mechanism:** Semisynthetic penicillins chemically interact with aminoglycosides forming biologically inactive amides.

**Detailed Information:** See *EDI*, 8/25.00

## Gentamicin-Cephalothin

**Significance:** 1—highly clinically significant

**Recommendations:** Patients receiving these drugs concurrently should be observed and monitored closely for signs of nephrotoxicity. High doses of either antibiotic given over an extended period should be avoided. If the concurrent use of these drugs is chosen, the dosage should be based on renal function.

**Summary:** Concurrent use of gentamicin and cephalothin have been associated with an increased risk of nephrotoxicity, acute renal failure and the development of an acquired Fanconi syndrome.

**Related Drugs:** Tobramycin and cephalothin have increased risks of nephrotoxicity. Tobramycin and moxalactam have resulted in a increase in tobramycin clearance. Gentamicin and cephalexin were shown to cause hypokalemia. Other aminoglycosides may interact similarly with cephalothin and other cephalosporins.

**Mechanism:** Gentamicin appears to affect the proximal tubule, and cephalothin may cause acute tubular necrosis. These actions may be additive or there may be a mutual enhancement of toxicity.

**Detailed Information:** See *EDI*, 8/27.00

## Gentamicin-Indomethacin

**Significance:** 2—moderately clinically significant

**Potential Effects:** Indomethacin may decrease the glomerular filtration rate, which may increase gentamicin levels and the risk of nephrotoxicity.

**Recommendations:** Aminoglycoside levels should be closely monitored during concomitant indomethacin therapy and the aminoglycoside dose decreased if necessary. It was suggested that the aminoglycoside dose be decreased prior to indomethacin administration.

**Summary:** There are data to show that administration of indomethacin may decrease the glomerular filtration rate, increasing gentamicin levels and the risk of nephrotoxicity.

**Related Drugs:** Amikacin and indomethacin were shown to exhibit a similar interaction. A similar interaction may occur between indomethacin and other aminoglycosides and between gentamicin and other NSAIAs.

**Mechanism:** Aminoglycoside elimination is dependent on glomerular filtration rate, and indomethacin has been shown to reduce this.

**Detailed Information:** See *EDI*, 8/28.10

## Gentamicin-Polymyxin B

**Significance:** 2—moderately clinically significant

**Recommendations:** With rare exception, the combination of these two drugs can, and should, be avoided because of the availability of safer, less toxic combinations. If the interaction does occur, the patient should be supported, as necessary, until the effects dissipate.

**Summary:** Both gentamicin and polymyxin B may cause nephrotoxicity and neuromuscular blockade; the combination of the two drugs may increase the risk of these side effects.

**Related Drugs:** Kanamycin and polymyxin resulted in an apneic episode. Neomycin, streptomycin, and kanamycin appear to have the greatest potential for causing neuromuscular blockade; gentamicin and tobramycin are less likely. The potential for other aminoglycosides to cause neuromuscular blockade and nephrotoxicity exists. The polypeptide antibiotics are nephrotoxic.

**Mechanism:** The toxicities of these two groups of drugs are additive.

**Detailed Information:** See *EDI*, 8/29.00

## Gentamicin-Vancomycin

**Significance:** 3—minimally clinically significant

**Potential Effects:** The concomitant use of these agents may result in increased nephrotoxicity. However, two studies found no increase in nephrotoxicity with concomitant administration.

**Recommendations:** Monitor drug levels and renal function closely during concurrent therapy with these agents. By proper dosing, it may be possible to avert, minimize or reverse nephrotoxicity. Further study of this interaction is needed.

**Summary:** Concurrent vancomycin and gentamicin have been shown to cause nephrotoxicity; however, not all data support this.

**Related Drugs:** Vancomycin with tobramycin or amikacin have shown a similar interaction. A similar interaction may occur between vancomycin and other parenteral aminoglycosides. There are no drugs related to vancomycin.

**Mechanism:** Nephrotoxicity is an additive or synergistic effect of vancomycin and the aminoglycoside.

**Detailed Information:** See *EDI*, 8/30.01

## Griseofulvin-Cyclosporine

**Significance:** 3—minimally clinically significant

**Potential Effects:** The addition of griseofulvin to a cyclosporine regimen may result in decreased cyclosporine blood levels.

**Recommendations:** Patients maintained on cyclosporine should be carefully monitored for changes in cyclosporine blood levels and possible precipitation of rejection events or toxicity if griseofulvin is added to therapy or discontinued. The dose of cyclosporine may need to be adjusted.

## Anti-infective

**Summary:** The addition of griseofulvin to a cyclosporine regimen resulted in decreased cyclosporine blood levels.
**Related Drugs:** There are no drugs related to cyclosporine or griseofulvin.
**Mechanism:** The mechanism of this interaction is not known.
**Detailed Information:** See *EDI*, 8/30.05

### Griseofulvin-Oral Contraceptive Agents

**Significance:** 2—moderately clinically significant
**Potential Effects:** Griseofulvin may increase the metabolism of oral contraceptive agents, leading to breakthrough bleeding and loss of contraceptive effectiveness.
**Recommendations:** The concomitant use of these agents need not be avoided. However, the potential for reduced contraceptive efficacy should be a consideration when these drugs are used concurrently.
**Summary:** Griseofulvin may increase the metabolism of oral contraceptive agents, leading to breakthrough bleeding and loss of contraceptive effectiveness.
**Related Drugs:** There are no drugs related to griseofulvin.
**Mechanism:** Griseofulvin may induce the metabolism of the oral contraceptive agents, with a corresponding decrease in estrogen concentration.
**Detailed Information:** See *EDI*, 8/30.10

### Griseofulvin-Phenobarbital

**Significance:** 3—minimally clinically significant
**Recommendations:** The clinical course of patients taking griseofulvin and phenobarbital concurrently should be closely followed. If the clinical response is inadequate, the dose of griseofulvin may need to be increased.
**Summary:** Administration of phenobarbital may decrease serum levels of griseofulvin.
**Related Drugs:** The effect of concurrent administration of other barbiturates on serum griseofulvin levels has not been studied.
**Mechanism:** Phenobarbital may induce enzymes, increasing the metabolism of the griseofulvin.
**Detailed Information:** See *EDI*, 8/31.00

### Imipenem, Cilastatin-Cyclosporine

**Significance:** 2—moderately clinically significant
**Potential Effects:** The concomitant administration of imipenem-cilastatin and cyclosporine may result in mental disturbances as well as changes in cyclosporine serum levels.
**Recommendations:** Patients receiving concomitant therapy with these agents should be monitored for disturbances of the central nervous system (CNS) and changes in cyclosporine levels. The dosage of cyclosporine may need to be adjusted, or imipenem-cilastatin may need to be discontinued.
**Summary:** The concomitant administration of imipenem-cilastatin and cyclosporine resulted in mental disturbances (including confused states, agitation, intensive tremor, seizures, myoclonus, and jacksonian fits) as well as increases in cyclosporine blood levels, although conflicting data in animals indicate concurrent administration results in decreasing cyclosporine levels. Another study showed that the administration of the imipenem-cilastatin with cyclosporine may result in a decrease in cyclosporine-related nephrotoxicity.
**Related Drugs:** There are no drugs related to imipenem-cilastatin or cyclosporine.

Anti-infective

**Mechanism:** The mechanism is unknown. However, both imipenem and cyclosporine alone are known to produce CNS disturbances, and it is possible the metabolism of cyclosporine is inhibited by imipenem, resulting in increased cyclosporine levels and side effects. The mechanism of decreased cyclosporine-related nephrotoxicity may be the result of a decrease in cyclosporine levels caused by imipenem-cilastatin or a decrease in tubular uptake of cyclosporine caused by cilastatin.

**Detailed Information:** See *EDI*, 8/32.10

## Isoniazid-Aluminum Hydroxide

**Significance:** 3—minimally clinically significant

**Recommendations:** Single high doses of isoniazid are more effective in arresting tuberculosis than the same amount of drug in divided doses. Although the clinical significance of this interaction is not known, high peak serum concentrations of isoniazid appear to be important in antitubercular therapy. Therefore, isoniazid should be administered at least one hour before antacid administration.

**Summary:** Administration of aluminum hydroxide may decrease the peak serum levels and delay or decrease the absorption of isoniazid.

**Related Drugs:** It is difficult to determine whether an interaction would occur between isoniazid and other antacids. There are no drugs related to isoniazid.

**Mechanism:** Aluminum hydroxide delays gastric emptying and causes retention of isoniazid in the stomach, causing lower peak serum concentrations.

**Detailed Information:** See *EDI*, 8/33.00

## Isoniazid-Chlorzoxazone

**Significance:** 3—minimally clinically significant

**Potential Effects:** Isoniazid increased the chlorzoxazone area-under-curve (AUC) and prolonged the chlorzoxazone elimination half-life.

**Recommendations:** Patients maintained on chlorzoxazone should be monitored for changes in chlorzoxazone serum levels if isoniazid is added to or discontinued from concurrent therapy. The dose of chlorzoxazone may need to be adjusted.

**Summary:** Isoniazid may increase the chlorzoxazone AUC and prolong the chlorzoxazone elimination half-life.

**Related Drugs:** There are no drugs related to isoniazid or chlorzoxazone.

**Mechanism:** It has been postulated that the inhibition of chlorzoxazone metabolism results from the effect of isoniazid on the cytochrome $P450_{2E1}$ isozyme.

**Detailed Information:** See *EDI*, 8/34.00

## Isoniazid-Disulfiram

**Significance:** 3—minimally clinically significant

**Recommendations:** Until further documentation is provided, patients receiving isoniazid and disulfiram concurrently should be monitored for the occurrence of central nervous system (CNS) effects such as dizziness, irritability, lethargy, and uncoordination. If these signs or symptoms occur, dosage reduction or discontinuation of disulfiram should be considered.

**Summary:** The concurrent use of isoniazid and disulfiram has been reported to result in adverse CNS effects.

**Related Drugs:** There are no drugs related to isoniazid or disulfiram.

**Mechanism:** The combination of isoniazid and disulfiram results in altered dopamine metabolism in the brain, resulting in an accumulation of methylated byproducts.

**Detailed Information:** See *EDI*, 8/35.00

Anti-infective

## Isoniazid-Meperidine

**Significance:** 3—minimally clinically significant

**Recommendations:** Patients should be monitored for adverse reactions during concurrent use of these agents. If lethargy or hypotension occurs, meperidine may need to be discontinued. Also, since morphine was shown not to interact in a particular patient, it may be considered as a suitable alternative to meperidine.

**Summary:** There are data to show that coadministration of these agents has caused lethargy and hypotension.

**Related Drugs:** There are no drugs related to isoniazid. Documentation is lacking regarding a similar interaction between isoniazid and other narcotic analgesics.

**Mechanism:** The mechanism of this interaction is unknown.

**Detailed Information:** See *EDI*, 8/37.00

## Isoniazid-Prednisolone

**Significance:** 3—minimally clinically significant

**Recommendations:** If concurrent administration of isoniazid and prednisolone is necessary, the dose of isoniazid may need to be increased.

**Summary:** There are data to show that administration of prednisolone lowered isoniazid plasma levels.

**Related Drugs:** A similar interaction may occur between isoniazid and other corticosteroids. There are no drugs related to isoniazid.

**Mechanism:** Prednisolone may increase the hepatic metabolism and/or renal clearance of isoniazid.

**Detailed Information:** See *EDI*, 8/39.00

## Isoniazid-Propranolol

**Significance:** 3—minimally clinically significant

**Potential Effects:** Propranolol may decrease the clearance of isoniazid.

**Recommendations:** Until further clinical studies are done, the concurrent administration of propranolol and isoniazid need not be avoided. However, patients should be monitored since a decreased dose of isoniazid may be necessary.

**Summary:** There are data to show that administration of propranolol may decrease the clearance of isoniazid.

**Related Drugs:** A similar interaction is expected to occur with the beta-blocking agents that are not extensively hepatically metabolized, if the mechanism involves inhibition of the metabolism of isoniazid by propranolol. It is not known if the other beta-blocking agents that are extensively metabolized in the liver would interact with isoniazid. There are no drugs related to isoniazid.

**Mechanism:** Propranolol may inhibit the acetylation of isoniazid in the liver.

**Detailed Information:** See *EDI*, 8/40.10

## Isoniazid-Pyridoxine

**Significance:** 3—minimally clinically significant

**Potential Effects:** Pyridoxine may reduce the antitubercular effects of isoniazid. Peripheral neuropathy may be increased.

**Recommendations:** Concurrent administration of pyridoxine and isoniazid does not reduce the effectiveness of isoniazid in eradicating tubercle bacilli. The use of concurrent pyridoxine-isoniazid therapy is currently advocated; however, caution should be observed for possible paradoxical vitamin $B_6$ deficiency.

**Summary:** There are data to show that pyridoxine may reduce the antitubercular effects of isoniazid. Peripheral neuropathy may be increased.

**Related Drugs:** There are no drugs related to isoniazid or pyridoxine.

## Anti-infective

**Mechanism:** An excess of the pyridoxine moiety may saturate the activating enzymes, resulting in paradoxical vitamin $B_6$ deficiency.
**Detailed Information:** See *EDI*, 8/41.00

## Isoniazid-Rifampin

**Significance:** 2—moderately clinically significant
**Potential Effects:** Incidence of hepatotoxicity may be increased when taking these agents together.
**Recommendations:** Patients should be aware of the signs and symptoms of hepatotoxicity when taking these agents concurrently. In children, limiting the isoniazid dose to 10 mg/kg and the rifampin dose to 15 mg/kg may help to minimize the toxicity.
**Summary:** Rifampin is frequently combined with isoniazid to treat tuberculosis; however, hepatotoxicity has been reported to occur more frequently.
**Related Drugs:** There are no drugs related to rifampin or isoniazid.
**Mechanism:** Liver damage caused by isoniazid is related to formation of hepatotoxic metabolites and is enhanced by enzyme-inducing drugs such as rifampin.
**Detailed Information:** See *EDI*, 8/43.00

## Isoniazid-Stavudine

**Significance:** 3—minimally clinically significant
**Potential Effects:** An increased incidence of sensory peripheral neuropathy may occur with concurrent stavudine and isoniazid.
**Recommendations:** It is recommended that when treating HIV and tuberculosis co-infection with isoniazid, the concomitant use of stavudine-containing regimens should be avoided. Patients receiving concurrent isoniazid and antiretroviral regimens should be monitored for distal sensory neuropathy (DSN).
**Summary:** An increased incidence of DSN occurred with concurrent stavudine and isoniazid. Symptoms included paresthesia, numbness, and tingling in the distal extremities with a diminished sensation to pinprick and vibration and loss of ankle jerks.
**Related Drugs:** It is not known whether a similar interaction would occur between isoniazid and the other nucleoside reverse transcriptase inhibitors. There are no drugs related to isoniazid.
**Mechanism:** Isoniazid can produce DSN, although this is rare with concurrent use of pyridoxine. Stavudine has been shown to produce DSN in up to 20% of patients at standard doses. There may be a synergistic effect on stavudine's potential to cause DSN.
**Detailed Information:** See *EDI*, 8/44.10

## Itraconazole-Buspirone

**Significance:** 3—minimally clinically significant
**Potential Effects:** Concurrent administration of buspirone and itraconazole may result in elevated levels of buspirone and a slight increase in buspirone-related adverse effects.
**Recommendations:** Although the pharmacodynamic changes in a single dose study were small, it would be prudent to reduce the dosage of buspirone during concomitant administration of itraconazole. Buspirone may exhibit nonlinear pharmacokinetics, thus elevations of buspirone during concomitant administration of itraconazole with multiple doses of buspirone may be more dramatic.
**Summary:** Concurrent administration of buspirone with itraconazole resulted in elevated buspirone maximum concentration by thirteenfold and a slight increase in buspirone-related adverse effects.
**Related Drugs:** Based on the proposed mechanism, an interaction would be expected to occur between buspirone and the other systemic azole antifungal agents.

## Anti-infective

**Mechanism:** Buspirone undergoes extensive first-pass metabolism. It is postulated that itraconazole inhibits the metabolism of buspirone at the cytochrome $P450_{3A4}$ isoenzyme.

**Detailed Information:** See *EDI*, 8/44.15

## Itraconazole-Didanosine

**Significance:** 2—moderately clinically significant

**Potential Effects:** Concurrent didanosine and itraconazole may result in decreased absorption of itraconazole.

**Recommendations:** It would be prudent to administer these two agents at least two hours apart. Itraconazole serum levels should be monitored to insure that levels remain within a range that will not lead to treatment failure.

**Summary:** Decreased itraconazole absorption occurred when coadministered with didanosine, resulting in decreased itraconazole levels and clinical effect.

**Related Drugs:** Ketoconazole has been reported to decrease the absorption of didanosine, but the reverse has not been shown. Based on structural and pharmacologic similarity and the postulated mechanism, an interaction would be expected to occur between didanosine and the other imidazole antifungal agents. It is unknown whether other antiretroviral agents will interact with itraconazole or the other imidazole antifungals.

**Mechanism:** Ketoconazole and itraconazole require an acidic media for predictable dissolution to occur, and solubility decreases as pH increases. Didanosine is formulated to prevent destruction by gastric acid. This formulation can cause an increase in gastric pH; thus a decrease in solubility and absorption of itraconazole may be expected.

**Detailed Information:** See *EDI*, 8/44.30

## Kanamycin-Ethacrynic Acid

**Significance:** 1—highly clinically significant

**Recommendations:** The concurrent use of these agents should be avoided whenever possible. Extreme caution as well as dose reduction and continuous monitoring of eighth cranial nerve function should be followed if concurrent administration is necessary.

**Summary:** Concurrent administration of kanamycin and ethacrynic acid may result in an increased incidence of ototoxic effects.

**Related Drugs:** Ethacrynic acid and other aminoglycoside antibiotics have been reported to interact in a similar manner. Bumetanide and furosemide have been reported to interact with the aminoglycosides, causing transient to permanent hearing problems.

**Mechanism:** A possible synergistic ototoxic effect may be involved with these two agents, or there may be a reduced antibiotic clearance.

**Detailed Information:** See *EDI*, 8/45.00

## Ketoconazole-Aluminum Hydroxide, Magnesium Hydroxide

**Significance:** 2—moderately clinically significant

**Potential Effects:** Concurrent administration of ketoconazole with an antacid may decrease ketoconazole absorption.

**Recommendations:** A prudent regimen would be to administer the two agents as far apart as possible. Since there is no information on how long antacids affect intragastric pH, antacids should be administered after ketoconazole dosages.

**Summary:** Concurrent administration of ketoconazole with an antacid decreased ketoconazole absorption. In one study, ketoconazole area-under-curve was decreased by 41% when given with the

Anti-infective

antacid combination compared with ketoconazole administration in the fasting state.

**Related Drugs:** The administration of sodium bicarbonate, alone and with aluminum hydroxide, has resulted in subtherapeutic concentrations of ketoconazole and treatment failure. Administration of a single dose of fluconazole with an antacid containing aluminum hydroxide and magnesium hydroxide resulted in no statistically significant changes in fluconazole pharmacokinetics when compared to fluconazole administration alone. Although other antacids may also interfere with the absorption of ketoconazole and fluconazole, documentation is lacking. It is not known if the other azole antifungal agents would interact with antacids.

**Mechanism:** Ketoconazole requires acidic media for predictable dissolution to occur, and solubility decreases as pH increases. The antacid presumably increases the intragastric pH, thereby decreasing dissolution and subsequent absorption.

**Detailed Information:** See *EDI*, 8/47.00

## Ketoconazole-Cimetidine

**Significance:** 2—moderately clinically significant

**Potential Effects:** Concurrent administration of ketoconazole with cimetidine may result in decreased absorption of ketoconazole.

**Recommendations:** In patients receiving concurrent therapy with ketoconazole and an $H_2$ receptor antagonist, consider monitoring ketoconazole levels. The dosage of ketoconazole may need to be increased or the $H_2$ receptor antagonist may need to be discontinued.

**Summary:** Concurrent administration of ketoconazole and cimetidine resulted in decreased absorption of ketoconazole. Administration of ketoconazole in an acidified solution two hours after cimetidine increased ketoconazole levels when compared to ketoconazole administration alone and with cimetidine.

**Related Drugs:** Ranitidine has shown a similar interaction with ketoconazole. An interaction between ketoconazole and the other $H_2$ receptor antagonists would be expected to occur. It is not known whether an interaction would occur between cimetidine and the other imidazole antifungal agents. The administration of fluconazole with cimetidine resulted in no significant interactions. It is not known whether an interaction would occur between the parenterally administered $H_2$ receptor antagonists and the imidazole antifungal agents.

**Mechanism:** Ketoconazole requires acidic media for predictable dissolution to occur, and solubility decreases as pH increases. The $H_2$ receptor antagonist increases the intragastric pH, thereby decreasing dissolution and subsequent absorption of ketoconazole.

**Detailed Information:** See *EDI*, 8/48.50

## Ketoconazole-Cyclosporine

**Significance:** 1—highly clinically significant

**Potential Effects:** Ketoconazole may cause an increase in cyclosporine levels.

**Recommendations:** Avoid using these agents together. If they are used together, monitor cyclosporine levels and renal function.

**Summary:** There are data to show that administration of ketoconazole may cause an increase in cyclosporine levels. Because cyclosporine alone is nephrotoxic, the combination of these agents may lead to an increased risk of nephrotoxicity.

**Related Drugs:** Similar interactions have been reported with itraconazole and fluconazole. A similar interaction may occur between other systemic imidazole antifungal agents and cyclosporine. There are no drugs related to cyclosporine.

## Anti-infective

**Mechanism:** This interaction may be due to an increase in cyclosporine absorption, competition for hepatic biotransformation, competition for cell-binding sites, ketoconazole-induced inhibition of hepatic metabolism, or competition for an excretion pathway.
**Detailed Information:** See *EDI*, 8/49.00

### Ketoconazole-Methylprednisolone

**Significance:** 2—moderately clinically significant
**Potential Effects:** Ketoconazole inhibits the metabolism of methylprednisolone, which may result in enhanced methylprednisolone side effects. Ketoconazole may also enhance the cortisol suppressive effects of methylprednisolone.
**Recommendations:** Patients should be monitored for enhanced adverse effects of methylprednisolone when receiving concurrent ketoconazole. The dose of methylprednisolone may need to be decreased. One report recommends reducing the methylprednisolone dose by 50% when used with ketoconazole.
**Summary:** There are data to show that administration of ketoconazole may inhibit the metabolism of methylprednisolone, resulting in enhanced methylprednisolone side effects.
**Related Drugs:** Ketoconazole was reported to increase plasma prednisolone. A similar interaction may occur with methylprednisolone and ketoconazole and other corticosteroids. There are no drugs related to ketoconazole.
**Mechanism:** Ketoconazole may inhibit the hepatic metabolism of methylprednisolone.
**Detailed Information:** See *EDI*, 8/50.01

### Ketoconazole-Omeprazole

**Significance:** 2—moderately clinically significant
**Potential Effects:** The concurrent administration of ketoconazole and omeprazole may result in decreased ketoconazole absorption.
**Recommendations:** Ketoconazole serum levels should be monitored in patients receiving concurrent ketoconazole and omeprazole. The dosage of ketoconazole may need to be increased or omeprazole may need to be discontinued. Administration of an acidic beverage with ketoconazole may improve ketoconazole absorption in some patients.
**Summary:** The concurrent administration of ketoconazole and a single dose of omeprazole resulted in decreased ketoconazole absorption. Area-under-curve and maximum concentration decreased by 98.9% and 99%, respectively, when compared to ketoconazole administration alone.
**Related Drugs:** The administration of a single dose of fluconazole on day seven of omeprazole treatment resulted in no significant changes in fluconazole. It is not known whether an interaction would be expected to occur between omeprazole and the other imidazole antifungal agents. An interaction between ketoconazole and the other proton pump inhibitors would be expected to occur.
**Mechanism:** Ketoconazole requires acidic media for predictable dissolution to occur, and solubility decreases as pH increases. Omeprazole increases the intragastric pH, thereby decreasing dissolution and subsequent absorption.
**Detailed Information:** See *EDI*, 8/50.06

### Ketoconazole-Rifampin

**Significance:** 2—moderately clinically significant
**Potential Effects:** Concurrent administration of ketoconazole and rifampin may result in decreased ketoconazole serum levels and efficacy.

**Recommendations:** It is important to monitor the patient for a decrease in ketoconazole efficacy when rifampin is added. Administering the two agents at separate times (at least 12 hours apart) appears to prevent the decrease in rifampin but not ketoconazole serum levels. Concurrent fluconazole and rifabutin may offer an alternative.

**Summary:** Concurrent rifampin and ketoconazole has been shown to result in a decrease in ketoconazole serum levels.

**Related Drugs:** Rifampin has been shown to cause a significant decrease in itraconazole serum levels with concurrent therapy. In spite of decreased itraconazole concentrations with rifabutin, this combination has been reported to be potentially synergistic when used to treat cryptococcoses. A similar interaction resulting in decreased fluconazole concentrations has been reported with concomitant rifampin. Patients receiving concurrent rifabutin and fluconazole showed a decrease in the incidence of *Mycobacterium avium* bacteremia. There was an increase in the incidence of leukopenia with combination therapy compared to rifabutin alone. Although no documentation exists, because of structural and pharmacological similarities an interaction may be expected to occur between rifampin or rifabutin and the other imidazole antifungal agents.

**Mechanism:** It has been suggested that rifampin increased the metabolism of ketoconazole. It is possible that ketoconazole interfered with the absorption of rifampin. Fluconazole is a potent inhibitor of cytochrome P450 hepatic enzyme systems. It has been noted to increase both the maximum concentration and area-under-curve of rifabutin and its D-acetyl metabolite.

**Detailed Information:** See *EDI*, 8/50.10

## Ketoconazole-Sucralfate

**Significance:** 3—minimally clinically significant

**Potential Effects:** Concurrent sucralfate and ketoconazole may decrease ketoconazole bioavailability.

**Recommendations:** It has been suggested that, in some patients, clinical failure of therapy may be associated with the concomitant administration of sucralfate and ketoconazole. It is recommended that the administration of sucralfate and ketoconazole be separated by as much time as possible to decrease the potential effect of sucralfate on ketoconazole bioavailability.

**Summary:** Concurrent sucralfate and ketoconazole resulted in decreased ketoconazole bioavailability.

**Related drugs:** It is not known whether an interaction would occur between sucralfate and other imidazole antifungal agents or between ketoconazole and other aluminum salts.

**Mechanism:** The mechanism of this interaction is not known, but it is not pH related.

**Detailed Information:** See *EDI*, 8/50.40

## Ketoconazole-Terfenadine

**Significance:** 1—highly clinically significant

**Potential Effects:** Concurrent use of ketoconazole (or itraconazole) and terfenadine will result in a decrease in the metabolism and clearance of terfenadine, resulting in increased levels and cardiotoxicity.

**Recommendations:** The concurrent use of terfenadine or astemizole with either ketoconazole or itraconazole is contraindicated according to the manufacturers' product information for these agents. Loratadine or cetirizine may be alternatives to terfenadine or astemizole.

## Anti-infective

**Summary:** The addition of ketoconazole to terfenadine therapy has resulted in elevations in levels of terfenadine. The resulting increase in terfenadine serum levels has been associated with occurrence of torsades de pointes arrhythmia and a risk of sudden cardiac death.

**Related Drugs:** Itraconazole and terfenadine have been reported to cause a similar arrhythmia. Ketoconazole was shown to be an inhibitor of *in vitro* astemizole metabolism. Based on the postulated mechanism, concurrent ketoconazole and loratadine may be expected to result in elevated levels of loratadine; however, no electrocardiographic changes have been reported. Fluconazole may not cause arrhythmias when combined with terfenadine. Although documentation is lacking regarding an interaction between the piperidine $H_1$ receptor antagonists and the other imidazole antifungal agents, an interaction may be expected to occur based on the postulated mechanism and structural similarity.

**Mechanism:** Ketoconazole has been shown to inhibit drug metabolism possibly by inhibition of the cytochrome P450 enzyme system. Terfenadine is metabolized to a great degree by the liver, presumably by cytochrome P450 oxidative metabolism. It is thought that the arrhythmia experienced by patients was due to an increase in serum concentration of either terfenadine or its acid metabolite.

**Detailed Information:** See *EDI*, 8/50.60

### Lincomycin-Erythromycin

**Significance:** 3—minimally clinically significant

**Recommendations:** Although there are insufficient data to conclude that an interaction occurs between lincomycin and erythromycin, the clinician should be aware of the possibility of the development of cross interference. This may offset any therapeutic advantage of combining these agents. If possible, concurrent use of lincomycin and erythromycin should be avoided.

**Summary:** Erythromycin can theoretically antagonize the activity of lincomycin by blocking access to ribosomal binding sites.

**Related Drugs:** Other macrolide antibiotics and chloramphenicol may also interfere with the activity of lincomycin.

**Mechanism:** Erythromycin has a greater affinity for the 50S ribosomal unit; therefore, erythromycin could block the effects of lincomycin by displacing it from the binding site or by preventing binding.

**Detailed Information:** See *EDI*, 8/51.00

### Lincomycin-Kaolin

**Significance:** 1—highly clinically significant

**Recommendations:** In patients receiving lincomycin who require antidiarrheal therapy, products that do not contain kaolin should be considered. When a kaolin-containing product must be used, it should be given at least two hours before lincomycin.

**Summary:** Kaolin reduces the gastrointestinal absorption of lincomycin.

**Related Drugs:** Kaolin had no effect on the extent of clindamycin absorption.

**Mechanism:** The physical coating action of kaolin on the intestinal mucosa and kaolin's adsorbent property may be responsible for this interaction.

**Detailed Information:** See *EDI*, 8/53.00

### Metronidazole-Chloroquine

**Significance:** 2—moderately clinically significant

**Potential Effects:** Concurrent use of these agents may result in acute dystonic reactions.

## Anti-infective

**Recommendations:** Concurrent used of these agents should be avoided. Sulfadoxine and pyrimethamine may be used in place of chloroquine for malaria if concurrent metronidazole is to be used.

**Summary:** There are data to show that coadministration of these agents has led to acute dystonic reactions—restlessness, facial grimacing, and coarse tremors.

**Related Drugs:** A similar interaction may occur between metronidazole and hydroxychloroquine or primaquine. There are no drugs related to metronidazole.

**Mechanism:** Chloroquine and metronidazole decrease neuronal calcium uptake/availability, which may decrease dopamine levels, resulting in dystonic reactions.

**Detailed Information:** See *EDI*, 8/54.05

## Metronidazole-Cimetidine

**Significance:** 3—minimally clinically significant

**Potential Effects:** Cimetidine may inhibit the metabolism of metronidazole.

**Recommendations:** The concurrent administration of metronidazole and cimetidine need not be avoided. However, monitor for metronidazole side effects (e.g., convulsive seizures, peripheral neuropathy). The dose of metronidazole may need to be adjusted.

**Summary:** There are data to show that administration of cimetidine may inhibit the metabolism of metronidazole; however, all data do not support the existence of this interaction.

**Related Drugs:** There are no drugs related to metronidazole. A similar interaction may occur between metronidazole and other $H_2$-receptor antagonists.

**Mechanism:** Cimetidine may inhibit the hepatic metabolism of metronidazole by interfering with the microsomal cytochrome P450 mono-oxygenase system.

**Detailed Information:** See *EDI*, 8/54.10

## Metronidazole-Disulfiram

**Significance:** 2—moderately clinically significant

**Potential Effects:** Concomitant metronidazole and disulfiram may result in an alternation of the effects of disulfiram, which may include acute psychosis, confusion, or visual and auditory hallucinations.

**Recommendations:** Concurrent administration of these agents should be avoided if possible. If concurrent use is necessary, one or both drugs may need to be discontinued if symptoms occur.

**Summary:** There are data to show that administration of metronidazole may result in an alteration of the effects of disulfiram, which may include acute psychosis, confusion, or visual and auditory hallucinations.

**Related Drugs:** A similar interaction may occur between metronidazole and calcium carbamide and monosulfiram and between disulfiram and anti-infective agents related to metronidazole.

**Mechanism:** Metronidazole may have an attenuated disulfiram effect.

**Detailed Information:** See *EDI*, 8/55.00

## Metronidazole-Phenobarbital

**Significance:** 2—moderately clinically significant

**Potential Effects:** Phenobarbital may increase the hepatic metabolism of metronidazole, resulting in decreased levels of metronidazole.

**Recommendations:** Patients receiving metronidazole therapy should be observed for a lack of, or a decrease in, antimicrobial response during the concurrent administration of phenobarbital. An increased dose of metronidazole may be necessary.

**Summary:** There are data to show that administration of phenobarbital may increase the hepatic metabolism of metronidazole, resulting in decreased levels of metronidazole.

**Related Drugs:** A similar interaction may occur between metronidazole and other barbiturates. There are no drugs related to metronidazole.

**Mechanism:** Phenobarbital, a known hepatic enzyme inducer, increases the hepatic metabolism of metronidazole.

**Detailed Information:** See *EDI*, 8/57.00

## Nitrofurantoin-Magnesium Trisilicate

**Significance:** 3—minimally clinically significant

**Recommendations:** Although concurrent use of these agents need not be avoided, it may be best to separate their administration by as much time as possible. The dose of nitrofurantoin may need to be increased.

**Summary:** Administration of magnesium trisilicate was shown to result in a decrease in both the rate and extent of nitrofurantoin absorption, and this may result in a decrease in antimicrobial effectiveness.

**Related Drugs:** Aluminum hydroxide, magnesium carbonate, and magnesium hydroxide decreased nitrofurantoin absorption. Because of variable results, it is difficult to determine whether an interaction would occur between nitrofurantoin and other antacids. There are no drugs related to nitrofurantoin.

**Mechanism:** The decreased gastrointestinal absorption of nitrofurantoin may be due to its subsequent slow and incomplete release from the antacid surface.

**Detailed Information:** See *EDI*, 8/58.10

## Nitrofurantoin-Probenecid

**Significance:** 3—minimally clinically significant

**Recommendations:** The significance of this interaction is difficult to determine for several reasons. Reports of a nitrofurantoin-probenecid interaction in clinical practice have been sparse. Second, the lower doses of probenecid frequently used in clinical practice would not exert as great an effect on nitrofurantoin excretion and systemic accumulation as the doses of 500 to 1000 mg every two hours used experimentally. An additional factor for consideration involves renal dysfunction. Systemic accumulation and decreased urinary excretion of nitrofurantoin occurred in patients in whom serum creatinine levels were greater than about 2.5 to 3 mg% (normal, 0.6 to 1.2 mg%). Thus, patients with decreased renal efficiency may not be good candidates for nitrofurantoin therapy. An increase in nitrofurantoin dosage in an attempt to enhance urine levels would only serve to increase the likelihood of systemic accumulation and the adverse effects associated with increased serum levels. Thus, concurrent administration of these drugs should be avoided whenever possible.

**Summary:** Concurrent administration of probenecid decreases the renal clearance of nitrofurantoin and increases the serum levels of the nitrofurantoin, and this has been associated with the onset of polyneuropathies.

**Related Drugs:** Sulfinpyrazone may have an effect on nitrofurantoin excretion similar to that of probenecid.

**Mechanism:** Probenecid is known to inhibit the tubular secretion of many compounds and presumably exerts the same effect with nitrofurantoin.

**Detailed Information:** See *EDI*, 8/59.00

Anti-infective

## Nitrofurantoin-Propantheline
**Significance:** 3—minimally clinically significant
**Recommendations:** The concurrent use of these agents need not be avoided. However, it is prudent to separate the administration of these drugs by as much time as possible.
**Summary:** The concurrent use of nitrofurantoin and propantheline causes an increase in nitrofurantoin absorption and excretion.
**Related Drugs:** There are no drugs related to nitrofurantoin. A similar interaction may occur with other anticholinergics.
**Mechanism:** It has been suggested that propantheline decreases gastric emptying time because of its ability to reduce gastric motility, increasing nitrofurantoin bioavailability.
**Detailed Information:** See *EDI*, 8/61.00

## Norfloxacin-Sucralfate
**Significance:** 2—moderately clinically significant
**Potential Effects:** Sucralfate may decrease norfloxacin absorption, resulting in decreased levels and efficacy.
**Recommendations:** Concurrent use of these agents should be avoided.
**Summary:** The bioavailability of norfloxacin is reduced in the presence of sucralfate.
**Related Drugs:** Sulcralfate was shown to decrease the bioavailability of ciprofloxacin. It is difficult to determine if an interaction would occur with cinoxacin or nalidixic acid. There are no drugs related to sucralfate.
**Mechanism:** Reduced levels of norfloxacin may occur because of reduced gastrointestinal absorption, possibly related to the formation of inactive norfloxacin aluminum chelates.
**Detailed Information:** See *EDI*, 8/62.10

## Penicillin-Aspirin
**Significance:** 3—minimally clinically significant
**Recommendations:** The limited clinical data prevent definite assessment of the clinical significance of this drug interaction. Concurrent use of high doses of aspirin has been suggested to increase the clinical benefits of penicillin, but the possible toxicities resulting discourage such therapy.
**Summary:** Aspirin significantly increases penicillin serum concentrations and half-life.
**Related Drugs:** Aspirin has reduced the serum protein binding of cloxacillin, dicloxacillin, nafcillin, and oxacillin. There appear to be no reports that the other salicylates affect the disposition of penicillin.
**Mechanism:** Aspirin may displace penicillin from its protein binding sites, or there may be competition of the two drugs for the same renal secretory sites in the proximal tubule.
**Detailed Information:** See *EDI*, 8/63.00

## Penicillin-Chloramphenicol
**Significance:** 4—not clinically significant
**Recommendations:** There is no unequivocal clinical evidence that chloramphenicol causes any significant antagonism of the bactericidal effect of penicillin. Therefore, concurrent use of these antibiotics need not be avoided in the limited circumstances where such therapy is indicated.
**Summary:** The bacteriostatic action of chloramphenicol may antagonize the bactericidal action of penicillin; however, several variables such as the organisms involved and the doses used can affect the potential interaction.

## Anti-infective

**Related Drugs:** Administration of chloramphenicol and ampicillin and chlor-amphenicol and procaine penicillin were found to be superior treatments to chloramphenicol alone. A similar interaction may occur between chloramphenicol and other penicillins. There are no drugs related to chloramphenicol.

**Mechanism:** Chloramphenicol inhibits protein synthesis, which may mask the bactericidal action of penicillin.

**Detailed Information:** See *EDI*, 8/65.00

### Penicillin-Chlortetracycline

**Significance:** 2—moderately clinically significant

**Recommendations:** Tetracycline may cause a clinically significant antagonism of penicillin in situations where rapid bactericidal activity is necessary (e.g., pneumococcal meningitis). There is no clinical evidence supporting a penicillin-tetracycline interaction with infections where rapid bacterial kill is not critical. Even in those cases where no antagonism occurs, there is no justification for concurrent use of penicillin and tetracycline.

**Summary:** Tetracycline derivatives may antagonize the bactericidal action of penicillin G under conditions where rapid bacterial kill is desired. Increased incidence of mortality and reinfection have been reported in patients receiving chlortetracycline and penicillin G.

**Related Drugs:** Antagonism of the action of all other penicillins may be expected based on their common mechanism of action. All tetracyclines may be expected to interact in a similar manner with penicillin.

**Mechanism:** Spheroplast formation, a preceding step in the lysis of bacteria exposed to penicillin, is inhibited by tetracyclines.

**Detailed Information:** See *EDI*, 8/67.00

### Penicillin-Erythromycin

**Significance:** 3—minimally clinically significant

**Recommendations:** Penicillins should not be used routinely in combination with erythromycin. Although concurrent administration has revealed synergism, indifference and antagonism have also been reported and are most likely the result of differences in microorganisms studied and their related susceptibilities to these antibiotics. If these drugs are used concurrently, both the minimum inhibitory concentration and the minimum bactericidal concentration should be checked to ensure a synergistic bactericidal effect.

**Summary:** Concomitant usage of penicillin and erythromycin may result in synergism, antagonism, or no alteration of the combined antibacterial effect.

**Related Drugs:** Penicillin G, penicillin V, ampicillin, and methicillin have been documented to interact with erythromycin. Cephalosporins may interact with erythromycin in a similar manner.

**Mechanism:** Erythromycin exerts a bacteriostatic effect resulting in decreased bacterial cytoplasmic growth and a decreased susceptibility to cellular lysis induced by bactericidal drugs such as penicillin.

**Detailed Information:** See *EDI*, 8/69.00

### Penicillin-Probenecid

**Significance:** 3—minimally clinically significant

**Recommendations:** Complications during concurrent administration of these drugs result from increased antibiotic levels and are encountered most frequently during long-term treatment. It may be advisable to reduce the dosage of penicillin when probenecid is combined with the antibiotic and to monitor the penicillin serum levels.

**Summary:** Concurrent administration of penicillin and probenecid results in higher and more sustained serum penicillin levels.

## Anti-infective

**Related Drugs:** All penicillins may interact in a similar manner with probenecid. There are many penicillin analogs that have been reported to interact with probenecid.

**Mechanism:** Probenecid may compete with other weak organic acids and diminish tubular secretion of such compounds, or it may decrease the apparent volume of distribution, resulting in a larger penicillin fraction in the central compartment.

**Detailed Information:** See *EDI*, 8/71.00

### Penicillin V-Guar Gum

**Significance:** 3—minimally clinically significant

**Potential Effects:** The concurrent use of penicillin V and guar gum may result in decreased absorption of penicillin V, which may lead to a decrease in serum levels.

**Recommendations:** The concurrent administration of penicillin V and guar gum is not recommended. Separating the dosing of penicillin V by two to four hours from that of guar gum may help reduce the potential for decreased absorption. Patients receiving penicillin V and guar gum concurrently should be monitored for decreased penicillin V levels as well as a possible decrease in efficacy. The dose of penicillin V may need to be increased or the guar gum discontinued until the course of penicillin V is finished.

**Summary:** Concurrent use of penicillin V and guar gum resulted in decreased absorption of penicillin V and a decrease in serum levels.

**Related Drugs:** The other orally administered penicillins may be expected to interact in a similar manner with guar gum. There are no agents related to guar gum. Other common names for guar gum include guar flour and jaguar gum.

**Mechanism:** Delayed gastric emptying, along with possible mechanical interference in the small intestine caused by the guar gum, may have some effect on the penicillin V absorption.

**Detailed Information:** See *EDI*, 8/70.00

### Polymyxin B-Prochlorperazine

**Significance:** 2—moderately clinically significant

**Recommendations:** Caution should be used when concurrently administering polymyxin B and prochlorperazine or other polypeptide antibiotics and phenothiazines. Ventilatory assistance should be made available.

**Summary:** In one case report, a patient who received intravenous polymyxin B experienced severe apnea after the administration of prochlorperazine.

**Related Drugs:** A similar interaction was documented after the concurrent administration of colistin and promethazine. A similar interaction may occur with other polypeptide antibiotics and other phenothiazines.

**Mechanism:** The development of apnea in these patients may result from a synergistic neuromuscular blockade.

**Detailed Information:** See *EDI*, 8/73.00

### Rifampin-Aminosalicylic Acid

**Significance:** 4—not clinically significant

**Recommendations:** It may not be possible to know if a granule formulation contains bentonite. However, it was demonstrated that separating the administration of these two agents by 8 to 12 hours prevented the interaction.

**Summary:** Aminosalicylic acid granules have been reported to decrease the bioavailability and pharmacologic activity of rifampin.

*Anti-infective*

Another study found that the reduction was caused by bentonite, an excipient in the aminosalicylic acid granules.
**Related Drugs:** There are no drugs related to rifampin or aminosalicylic acid.
**Mechanism:** Physical adsorption of rifampin is the likely mechanism in this interaction.
**Detailed Information:** See *EDI*, 8/75.00

## Rifampin-Amiodarone

**Significance:** 2—moderately clinically significant
**Potential Effects:** The concurrent administration of rifampin and amiodarone may result in decreased levels and clinical effects of amiodarone.
**Recommendations:** Use of rifampin and amiodarone together should be avoided, if possible. If co-administration is necessary, amiodarone and desethylamiodarone levels should be carefully monitored before, during, and following concurrent therapy with rifampin and amiodarone.
**Summary:** Concurrent administration of rifampin and amiodarone resulted in decreased levels and clinical effects of amiodarone.
**Related Drugs:** A similar interaction may occur between the other rifamycins and amiodarone. There are no drugs related to amiodarone.
**Mechanism:** Rifampin induces cytochrome P450 isozymes, increasing the metabolism and clearance of amiodarone.
**Detailed Information:** See *EDI*, 8/75.10

## Rifampin-Buspirone

**Significance:** 3—minimally clinically significant
**Potential Effects:** The concurrent administration of rifampin and buspirone resulted in decreased levels and clinical effects of buspirone.
**Recommendations:** Patients receiving concurrent therapy with buspirone and rifampin should be monitored for possible decreased effects of buspirone. The dosage of buspirone may need to be adjusted.
**Summary:** The concurrent administration of rifampin and buspirone resulted in decreased levels and clinical effects of buspirone. Pretreatment with rifampin decreased buspirone half-life and maximum concentration. There were significant decreases in the effects of buspirone with concurrent therapy.
**Related Drugs:** Based on the postulated mechanism, a similar interaction would be expected to occur between the other rifamycins and buspirone. There are no drugs related to buspirone.
**Mechanism:** It has been postulated that rifampin induced the metabolism of buspirone at the cytochrome $P450_{3A4}$ isozyme.
**Detailed Information:** See *EDI*, 8/75.30

## Rifampin-Clofibrate

**Significance:** 3—minimally clinically significant
**Recommendations:** In order to achieve therapeutic plasma concentrations of clofibrate, it may be necessary to increase the dose of clofibrate when it is administered concomitantly with rifampin.
**Summary:** There are data to show that administration of rifampin significantly reduces the plasma levels of clofibric acid.
**Related Drugs:** There are no drugs related to clofibrate or rifampin.
**Mechanism:** Rifampin may enhance the hepatic metabolism of clofibrate and the renal excretion of its metabolite.
**Detailed Information:** See *EDI*, 8/76.10

Anti-infective

## Rifampin-Cyclosporine

**Significance:** 1—highly clinically significant

**Potential Effects:** Rifampin causes a decrease in cyclosporine levels which may lead to graft rejections. Avoid using these agents together.

**Recommendations:** If they must be given together, cyclosporine levels should be monitored frequently.

**Summary:** There are data to show that administration of rifampin causes a decrease in cyclosporine levels, which may lead to graft rejections. When rifampin was discontinued, cyclosporine levels were shown to increase dramatically.

**Related Drugs:** There are no drugs related to cyclosporine or rifampin.

**Mechanism:** Rifampin, a known inducer of hepatic microsomal enzymes, increases the metabolism and clearance of cyclo-sporine.

**Detailed Information:** See *EDI,* 8/76.30

## Rifampin-Oral Contraceptive Agents

**Significance:** 1—highly clinically significant

**Potential Effects:** Concurrent rifampin may increase the metabolism of oral contraceptive agents, leading to breakthrough bleeding and loss of contraceptive effectiveness.

**Recommendations:** Although some women may take these agents concomitantly without risk, there is no way to predict who will be affected. Some prescribers may choose to warn patients that spotting and breakthrough bleeding are signs of diminished contraceptive effectiveness, and alternative forms of contraception should be used. Others may choose to recommend an alternative contraception method.

**Summary:** Concurrent administration of rifampin and oral contraceptive agents have been shown to result in an increased incidence of menstrual disorders and pregnancies.

**Related Drugs:** A similar interaction may occur between oral contraceptive agents and rifabutin.

**Mechanism:** Antibiotics destroy gut flora and may prevent steroid reabsorption, resulting in lower than normal concentrations of the contraceptive. Rifampin is a microsomal enzyme inducer, increasing the hydroxylation of estrogens.

**Detailed Information:** See *EDI,* 8/77.00

## Rifampin-Prednisolone

**Significance:** 2—moderately clinically significant

**Recommendations:** A reduced corticosteroid activity may be expected when rifampin is coadministered, necessitating an increased steroid dose. One approximation is to double the daily steroid dose when rifampin therapy is initiated. Patients stabilized on both agents may require a steroid dosage decrease when rifampin is discontinued.

**Summary:** Prednisolone disposition is altered by rifampin, resulting in a decreased corticosteroid activity. Rifampin was further implicated in the decreased serum area-under-curve and increased clearance of prednisolone.

**Related Drugs:** Similar changes in corticosteroid disposition have been reported for cortisone acetate, fludrocortisone, cortisol (hydrocortisone), and methylprednisolone. A similar interaction may occur with other corticosteroids. There are no drugs related to rifampin.

**Mechanism:** Rifampin induces hepatic metabolizing enzymes, leading to an increased metabolism of the steroid.

**Detailed Information:** See *EDI,* 8/79.00

Anti-infective

## Rifampin-Probenecid
**Significance:** 4—not clinically significant
**Recommendations:** At this point, there appears to be no advantage of adding probenecid to rifampin therapy with the goal of increasing rifampin's plasma levels or decreasing its rate of metabolism.
**Summary:** Rifampin and probenecid have been the subject of conflicting data designed to evaluate whether the addition of probenecid to rifampin therapy would add any therapeutic benefit.
**Related Drugs:** There are no drugs related to rifampin. It is not known if an interaction occurs between rifampin and sulfinpyrazone.
**Mechanism:** Both agents may compete at the plasma membrane, increasing peak serum rifampin levels, or individual patient variations could cause the serum levels of rifampin to increase.
**Detailed Information:** See *EDI*, 8/81.00

## Sulfadiazine-Cyclosporine
**Significance:** 2—moderately clinically significant
**Potential Effects:** The addition of sulfadiazine to cyclosporine therapy may result in decreased cyclosporine levels.
**Recommendations:** The addition of sulfadiazine to the therapy of a patient maintained on cyclosporine requires close monitoring of cyclosporine levels. The dose of cyclosporine may need to be adjusted, especially when high daily sulfonamide doses are required.
**Summary:** Sulfadiazine therapy may result in a decreased cyclosporine concentration.
**Related Drugs:** Sulfamethoxydiazine was shown to decrease cyclosporine levels. It is not known whether an interaction would occur between cyclosporine and other sulfonamides, but one may occur.
**Mechanism:** The different effects of the related sulfonamides on cyclosporine levels are dependent on the absolute dosage used.
**Detailed Information:** See *EDI*, 8/82.50

## Sulfamethazine/Trimethoprim-Cyclosporine
**Significance:** 3—minimally clinically significant
**Recommendations:** Patients should be observed for a decrease in cyclosporine serum levels. Until further studies are done, an increase in the cyclosporine dose, use of an alternative antibiotic, or use of the oral rather than the intravenous route of administration for the antibiotics may be necessary.
**Summary:** Administration of trimethoprim and sulfamethazine may result in undetectable cyclosporine serum levels, potentiating graft rejection.
**Related Drugs:** There are no drugs related to cyclosporine. It is not known whether other sulfonamides would interact similarly with cyclosporine.
**Mechanism:** The mechanism of this interaction is unknown.
**Detailed Information:** See *EDI*, 8/83.00

## Sulfamethoxazole/Trimethoprim-Oral Contraceptive Agents
**Significance:** 3—minimally clinically significant
**Potential Effects:** The estrogenic effects of oral contraceptives may be increased in women receiving sulfamethoxazole-trimethoprim.
**Recommendations:** It is unlikely that clinical problems will arise in women taking long-term oral contraceptive agents who are given short courses of sulfamethoxazole-trimethoprim.
**Summary:** There are data to show that administration of sulfamethoxazole-trimethoprim may increase the estrogenic effects of oral contraceptives; however, all data do not support this interaction.

# Anti-infective

**Related Drugs:** Documentation is lacking regarding an interaction between oral contraceptive agents and other sulfonamides.
**Mechanism:** The enhanced effects of ethinylestradiol may be due to the inhibition of steroid microsomal hydroxylation enzymes in the liver by sulfamethoxazole.
**Detailed Information:** See *EDI*, 8/84.10

## Sulfasalazine-Ampicillin

**Significance:** 3—minimally clinically significant
**Recommendations:** Sulfasalazine is often used in the management of inflammatory bowel disease. Patients receiving this drug should be monitored for loss of therapeutic efficacy when ampicillin is added to their therapy.
**Summary:** Ampicillin was shown to affect the extent of absorption, reducing the availability of sulfasalazine.
**Related Drugs:** There is no documentation regarding an interaction between sulfasalazine and the other penicillins. It is difficult to determine whether an interaction would occur between ampicillin and the other sulfonamides.
**Mechanism:** The mechanism of this interaction is unknown.
**Detailed Information:** See *EDI*, 8/85.00

## Terbinafine-Cyclosporine

**Significance:** 2—moderately clinically significant
**Potential Effects:** Concurrent terbinafine and cyclosporine administration may result in a decrease in cyclosporine trough blood levels.
**Recommendations:** Cyclosporine blood levels should be monitored whenever terbinafine is added to or discontinued from concurrent therapy. Cyclosporine levels should be closely monitored in patients whose levels are at the lower end of the therapeutic range.
**Summary:** The addition of terbinafine to the therapy of several patients maintained on cyclosporine resulted in a decrease in mean cyclosporine trough blood levels. However, conflicting data are available.
**Related Drugs:** There are no drugs related to terbinafine or cyclosporine.
**Mechanism:** Terbinafine may induce cyclosporine metabolism even though studies have shown that terbinafine is not a significant enzyme inducer *in vitro*.
**Detailed Information:** See *EDI*, 8/86.00

## Tetracycline-Aluminum Hydroxide

**Significance:** 1—highly clinically significant
**Potential Effects:** Concurrent used may decrease absorption of tetracycline because of chelation.
**Recommendations:** If these agents must be used together, separate the administration by at least two hours.
**Summary:** Concurrent administration of aluminum hydroxide containing antacids or products containing divalent ions and tetracycline significantly decreases the gastrointestinal absorption of tetracycline.
**Related Drugs:** Most tetracycline analogs may interact in a similar manner with aluminum hydroxide and/or dairy products. Minocycline absorption is not notably influenced by food and dairy products, but aluminum, calcium, and magnesium ions may impair absorption. Sucralfate may prevent absorption of tetracycline. Bismuth subsalicylate has been shown to decrease tetracycline absorption and decrease the bioavailability of doxycycline.

## Anti-infective

**Mechanism:** Tetracycline forms relatively insoluble chelates with divalent and trivalent metallic ions.
**Detailed Information:** See *EDI*, 8/87.00

### Tetracycline-Cimetidine

**Significance:** 3—minimally clinically significant
**Recommendations:** Further studies are needed to elucidate this interaction; however, patients should be monitored for a decrease in the efficacy of tetracycline. The dose of tetracycline may need to be increased. Alternatively, the use of the oral solution of tetracycline, which was shown not to interact, might be considered.
**Summary:** The concurrent use of tetracycline and cimetidine resulted in a reduction in the tetracycline plasma concentration, a decrease in the area-under-curve, and a reduction in excretion.
**Related Drugs:** A similar interaction may occur between cimetidine and other tetracyclines or between tetracycline and other $H_2$-receptor antagonists, if the mechanism involves an increased gastric pH.
**Mechanism:** Dissolution of the capsule form of tetracycline depends on gastric acidity, and cimetidine raises gastric pH.
**Detailed Information:** See *EDI*, 8/89.00

### Tetracycline-Ferrous Sulfate

**Significance:** 1—highly clinically significant
**Recommendations:** Ferrous sulfate should not be given simultaneously with tetracycline or tetracycline analogs. When it is necessary for patients to receive both agents orally, this interaction may be avoided by administering the ferrous sulfate not less than three hours before or two hours after the tetracycline.
**Summary:** The concurrent oral administration of ferrous sulfate and tetracycline causes an interference with the absorption of tetracycline and the ferrous ion.
**Related Drugs:** The absorption of most tetracycline analogs will be decreased with concurrent administration of ferrous salts. Ferrous gluconate and fumarate have been shown to interact with the tetracyclines, and ferrous lactate may also interact in a similar manner.
**Mechanism:** Ferric and ferrous ions have been shown to form chelates with tetracyclines.
**Detailed Information:** See *EDI*, 8/91.00

### Tetracycline-Oral Contraceptive Agents

**Significance:** 2—moderately clinically significant
**Potential Effects:** The concurrent use of these agents may result in loss of contraceptive efficacy.
**Recommendations:** The majority of women may take these agents concomitantly without risk, but there seems no way to predict who will be affected. Some prescribers may choose to warn patients that spotting and breakthrough bleeding are signs of diminished contraceptive effectiveness, and alternative forms of contraception should be used. Others may choose to recommend an alternative contraceptive method.
**Summary:** The concurrent use of tetracycline and oral contraceptive agents has led to contraceptive failure.
**Related Drugs:** Oxytetracycline has been reported to exhibit a similar interaction. The other tetracycline derivatives may interact with oral contraceptive agents.
**Mechanism:** Antibiotics destroy the gut flora and prevent steroid reabsorption, resulting in lower than normal concentrations of the contraceptive.
**Detailed Information:** See *EDI*, 8/93.00

## Anti-infective

### Tetracycline-Sodium Bicarbonate
**Significance:** 4—not clinically significant
**Recommendations:** The incidence of the tetracycline-sodium bicarbonate interaction is not known, and there is conflicting evidence regarding the occurrence of adverse effects. A cautious regimen would be to administer the drugs as far apart as possible. There is no documentation whether this interaction will occur when tetracycline is administered in a liquid dosage form.
**Summary:** There are data to show that administration of sodium bicarbonate will reduce tetracycline absorption; however, all data do not support this.
**Related Drugs:** There appear to be no reports on the effect of sodium bicarbonate on any other tetracycline analog.
**Mechanism:** Tetracycline dissolves slower at a higher intragastric pH.
**Detailed Information:** See *EDI*, 8/95.00

### Tetracycline-Thimerosal
**Significance:** 3—minimally clinically significant
**Recommendations:** Reactions to thimerosal-containing contact lens solution are common. Delayed hypersensitivity reactions have also been reported. However, when patients develop a reaction after long-term use, another explanation for the reaction is necessary. Until additional cases are reported in the literature, the concurrent use of these agents need not be avoided. Should an ocular reaction occur, one or both drugs may have to be withdrawn.
**Summary:** Tetracycline appears to potentiate ocular reactions when thimerosal-containing contact lens solution is being used.
**Related Drugs:** Other tetracyclines may interact similarly with thimerosal.
**Mechanism:** Tetracyclines are known to penetrate into ocular fluid and may chelate the mercury in thimerosal.
**Detailed Information:** See *EDI*, 8/96.10

### Tobramycin-Miconazole
**Significance:** 3—minimally clinically significant
**Potential Effects:** Intravenously administered miconazole may cause a decrease in tobramycin levels.
**Recommendations:** Closely monitor tobramycin levels when these agents are used together.
**Summary:** There are data to show that administration of miconazole may cause a decrease in tobramycin levels.
**Related Drugs:** It is not known if miconazole would interact similarly with other aminoglycosides. There are no drugs related to miconazole.
**Mechanism:** The miconazole vehicle may cause an increased cellular uptake of tobramycin, leading to an increased volume of distribution.
**Detailed Information:** See *EDI*, 8/96.21

### Troleandomycin-Methylprednisolone
**Significance:** 2—moderately clinically significant
**Potential Effects:** Troleandomycin may inhibit the metabolism of methylprednisolone, leading to increased levels and possible adverse steroid effects.
**Recommendations:** Patients should be monitored for corticosteroid toxicity during concomitant use. Erythromycin may be an alternate to troleandomycin because it interacts to a lesser extent. The concurrent use of these agents may be beneficial for some patients.

**Summary:** There are data to show that administration of troleandomycin may inhibit the metabolism of methylprednisolone, leading to increased levels and increased adverse effects.
**Related Drugs:** Erythromycin and oleandomycin alter methylprednisolone disposition. Prednisolone is unaffected by troleandomycin. A similar interaction may occur with other corticosteroids and troleandomycin.
**Mechanism:** The interaction may result from a macrolide antibiotic inhibition of methylprednisolone metabolism.
**Detailed Information:** See *EDI*, 8/96.30

## Troleandomycin-Oral Contraceptive Agents

**Significance:** 2—moderately clinically significant
**Recommendations:** The large number of cases of cholestasis in women taking both troleandomycin and oral contraceptives strongly suggests a marked cholestatic effect from this association; therefore, women taking oral contraceptives should avoid taking troleandomycin.
**Summary:** The use of troleandomycin in women taking oral contraceptive agents has caused jaundice.
**Related Drugs:** Documentation is lacking describing a similar interaction with the other macrolide antibiotics.
**Mechanism:** The explanation for jaundice associated with troleandomycin is not known.
**Detailed Information:** See *EDI*, 8/97.00

## Vidarabine-Allopurinol

**Significance:** 2—moderately clinically significant
**Recommendations:** Until further information concerning this interaction is available, caution is warranted when these two drugs are used simultaneously.
**Summary:** There are data to show that coadministration of allopurinol and vidarabine may cause severe neurotoxicity.
**Related Drugs:** There are no drugs related to allopurinol or vidarabine.
**Mechanism:** Inhibition of xanthine oxidase by allopurinol could increase the drug levels of vidarabine, producing adverse effects.
**Detailed Information:** See *EDI*, 8/99.00

## Zidovudine-Acetaminophen

**Significance:** 3—minimally clinically significant
**Potential Effects:** Concomitant use of these agents may result in neutropenia and/or changes in zidovudine serum levels.
**Recommendations:** Patients on zidovudine therapy should be closely monitored for symptoms of toxicity when acetaminophen is added to the regimen. The dosage of zidovudine may have to be adjusted.
**Summary:** There are data to show that concomitant use of these agents may result in neutropenia and changes in zidovudine serum levels. There are no significant changes in acetaminophen serum levels.
**Related Drugs:** There are no drugs related to zidovudine or acetaminophen.
**Mechanism:** Acetaminophen and zidovudine are both metabolized by hepatic glucuronidation, and this could explain the decreased zidovudine plasma levels after acetaminophen administration.
**Detailed Information:** See *EDI*, 8/100.10

## Anti-infective

### Zidovudine-Acyclovir

**Significance:** 3—minimally clinically significant

**Potential Effects:** The concurrent use of zidovudine and acyclovir may result in increased lethargy and decreased alertness.

**Recommendations:** Since it is likely these two agents will be administered concurrently because herpes simplex infections are common in AIDS patients, patients should be observed for increased lethargy and decreased alertness. If this effect occurs, acyclovir may need to be discontinued.

**Summary:** There are data to show that coadministration of these agents can produce dramatic lethargy and fatigue.

**Related Drugs:** There are no drugs related to zidovudine or acyclovir.

**Mechanism:** The mechanism of this interaction is not known.

**Detailed Information:** See *EDI*, 8/101.00

### Zidovudine-Probenecid

**Significance:** 2—moderately clinically significant

**Potential Effects:** Probenecid will decrease the metabolism of zidovudine, resulting in increased zidovudine levels.

**Recommendations:** The use of concomitant zidovudine and probenecid should be approached with caution. The patient should be monitored for increased levels of zidovudine and its active metabolite. The dose of zidovudine may need to be reduced.

**Summary:** Probenecid may inhibit the metabolism of zidovudine, causing increased zidovudine levels.

**Related Drugs:** It is not known whether a similar interaction would occur between zidovudine and sulfinpyrazone. There are no drugs related to zidovudine.

**Mechanism:** The mechanism may be due to inhibition of zidovudine glucuronidation by probenecid.

**Detailed Information:** See *EDI*, 8/105.00

# Chapter Nine

# Antineoplastic Drug Interactions

## Antineoplastic

### Bleomycin-Cisplatin

**Significance:** 3—minimally clinically significant

**Potential Effects:** Bleomycin total clearance may decrease during successive cycles of concurrent administration with cisplatin as cumulative doses of cisplatin increase.

**Recommendations:** Patients receiving concurrent therapy with bleomycin and cisplatin should be monitored closely for cisplatin-induced changes in renal function, which may alter the clearance of bleomycin. The bleomycin dosage may need to be adjusted.

**Summary:** Bleomycin total clearance decreased during successive cycles of concurrent administration with cisplatin as cumulative doses of cisplatin increased. Greater effects appeared to occur at cisplatin doses greater than 300 mg/m, although this relationship was not proven to be statistically significant. Bleomycin toxicity was not observed.

**Related Drugs:** It is not known if a similar interaction would be expected to occur between bleomycin and carboplatin. There are no drugs related to bleomycin.

**Mechanism:** It is postulated that cisplatin administration results in changes in renal function that alter the elimination of bleomycin, although nonrenal mechanisms for the decrease are not ruled out. It has been shown that cisplatin-induced renal damage persists even when serum creatinine values return to normal. Also, serious renal dysfunction has reportedly occurred in children who receive long-term therapy with cisplatin.

**Detailed Information:** See *EDI*, 9/0.50

### Carmustine-Cimetidine

**Significance:** 3—minimally clinically significant

**Recommendations:** Patients receiving these agents concurrently should be monitored for the appearance of bone marrow suppression. If suppression is detected, cimetidine should be discontinued.

**Summary:** There are data to show that concomitant cimetidine and carmustine have an additive bone marrow depressant effect.

**Related Drugs:** There are no published reports of an additive effect between other antineoplastic nitrosoureas and cimetidine. It is unknown whether ranitidine would interact similarly.

**Mechanism:** Both drugs have bone marrow suppressant properties which would appear to be additive during cotherapy.

**Detailed Information:** See *EDI*, 9/1.00

### Cyclophosphamide-Allopurinol

**Significance:** 2—moderately clinically significant

**Recommendations:** The routine prophylactic use of allopurinol to prevent hyperuricemia may not be advisable during chemotherapy with alkylating agents. Patients who receive these drugs concurrently should be monitored for signs of bone marrow depression (leukopenia, thrombocytopenia, and pancytopenia).

**Summary:** The concurrent administration of cyclophosphamide and allopurinol may enhance the bone marrow depression induced by cyclophosphamide; however, all data do not support this.

**Related Drugs:** No specific interactions have been reported with other alkylating agents. There are no drugs related to allopurinol.

**Mechanism:** The mechanism is unknown; however, allopurinol does affect liver enzyme systems, and cyclophosphamide undergoes hepatic oxidation.

**Detailed Information:** See *EDI*, 9/3.00

Antineoplastic

### Cyclophosphamide-Chloramphenicol
**Significance:** 2—moderately clinically significant
**Recommendations:** Cyclophosphamide must be converted to active metabolites to produce its antineoplastic activity. Therefore, concomitant administration with chloramphenicol may delay or partially inhibit cyclophosphamide's antineoplastic activity. This interaction is clinically significant and should be avoided.
**Summary:** Chloramphenicol has been shown to inhibit the metabolism of cyclophosphamide.
**Related Drugs:** There are no drugs related to cyclophosphamide or chloramphenicol.
**Mechanism:** Chloramphenicol is thought to inhibit the hepatic biotransformation of cyclophosphamide.
**Detailed Information:** See *EDI*, 9/4.10

### Cyclophosphamide-Indomethacin
**Significance:** 3—minimally clinically significant
**Potential Effects:** Concurrent use of these agents may result in water intoxication.
**Recommendations:** Concurrent indomethacin and low-dose cyclophosphamide therapy should be approached with caution because of the possibility of acute water intoxication. Appropriate supportive measures should be employed if water intoxication occurs.
**Summary:** Concurrent administration of indomethacin and cyclophosphamide induced acute water intoxication.
**Related Drugs:** An interaction may occur between cyclophosphamide and other NSAIAs. It is not known whether an interaction may occur between indomethacin and other antineoplastic alkylating agents.
**Mechanism:** Inhibition of prostaglandins may result in an increase in anti-diuretic hormone, which may have precipitated the water intoxication.
**Detailed Information:** See *EDI*, 9/5.10

### Cyclophosphamide Fluorouracil-Hydrochlorothiazide Methotrexate
**Significance:** 3—minimally clinically significant
**Recommendations:** Patients' neutrophil counts should be monitored closely during concurrent use of these agents. If neutropenia develops, the dose of the thiazide diuretic may need to be lowered or the drug discontinued.
**Summary:** The concurrent use of hydrochlorothiazide and cancer chemotherapy combinations have resulted in granulocytopenia.
**Related Drugs:** The same interaction was shown to occur with chlorothiazide and trichlormethiazide. A similar interaction may occur with all thiazide diuretics and thiazide-related diuretics.
**Mechanism:** The mechanism is unknown.
**Detailed Information:** See *EDI*, 9/5.00

### Cyclophosphamide-Methotrexate
**Significance:** 3—minimally clinically significant
**Recommendations:** Although further clinical studies are necessary, clinicians should be aware of the possibility of decreased levels of the active metabolites of cyclophosphamide.
**Summary:** The concurrent administration of methotrexate and cyclophosphamide may result in the inhibition of the metabolism of cyclophosphamide.

## Antineoplastic

**Related Drugs:** There are no drugs related to cyclophosphamide or methotrexate.
**Mechanism:** Methotrexate may inhibit the metabolism of cyclophosphamide, decreasing the formation of the active metabolites of cyclophosphamide.
**Detailed Information:** See *EDI*, 9/6.01

### Cyclophosphamide-Prednisone

**Significance:** 3—minimally clinically significant
**Recommendations:** Administration of concomitant prednisolone and cyclophosphamide appears not to significantly alter the metabolism of cyclophosphamide. Although the concurrent administration of these agents is often utilized as therapy for various malignancies, concomitant prednisone use may necessitate an increase in cyclophosphamide dosage.
**Summary:** The concurrent administration of oral cyclophosphamide and prednisone resulted in no difference in cyclophosphamide half-life when used for five days. Pretreatment for 12-15 days resulted in a 20% decrease in cyclophosphamide half-life.
**Related Drugs:** The metabolism of cyclophosphamide was not altered by the concomitant administration of prednisolone; however, it has also been shown to immediately prolong cyclophosphamide half-life in a patient pretreated with prednisone. It is difficult to determine the influence of other corticosteroids on cyclophosphamide disposition.
**Mechanism:** The increased metabolism of cyclophosphamide is thought to result from the induction of hepatic enzymes by prednisone.
**Detailed Information:** See *EDI*, 9/6.10

### Doxorubicin-Phenobarbital

**Significance:** 3—minimally clinically significant
**Recommendations:** Although it was not determined if the efficacy of doxorubicin was decreased with concurrent phenobarbital, patients should be monitored, as the dose of doxorubicin may need to be increased to obtain optimal drug efficacy.
**Summary:** There are data to show that coadministration of these agents may potentially result in a decrease in the therapeutic effect of doxorubicin.
**Related Drugs:** It may be expected that all barbiturates would interact similarly with doxorubicin. Daunorubicin may be expected to interact also.
**Mechanism:** Phenobarbital, because of hepatic microsomal enzyme induction, may affect the metabolism of doxorubicin.
**Detailed Information:** See *EDI*, 9/6.21

### Etoposide-Cyclosporine

**Significance:** 2—moderately clinically significant
**Potential Effects:** Concurrent administration of cyclosporine and etoposide may result in a decrease in etoposide clearance and an increase in etoposide levels. Cyclosporine may also increase the sensitivity of certain multidrug-resistant cell lines to etoposide.
**Recommendations:** In patients receiving concurrent therapy with etoposide and high-dose cyclosporine, etoposide dosages should be reduced 50%. Dosages may need further adjustment in patients with renal or hepatic impairment.
**Summary:** Concurrent administration of cyclosporine resulted in a decrease in etoposide clearance and an increase in etoposide levels. Cyclosporine may increase the etoposide sensitivity of certain multidrug-resistant cell lines.

**Related Drugs:** A similar interaction has occurred with the concomitant administration of cyclosporine and teniposide; however, there was significant interpatient variation. There are no drugs related to cyclosporine.

**Mechanism:** It is postulated that cyclosporine decreases etoposide P-gp-mediated excretion in the brush border of the proximal renal tubule and luminal surface of the biliary tract in the liver, thus explaining the decrease in both renal and nonrenal clearance of etoposide. Cyclosporine may also inhibit etoposide metabolism at the P450 isoenzyme system.

**Detailed Information:** See *EDI,* 9/6.26

## Fluorouracil-Cimetidine

**Significance:** 1—highly clinically significant

**Recommendations:** Until further clinical studies are done, the concurrent administration of these two agents should be used with caution. If signs of 5-fluorouracil toxicity develop (e.g., stomatitis or esophagopharyngitis, rapidly falling white blood cell count, leukopenia, gastrointestinal effects), the dose of 5-fluorouracil may need to be decreased.

**Summary:** There are data to show that coadministration of these agents did not exhibit any significant pharmacokinetic alterations; however, use of these agents concomitantly should be done with caution.

**Related Drugs:** A similar interaction may occur with floxuridine. A similar interaction is not expected to occur between 5-fluorouracil and other $H_2$-receptor antagonists, if the mechanism involves hepatic enzyme inhibition by cimetidine.

**Mechanism:** The interaction between 5-fluorouracil and cimetidine may result from a reduction in liver blood flow caused by cimetidine or from cimetidine's inhibition of the hepatic metabolism of 5-fluorouracil.

**Detailed Information:** See *EDI,* 9/6.30

## Fluorouracil-Metronidazole

**Significance:** 2—moderately clinically significant

**Potential Effects:** The concurrent administration of fluorouracil and metronidazole resulted in decreased clearance and increased toxicity of fluorouracil.

**Recommendations:** It is recommended that patients receiving fluorouracil therapy avoid concurrent metronidazole. Patients receiving fluorouracil should be monitored for toxicity if metronidazole is added to therapy.

**Summary:** The concurrent administration of fluorouracil and metronidazole resulted in decreased fluorouracil clearance and increased toxicity of fluorouracil.

**Related Drugs:** There are no drugs related to metronidazole or fluorouracil.

**Mechanism:** Misonidazole (a radiosensitizer of hypoxic cells structurally similar to metronidazole) may inhibit the initial catabolic step of fluorouracil metabolism. An aspect of renal clearance is also involved, indicating that another mechanism of inhibition of fluorouracil clearance may need to be considered.

**Detailed Information:** See *EDI,* 9/6.40

## Interleukin-2–Dexamethasone

**Significance:** 2—moderately clinically significant

**Potential Effects:** Concurrent use of these agents may result in a decrease in the antitumor effectiveness of interleukin-2.

Antineoplastic

**Recommendations:** Because concurrent use of dexamethasone with interleukin-2 may reduce the antitumor effectiveness of interleukin-2, the concurrent use of these agents should be avoided.
**Summary:** Concurrent interleukin-2 and dexamethasone may result in a decreased interleukin-2 antineoplastic effect.
**Related Drugs:** A similar interaction may occur between interleukin-2 and other corticosteroids. There are no drugs related to interleukin-2.
**Mechanism:** The mechanism of this interaction is not known, but it may be related to the immunosuppressive effects of dexamethasone on interleukin-2-induced tumor necrosis factor synthesis.
**Detailed Information:** See *EDI*, 9/6.60

## Lomustine-Theophylline

**Significance:** 3—minimally clinically significant
**Recommendations:** Evidence is insufficient to indicate that theophylline should not be used concurrently with lomustine, although one should be aware that thrombocytopenia and myelotoxicity are possible during combined therapy with these agents.
**Summary:** A patient receiving theophylline and lomustine for medulloblastoma developed epistaxis and thrombocytopenia.
**Related Drugs:** There have been no reports of similar interactions with theophylline and other alkylating agents. A synergistic effect was seen with theophylline and carmustine in mice. A similar interaction is expected to occur with other theophylline derivatives. Dyphylline may also be expected to interact with lomustine.
**Mechanism:** The mechanism is unknown, but it has been suggested that theophylline may disrupt normal platelet function.
**Detailed Information:** See *EDI*, 9/7.00

## Melphalan-Cyclosporine

**Significance:** 2—moderately clinically significant
**Recommendations:** Since renal impairment may occur with the concomitant use of cyclosporine and melphalan, patients' renal function should be closely monitored when these agents are administered concurrently.
**Summary:** There are data to show that coadministration of cyclosporine and melphalan may lead to the development of severe renal failure; however, some patients experienced mild, or no, renal failure.
**Related Drugs:** There are no drugs related to melphalan or cyclosporine.
**Mechanism:** The mechanism of this interaction is unknown; however, it may involve a direct effect on the kidney rather than an effect on the absorption or metabolism of cyclosporine. Both of these agents have been documented to cause renal impairment alone.
**Detailed Information:** See *EDI*, 9/8.10

## Mercaptopurine-Allopurinol

**Significance:** 1—highly clinically significant
**Potential Effects:** Allopurinol decreases the first-pass metabolism of mercaptopurine, resulting in an increase in mercaptopurine serum levels and toxic effects.
**Recommendations:** The initial dose of oral mercaptopurine should be reduced to one-third or one-fourth of the presently recommended dosage level when allopurinol is administered concurrently. Subsequent adjustments of mercaptopurine dosages should be made on the basis of clinical response and/or toxicity.

## Antineoplastic

**Summary:** The concurrent administration of mercaptopurine and allopurinol has been shown to result in a clinically significant increase in the pharmacologic and toxic effects of mercaptopurine.
**Related Drugs:** Azathioprine has been shown to interact with allopurinol. There are no drugs related to allopurinol.
**Mechanism:** Mercaptopurine metabolite is catalyzed by the enzyme xanthine oxidase, and allopurinol inhibits the action of xanthine oxidase, reducing the rate of mercaptopurine inactivation and resulting in higher blood levels.
**Detailed Information:** See *EDI,* 9/9.00

## Methotrexate-Alcohol, Ethyl

**Significance:** 3—minimally clinically significant
**Recommendations:** Because of the possibility that ethyl alcohol may increase the hepatotoxic potential of methotrexate, patients receiving this drug should be advised to minimize consumption of products containing ethyl alcohol.
**Summary:** Concurrent methotrexate therapy and ethyl alcohol consumption may lead to greater incidence of hepatotoxicity.
**Related Drugs:** Benzyl alcohol, a preservative in some methotrexate preparations, has been implicated as a contributor to neurologic side effects when methotrexate is administered intrathecally. Preservative-free parenteral preparations should be used for the intrathecal route of administration.
**Mechanism:** A specific mechanism for a methotrexate and ethyl alcohol interaction is not known. It has been observed that high concentrations of ethyl alcohol weakly inhibit transport and may lead to higher intrahepatic concentrations of methotrexate.
**Detailed Information:** See *EDI,* 9/11.00

## Methotrexate-Aspirin

**Significance:** 1—highly clinically significant
**Recommendations:** Administration of aspirin should be avoided in patients receiving methotrexate when an acceptable alternative drug is available. Acetaminophen has been used concurrently with methotrexate without causing an increase in methotrexate toxicity. If concurrent administration is necessary, the patient should be observed closely for methotrexate toxicity.
**Summary:** The concurrent administration of methotrexate and aspirin may result in elevated or prolonged serum concentrations of methotrexate, increasing toxicity.
**Related Drugs:** All salicylates and their combination products may interact with methotrexate. There are no drugs related to methotrexate.
**Mechanism:** Aspirin is capable of displacing methotrexate from plasma proteins *in vitro,* and methotrexate and aspirin have a common elimination pathway. Aspirin may compete with, and inhibit, methotrexate elimination.
**Detailed Information:** See *EDI,* 9/13.00

## Methotrexate-Cisplatin

**Significance:** 2—moderately clinically significant
**Potential Effects:** Pretreatment with cisplatin may increase the incidence of methotrexate toxicity.
**Recommendations:** Because of the possible serious nature of this interaction, extreme caution should be exercised when using these agents concurrently. Methotrexate levels and blood counts should be carefully monitored.

Antineoplastic

**Summary:** Administration of methotrexate following pretreatment with cisplatin resulted in methotrexate toxicity and death. Severe stomatitis, myelosuppression and renal failure were observed.
**Related Drugs:** It is not known if cisplatin would interact with the other antineoplastic antimetabolites. There are no drugs related to cisplatin.
**Mechanism:** The mechanism is not known.
**Detailed Information:** See *EDI*, 9/14.10

## Methotrexate-Cytarabine

**Significance:** 3—minimally clinically significant
**Potential Effects:** Concurrent use of these agents may result in enhanced cell-kill. Methotrexate may also increase mercaptopurine levels.
**Recommendations:** Although there are inconclusive reports regarding this interaction, patients receiving concurrent methotrexate and cytarabine should be closely monitored. Concurrent methotrexate and topical fluorouracil should be avoided.
**Summary:** Administration of cytarabine before initiation of methotrexate therapy enhances methotrexate. Conversely, the cytarabine can be enhanced when methotrexate is administered before the initiation of cytarabine therapy.
**Related Drugs:** Methotrexate was found to increase mercaptopurine's area-under-curve and levels. Fluorouracil 2% cream was shown to cause erythema, blisters and necrosis when administered with methotrexate. It is not known if methotrexate would enhance the cell-kill of the other antineoplastic antimetabolites.
**Mechanism:** Many factors are involved in the mechanism of the interaction of these two chemotherapeutic agents. These include the order of administration of the agents, the time interval between administration and the complexities of the enzyme-substrate system within a given patient. Thus the exact outcome of the interaction can be variable from patient to patient.
**Detailed Information:** See *EDI*, 9/15.00

## Methotrexate-Etretinate

**Significance:** 2—moderately clinically significant
**Potential Effects:** Concurrent use of these agents may result in hepatotoxicity.
**Recommendations:** Monitor drug levels and hepatic function when these agents are coadministered. The dosage of one or both agents may need to be changed.
**Summary:** There are data to show that coadministration of these agents results in hepatotoxicity; however, not all data support this. An absence of significant side effects and no evidence of hepatotoxicity have been documented.
**Related Drugs:** A similar interaction may occur between methotrexate and isotretinoin.
**Mechanism:** Increased hepatotoxicity may be due to an additive effect of these two potentially hepatotoxic agents. Etretinate may also interfere with the metabolism or excretion of methotrexate.
**Detailed Information:** See *EDI*, 9/16.05

## Methotrexate-Ketoprofen

**Significance:** 2—moderately clinically significant
**Potential Effects:** Ketoprofen may increase methotrexate levels, leading to serious methotrexate toxicity.

## Antineoplastic

**Recommendations:** Avoid using these agents together. If ketoprofen is to be administered, it should not be given for at least 24 hours after the last methotrexate dose.

**Summary:** Simultaneous administration of ketoprofen was associated with prolonged and striking enhancement of serum methotrexate levels.

**Related Drugs:** Indomethacin, ibuprofen and diclofenac were shown to increase methotrexate levels, potentiating toxicity. Phenylbutazone therapy has been shown to cause fever, oral ulcerations, severe bone marrow suppression, and septicemia when given with methotrexate. A similar interaction may occur between methotrexate and the other NSAIAs. There are no drugs related to methotrexate.

**Mechanism:** This interaction may be explained by the inhibition of renal prostaglandin synthesis by ketoprofen, which decreases renal perfusion rate and inhibits methotrexate clearance. Competitive renal secretion of these two drugs may be another explanation.

**Detailed Information:** See *EDI,* 9/16.10

## Methotrexate-Leucovorin

**Significance:** 1—highly clinically significant

**Recommendations:** The evidence shows that leucovorin reverses methotrexate-induced inhibition of folic acid antagonism. Beneficial results in some diseases are obtained by intramuscular or intravenous methotrexate administration followed by intramuscular leucovorin. The optimal interval between the administration of the two drugs is six hours or less. Effective leucovorin doses have ranged from 4 to 12 mg. Methotrexate dosage can be greater than usual (up to 600 mg/kg) when consecutive leucovorin administration is used.

**Summary:** Methotrexate toxicity can be greatly reduced by consecutive administration of leucovorin within six hours. "Leucovorin rescue" can be accomplished while maintaining the therapeutic effectiveness of methotrexate against tumors.

**Related Drugs:** There are no drugs related to methotrexate or leucovorin.

**Mechanism:** Methotrexate is a folic acid antagonist. Leucovorin is an active metabolite of folic acid.

**Detailed Information:** See *EDI,* 9/17.00

## Methotrexate-Neomycin

**Significance:** 2—moderately clinically significant

**Recommendations:** Patients should be monitored during concurrent use of these agents. An increased dose of methotrexate may be necessary, or, in the case of kanamycin, the dose of methotrexate may need to be reduced.

**Summary:** The concurrent use of oral neomycin and methotrexate has resulted in a reduced methotrexate absorption, necessitating an increased methotrexate dose.

**Related Drugs:** Paromomycin also reduced the absorption of methotrexate. Kanamycin has been reported to increase methotrexate plasma levels. There are no drugs related to methotrexate.

**Mechanism:** Neomycin is known to produce malabsorption of many drugs, and this may be the mechanism here; however, further study is needed.

**Detailed Information:** See *EDI,* 9/19.00

## Antineoplastic

### Methotrexate-Omeprazole

**Significance:** 2—moderately clinically significant

**Potential Effects:** Increased methotrexate levels may result with concurrent administration of omeprazole.

**Recommendations:** Omeprazole should be withdrawn in patients several days prior to methotrexate therapy to avoid methotrexate toxicity.

**Summary:** Increased methotrexate levels may result with concurrent administration of omeprazole, a case report suggested.

**Related Drugs:** Although documentation is lacking, based on the proposed mechanism a similar interaction may be expected to occur between methotrexate and lansoprazole. It is not known whether a similar interaction would occur between omeprazole and other folic acid antagonists related to methotrexate (trimetrexate and aminopterin).

**Mechanism:** It is postulated that omeprazole may inhibit the active secretion of methotrexate from the kidney.

**Detailed Information:** See *EDI*, 9/20.00

### Methotrexate-Piperacillin

**Significance:** 2—moderately clinically significant

**Potential Effects:** The concurrent administration of methotrexate and piperacillin resulted in elevated and prolonged levels of methotrexate.

**Recommendations:** Patients receiving concurrent therapy with methotrexate and piperacillin should be monitored closely for methotrexate toxicity. Leucovorin-rescue therapy may need to be increased in dosage and duration. Piperacillin may need to be discontinued.

**Summary:** Concurrent administration of methotrexate and piperacillin has resulted in elevated and prolonged levels of methotrexate in several patients.

**Related Drugs:** A significant decrease in the clearance of methotrexate has been observed when amoxicillin (with and without clavulanic acid), mezlocillin, penicillin, ticarcillin, flucloxacillin, and dicloxacillin were administered concomitantly; methotrexate toxicity occurred in many cases. A similar interaction may occur between methotrexate and the other penicillin derivatives. There are no drugs related to methotrexate.

**Mechanism:** Penicillins are weak organic acids and compete with the renal tubular secretion of methotrexate to decrease the clearance of methotrexate and 7-hydroxymethotrexate. Penicillin blocks methotrexate secretion in the kidney by inhibiting cellular uptake and stimulating efflux.

**Detailed Information:** See *EDI*, 9/20.50

### Methotrexate-Probenecid

**Significance:** 1—highly clinically significant

**Recommendations:** Although the concurrent use of these agents need not be avoided, it is important to monitor methotrexate plasma levels and lower the dose of methotrexate when necessary.

**Summary:** The concurrent use of methotrexate and probenecid leads to a marked increase in serum methotrexate levels.

**Related Drugs:** There are no drugs related to methotrexate. A similar interaction may occur between methotrexate and sulfinpyrazone if the mechanism involves inhibition of renal tubular transport.

**Mechanism:** Probenecid may inhibit the excretion of methotrexate by the renal and biliary routes, and displacement of methotrexate from plasma albumin binding sites by probenecid may also contribute.

**Detailed Information:** See *EDI*, 9/21.00

Antineoplastic

## Methotrexate-Procarbazine

**Significance:** 2—moderately clinically significant

**Potential Effects:** Procarbazine may predispose patients to nephrotoxicity with concurrent methotrexate.

**Recommendations:** Consideration should be given to allowing an interval of at least 72 hours between the administration of the final dose of procarbazine and the initiation of high-dose methotrexate therapy. Renal function should be closely monitored, and methotrexate therapy may need to be modified or discontinued.

**Summary:** Concurrent therapy with high-dose methotrexate and procarbazine may increase the nephrotoxicity of methotrexate.

**Related Drugs:** It is not known if an interaction would occur between metho-trexate and other MAOIs. There are no drugs related to methotrexate.

**Mechanism:** Procarbazine may have a transient effect on the kidneys and alter the renal excretion of methotrexate. If the excretion of methotrexate is delayed, there will be further impairment of renal function.

**Detailed Information:** See *EDI*, 9/22.10

## Methotrexate-Sodium Bicarbonate

**Significance:** 3—minimally clinically significant

**Recommendations:** Although urinary alkalinization with an agent such as sodium bicarbonate is used in high-dose methotrexate therapy, it is important to monitor the patient for decreased methotrexate levels.

**Summary:** Sodium bicarbonate has been shown to increase the renal elimination of methotrexate.

**Related Drugs:** There are no drugs related to methotrexate. If the mechanism deals with urinary alkalinization, then other agents capable of alkalinizing the urine may be expected to interact similarly.

**Mechanism:** A urinary pH greater than 8.0 may result in a significant increase in the urinary elimination rate of methotrexate.

**Detailed Information:** See *EDI*, 9/23.00

## Methotrexate-Sulfamethoxazole, Trimethoprim

**Significance:** 1—highly clinically significant

**Potential Effects:** The use of these agents together can induce folate deficiency, leading to megaloblastic anemia.

**Recommendations:** If these agents are used together, the patient's hematologic status should be monitored closely for signs of folate deficiency anemia. The administration of folic acid may be considered.

**Summary:** There are data to show that coadministration of these agents can induce folate deficiency, leading to megaloblastic anemia. Sulfamethoxazole and trimethoprim have been shown to alter the pharmacokinetics of methotrexate; however, all data do not support this.

**Related Drugs:** Methotrexate plasma protein binding and renal clearance have been shown to be decreased by sulfisoxazole. A similar interaction may occur between methotrexate and other sulfonamides. There are no drugs related to methotrexate.

**Mechanism:** Methotrexate and cotrimoxazole act synergistically to produce significant folate deficiency, leading to megaloblastic changes.

**Detailed Information:** See *EDI*, 9/25.00

Antineoplastic

## Mitomycin-Etoposide
**Significance:** 3—minimally clinically significant
**Potential Effects:** The concurrent use of these agents may result in dyspnea, tachycardia, and diaphoresis.
**Recommendations:** Until further studies are done to confirm the occurrence of this interaction, no specific recommendations can be made with regard to this therapy. However, it is prudent to be aware of the possible sudden dyspnea that may occur with concurrent mitomycin and etoposide.
**Summary:** There are data to show that coadministration of these agents may lead to dyspnea, tachycardia, diaphoresis, and the absence of bronchospasm or rales.
**Related Drugs:** There are no drugs related to mitomycin or etoposide.
**Mechanism:** The mechanism of this interaction is not known.
**Detailed Information:** See *EDI*, 9/26.01

## Mitomycin-Vinblastine
**Significance:** 2—moderately clinically significant
**Potential Effects:** The concomitant use of these agents may result in pulmonary toxicity. It has been stated that the incidence of abrupt pulmonary toxicity with this combination is 3% to 6%.
**Recommendations:** Patients receiving these agents should be closely monitored for pulmonary toxicity. If this occurs, bronchodilators or mechanical support may be required. Continuing concomitant therapy in these patients should be avoided.
**Summary:** Several case studies have reported the occurrence of pulmonary toxicity in patients receiving combination therapy with mitomycin and vinblastine for lung cancer.
**Related Drugs:** A similar interaction may occur between mitomycin and vincristine. There are no drugs related to mitomycin.
**Mechanism:** Pulmonary edema resulting from the administration of mitomycin and vinblastine may be the underlying mechanism.
**Detailed Information:** See *EDI*, 9/27.00

## Mitotane-Spironolactone
**Significance:** 2—moderately clinically significant
**Potential Effects:** Concurrent mitotane and spironolactone administration may result in antagonism of the therapeutic effectiveness of mitotane.
**Recommendations:** The therapeutic effectiveness of mitotane should be closely monitored in patients receiving these agents concurrently. Alternative therapy may need to be considered.
**Summary:** Concurrent mitotane and spironolactone administration resulted in antagonism of the therapeutic effectiveness of mitotane.
**Related Drugs:** An interaction may be expected to occur between mitotane and the other potassium-sparing diuretics.
**Mechanism:** The mechanism is not known, but it has been postulated that spironolactone may reverse patients' hypokalemia with probable adrenocortical hyperplasia.
**Detailed Information:** See *EDI*, 9/28.30

## Paclitaxel-Cisplatin
**Significance:** 2—moderately clinically significant
**Potential Effects:** The sequence of administration of paclitaxel and cisplatin may affect efficacy and the severity of neutropenic side effects.

## Antineoplastic

**Recommendations:** In chemotherapy regimens that include both paclitaxel and cisplatin, paclitaxel should be administered prior to cisplatin. Consideration should be given to administering paclitaxel prior to the concurrent administration of paclitaxel and cisplatin.

**Summary:** The sequence of administration of paclitaxel and cisplatin may affect efficacy and the severity of neutropenic side effects. Additive cytotoxic effects were seen *in vitro* when paclitaxel was administered prior to cisplatin. Antagonistic effects were seen when cisplatin was administered prior to paclitaxel. Synergistic cell kills may occur when paclitaxel is administered before concurrent administration of paclitaxel and cisplatin. In one *in vitro* study, the administration of combination paclitaxel and cisplatin significantly increased cell kills over those produced by cisplatin alone only when cisplatin followed paclitaxel, not when paclitaxel followed cisplatin. In an *in vivo* dose escalating study, the administration of cisplatin prior to paclitaxel resulted in more profound neutropenia than when the order was reversed. Paclitaxel clearance was 20% lower when paclitaxel was administered following cisplatin than prior to cisplatin.

**Related Drugs:** Concurrent administration of carboplatin and paclitaxel or the administration of paclitaxel followed by carboplatin has been shown to be more effective than the administration of carboplatin followed by paclitaxel. However, conflicting data are available. Based on the proposed mechanism and pharmacologic similarity, a similar interaction may be expected to occur between docetaxol and cisplatin.

**Mechanism:** Paclitaxel's cytotoxic effects are thought to result from its effects on the microtubules that are present during mitosis. Administration of cisplatin prior to paclitaxel is thought to decrease the number of cells entering mitosis, thereby decreasing the cytotoxic effects of paclitaxel. Administration of paclitaxel following cisplatin has been shown to result in a decrease in paclitaxel clearance, which may be responsible for the increase in severity of neutropenia.

**Detailed Information:** See *EDI,* 9/28.50

## Vinblastine-Erythromycin

**Significance:** 3—minimally clinically significant

**Potential Effects:** The concurrent administration of these agents may lead to increased vinblastine toxicity.

**Recommendations:** It is recommended that patients receiving vinblastine therapy should not be administered concurrent erythromycin. If these agents are given together, the toxicity observed may be typical of much higher doses of vinblastine.

**Summary:** Concurrent vinblastine and erythromycin resulted in severe neutropenia and myalgia.

**Related Drugs:** It is not known whether an interaction would occur between vinblastine and the other macrolide antibiotic agents. A similar interaction may be expected to occur between erythromycin and the other vinca alkaloids.

**Mechanism:** Erythromycin has been reported to potentiate a number of drugs by interference with cytochrome P450-mediated metabolism, and vinblastine or vindesine metabolism has been shown to be mediated by cytochrome P450 isozymes. Inhibition of the cytochrome P450-mediated metabolism of vinblastine by erythromycin is likely the mechanism for the observed interaction.

**Detailed Information:** See *EDI,* 9/30.00

Antineoplastic

## Vincristine-Carbamazepine

**Significance:** 2—moderately clinically significant

**Potential Effects:** The concurrent administration of vincristine and carbamazepine may result in decreased vincristine plasma levels and a possible decrease in antineoplastic activity.

**Recommendations:** Caution is advised with the concurrent administration of vincristine and carbamazepine. Patients should be monitored for possible decreased antineoplastic activity. Although the clinical significance has not been determined, results suggest that the efficacy of vincristine may be decreased. Because decreased vincristine efficacy may be difficult to assess in a clinical setting, an alternative to carbamazepine should be considered.

**Summary:** Concurrent administration of vincristine and carbamazepine resulted in decreased vincristine plasma levels and a possible decrease in antineoplastic activity.

**Related Drugs:** A similar interaction may occur between carbamazepine and the other vinca alkaloids. An interaction would not be expected to occur between vincristine and oxcarbazepine, although it is structurally related to carbamazepine.

**Mechanism:** Carbamazepine induces cytochrome $P450_{3A4}$ isozymes, which mediate the metabolism of vindesine, vinblastine, and vincristine. It is postulated that carbamazepine induced the metabolism of vincristine.

**Detailed Information:** See *EDI*, 9/31.00

# Chapter Ten

# Antipsychotic and Antianxiety Drug Interactions

## Alprazolam-Fluoxetine

**Significance:** 2—moderately clinically significant

**Potential Effects:** Fluoxetine may decrease the metabolism of alprazolam, resulting in increased effects of alprazolam.

**Recommendations:** The dose of benzodiazepines which undergo extensive phase I hepatic metabolism may need to be lowered in patients receiving therapy with selective serotonin reuptake inhibitors or nefazodone.

**Summary:** Concurrent administration of alprazolam and fluoxetine resulted in decreased clearance and increased effects of alprazolam.

**Related Drugs:** Fluoxetine has been reported to interact with diazepam and clonazepam. Fluvoxamine significantly interacted with diazepam and alprazolam. A study with triazolam and fluoxetine could not be evaluated for an interaction. Paroxetine has been reported to not significantly interact with oxazepam. Sertraline decreased diazepam clearance in one report by 13%. Nefazodone interacted with both alprazolam and triazolam, while venlafaxine did not interact with diazepam. If the mechanism involves inhibition of benzodiazepine metabolism, then the benzodiazepines metabolized by phase I reactions would be expected to interact similarly. An interaction with the benzodiazepines metabolized by phase II reactions is not likely to occur.

**Mechanism:** It is thought that fluoxetine decreased the hepatic metabolism of diazepam, decreasing the clearance and increasing the half-life. The selective-serotonin reuptake inhibitors and nefazodone may decrease the metabolism of phase I hepatically metabolized benzodiazepines through competitive inhibition at the cytochrome P450 site.

**Detailed Information:** See *EDI*, 10/0.04

## Alprazolam-Kava

**Significance:** 3—minimally clinically significant

**Potential Effects:** The addition of kava to the therapy of a patient maintained on alprazolam may result in lethargy and disorientation.

**Recommendations:** Patients taking concurrent alprazolam and kava should be monitored for possible increased pharmacologic effects of these agents. The dose of one or both of these agents may need to be reduced or one of these agents may need to be discontinued.

**Summary:** The addition of kava to a patient maintained on alprazolam resulted in lethargy, disorientation, and hospitalization.

**Related Drugs:** A similar interaction may occur between kava and the other benzodiazepines. There are no agents related to kava, the dried rhizome and roots of *Piper methysticum*. Other common names for kava include awa, kava-kava, kew, and tonga.

**Mechanism:** It has been postulated that the a-pyrones found in kava may have a synergistic effect on other sedatives that mediate $\gamma$-amino butyric acid (GABA) receptors by increasing the number of GABA binding sites.

**Detailed Information:** See *EDI*, 10/0.05

## Buspirone-Cimetidine

**Significance:** 4—not clinically significant

**Potential Effects:** Cimetidine does not markedly alter any pharmacokinetic parameters of buspirone.

**Recommendations:** Since a clinically significant interaction between buspirone and cimetidine is unlikely, buspirone may be considered as an alternative antianxiety agent.

**Summary:** In one study, concurrent administration of cimetidine and buspirone did not alter the pharmacokinetic profile of buspirone.
**Related Drugs:** Although documentation is lacking, buspirone would also not be expected to interact with the other $H_2$ receptor antagonists.
**Mechanism:** The administration of cimetidine did not markedly alter any pharmacokinetic parameters of buspirone.
**Detailed Information:** See *EDI*, 10/0.07

## Buspirone-Ritonavir

**Significance:** 3—minimally clinically significant
**Potential Effects:** The addition of ritonavir to the therapy of a patient maintained on buspirone resulted in severe Parkinson's disease-like symptoms.
**Recommendations:** If ritonavir and buspirone are given concurrently, the patient should be carefully monitored for signs of buspirone toxicity. The dose of buspirone may need to be decreased or the ritonavir may need to be replaced by other antiretroviral therapy.
**Summary:** The addition of ritonavir to the therapy of a patient maintained on buspirone may result in severe Parkinson's disease-like symptoms including resting tremor, blank facial expression, ataxia, and shuffling gait.
**Related Drugs:** A similar interaction might occur between buspirone and the other protease inhibitors that inhibit the cytochrome $P450_{3A4}$. Buspirone is chemically and pharmacologically unrelated to the benzodiazepines, barbiturates, or other sedative/anxiolytic agents.
**Mechanism:** Ritonavir may inhibit the metabolism of buspirone; both are metabolized by cytochrome $P450_{3A4}$. Ritonavir is a potent inhibitor of cytochrome $P450_{3A4}$.
**Detailed Information:** See *EDI*, 10/0.15

## Chlorpromazine-Alcohol, Ethyl

**Significance:** 2—moderately clinically significant
**Recommendations:** Patients receiving chlorpromazine should be warned that alcohol ingestion may produce enhanced CNS depression. Concurrent use may impair their ability to drive an automobile and operate hazardous machinery. Oral prescription and nonprescription products containing alcohol, as well as alcoholic beverages, should be used with caution.
**Summary:** Concurrent use of chlorpromazine and alcohol may cause an intensification of the CNS depression of each drug. Alcohol may precipitate extrapyramidal reactions.
**Related Drugs:** Thioridazine may produce less CNS depression in combination with alcohol. Other phenothiazines, thioxanthenes, butyrophenones, dihydroindolones and dibenzoxazepines may interact in a similar manner.
**Mechanism:** Alcohol may precipitate extrapyramidal reactions in patients on phenothiazines by inducing a temporary brain dysfunction.
**Detailed Information:** See *EDI*, 10/1.00

## Chlorpromazine-Aluminum Hydroxide, Magnesium Hydroxide

**Significance:** 3—minimally clinically significant
**Recommendations:** It is not known whether magnesium hydroxide and aluminum hydroxide alone have an effect on chlorpromazine absorption, but documentation indicates the combination of ingredients did alter chlorpromazine absorption. Therefore, until further clinical evidence is available, antacid products containing alu-

## Antipsychotic

minum hydroxide and magnesium hydroxide, or those containing magnesium trisilicate, should be administered one hour before or two hours after chlorpromazine administration.

**Summary:** Chlorpromazine absorption from the gastrointestinal tract may be altered by the simultaneous administration of antacids.

**Related Drugs:** Other phenothiazines, thioxanthenes, butyrophenones, dihydroindolones and dibenzoxazepines may interact. Trisilicate gel antacids have been shown to decrease chlorpromazine levels, whereas calcium carbonate-glycine antacids do not.

**Mechanism:** Administration of aluminum and magnesium containing antacids decreases the gastrointestinal absorption and serum levels of chlorpromazine.

**Detailed Information:** See *EDI*, 10/3.00

## Chlorpromazine-Amphetamine

**Significance:** 2—moderately clinically significant

**Potential Effects:** These agents may exert opposing effects on monoaminergic function in the central and peripheral nervous system if used concurrently.

**Recommendations:** Simultaneous use of chlorpromazine and amphetamine should be restricted to treating amphetamine overdose cases. A chlorpromazine dose of 1 mg/kg intramuscularly has been recommended. This may be followed by 0.5 mg/kg intramuscularly after 30 minutes if necessary to control recurrence of excitement. Conversely, overdosage with chlorpromazine generally is best managed with supportive measures alone.

**Summary:** Chlorpromazine and amphetamine are pharmacologic antagonists. These two drugs exert opposing effects on monoaminergic function in the central and peripheral nervous system. This antagonistic relationship has been utilized clinically in the management of amphetamine overdosage. Inclusion of either agent in a therapeutic regimen of the other could prove counterproductive. The amphetamines may antagonize the antipsychotic effect of the phenothiazine.

**Related Drugs:** Chlorpromazine is a multifunctional antagonist to several neurotransmitters. Other phenothiazines exhibit somewhat different potencies in their ability to interfere with the actions of norepinephrine or dopamine, the neurotransmitters generally believed involved in the stimulatory actions of amphetamine. Thus one would presume that other phenothiazine derivatives such as the thioxanthenes as well as the dihydroindolone and dibenzoxazepine would also exhibit antagonism of amphetamine actions with varying degrees of potency. Other antipsychotic agents such as haloperidol, a butyrophenone that possesses dopamine blocking activity and significant alpha-adrenergic blocking activity, may also effectively antagonize the actions of amphetamine. Other indirect-acting sympathomimetics as well as direct and mixed-acting sympathomimetics, which characteristically produce central and peripheral stimulation, would logically be expected to undergo antagonism by chlorpromazine.

**Mechanism:** The precise mechanism involved in the antagonism of amphet-amine by chlorpromazine is not known, but it appears to involve quite complex pharmacodynamic interplay with monoaminergic effector and control. Thioridazine has been associated with electrocardiogram repolarization abnormalities more frequently than other neuroleptics, and it has been reported to have induced ventricular arrhythmias and fatalities in some cases.

**Detailed Information:** See *EDI*, 10/5.00

Antipsychotic

### Chlorpromazine-Benztropine
**Significance:** 2—moderately clinically significant
**Recommendations:** Use of benztropine should probably be reserved to treat those responsive aspects of extrapyramidal syndrome (EPS) that can arise during chlorpromazine therapy. Clinical evidence suggests that relatively short-term treatment (three to four months) with benztropine may suffice to effectively deal with drug-induced parkinsonism. Refractory EPS cases may be a result of suboptimal serum concentrations of anticholinergic medication. Additive anticholinergic actions of benztropine and chlorpromazine may be hazardous in angle closure glaucoma or in individuals hyperresponsive to parasympathetic blockade.
**Summary:** The interaction between chlorpromazine and benztropine is used in managing certain movement disorders resulting from the antipsychotic-induced extrapyramidal syndrome (EPS).
**Related Drugs:** Virtually all antipsychotic drugs are able to induce EPS to varying extents. Other phenothiazines, thioxanthenes, dihydroindolones and dibenzoxazepines are expected to interact in a similar manner with benztropine. Other anticholinergic drugs commonly used in the treatment of parkinsonism may be effective in treating chlorpromazine-induced parkinsonism.
**Mechanism:** Chlorpromazine-induced parkinsonism appears to arise from a functional increase of cholinergic activity secondary to dopamine receptor blockade.
**Detailed Information:** See *EDI*, 10/7.00

### Chlorpromazine-Diazoxide
**Significance:** 2—moderately clinically significant
**Recommendations:** Patients' blood glucose should be closely monitored if chlorpromazine and diazoxide are to be used concurrently. The dose of diazoxide may need to be decreased.
**Summary:** A child on long-term diazoxide and bendroflumethiazide treatment developed severe hyperglycemia after administration of chlorpromazine.
**Related Drugs:** There are no drugs related to diazoxide. The phenothiazines, thioxanthenes, butyrophenones, dihydroindolones and dibenzoxazepines may interact in a similar manner with diazoxide.
**Mechanism:** The mechanism of this interaction is unknown; however, chlorpromazine has been reported to result in hyperglycemia.
**Detailed Information:** See *EDI*, 10/9.00

### Chlorpromazine-Levodopa
**Significance:** 3—minimally clinically significant
**Recommendations:** The effect of levodopa and chlorpromazine on each other is unpredictable. In instances where no alternative drugs are available and both drugs must be used, the patient should be observed closely for a deterioration in levodopa's growth hormone stimulating or antiparkinsonian effects, or a decrease in the therapeutic effect of chlorpromazine.
**Summary:** Levodopa and chlorpromazine may antagonize each other when these drugs are administered together.
**Related Drugs:** Other phenothiazines, thioxanthenes, butyrophenones, dihydroindolones and dibenzoxazepines may interact in a similar manner with levodopa. There are no drugs related to levodopa.
**Mechanism:** Chlorpromazine and levodopa have opposing actions at central dopaminergic receptor sites.
**Detailed Information:** See *EDI*, 10/11.00

## Antipsychotic

### Chlorpromazine-Lithium Carbonate
**Significance:** 2—moderately clinically significant
**Potential Effects:** Lithium carbonate may cause a decrease in chlorpromazine levels. Neurotoxicity may also occur when these agents are used together.
**Recommendations:** Monitor patients for decreased chlorpromazine levels or neurotoxicity when these agents are used together. Dosage adjustments or discontinuation of one or both agents may be necessary.
**Summary:** Concurrent administration of chlorpromazine and lithium carbonate has been shown to decrease plasma chlorpromazine levels, and neurotoxic and/or somnambulistic episodes have been reported.
**Related Drugs:** There are no drugs related to lithium carbonate. Interactions between lithium carbonate and other antipsychotics are discussed in other monographs (see Lithium Carbonate-Haloperidol, page 248, and Lithium Carbonate-Thioridazine, page 253).
**Mechanism:** The decreased chlorpromazine levels may be due to a lithium-induced delay in gastric emptying, decreasing bioavailability of chlorpromazine, or to a decreased chlorpromazine absorption.
**Detailed Information:** See *EDI*, 10/13.00

### Chlorpromazine-Phenobarbital
**Significance:** 3—minimally clinically significant
**Recommendations:** Since long-term administration of barbiturates might decrease the effectiveness of chlorpromazine by decreasing serum levels, the dosage of chlorpromazine may need to be increased. However, if the barbiturate is discontinued, chlorpromazine toxicity might result, and the dose would have to be readjusted.
**Summary:** The long-term administration of phenobarbital may decrease serum chlorpromazine levels, but no change in therapeutic response is documented.
**Related Drugs:** Chlorpromazine may enhance the action of some barbiturates. Other phenothiazines, thioxanthenes, butyrophenones, dihydroindolones and dibenzoxazepines may interact in a similar manner with phenobarbital.
**Mechanism:** Phenobarbital may increase the induction of hepatic microsomal enzymes, decreasing serum chlorpromazine levels. The sedative action of barbiturates is primarily the result of depression on the arousal system.
**Detailed Information:** See *EDI*, 10/15.00

### Chlorpromazine-Piperazine
**Significance:** 3—minimally clinically significant
**Recommendations:** From analysis of the data available regarding the potential interaction between chlorpromazine and piperazine, this combination appears devoid of serious risk. Individuals receiving this combined therapy should be carefully monitored for any manifestations of seizure disorders. Renal dysfunction may impair elimination of piperazine and potentially enhance the ability of this drug to elicit toxicity or interact with chlorpromazine.
**Summary:** There has been a report of the concurrent use of chlorpromazine and piperazine leading to convulsions.
**Related Drugs:** There is a lack of documentation concerning a similar interaction with other phenothiazines, thioxanthenes, butyrophenones, dihydroindolones and dibenzoxazepines. There are no drugs related to piperazine.
**Mechanism:** Chlorpromazine alone lowers the seizure threshold and, given in combination with piperazine, it may cause convulsions.
**Detailed Information:** See *EDI*, 10/17.00

Antipsychotic

### Chlorpromazine-Tobacco
**Significance:** 3—minimally clinically significant
**Recommendations:** Patients stabilized on chlorpromazine may exhibit altered responses to the drug if they change their smoking habits. Cessation of smoking may require decreased drug dosage to minimize sedation.
**Summary:** Smoking causes a decrease in chlorpromazine-induced drowsiness, sedation and hypotension.
**Related Drugs:** A similar interaction may occur with other phenothiazines, thioxanthenes, butyrophenones, dihydroindolones and dibenzoxazepines.
**Mechanism:** An increased dosage requirement in smokers could result from induction of chlorpromazine metabolism.
**Detailed Information:** See *EDI*, 10/18.01

### Clorazepate-Aluminum Hydroxide, Magnesium Hydroxide
**Significance:** 3—minimally clinically significant
**Recommendations:** Although concurrent use of these agents need not be avoided, it may be best to separate their administration by as much time as possible to avoid any possible interaction.
**Summary:** These agents have been shown to reduce the rate and extent of desmethyldiazepam, the metabolite of clorazepate; however, all data do not support this interaction.
**Related Drugs:** It is difficult to determine whether clorazepate would interact with other antacids or if an interaction would occur between aluminum hydroxide-magnesium hydroxide antacids and other benzodiazepines due to conflicting results.
**Mechanism:** The rate of clorazepate conversion to desmethyldiazepam depends on the presence of strong acid and may be decreased by the presence of the antacid.
**Detailed Information:** See *EDI*, 10/18.10

### Clorazepate-Influenza Virus Vaccine
**Significance:** 3—minimally clinically significant
**Potential Effects:** Influenza virus vaccine may inhibit the metabolism of clorazepate, leading to increased side effects.
**Recommendations:** The concurrent use of these agents need not be avoided; however, patients should be monitored for disorientation. The dose of clorazepate may need to be decreased or the clorazepate discontinued.
**Summary:** There are data to show that coadministration of these agents may lead to disorientation and lethargy.
**Related Drugs:** It is not known if an interaction would occur between influenza virus vaccine and other benzodiazepines due to conflicting results.
**Mechanism:** Influenza virus vaccine may inhibit the hepatic metabolism of clorazepate.
**Detailed Information:** See *EDI*, 10/18.30

### Clozapine-Caffeine
**Significance:** 3—minimally clinically significant
**Potential Effects:** Concurrent clozapine and caffeinated beverages may result in exacerbation of psychotic episodes, increased clozapine levels, and tachycardia.
**Recommendations:** Patients receiving therapy with clozapine who ingest caffeine should be monitored for exacerbation of psychotic symptoms and increased clozapine levels and adverse effects. Although the manufacturer states that the use of caffeine may help decrease the sedative effects of clozapine, some patients may

## Antipsychotic

need to be instructed to avoid caffeine-containing beverages and medications.

**Summary:** The concurrent use of clozapine with caffeinated beverages may result in exacerbation of psychotic episodes, increased clozapine levels, or tachycardia.

**Related Drugs:** There are no drugs related to clozapine. Documentation is lacking regarding a similar interaction between clozapine and the other xanthine derivatives.

**Mechanism:** Although the exact mechanism of this interaction is unknown, it is speculated that adenosine A2a receptor antagonism by caffeine results in increased dopamine activation at the $D_2$ receptor site. It has been postulated that the combination of clozapine, caffeine, and electroconvulsive therapy (ECT) may result in supraventricular tachycardia, although there are reports of caffeine-associated cardiac rhythm disturbances during ECT and tachycardia has been reported during clozapine use alone.

**Detailed Information:** See *EDI*, 10/18.45

## Clozapine-Carbamazepine

**Significance:** 1—highly clinically significant

**Potential Effects:** The concurrent use of carbamazepine and clozapine may result in decreased levels of clozapine, which may result in decreased antipsychotic control. Concurrent use may also result in ataxia. Additionally, both agents may increase the risk of agranulocytosis.

**Recommendations:** The potential for severe bone marrow depression by either clozapine or carbamazepine alone indicates that this combination should only be used with appropriate monitoring and when absolutely necessary. A clozapine dosage adjustment may be necessary to avoid subtherapeutic or toxic levels when carbamazepine is added to or discontinued from concurrent therapy.

**Summary:** The concurrent use of carbamazepine and clozapine resulted in decreased levels of clozapine by as much as 75%, which may have resulted in decreased antipsychotic control. Concurrent use may have also resulted in ataxia. Additionally, both agents have been shown to increase the risk of agranulocytosis.

**Related Drugs:** There are no drugs related to clozapine or carbamazepine.

**Mechanism:** Carbamazepine is known to be an inducer of liver microsomal enzyme systems regulating the inactivation of a variety of drugs, and it has been shown to substantially decrease the plasma levels of other neuroleptics. Similarly, the abrupt discontinuation of carbamazepine can markedly increase the plasma levels of concomitantly used neuroleptics. Carbamazepine has been reported to cause neutropenia, agranulocytosis, and aplastic anemia. Clozapine may also cause neutropenia, leukopenia, and granulocytopenia. It is not known if the bone marrow toxicity is an additive or synergistic effect due to the interaction between clozapine and carbamazepine.

**Detailed Information:** See *EDI*, 10/18.47

## Clozapine-Cimetidine

**Significance:** 2—moderately clinically significant

**Potential Effects:** Cimetidine may decrease the metabolism of clozapine, resulting in increased levels and toxicity.

**Recommendations:** Concurrent use of clozapine and cimetidine should be approached with caution. The patient should be monitored for symptoms of clozapine toxicity, and the clozapine dose may need to be reduced. Ranitidine may be an alternative to cimetidine.

**Summary:** Increased clozapine serum levels may result if cimetidine is added to therapy, thereby increasing adverse reactions to clozapine.

**Related Drugs:** Although ranitidine binds readily to clozapine P450 *in vitro*, doses of 300 mg/day have shown no similar effect on clozapine levels. The addition of cimetidine has resulted in excessive sedation, necessitating a reduction in chlorpromazine dosage in schizophrenic patients. Chronic administration of cimetidine may produce a fall in steady-state plasma chlorpromazine percent ratios. Conflicting studies with concurrent cimetidine and haloperidol in animal models have reported that cimetidine does not affect haloperidol-induced catalepsy and that cimetidine blocks the cataleptogenic effect of chlorpromazine. It is difficult to determine whether the other phenothiazines as well as molindone, loxapine, or pimozide would interact with cimetidine. It is also not known if an interaction would be expected to occur between clozapine and the other $H_2$-receptor antagonists.

**Mechanism:** It has been postulated that cimetidine may decrease the metabolism of clozapine due to cimetidine's cytochrome P450 inhibitory effect.

**Detailed Information:** See *EDI*, 10/18.50

## Clozapine-Erythromycin

**Significance:** 2—moderately clinically significant

**Potential Effects:** The addition of erythromycin to clozapine therapy may result in increased clozapine levels and tonic-clonic seizure.

**Recommendations:** Patients receiving clozapine and erythromycin concurrently should be monitored for signs of clozapine toxicity. Alternative antibiotic therapy may need to be instituted or the dose of clozapine may need to be reduced.

**Summary:** The addition of erythromycin to clozapine therapy may have resulted in increased clozapine levels and tonic-clonic seizure activity in a patient.

**Related Drugs:** It is expected that if the mechanism of the interaction is secondary to hepatic microsomal inhibition, clarithromycin and troleandomycin would interact and azithromycin, dirithromycin, and spiramycin would not. Documentation of this is lacking.

**Mechanism:** The mechanism of this interaction is unknown. Both clozapine and erythromycin are metabolized by the hepatic microsomal enzyme system. Erythromycin may have inhibited the metabolism of clozapine, resulting in increased clozapine levels.

**Detailed Information:** See *EDI*, 10/18.60

## Clozapine-Fluvoxamine

**Significance:** 2—moderately clinically significant

**Potential Effects:** Concurrent therapy with clozapine and fluvoxamine may result in increased clozapine and clozapine-related side effects.

**Recommendations:** Concurrent therapy with clozapine and a selective serotonin reuptake inhibitor (SSRI) need not be avoided. However, clozapine levels should be monitored and the patient should be monitored for signs of clozapine toxicity. The dosage of either clozapine or the SSRI may need to be adjusted or one or both agents may need to be discontinued.

**Summary:** Concurrent therapy with clozapine and fluvoxamine resulted in increased clozapine levels by as much as 269% and, in some reports, clozapine-related side effects.

**Related Drugs:** Paroxetine and sertraline have also been shown to increase clozapine levels. There are no drugs related to clozapine.

**Mechanism:** It is postulated that the metabolism of clozapine is inhibited by fluoxetine, fluvoxamine, paroxetine, and sertraline. Clozapine is metabolized at multiple cytochrome P450 isoenzymes, including $P450_{1A2}$.

**Detailed Information:** See *EDI*, 10/18.80

## Antipsychotic

### Clozapine-Rifampin

**Significance:** 2—moderately clinically significant

**Potential Effects:** Concurrent administration of rifampin and clozapine resulted in decreased clozapine levels and clinical effects.

**Recommendations:** The concurrent use of rifampin and clozapine should be approached with caution. Patients maintained on clozapine in whom rifampin is initiated should be monitored for decreased levels and therapeutic effectiveness of clozapine. Clozapine dosage adjustments or discontinuation of rifampin may be necessary. Clozapine dosage adjustments may be needed in patients who have been receiving concomitant clozapine and rifampin if rifampin is discontinued.

**Summary:** Concurrent administration of rifampin and clozapine resulted in decreased clozapine levels and clinical effects. Two to three weeks after the addition of rifampin to a clozapine regimen, clozapine levels decreased and did not increase despite an increase in clozapine dosage. Clozapine levels returned to therapeutic ranges within three days of discontinuing rifampin.

**Related Drugs:** If the other rifamycins (rifabutin, rifapentine) are also inducers of cytochrome $P450_{3A4}$ and $P450_{1A2}$, then a similar interaction would be expected to occur with these agents and clozapine, although documentation is lacking. There are no drugs related to clozapine.

**Mechanism:** It has been postulated that rifampin induces the metabolism of clozapine at the cytochrome $P450_{1A2}$ and $P450_{3A}$ isozymes. Rifampin has been shown to be a potent inducer of cytochrome $P450_{3A4}$ in both the liver and the intestine and an inducer of cytochrome $P450_{1A2}$. Clozapine has been shown to be metabolized by multiple P450 cytochromes, including $P450_{3A4}$ and $P450_{1A2}$.

**Detailed Information:** See *EDI*, 10/18.90

### Diazepam-Alcohol, Ethyl

**Significance:** 2—moderately clinically significant

**Potential Effects:** Concurrent use of diazepam with alcohol causes increased central nervous system (CNS) depression.

**Recommendations:** Patients receiving diazepam should be informed of the potentially serious effects of concomitant use of alcohol.

**Summary:** Diazepam and ethyl alcohol will lead to enhanced disruption of psychomotor performance and increased CNS depression.

**Related Drugs:** Temazepam and the other short-acting or intermediate-acting benzodiazepines tend to result in fewer alcohol interactions. Midazolam with alcohol results in impairment of immediate recall. Reports have been conflicting regarding the actions of chlordiazepoxide. An interaction may occur between alcohol and other benzodiazepines, although the extent of the interaction is difficult to determine.

**Mechanism:** There appears to be an unknown pharmacodynamic mechanism causing additive CNS depressant effect.

**Detailed Information:** See *EDI*, 10/19.00

### Diazepam-Aminophylline

**Significance:** 3—minimally clinically significant

**Potential Effects:** Aminophylline may decrease the sedative effects of diazepam.

**Recommendations:** If diazepam is being used for its sedative effects, the dose may need to be increased during concomitant aminophylline therapy.

**Summary:** Aminophylline has been shown to antagonize diazepam-induced anesthesia, sedation, somnolence, and impairment in thinking and psychomotor performance.

Antipsychotic

**Related Drugs:** A similar interaction may occur between diazepam and other theophylline derivatives. Caffeine has also been shown to antagonize the effects of diazepam and lorazepam.
**Mechanism:** Aminophylline and other xanthines may compete with diazepam at receptor sites, may depress GABA transmission or may interfere with adenosine receptors.
**Detailed Information:** See *EDI*, 10/20.10

## Diazepam-Cimetidine

**Significance:** 2—moderately clinically significant
**Potential Effects:** Cimetidine may decrease the metabolism of diazepam, leading to increased side effects such as sedation, fatigue, or drowsiness.
**Recommendations:** If these agents are given together, the patient should be monitored for increased side effects. A noninteracting benzodiazepine or famotidine or ranitidine may be considered.
**Summary:** Cimetidine has been found to increase the absorption and to significantly impair the elimination of diazepam, resulting in a potentiation of the sedative effects of diazepam.
**Related Drugs:** Chlordiazepoxide, alprazolam, triazolam, nitrazepam and midazolam have all been shown to interact with cimetidine in varying degrees. Other benzodiazepines dependent on phase I reactions would be expected to interact with cimetidine. Cimetidine does not alter the elimination of oxazepam, lorazepam or temazepam; lorazepam absorption is enhanced with concomitant cimetidine. Ranitidine has been shown to reduce diazepam's steady-state plasma levels and increase plasma clearance. Famotidine has been shown to have no effect on any pharmacokinetic parameters of diazepam.
**Mechanism:** Cimetidine may inhibit hepatic microsomal drug metabolism, causing a reduction in the hepatic elimination of diazepam.
**Detailed Information:** See *EDI*, 10/21.00

## Diazepam-Disulfiram

**Significance:** 3—minimally clinically significant
**Potential Effects:** Concurrent use of diazepam in patients receiving disulfiram may lead to enhanced sedation.
**Recommendations:** Present documentation suggests that the benzodiazepines that undergo N-demethylation, including diazepam, will be affected by disulfiram. It may be necessary to reduce the dosage of these particular benzodiazepines if concurrent use with disulfiram is required. An alternative may be to use oxazepam, lorazepam, or any other benzodiazepine that does not undergo N-demethylation. It is also important to realize that drowsiness is one of the most common side effects of disulfiram, and this may lead to an additive effect with use of benzodiazepines.
**Summary:** Concurrent use of diazepam in patients receiving disulfiram may lead to enhanced sedation.
**Related Drugs:** Chlordiazepoxide, oxazepam and lorazepam have been shown to interact with disulfiram in varying degrees. A similar interaction may occur between diazepam and other antialcoholic agents. A similar interaction is expected to occur with those benzodiazepines whose metabolic pathway is dependent on phase I reactions.
**Mechanism:** Disulfiram inhibits N-demethylation and C-hydroxylation of diazepam and the glucuronidation of the metabolites so formed.
**Detailed Information:** See *EDI*, 10/25.00

## Antipsychotic

### Diazepam-Isoniazid
**Significance:** 3—minimally clinically significant
**Recommendations:** The reduction in diazepam clearance is small but may necessitate a decreased diazepam dosage in some patients.
**Summary:** Isoniazid has been shown to prolong diazepam half-life and decrease diazepam clearance.
**Related Drugs:** There are no drugs related to isoniazid. A similar interaction is expected to occur with other benzodiazepines metabolized by phase I reactions, if the mechanism involves inhibition of hepatic enzymes by isoniazid.
**Mechanism:** Isoniazid inhibits hepatic microsomal drug metabolism, and this may cause a decrease in diazepam clearance.
**Detailed Information:** See *EDI*, 10/27.00

### Diazepam-Levodopa
**Significance:** 3—minimally clinically significant
**Recommendations:** Clinical data about this drug interaction are insufficient to recommend avoiding the concurrent use of levodopa and benzodiazepines. However, one should be alert for evidence of worsening parkinsonism in patients previously stabilized on levodopa who are receiving this drug combination.
**Summary:** Concurrent administration of diazepam and levodopa may result in a diminished antiparkinson effect of levodopa.
**Related Drugs:** Chlordiazepoxide, nitrazepam, flurazepam and oxazepam have been used with levodopa without any significant loss in antiparkinson activity. It is difficult to predict possible interactions of other benzodiazepines with levodopa. Levodopa-carbidopa may interact with benzodiazepines in a similar manner.
**Mechanism:** Benzodiazepines are known to increase the brain's acetylcholine content, possibly antagonizing the beneficial dopamine-mediated response to levodopa.
**Detailed Information:** See *EDI*, 10/29.00

### Diazepam-Omeprazole
**Significance:** 3—minimally clinically significant
**Potential Effects:** Concurrent administration of diazepam and omeprazole may result in a decrease in the mean clearance of diazepam.
**Recommendations:** Patients maintained on omeprazole should be monitored for enhanced diazepam response with concurrent administration of these agents.
**Summary:** Concurrent administration of diazepam and omeprazole resulted in a decrease in the mean clearance of diazepam by up to 54% and an increase in diazepam half-life by as much as 130%.
**Related Drugs:** When added to triazolam and lorazepam therapy, omeprazole has caused gait disturbance. Dizziness and difficulty walking have also been reported when omeprazole was added to flurazepam therapy. *In vitro*, omeprazole has inhibited the metabolism of midazolam. The other benzodiazepines metabolized by N-demethylation or hydroxylation may be expected to interact similarly; however, it is not known if those dependent on glucuronidation would interact. Lansoprazole and pantoprazole have shown no significant effects on diazepam pharmacokinetics.
**Mechanism:** It is postulated that the decrease in diazepam clearance is an effect of omeprazole's inhibition of the cytochrome P450 enzyme system. Diazepam is metabolized by the $P450_{2C19}$ and $P450_{3A}$ isozymes. Lansoprazole, pantoprazole, and omeprazole are also metabolized by the $P450_{2C19}$ and $P450_{3A}$ isozymes and inhibit these isozymes. Pantoprazole is also metabolized by a cytosolic sulfotransferase, a conjugating enzyme.
**Detailed Information:** See *EDI*, 10/30.10

Antipsychotic

### Diazepam-Oral Contraceptive Agents
**Significance:** 3—minimally clinically significant
**Potential Effects:** Oral contraceptive agents may alter the metabolism of diazepam, resulting in increased diazepam levels.
**Recommendations:** Although a direct relationship between the plasma concentration of diazepam and its clinical effect is not clearly established, patients who are taking oral contraceptives should be closely monitored for increased diazepam effects. A dosage adjustment may be necessary in some patients.
**Summary:** There are data to show that coadministration of these agents may lead to an increased diazepam effect.
**Related Drugs:** The data regarding the coadministration of oral contraceptives and benzodiazepines are very conflicting.
**Mechanism:** Estrogens may bind to cytochrome P450 and decrease the amount of the hepatic oxidative drug-metabolizing enzyme system necessary in diazepam oxidation.
**Detailed Information:** See *EDI*, 10/31.00

### Diazepam-Propranolol
**Significance:** 3—minimally clinically significant
**Potential Effects:** Propranolol may inhibit the metabolism of diazepam.
**Recommendations:** If increased effects of diazepam are observed during concurrent administration with propranolol, the dose of diazepam may need to be decreased.
**Summary:** There are data to show that coadministration of these agents may lead to the increased effects of diazepam, and it has been documented that these agents did impair measures of subjective arousal and mood.
**Related Drugs:** The data regarding the use of the benzodiazepines and beta-blockers are conflicting, and it is suggested that the use of these agents be monitored closely and dosage adjustments made when required.
**Mechanism:** Propranolol may inhibit the metabolism of diazepam, and the inhibition of diazepam's metabolism has been found to be proportional to the degree of lipid solubility of the beta-blocking agent.
**Detailed Information:** See *EDI*, 10/32.10

### Diazepam-Rifampin
**Significance:** 3—minimally clinically significant
**Potential Effects:** Rifampin may induce the metabolism of diazepam, resulting in decreased levels.
**Recommendations:** Patients receiving rifampin, either alone or in combination therapy, may have markedly enhanced diazepam clearance, and may therefore require higher doses of diazepam.
**Summary:** There are data to show that administration of rifampin may lead to an enhanced diazepam clearance and a reduced half-life, maximum concentration and area-under-curve, and this may necessitate higher doses of diazepam.
**Related Drugs:** A similar interaction is expected to occur with the other benzodiazepines metabolized by phase I and rifampin, if the mechanism involves induction of hepatic enzymes by rifampin. There are no drugs related to rifampin.
**Mechanism:** Rifampin, a known enzyme inducer, may be the primary cause of this interaction.
**Detailed Information:** See *EDI*, 10/33.00

# Antipsychotic

## Diazepam-Tobacco

**Significance:** 3—minimally clinically significant

**Potential Effects:** Tobacco may decrease the sedative effect of diazepam. The dose of diazepam, in most cases, need not be changed in patients who use tobacco.

**Recommendations:** However, in some patients, the dose of diazepam may need to be increased.

**Summary:** There are data to show that smokers who were administered diazepam experienced less sedation.

**Related Drugs:** The data regarding smokers who use benzodiazepines are conflicting, and it is suggested that the use of these agents be monitored closely and dosage adjustments made when required.

**Mechanism:** The constituents of cigarette smoke may stimulate a more rapid metabolism of diazepam and other benzodiazepines.

**Detailed Information:** See *EDI*, 10/34.10

## Fluphenazine-Clonidine

**Significance:** 3—minimally clinically significant

**Recommendations:** Since the discontinuation of clonidine causes neurologic symptoms to disappear, this is the course of action suggested in patients developing such symptoms. Hydralazine has been substituted for clonidine with no similar interaction.

**Summary:** In one patient receiving clonidine and chlorthalidone, administration of fluphenazine led to acute organic brain syndrome.

**Related Drugs:** There are no drugs related to clonidine. Other phenothiazines, thioxanthenes, butyrophenones, dihydroindolones and dibenzoxazepines may interact in a similar manner.

**Mechanism:** Clonidine, a potent alpha-adrenergic agonist, when combined with fluphenazine, a potent dopamine blocker, may result in a relative adrenergic dominance.

**Detailed Information:** See *EDI*, 10/35.00

## Haloperidol-Carbamazepine

**Significance:** 2—moderately clinically significant

**Potential Effects:** Carbamazepine may cause a decrease in haloperidol levels.

**Recommendations:** Monitor the patient's mental status and haloperidol levels if carbamazepine is added to, or withdrawn from, therapy.

**Summary:** There are data to show that administration of carbamazepine may cause a decrease in haloperidol levels; however, all data do not support this interaction.

**Related Drugs:** Because the mechanism of this interaction is unclear, it is not known if the phenothiazines, thioxanthenes, butyrophenones, dihydroindolones and dibenzoxazepines would interact with carbamazepine. There are no drugs related to carbamazepine.

**Mechanism:** Carbamazepine may increase haloperidol's metabolism, or haloperidol may facilitate intracellular transport of carbamazepine; however, this is not documented.

**Detailed Information:** See *EDI*, 10/36.10

## Haloperidol-Fluoxetine

**Significance:** 3—minimally clinically significant

**Potential Effects:** Addition of fluoxetine to haloperidol therapy may cause extrapyramidal symptoms.

## Antipsychotic

**Recommendations:** Patients maintained on haloperidol should be carefully monitored for extrapyramidal symptoms if fluoxetine is added to therapy. One or both agents may need to be discontinued.

**Summary:** There are data to show that a patient maintained on haloperidol developed extrapyramidal symptoms when administered fluoxetine.

**Related Drugs:** It is not known if an interaction would occur between fluoxetine and other antipsychotic agents such as the phenothiazines, thioxanthenes, butyrophenones, dihydroindolones and dibenzoxazepines. There are no drugs related to fluoxetine.

**Mechanism:** The mechanism of this interaction is not known.

**Detailed Information:** See *EDI*, 10/36.30

### Haloperidol-Itraconazole

**Significance:** 3—minimally clinically significant

**Potential Effects:** The concurrent use of haloperidol and itraconazole resulted in elevated levels of haloperidol and "reduced haloperidol" (RHAL), a major metabolite of haloperidol, and an increase in haloperidol-related side effects.

**Recommendations:** Patients receiving concurrent therapy with haloperidol and itraconazole should be observed for increased haloperidol-related side effects. The dosage of haloperidol may need to be reduced. Haloperidol and/or itraconazole may need to be discontinued.

**Summary:** Concurrent use of haloperidol and itraconazole has resulted in elevated levels of haloperidol and RHAL, a major metabolite of haloperidol, and an increase in haloperidol-related side-effects.

**Related Drugs:** Bromperidol levels increased 87.6% and reduced bromperidol (RBRM), a major metabolite of bromperidol, levels increased 100% during itraconazole administration in one study. An interaction may occur between ketoconazole and haloperidol. It is not known if an interaction would occur between haloperidol and other imidazole antifungal agents. There are no other agents related to haloperidol.

**Mechanism:** Itraconazole may inhibit the metabolism of haloperidol and bromperidol by the cytochrome $P450_{3A4}$ isoenzyme. Ketoconazole inhibits the metabolism of haloperidol and RHAL by the cytochrome $P450_{3A4}$ isoenzyme *in vitro*.

**Detailed Information:** See *EDI*, 10/36.36

### Haloperidol-Rifampin

**Significance:** 2—moderately clinically significant

**Potential Effects:** Concurrent administration of haloperidol and rifampin may result in decreased levels of haloperidol.

**Recommendations:** Patients receiving haloperidol who are started on rifampin should be monitored for decreased haloperidol levels and decreased effectiveness of haloperidol. Patients maintained on haloperidol in whom rifampin is discontinued should be monitored for increased haloperidol levels and possible adverse effects. The dose of haloperidol may need to be adjusted.

**Summary:** Concurrent administration of haloperidol and rifampin resulted in decreased levels of haloperidol. Discontinuation of rifampin from concurrent therapy with haloperidol resulted in increased haloperidol levels.

**Related Drugs:** An interaction would be expected to occur between the other butyrophenones and rifampin as well as between haloperidol and rifabutin.

# Antipsychotic

**Mechanism:** Rifampin has been shown to induce the cytochromes $P450_{3A}$, $P450_{2C}$, and $P450_{2D6}$. Haloperidol is metabolized by several cytochrome P450 isozymes, including $P450_{2D6}$ and $P450_{1A2}$. Rifampin may induce the metabolism of haloperidol at the $P450_{2D6}$ isozyme site.

**Detailed Information:** See *EDI*, 10/36.45

## Haloperidol-Tacrine

**Significance:** 2—moderately clinically significant

**Potential Effects:** Concurrent administration of haloperidol and tacrine may result in parkinsonian symptoms.

**Recommendations:** Patients receiving concurrent therapy with haloperidol and tacrine should be monitored for parkinsonian symptoms. One or both agents may need to be discontinued.

**Summary:** Concurrent administration of haloperidol and tacrine resulted in parkinsonian symptoms. After discontinuation and resolution of symptoms, rechallenge with the two drugs produced the same adverse effects.

**Related Drugs:** It is not known if the other antipsychotic agents such as the phenothiazines, thioxanthenes, as well as molindone, loxapine, clozapine, risperidone, and pimozide would interact with tacrine. There are no drugs related to tacrine.

**Mechanism:** It is postulated that a tacrine-induced increase in cholinergic activity enhances basal ganglia sensitivity to haloperidol's dopamine-blocking ability. Concurrent administration may result in increased striatal acetylcholine activity, resulting in parkinsonian symptoms.

**Detailed Information:** See *EDI*, 10/36.60

## Hypericum-Hormonal Contraceptive Agents

**Significance:** 2—moderately clinically significant

**Potential Effects:** Concurrent administration of hypericum (*Hypericum perforatum L*) and progestin/estrogen oral contraceptive agents may result in breakthrough bleeding and a possible decrease in contraceptive effectiveness.

**Recommendations:** In patients receiving concurrent hypericum and hormonal contraceptive agents, there is a possibility of induced metabolism of the estrogen and a possible resultant reduced contraceptive effect. Until more studies are done, it would seem prudent to advise women of this possibility and suggest that they consider an alternative method of contraception or an alternative to St. John's wort.

**Summary:** Concurrent administration of hypericum and progestin/estrogen oral contraceptive agents has resulted in breakthrough bleeding and a possible decrease in contraceptive effectiveness.

**Related Drugs:** It is not known whether a similar interaction would occur between hypericum and other estrogenic substances.

**Mechanism:** St. John's wort induces cytochrome $P450_{3A4}$ and may induce P-glycoprotein transport. Cytochrome $P450_{3A4}$ inducers such as rifampin and rifabutin may cause breakthrough bleeding when given with oral contraceptives. This may be related to induction of metabolism of the estrogen component.

**Detailed Information:** See *EDI*, 10/36.80

## Lithium Carbonate-Acetazolamide

**Significance:** 1—highly clinically significant

**Recommendations:** It is important to measure lithium serum levels during concurrent use of these agents. A higher dose of lithium carbonate may be necessary.

**Summary:** There are data to show that the administration of acetazolamide causes an increase in the excretion of lithium, necessitating an increase in lithium dosages.
**Related Drugs:** A similar interaction is expected to occur between lithium carbonate and other carbonic anhydrase inhibitors.
**Mechanism:** Acetazolamide may increase the renal excretion of lithium by alkalinization of the urine or by impairing the proximal tubular reabsorption of lithium.
**Detailed Information:** See *EDI*, 10/37.00

## Lithium Carbonate-Acyclovir

**Significance:** 3—minimally clinically significant
**Potential Effects:** The addition of acyclovir to a lithium carbonate regimen may result in increased lithium levels and toxicity.
**Recommendations:** Patients should be carefully monitored for increased serum lithium levels and toxicity with concurrent administration of lithium carbonate and high-dose intravenous acyclovir. Further studies are needed.
**Summary:** The addition of intravenous acyclovir to a lithium carbonate regimen resulted in increased serum lithium levels from 0.8 meq/L to 3.4 meq/L (normal range: 0.6–1.2 meq/L) and lithium toxicity.
**Related Drugs:** It is not known whether an interaction would be expected to occur between lithium and the other nucleoside analogues. There are no drugs related to lithium.
**Mechanism:** Since both of these agents are primarily eliminated unchanged in the kidneys and the percentage of acyclovir excreted increases with increasing dose, acyclovir serum concentrations attained following intravenous acyclovir doses of 10 mg/kg may impair the clearance of lithium. Further studies are needed to validate this hypothesis. The bioavailability of oral acyclovir ranges from 15–30%; it has been postulated that it may be unlikely that increased serum lithium levels will occur with concurrent lithium carbonate and oral acyclovir.
**Detailed Information:** See *EDI*, 10/37.50

## Lithium Carbonate-Alcohol, Ethyl

**Significance:** 3—minimally clinically significant
**Potential Effects:** Alcohol may cause an increase in lithium levels.
**Recommendations:** The use of these agents together need not be avoided; however, lithium levels should be closely monitored in patients who use alcohol.
**Summary:** There are data to show that alcohol may cause an increase in lithium levels; however, all data do not support this, and there are conflicting reports.
**Related Drugs:** There are no drugs related to lithium carbonate.
**Mechanism:** The mechanism of this interaction is not known.
**Detailed Information:** See *EDI*, 10/38.10

## Lithium Carbonate-Carbamazepine

**Significance:** 2—moderately clinically significant
**Potential Effects:** Neurotoxicity may occur when these agents are used together.
**Recommendations:** Monitor patients for neurotoxicity when these agents are used concurrently. One or both agents may need to be discontinued.
**Summary:** There are data to show that coadministration of these agents may cause neurotoxicity; however, data have shown that use of these agents does not potentiate neurotoxicity.

# Antipsychotic

**Related Drugs:** There are no drugs related to lithium carbonate or carbamazepine.

**Mechanism:** This interaction may be related to the combined, mutual effects of lithium carbonate and carbamazepine on sodium metabolism or on nerve conduction velocity.

**Detailed Information:** See *EDI*, 10/39.00

## Lithium Carbonate-Chlorothiazide

**Significance:** 1—highly clinically significant

**Recommendations:** Although several studies have pointed out specific instances in which lithium and chlorothiazide are useful (e.g., lithium polyuria and lithium-induced nephrogenic diabetes insipidus) when given concurrently, in general they should not be used together. If these drugs must be given simultaneously, the patient should be observed closely for signs and symptoms of lithium-induced neurotoxicity or cardiotoxicity, and a lower dose of lithium may be required. The potassium-sparing diuretics, spironolactone and triamterene, did not affect serum lithium concentrations in a small group of patients and may be safer diuretics to use concurrently with lithium. Amiloride, another potassium-sparing diuretic, may also be considered.

**Summary:** Concurrent administration of chlorothiazide may result in enhanced cardiotoxicity and neurotoxicity secondary to lithium.

**Related Drugs:** Any thiazide diuretic that promotes or enhances the excretion of both sodium and potassium may interact with lithium. The loop diuretics, the mercurial diuretics, other thiazides and other thiazide-related diuretics may interact with lithium.

**Mechanism:** Long-term thiazide administration may lead to an increase in the reabsorption of lithium and a subsequent decrease in lithium clearance.

**Detailed Information:** See *EDI*, 10/41.00

## Lithium Carbonate-Cisplatin

**Significance:** 3—minimally clinically significant

**Potential Effects:** Cisplatin therapy may temporarily decrease lithium levels.

**Recommendations:** Monitor lithium levels when cisplatin therapy (cisplatin and fluid load) are added to lithium therapy. The decrease in lithium levels should return to baseline shortly after completion of therapy.

**Summary:** There are data to show that cisplatin therapy may temporarily decrease lithium levels; however, fluid load, which is part of cisplatin therapy, may be responsible for the decreased lithium levels.

**Related Drugs:** There are no drugs related to lithium or cisplatin.

**Mechanism:** The decreased lithium levels occurred because of enhanced renal elimination of lithium.

**Detailed Information:** See *EDI*, 10/42.10

## Lithium Carbonate-Diazepam

**Significance:** 3—minimally clinically significant

**Potential Effects:** The use of these agents together may result in hypothermia associated with coma, reduced pulse rates, and lowering of systolic blood pressure.

**Recommendations:** The use of these agents together need not to be avoided. If hypothermia occurs, one or both drugs may need to be discontinued.

**Summary:** The concurrent use of lithium carbonate and diazepam has been shown to result in hypothermia associated with coma, reduced reflexes, decreased pulse and a low systolic blood pressure.

## Antipsychotic

**Related Drugs:** There is no documentation regarding a similar interaction between lithium carbonate and the other benzodiazepines. There are no drugs related to lithium carbonate.
**Mechanism:** The mechanism of this interaction is unknown.
**Detailed Information:** See *EDI*, 10/43.00

### Lithium Carbonate-Enalapril

**Significance:** 2—moderately clinically significant
**Potential Effects:** Enalapril may increase lithium levels, leading to toxicity.
**Recommendations:** Patients should be monitored for signs of lithium toxicity, increased lithium levels, and a decrease in renal function when concurrent enalapril is administered. The dose of lithium may need to be decreased or enalapril may need to be discontinued.
**Summary:** The addition of lithium carbonate to the therapy of a patient maintained on enalapril resulted in increased serum lithium levels.
**Related Drugs:** Lisinopril has been shown to potentiate lithium carbonate toxicity. A similar interaction may occur between lithium carbonate and other ACE inhibitors. A similar interaction would be expected to occur between enalapril and lithium citrate.
**Mechanism:** The increase in lithium serum concentration may be because of the loss of sodium ions and decreased fluid volume.
**Detailed Information:** See *EDI*, 10/44.10

### Lithium Carbonate-Fluoxetine

**Significance:** 2—moderately clinically significant
**Potential Effects:** Fluoxetine may increase lithium levels, resulting in toxicity.
**Recommendations:** Patients on lithium therapy should be closely monitored for increased lithium levels if fluoxetine is administered. The dose of lithium may need to be decreased or fluoxetine may need to be discontinued. Paroxetine may be a potential agent for alternative therapy.
**Summary:** Increased lithium levels may occur when coadministered with fluoxetine.
**Related Drugs:** Sertraline and lithium carbonate exhibited a similar interaction. Fluvoxamine and lithium therapy resulted in somnolence.
**Mechanism:** Fluoxetine has been reported to cause mania, and manic patients have a greater vulnerability to neurotoxicity associated with lithium. There may be a possible synergistic antidepressant effect between lithium and fluoxetine.
**Detailed Information:** See *EDI*, 10/44.30

### Lithium Carbonate-Haloperidol

**Significance:** 2—moderately clinically significant
**Recommendations:** Lithium's onset of action occurs several days after therapy is begun. Therefore, haloperidol is usually added during the acute manic phase and then its dose is tapered and finally discontinued. It is preferable to avoid using these agents together during the acute manic phase since there is a higher risk of combined toxicity at that time. If this combination of drugs is to be used during the acute manic symptoms, a conservative lithium dosage is recommended.
**Summary:** Concomitant administration of lithium carbonate and haloperidol has been reported to cause confusion, extrapyramidal and cerebellar dysfunction, and, in some cases, permanent brain damage and irreversible dyskinesias.

Antipsychotic

**Related Drugs:** There are no drugs related to lithium carbonate. The interactions between lithium carbonate and other antipsychotics are discussed in other monographs (see Chlorpromazine-Lithium Carbonate, page 235, and Lithium Carbonate-Thioridazine, page 253).

**Mechanism:** The mechanism is not known. It has been suggested that this interaction may be dose related.

**Detailed Information:** See *EDI*, 10/45.00

## Lithium Carbonate-Indomethacin

**Significance:** 2—moderately clinically significant

**Potential Effects:** Indomethacin may cause an increase in lithium levels, possibly resulting in lithium toxicity.

**Recommendations:** Monitor patients and lithium levels carefully if these agents are used together. The dose of lithium may need to be decreased or sulindac may possibly be used instead of indomethacin.

**Summary:** The addition of indomethacin to a stable lithium carbonate regimen resulted in increased lithium plasma levels and toxicity (e.g., polyuria, delirium, lethargy).

**Related Drugs:** Other nonsteroidal anti-inflammatory drugs (NSAIDs) that have been reported to interact with lithium carbonate resulting in increased lithium levels include ibuprofen, diclofenac, piroxicam, phenylbutazone, mefenamic acid, tiaprofenic acid, naproxen, and ketorolac. Although the interaction with sulindac is conflicting (causing both increased and decreased serum lithium levels), an interaction between lithium and other NSAIDs would be expected to occur. There are no drugs related to lithium.

**Mechanism:** Prostaglandins may play an important role in renal lithium clearance. Concurrent administration of NSAIDs (prostaglandin synthesis inhibitors) with lithium reduces renal lithium clearance, causing an increase in plasma lithium concentrations. Enhanced renal reabsorption of lithium induced by indomethacin is another possible explanation. The mechanism of action of sulindac's paradoxical effect on lithium is not known. However, it has been suggested that sulindac has a sparing effect on renal prostaglandin synthesis. A possible mechanism may be a sparing effect on intrarenal cyclooxygenase since sulindac is broken down into inactive metabolites (sulindac sulfoxide and sulindac sulfone) in the kidney. Since lithium is approximately 80% reabsorbed in the proximal tubule, the addition of tiaprofenic acid may result in enhanced tubular lithium reabsorption.

**Detailed Information:** See *EDI*, 10/47.00

## Lithium Carbonate-Ispaghula (Psyllium Hydrophilic Mucilloid)

**Significance:** 3—minimally clinically significant

**Potential Effects:** The concurrent administration of lithium carbonate and ispaghula husk (psyllium hydrophilic mucilloid) may result in decreased plasma lithium concentrations.

**Recommendations:** Patients receiving lithium compounds should be carefully monitored to ensure therapeutic plasma lithium levels when receiving concurrent ispaghula husk or other psyllium hydrophilic mucilloid-type bulk-forming laxatives. An alternate laxative choice may need to be considered.

**Summary:** Concurrent administration of lithium carbonate and ispaghula husk resulted in decreased plasma lithium concentrations in a single case report.

**Related Drugs:** There are no drugs related to lithium or ispaghula husk.

**Mechanism:** Ispaghula husk may inhibit lithium absorption from the GI tract. This hydrophilic mucilloid bulk-forming laxative maintains hydrated feces; therefore, a greater amount of ingested lithium may remain ionized, unabsorbed from the gut, and excreted.
**Detailed Information:** See *EDI*, 10/60.00

## Lithium Carbonate-Losartan
**Significance:** 3—minimally clinically significant
**Potential Effects:** Concurrent administration of lithium carbonate and losartan may result in increased serum lithium levels and toxicity.
**Recommendations:** A case report suggests a potential risk of lithium toxicity in elderly patients receiving concurrent lithium carbonate and losartan. Prudence would indicate careful monitoring of lithium serum levels.
**Summary:** The addition of losartan to the therapy of a patient stabilized on lithium carbonate resulted in increased serum lithium levels and resultant toxicity, including ataxia, dysarthria, and confusion.
**Related Drugs:** A similar interaction may occur between lithium carbonate and the other angiotensin-II-receptor antagonists. There are no drugs related to lithium carbonate.
**Mechanism:** Increased lithium levels may have been the result of an increase in renal lithium reabsorption. Renal lithium reabsorption occurs primarily at a proximal tubular site and may have been triggered by natriuresis associated with inhibition of aldosterone secretion induced by losartan.
**Detailed Information:** See *EDI*, 10/48.00

## Lithium Carbonate-Mazindol
**Significance:** 2—moderately clinically significant
**Recommendations:** When an anorexic agent such as mazindol is used concurrently with lithium therapy, care should be taken to assure that sodium intake remains adequate so that increased serum lithium concentrations and possible toxicity are avoided. It may be necessary to lower the dose of lithium during concurrent administration of mazindol.
**Summary:** Lithium intoxication has been observed in a case where lithium carbonate and mazindol were administered simultaneously.
**Related Drugs:** Other anorexic agents should be used cautiously. There are no drugs related to lithium carbonate.
**Mechanism:** A compensatory increase in lithium reabsorption may occur, resulting in a decreased lithium clearance. Dieting and a decrease in sodium intake may induce lithium intoxications.
**Detailed Information:** See *EDI*, 10/49.00

## Lithium Carbonate-Methyldopa
**Significance:** 2—moderately clinically significant
**Potential Effects:** The use of these agents together may result in lithium toxicity despite normal lithium levels.
**Recommendations:** If toxicity occurs, the dose of lithium should be decreased or another antihypertensive used.
**Summary:** Several case reports have shown that the concurrent administration of lithium carbonate and methyldopa may result in signs of lithium toxicity despite the presence of therapeutic serum lithium levels.
**Related Drugs:** There are no drugs related to lithium carbonate or methyldopa.
**Mechanism:** Methyldopa may exacerbate the CNS response to lithium or may increase the brain uptake of lithium.
**Detailed Information:** See *EDI*, 10/51.00

## Lithium Carbonate-Metoprolol

**Significance:** 2—moderately clinically significant

**Recommendations:** Because all beta-blocking agents can improve lithium-induced tremors, it is advisable to use a cardioselective agent such as metoprolol in patients with bronchospastic problems.

**Summary:** In two patients with a history of bronchospastic disease, the use of metoprolol produced objective and subjective improvement of lithium carbonate-induced tremors.

**Related Drugs:** Propranolol, pindolol and nadolol have been shown to act like metoprolol, but these are contraindicated in bronchospastic disease. A similar interaction may occur with other non-cardioselective beta-blocking agents. The other cardioselective beta-blocking agents would act like metoprolol.

**Mechanism:** The mechanism of this interaction is not fully known; however, both $beta_1$ and $beta_2$ receptors have been implicated in essential tremor.

**Detailed Information:** See *EDI*, 10/53.00

## Lithium Carbonate-Metronidazole

**Significance:** 2—moderately clinically significant

**Potential Effects:** Metronidazole may increase the incidence of lithium nephrotoxicity.

**Recommendations:** Patients should be closely monitored for the development of renal complications during concurrent use of these agents. Also, lithium, creatinine, and electrolyte levels should be monitored. Lithium may need to be discontinued or the dosage tapered.

**Summary:** The administration of metronidazole and lithium carbonate has resulted in toxic reactions to lithium.

**Related Drugs:** There are no drugs related to lithium carbonate or metronidazole.

**Mechanism:** The mechanism of this interaction is not known.

**Detailed Information:** See *EDI*, 10/54.10

## Lithium Carbonate-Norepinephrine

**Significance:** 3—minimally clinically significant

**Recommendations:** If a patient on lithium carbonate is to receive norepinephrine, a higher dose of norepinephrine may be necessary to achieve the desired pressor response.

**Summary:** Lithium carbonate has been shown to decrease the pressor response to norepinephrine.

**Related Drugs:** A similar interaction may be expected between lithium carbonate and other direct acting sympathomimetics. Documentation is lacking regarding a similar interaction with other mixed acting sympathomimetics. Tyramine has been shown to not alter lithium carbonate. The indirect acting sympathomimetics have been reported to increase lithium levels (see also Lithium Carbonate-Mazindol, page 250). There is no documentation regarding a similar interaction between lithium carbonate and other indirect acting sympathomimetics. There are no drugs related to lithium carbonate.

**Mechanism:** The mechanism of this interaction is unknown.

**Detailed Information:** See *EDI*, 10/55.00

## Lithium Carbonate-Phenytoin

**Significance:** 3—minimally clinically significant

**Recommendations:** Until further documentation is available, patients receiving concurrent therapy of lithium and phenytoin should be observed for clinical signs of lithium toxicity. Since toxicity has been reported in the presence of normal therapeutic levels, therapy should be closely supervised. Dosing adjustments of lithium may be required.

Antipsychotic

**Summary:** There are data to show that administration of phenytoin may potentiate clinical signs of lithium toxicity, and toxicity has been reported in the presence of normal therapeutic levels.
**Related Drugs:** There is a lack of documentation regarding an interaction between lithium and other hydantoin derivatives. There are no drugs related to lithium carbonate.
**Mechanism:** The mechanism of this interaction is unknown.
**Detailed Information:** See *EDI*, 10/57.00

## Lithium Carbonate-Potassium Iodide

**Significance:** 2—moderately clinically significant
**Recommendations:** Patients receiving lithium carbonate should avoid taking nonprescription or prescription iodine-containing preparations. The appearance of goiter or detection of abnormal chemical thyroid tests is not an indication to discontinue lithium therapy. However, it is appropriate to discontinue any iodine-containing drugs and to stabilize thyroid status with appropriate drugs.
**Summary:** The concurrent administration of lithium carbonate and potassium iodide or other iodine-containing compounds may enhance the hypothyroid and goitrogenic effects of either drug.
**Related Drugs:** An interaction between lithium carbonate and isopropamide iodide has been reported. All prescription, nonprescription and radiographic products containing iodine may enhance lithium's antithyroid effects. There are no drugs related to lithium carbonate.
**Mechanism:** Concurrent use of these compounds could have additive or synergistic hypothyroid effects.
**Detailed Information:** See *EDI*, 10/59.00

## Lithium Carbonate-Tetracycline

**Significance:** 2—moderately clinically significant
**Potential Effects:** Concurrent use of these agents may lead to lithium toxicity or a decrease in lithium levels.
**Recommendations:** Caution should be used when concurrently administering lithium and tetracycline, since lithium levels may be increased or decreased by tetracycline. Serum lithium concentrations should be determined routinely, and the dose of lithium adjusted accordingly.
**Summary:** The concurrent administration of lithium carbonate and tetracycline may cause serum concentrations of lithium to increase and may lead to lithium toxicity; however, there are conflicting data.
**Related Drugs:** Documentation is lacking regarding an interaction between lithium carbonate and other tetracyclines.
**Mechanism:** The mechanism of this interaction is unknown.
**Detailed Information:** See *EDI*, 10/61.00

## Lithium Carbonate-Theophylline

**Significance:** 2—moderately clinically significant
**Potential Effects:** Theophylline and caffeine may increase lithium clearance, resulting in decreased lithium levels.
**Recommendations:** Monitor lithium levels closely if theophylline or caffeine is added to or withdrawn from cotherapy. The dosage of lithium may need to be changed.
**Summary:** Theophylline and caffeine may increase lithium clearance, resulting in increased lithium clearances by 51%. It has been suggested that theophylline infusions might be an alternative to hemodialysis in lithium intoxications requiring an immediate reduction in lithium concentration.

**Related Drugs:** It has been shown that aminophylline increases the lithium/creatinine clearance ratio, which may result in decreased serum lithium below the therapeutic level. Lithium levels increased 23.9% from baseline following caffeine withdrawal and returned to baseline following resumption of caffeine. A similar interaction may be expected between lithium carbonate and the other theophylline derivatives. There are no drugs related to lithium carbonate.

**Mechanism:** The mechanism of this interaction is related to an increase in the renal excretion of lithium by the theophylline derivative aminophylline.

**Detailed Information:** See *EDI*, 10/63.00

## Lithium Carbonate-Thioridazine

**Significance:** 2—moderately clinically significant

**Recommendations:** Plasma level monitoring of either agent is of questionable value in preventing the occurrence of neurotoxic symptoms, since many patients experienced neurotoxic symptoms with plasma concentrations within the therapeutic range. Routine electroencephalogram monitoring may aid in the detection or prevention of neurotoxicity; however, it is recommended that therapy be based on the total clinical picture. Conservative use of both agents is warranted, and dosage adjustments of one or both agents may be necessary. If possible, it would be preferable to use only one agent.

**Summary:** Neurotoxic symptoms and somnambulistic episodes have been observed in patients simultaneously receiving lithium carbonate and thioridazine.

**Related Drugs:** Neurotoxic or somnambulistic episodes have also been reported when lithium was coadministered with thiothixene, fluphenazine, perphenazine, and chlorpromazine (see Chlorpromazine-Lithium Carbonate, page 235). Other phenothiazines, thioxanthenes, dihydroindolones and dibenzoxazepines may interact similarly with lithium. Haloperidol may also interact with lithium carbonate (see Lithium Carbonate-Haloperidol, page 248). There are no drugs related to lithium carbonate.

**Mechanism:** The neurotoxicity-type symptoms may be a potentiation or a pharmacologic summation of the antipsychotic agents and lithium.

**Detailed Information:** See *EDI*, 10/65.00

## Lithium Carbonate-Verapamil

**Significance:** 2—moderately clinically significant

**Potential Effects:** Concurrent lithium and calcium channel blockers may result in signs of neurotoxicity or decreased lithium levels with or without manic symptoms.

**Recommendations:** Patients receiving concurrent therapy with lithium and calcium channel blockers should be monitored for development of manic symptoms or neurotoxicity. Lithium levels should be monitored if calcium channel blockers are added to or withdrawn from therapy; however, neurotoxicity may develop at therapeutic or subtherapeutic lithium levels.

**Summary:** In case reports, concurrent lithium and verapamil resulted in symptoms of neurotoxicity or decreased lithium levels with or without manic symptoms.

**Related Drugs:** Patients receiving diltiazem and lithium have been reported to have similar reactions. Nifedipine was reported not to interact with lithium in one case report. Documentation is lacking regarding a similar interaction between lithium carbonate and the other calcium channel blockers; however, based on the proposed mechanism an interaction may be expected to occur.

## Antipsychotic

**Mechanism:** It has been postulated that the decrease in serum lithium concentration by verapamil results from (1) enhancement of lithium excretion from improved cardiac output due to correction of arrhythmias or (2) a shift of extracellular lithium to an intracellular compartment because of calcium slow channel blocker inhibition of the sodium-potassium ATPase pump. The neurotoxicity that was induced by concurrent lithium and calcium channel blockers may result from similar effects of both agents on neurosecretory processes. Concurrent use may also result in an acute increase in dopamine availability secondary to an increase in dopamine synthesis triggered by lithium and verapamil-induced blockade of dopamine autoreceptors.
**Detailed Information:** See *EDI*, 10/66.10

### Lorazepam-Probenecid

**Significance:** 3—minimally clinically significant
**Potential Effects:** Probenecid may decrease the metabolism of lorazepam, leading to increased lorazepam plasma concentrations and potentiated side effects.
**Recommendations:** If these agents are used together, the patient should be monitored for an increase in lorazepam side effects (e.g., sedation).
**Summary:** There are data to show that administration of probenecid decreases clearance and prolongs the mean elimination half-life, creating a potential for increased adverse effects.
**Related Drugs:** The other benzodiazepines with primary metabolic pathways dependent on phase II reactions may interact similarly with probenecid. It is not known if other benzodiazepines metabolized by phase I reactions would interact with probenecid. It is not known if an interaction would occur between lorazepam and sulfinpyrazone.
**Mechanism:** Probenecid may reduce lorazepam clearance by inhibiting glucuronyl transferase activity, decreasing the formation of lorazepam glucuronide.
**Detailed Information:** See *EDI*, 10/66.30

### Loxapine-Sumatriptan

**Significance:** 3—minimally clinically significant
**Potential Effects:** Concurrent administration of loxapine and sumatriptan may result in a dystonic reaction or other extrapyramidal side effects.
**Recommendations:** Concurrent use of sumatriptan and antipsychotics should be approached with caution. Patients receiving antipsychotics should be monitored for extrapyramidal side effects following sumatriptan administration.
**Summary:** In a single case report, a patient being treated with loxapine developed a dystonic reaction within 15 minutes of sumatriptan administration.
**Related Drugs:** Although documentation is lacking, based on the postulated mechanism a similar interaction may be expected to occur between sumatriptan and the phenothiazines, the thioxanthines, as well as haloperidol and molindone.
**Mechanism:** Concurrent administration of loxapine and sumatriptan may predispose the patient to a dystonic reaction because of an additive pharmacologic effect.
**Detailed Information:** See *EDI*, 10/66.35

### Midazolam-Erythromycin

**Significance:** 2—moderately clinically significant
**Potential Effects:** Erythromycin may inhibit the metabolism of midazolam, possibly leading to increased effects of midazolam.

## Antipsychotic

**Recommendations:** Patients should be observed for increased midazolam effect, especially drowsiness, when erythromycin is administered concurrently. The dose of midazolam may need to be lowered.

**Summary:** Concurrent midazolam and erythromycin resulted in increased midazolam levels.

**Related Drugs:** Erythromycin, roximthromycin, and troleandomyin have been shown to interact with triazolam, while azithromycin has been shown not to interact. If the mechanism involves inhibition of the metabolism of triazolam by erythromycin, then a similar interaction may be expected to occur between erythromycin and the other benzodiazepines metabolized by phase I reactions; however, documentation is lacking. Although there is no documentation, erythromycin would not be expected to interact with the other benzodiazepines metabolized by phase II reactions.

**Mechanism:** The proposed mechanism is one of hepatic microsomal inhibition, causing elevated midazolam concentrations.

**Detailed Information:** See *EDI*, 10/66.42

## Midazolam-Thiopental

**Significance:** 3—minimally clinically significant

**Potential Effects:** Concurrent use of these agents may result in a synergistic anesthetic effect.

**Recommendations:** Patients receiving concurrent midazolam and thiopental should be monitored for a possible synergistic effect. The dose of one or both agents may need to be reduced.

**Summary:** There are data to show that coadministration of the agents may cause a supra-additive anesthesia effect.

**Related Drugs:** A similar reaction may occur between thiopental and other benzodiazepines and between midazolam and other barbiturates.

**Mechanism:** This interaction involves the GABA receptor and the barbiturate binding sites. Binding to these sites can allosterically modify the benzodiazepine receptor. Barbiturates may enhance the binding of benzodiazepines.

**Detailed Information:** See *EDI*, 10/66.45

## Olanzapine-Fluvoxamine

**Significance:** 3—minimally clinically significant

**Potential Effects:** Concurrent administration of fluvoxamine and olanzapine may result in a decrease in olanzapine clearance and increased olanzapine levels.

**Recommendations:** Patients receiving concurrent therapy with olanzapine and fluvoxamine should be monitored for increased olanzapine effects. The dosage of olanzapine may need to be adjusted, or fluvoxamine may need to be discontinued.

**Summary:** Concurrent administration of fluvoxamine and olanzapine resulted in a decrease in olanzapine clearance and increased olanzapine levels. In one study, olanzapine maximum concentration and area-under-curve increased by 84% and 119%, respectively.

**Related Drugs:** A similar interaction would be expected to occur between olanzapine and the other selective serotonin reuptake inhibitors and the nonselective serotonin reuptake inhibitors. It is not known whether fluvoxamine would interact with the other antipsychotic agents chemically unrelated to olanzapine.

**Mechanism:** It is postulated that olanzapine's metabolism is mediated by the cytochrome $P450_{1A2}$ isozyme system and that fluvoxamine inhibits this same system. It is thus speculated that fluvoxamine inhibits the metabolism of olanzapine.

**Detailed Information:** See *EDI*, 10/66.47

## Oxazepam-Diflunisal

**Significance:** 3—minimally clinically significant

**Potential Effects:** Diflunisal may decrease oxazepam levels.

**Recommendations:** The dose of oxazepam may need to be increased if these agents are used together.

**Summary:** In one study, concurrent administration of diflunisal and oxazepam resulted in decreased oxazepam concentrations.

**Related Drugs:** Aspirin has been reported to increase the activity of midazolam. Midazolam has been reported to have no interaction with diflunisal. The other benzodiazepines with primary metabolic pathways dependent on phase II reactions may interact similarly with diflunisal based on the proposed mechanism; however, documentation is lacking. It is not known if a similar interaction would occur between oxazepam and the other salicylates; however, they may also interact because salicylates compete for protein binding with oxazepam.

**Mechanism:** It has been suggested that this interaction results from a presystemic displacement of oxazepam from its plasma protein binding sites by diflunisal. Also, inhibition of the tubular secretion of oxazepam glucuronide by the glucuronides of diflunisal may be involved.

**Detailed Information:** See *EDI*, 10/66.50

## Perphenazine-Disulfiram

**Significance:** 3—minimally clinically significant

**Potential Effects:** Disulfiram may decrease perphenazine plasma concentration levels along with its sulfoxide metabolite.

**Recommendations:** Patients receiving oral perphenazine and disulfiram concurrently should be observed for exacerbated psychotic symptoms. The dosage of disulfiram and the oral form of perphenazine may need to be adjusted.

**Summary:** There are data to show that administration of disulfiram may decrease perphenazine plasma concentration levels along with its sulfoxide metabolite.

**Related Drugs:** A similar interaction may occur between disulfiram and other phenothiazines, thioxanthenes, butyrophenones, dihydroindolones, and dibenzoxazepines. A similar interaction is not expected to occur between perphenazine and other antialcoholic agents.

**Mechanism:** Disulfiram may activate the liver enzymes inactivating perphenazine.

**Detailed Information:** See *EDI*, 10/67.00

## Pimozide-Fluoxetine

**Significance:** 3—minimally clinically significant

**Potential Effects:** The addition of fluoxetine to the therapy of a patient maintained on pimozide may result in an increase in pimozide adverse effects.

**Recommendations:** Patients should be monitored for bradycardia, changes in sensorium, or other signs of pimozide side effects when fluoxetine or pimozide is added to a regimen including the other. The dosage of one or both drugs may need to be adjusted.

**Summary:** Increased pimozide adverse effects were seen when fluoxetine was added to the therapy of patients maintained on pimozide. Effects included bradycardia, galactorrhea, and a change in sensorium.

**Related Drugs:** An oculogyric crisis occurred in a nine-year-old after paroxetine was added to pimozide therapy and reoccurred upon rechallenge with the two drugs. It is not known if a similar interaction would occur between pimozide and the other selective serotonin reuptake inhibitors, though this may be possible based on the proposed mechanism of action.

# Antipsychotic

**Mechanism:** It is hypothesized that fluoxetine may decrease the plasma clearance of pimozide, increasing plasma levels of pimozide, possibly because of impaired hepatic microsomal activity. It is also possible that the two drugs, which both can cause bradycardia, exert additive effects in the patient.

**Detailed Information:** See *EDI*, 10/68.50

## Promazine-Charcoal

**Significance:** 3—minimally clinically significant

**Recommendations:** Activated charcoal may be an effective treatment in an acute promazine overdose. It should be administered as soon as possible, and subsequent doses should be given to increase promazine elimination. However, if charcoal is not used for promazine overdose, the administration of these agents should be separated by as much time as possible.

**Summary:** The concomitant administration of activated charcoal and promazine decreases the rate and extent of promazine absorption.

**Related Drugs:** It is expected that the other phenothiazines will also be adsorbed to charcoal. There are no drugs related to charcoal.

**Mechanism:** It has been suggested that activated charcoal adsorbs promazine.

**Detailed Information:** See *EDI*, 10/69.00

## Temazepam-Diphenhydramine

**Significance:** 2—moderately clinically significant

**Potential Effects:** In one case report, the concurrent use of these agents in a pregnant patient resulted in the delivery of a stillborn infant.

**Recommendations:** These agents should not be used together in pregnant patients because of the potentially serious consequences.

**Summary:** There are data to show that coadministration of diphenhydramine and temazepam resulted in violent intrauterine fetal movements leading to the delivery of a stillborn infant.

**Related Drugs:** It is difficult to determine if a similar interaction would occur between temazepam and other antihistamines or between diphenhydramine and other benzodiazepines.

**Mechanism:** Both drugs cross the placenta. Antihistamines cause vasoconstriction of the placenta, increasing the maternal-fetal exchange, and antihistamines also have an embryotoxic effect. Diphenhydramine may affect the metabolism of temazepam.

**Detailed Information:** See *EDI*, 10/70.10

## Thioridazine-Bromocriptine

**Significance:** 2—moderately clinically significant

**Recommendations:** The concurrent use of thioridazine and bromocriptine should be used with caution, and patients should be monitored for increased prolactin levels. Thioridazine may need to be discontinued, as this interaction appears to be reversible.

**Summary:** There are data to show that coadministration of these agents will increase prolactin levels. A temporary loss of vision was documented to occur with coadministration of these therapies.

**Related Drugs:** A similar interaction may occur between bromocriptine and other phenothiazines, thioxanthenes, butyrophenones, dihydroindolones, and dibenzoxazepines. There are no drugs related to bromocriptine.

**Mechanism:** It has been suggested that thioridazine diminishes the prolactin-lowering ability of bromocriptine.

**Detailed Information:** See *EDI*, 10/71.00

Antipsychotic

## Triazolam-Ketoconazole

**Significance:** 1—highly clinically significant

**Potential Effects:** Concurrent administration of imidazole antimycotics with phase I metabolized benzodiazepines may result in decreased clearance of benzodiazepines and increased levels and clinical effects of benzodiazepines.

**Recommendations:** The concurrent administration of either alprazolam or triazolam with either itraconazole or ketoconazole is contraindicated according to the manufacturer's product labeling. The concurrent administration of other combinations of imidazole antifungals and phase I metabolized benzodiazepines need not be avoided. However, patients should be observed for an increase in the effects of the benzodiazepines. The dose of the benzodiazepine may need to be decreased.

**Summary:** Concurrent administration of imidazole antimycotics with phase I metabolized benzodiazepines may result in decreased clearance of benzodiazepines and increased levels, clinical effects, and adverse effects of benzodiazepines including increased sedation and amnesiac effects.

**Related Drugs:** Based on the postulated mechanism, benzodiazepines that are metabolized by phase I (N-dealkylation or hydroxylation) may be expected to interact with fluconazole, itraconazole, and ketoconazole. It is not known if these imidazole antifungal agents would interact with the benzodiazepines. Alprazolam, chlordiazepoxide, midazolam, and triazolam may be expected to interact with the other imidazole antifungals.

**Mechanism:** It is believed that the imidazole antifungals inhibit the metabolism of the benzodiazepines by inhibition of the cytochrome $P450_{3A4}$ enzyme system.

**Detailed Information:** See *EDI*, 10/73.00

# Chapter Eleven

# Beta-Adrenergic Blocking Agents' Drug Interactions

## Atenolol-Ampicillin

**Significance:** 3—minimally clinically significant

**Potential Effects:** Ampicillin may decrease the effects of atenolol. Also, beta-blockers may increase the risk of anaphylactic reactions to the penicillins.

**Recommendations:** Monitor patients for lack of atenolol's effects when administered with ampicillin. Observe patients for signs of anaphylactic reactions when taking beta-blocking agents and penicillins together.

**Summary:** There are data to show that ampicillin administration may decrease the effects of atenolol.

**Related Drugs:** It is not known if a similar interaction would occur between atenolol and other penicillins or between ampicillin and other beta-blocking agents. There is an increased risk of penicillin anaphylactic reactions with beta-blocking agents (see also Propranolol-Allergenic Extracts, page 264).

**Mechanism:** The mechanism of this interaction is unknown.

**Detailed Information:** See *EDI*, 11/1.00

## Atenolol-Calcium Carbonate

**Significance:** 3—minimally clinically significant

**Recommendations:** The patient's response to atenolol should be monitored during administration of concurrent calcium salts, and the atenolol dose may need to be adjusted.

**Summary:** The administration of calcium carbonate was shown to reduce the peak plasma concentration and decrease the area-under-curve of atenolol. A reduction in beta-blockade was demonstrated, but blood pressure response did not significantly change.

**Related Drugs:** A similar interaction would be expected to occur with the other calcium salts. There is no documentation regarding a similar interaction with the other beta-blocking agents.

**Mechanism:** The gastrointestinal absorption of atenolol is impaired by calcium salts, although other mechanisms may exist.

**Detailed Information:** See *EDI*, 11/3.00

## Atenolol-Propantheline

**Significance:** 3—minimally clinically significant

**Recommendations:** Although the concurrent use of these agents need not be avoided, it may be necessary to decrease the dose of atenolol or separate the administration of the drugs by as much time as possible.

**Summary:** Propantheline was shown to prolong the absorption and the time to peak, and to increase the area-under-curve, of atenolol.

**Related Drugs:** Metoprolol and propranolol exhibited similar interactions with propantheline. A similar interaction is expected to occur between propantheline and other beta-blocking agents and between atenolol and other anticholinergics.

**Mechanism:** Propantheline, by decreasing gastrointestinal motility, increases the absorption of atenolol.

**Detailed Information:** See *EDI*, 11/4.01

## Carvedilol-Cyclosporine

**Significance:** 3—minimally clinically significant

**Potential Effects:** The concurrent administration of carvedilol and cyclosporine may result in an increase in cyclosporine levels.

**Recommendations:** Patients should be carefully monitored for changes in cyclosporine levels and effects if carvedilol is added to or removed from the therapy of a patient maintained on cyclosporine. The dose of cyclosporine may need to be adjusted.

**Summary:** Concurrent administration of cyclosporine and carvedilol resulted in increased cyclosporine levels.

**Related Drugs:** A similar interaction may occur between cyclosporine and other beta-adrenergic blockers that are primarily metabolized by the cytochrome $P450_{3A4}$ isozyme (e.g., bisoprolol). It is not known whether an interaction would occur between cyclosporine and other beta-adrenergic-blockers. There are no drugs related to cyclosporine.

**Mechanism:** Carvedilol is primarily metabolized by the cytochrome P450 isozymes 2D6 and 2C9 and, to a lesser extent, by 3A4, 2C19, 1A2, and 2E1. Cyclosporine is primarily metabolized by cytochrome $P450_{3A4}$. Competitive inhibition at the cytochrome $P450_{3A4}$ isozyme may decrease cyclosporine metabolism and increase cyclosporine serum levels.

**Detailed Information:** See *EDI*, 11/4.06

## Labetalol-Glutethimide

**Significance:** 3—minimally clinically significant

**Recommendations:** If a decreased response to labetalol occurs during concurrent administration of glutethimide, the dose of labetalol may need to be increased or the glutethimide discontinued.

**Summary:** The administration of glutethimide resulted in a significant reduction in labetalol area-under-curve and systemic bioavailability, necessitating a possible increase in labetalol dosage.

**Related Drugs:** A similar interaction is expected to occur between glutethimide and other hepatically metabolized beta-blocking agents if the mechanism involves enzyme induction by glutethimide. The agents that are not extensively metabolized by the liver would not be expected to interact with glutethimide. There are no drugs related to glutethimide.

**Mechanism:** Glutethimide, a known hepatic microsomal oxidative enzyme inducer, increases the metabolism of labetalol.

**Detailed Information:** See *EDI*, 11/4.10

## Labetalol-Halothane

**Significance:** 2—moderately clinically significant

**Recommendations:** The interaction may be of benefit in some patients since hypotension may be induced, causing a decrease in arterial pressure unaccompanied by tachycardia, thereby reducing blood loss during surgery. However, if this effect is not desired, the concentration of halothane may need to be decreased or the use of another anesthetic considered. It was reported that dopamine, a beta agonist acting on different receptors in the myocardium than either epinephrine or isoproterenol, may be useful as an inotropic agent in patients experiencing this interaction.

**Summary:** The administration of halothane and labetalol has been shown to result in myocardial depression, a decrease in arterial blood pressure, cardiac output, peripheral resistance, a fall in heart rate and an increase in central venous pressure.

**Related Drugs:** A similar interaction may occur between halothane and other beta-blocking agents; however, it is difficult to determine the extent of the interaction. The other halogenated inhalation anesthetics may interact with labetalol.

**Mechanism:** A synergism between labetalol's alpha and beta receptor blockade and halothane's myocardial depressant activity has been revealed.

**Detailed Information:** See *EDI*, 11/4.30

Beta-Adrenergic Blocker

## Metoprolol-Amiodarone
**Significance:** 2—moderately clinically significant
**Potential Effects:** Concurrent use of the agents results in severe bradycardia.
**Recommendations:** Monitor patients closely for bradycardia during concurrent use. If this occurs, metoprolol should be discontinued, and a sympathomimetic agent may be required. Atenolol might be an alternative to metoprolol.
**Summary:** Metoprolol may interact with amiodarone by producing severe bradycardia.
**Related Drugs:** There has been documentation of an interaction between amiodarone and propranolol. Because of conflicting results, it is not known whether an interaction would occur between amiodarone and other beta-adrenergic blocking agents.
**Mechanism:** The mechanism by which metoprolol and amiodarone produce severe bradycardia and hypotension has not been established.
**Detailed Information:** See *EDI*, 11/4.50

## Metoprolol-Oral Contraceptive Agents
**Significance:** 3—minimally clinically significant
**Potential Effects:** Oral contraceptives may decrease the metabolism of metoprolol.
**Recommendations:** Although concurrent use of these agents need not be avoided, patients should be monitored for a possible increase in the effects of metoprolol.
**Summary:** There are data to show that oral contraceptive agents may decrease the metabolism and increase the effects of metoprolol.
**Related Drugs:** Propranolol and acebutolol have been shown to interact with oral contraceptive agents. Because of conflicting results, it is not known if an interaction would occur between oral contraceptive agents and other hepatically metabolized beta-blocking agents. A similar interaction is not expected to occur with beta-blocking agents that do not undergo significant hepatic metabolism.
**Mechanism:** Oral contraceptive agents inhibit hepatic microsomal enzymes, leading to a reduction in first-pass hepatic metabolism of metoprolol and propranolol.
**Detailed Information:** See *EDI*, 11/5.00

## Metoprolol-Pentobarbital
**Significance:** 2—moderately clinically significant
**Recommendations:** The dosage regimen of orally administered metoprolol may have to be increased if prescribed concomitantly with long-term (longer than ten days) pentobarbital therapy. The barbiturates do not seem to change the bioavailability of beta-blockers administered intravenously. Patients should be observed for a less than optimal therapeutic effect. Alternatively, timolol or one of the beta-blockers not dependent on hepatic first-pass metabolism (atenolol, nadolol, and pindolol) may be substituted.
**Summary:** Pentobarbital has been reported to reduce the plasma concentration and bioavailability of metoprolol.
**Related Drugs:** Phenobarbital has been shown to increase the clearance of propranolol. Pentobarbital has reduced the plasma concentrations and bioavailability of alprenolol. Timolol or the beta-blocking agents not dependent on first-pass hepatic metabolism have been shown not to interact. A similar interaction may occur between metoprolol and other barbiturates.

**Mechanism:** Pentobarbital and phenobarbital have been reported to induce liver enzymes, reducing the plasma concentrations of the beta-blocking agents dependent on hepatic metabolism.
**Detailed Information:** See *EDI,* 11/7.00

## Metoprolol-Rifampin

**Significance:** 2—moderately clinically significant
**Recommendations:** During concurrent use of these agents, blood pressure changes should be carefully monitored as the dose of metoprolol may need to be increased.
**Summary:** Rifampin, when administered concurrently with metoprolol, reduced the area-under-curve of metoprolol.
**Related Drugs:** There are no drugs related to rifampin. Propranolol has been shown to interact with rifampin. A similar interaction is not expected to occur with other beta-blocking agents that are not extensively metabolized by first-pass hepatic metabolism.
**Mechanism:** Induction of hepatic microsomal enzymes by rifampin is probably responsible for this interaction.
**Detailed Information:** See *EDI,* 11/9.00

## Nadolol-Phenelzine

**Significance:** 3—minimally clinically significant
**Potential Effects:** Bradycardia and a decrease in the pulse rate may occur with concurrent administration of nadolol and phenelzine.
**Recommendations:** A careful observation should be made of the pulse rates with coadministration of nadolol and phenelzine. One review suggests that monoamine oxidase inhibitor therapy should be discontinued at least two weeks prior to the institution of propranolol therapy.
**Summary:** A patient on nadolol therapy experienced bradycardia when phenelzine was added to the regimen.
**Related Drugs:** Metoprolol with phenelzine has been shown to cause changes in pulse. Documentation is lacking regarding an interaction between other monoamine oxidase inhibitors and other beta-blocking agents and with furazolidone and procarbazine.
**Mechanism:** The mechanism of this interaction is unknown.
**Detailed Information:** See *EDI,* 11/10.50

## Propranolol-Alcohol, Ethyl

**Significance:** 3—minimally clinically significant
**Recommendations:** Alcohol alone may lead to incidences of angina and tachycardia. It is possible that the concomitant use of these agents potentiates these adverse reactions as well as other side effects involving neurologic functions. It is prudent to caution patients regarding the concurrent use of propranolol and alcohol.
**Summary:** The elimination of propranolol is increased by concomitant administration of alcohol, and the blood pressure reducing effect of propranolol may be diminished.
**Related Drugs:** The beta-blocking agents that undergo extensive hepatic metabolism may be affected by concurrent alcohol ingestion. The beta-blocking agents that are not extensively metabolized by the liver are expected to interact similarly with alcohol.
**Mechanism:** Blood flow to the liver is increased by alcohol through vascular dilation, resulting in an increased amount of propranolol presented to the liver for metabolism.
**Detailed Information:** See *EDI,* 11/11.00

## Propranolol-Allergenic Extracts
**Significance:** 3—minimally clinically significant
**Recommendations:** Although anaphylaxis may occur with the use of the allergenic extract alone, patients receiving a beta-blocking agent who are given immunotherapy may experience an exaggerated anaphylactic reaction. Aggressive therapy may be required if such an interaction occurs. Further documentation of the extent of such an interaction is necessary.
**Summary:** A patient experienced an anaphylactic reaction to a monthly allergenic extract injection after being started on propranolol therapy. Severe hypertension was also reported in this patient.
**Related Drugs:** Other beta-blocking agents may have the same ability to potentiate anaphylactic reactions as propranolol.
**Mechanism:** Beta receptor blockade may potentiate anaphylactic reactions by decreasing intracellular cyclic AMP, lowering the threshold for mediator release by mast cells.
**Detailed Information:** See *EDI*, 11/12.10

## Propranolol-Aluminum Hydroxide
**Significance:** 3—minimally clinically significant
**Recommendations:** The clinical significance of the changes in bioavailability have not been determined for any of the beta-blocking agents. Until such data are available, it would seem prudent to separate the dosages of the antacid and beta-blockers by as much time as possible.
**Summary:** Concomitant administration of propranolol and aluminum hydroxide gel resulted in a decrease in propranolol bioavailability.
**Related Drugs:** Because of conflicting results, it is difficult to determine whether an interaction would occur between aluminum hydroxide and other beta-blockers.
**Mechanism:** The proposed mechanisms involve propranolol being adsorbed to, or complexing with, the antacid compound, inhibiting gastrointestinal absorption.
**Detailed Information:** See *EDI*, 11/13.00

## Propranolol-Aminoglutethimide
**Significance:** 3—minimally clinically significant
**Recommendations:** Although no special precautions are necessary at this time, the patient's blood pressure should still be periodically monitored following the concomitant use of propranolol and aminoglutethimide.
**Summary:** A case of lethargy, skin rash, and hypotension was reported in a patient with metastatic cancer taking propranolol following the addition of aminoglutethimide.
**Related Drugs:** An interaction may occur between aminoglutethimide and other beta-blocking agents. Glutethimide has been shown to interact in a different manner with labetalol (see Labetalol-Glutethimide, page 261).
**Mechanism:** Aminoglutethimide may exert an antithyroid-like effect, and propranolol may enhance this effect. Propranolol may cause vasodilation and hypotension.
**Detailed Information:** See *EDI*, 11/14.01

## Propranolol-Aspirin
**Significance:** 3—minimally clinically significant
**Recommendations:** Patients' blood pressure should be monitored closely during concurrent use of these agents. If a loss of blood pressure control is noted, the dose of propranolol may need to be increased or aspirin may need to be discontinued. Further studies are needed.

# Beta-Adrenergic Blocker

**Summary:** Administration of aspirin with propranolol has been shown to increase diastolic blood pressure.

**Related Drugs:** A similar interaction may occur between aspirin and other beta-blocking agents. An interaction may occur between propranolol and other salicylates; however, documentation is lacking.

**Mechanism:** Aspirin may inhibit the prostaglandins responsible for vasodilation, resulting in an increase in blood pressure.

**Detailed Information:** See *EDI*, 11/14.10

## Propranolol-Chlorpheniramine

**Significance:** 4—not clinically significant

**Recommendations:** The possibility of an interaction between these agents, though remote, should be considered when they are coadministered.

**Summary:** Chlorpheniramine could theoretically inhibit the beta-adrenergic blocking effect of propranolol and enhance its quinidine-like effect.

**Related Drugs:** Other beta-adrenergic blocking agents could also be affected by the antihistamines.

**Mechanism:** Chlorpheniramine has been shown to prevent the uptake of catecholamines at the adrenergic nerve terminal, raising the concentration at the adrenergic receptor sites.

**Detailed Information:** See *EDI*, 11/15.00

## Propranolol-Chlorpromazine

**Significance:** 2—moderately clinically significant

**Potential Effects:** The concomitant administration of these agents may result in increased levels of either agent.

**Recommendations:** Patients receiving chlorpromazine and propranolol concurrently should be monitored for increased levels of both agents, as well as for symptoms of chlorpromazine toxicity (e.g., delirium, grand mal seizure). The dose of either agent may need to be decreased.

**Summary:** The concurrent administration of propranolol and chlorpromazine has been shown to increase levels of each other.

**Related Drugs:** A similar interaction is expected to occur between phenothiazines, thioxanthenes, butyrophenones, dihydroindolones and dibenzoxazepines and propranolol. A similar interaction is expected to occur with other beta-blocking agents extensively metabolized by the liver, if the mechanism involves a decreased first-pass hepatic metabolism. It is not known if the beta-blocking agents that do not exhibit an extensive first-pass metabolism would be expected to interact with chlorpromazine.

**Mechanism:** The bioavailability of propranolol is increased as a result of a decrease in the first-pass hepatic metabolism by chlorpromazine.

**Detailed Information:** See *EDI*, 11/17.00

## Propranolol-Cholestyramine

**Significance:** 3—minimally clinically significant

**Recommendations:** Concomitant administration of cholestyramine and propranolol need not be avoided; however, patients receiving long-term propranolol therapy who have cholestyramine added to, or withdrawn from, their therapy may require an adjustment in the propranolol dosage.

**Summary:** Cholestyramine administration may necessitate an adjustment in propranolol dosage in some patients.

**Related Drugs:** Other beta-blocking agents may interact similarly with cholestyramine.

**Mechanism:** This interaction may result from the formation of a non-absorbable complex by propranolol and cholestyramine.
**Detailed Information:** See *EDI*, 11/18.10

## Propranolol-Cimetidine

**Significance:** 1—highly clinically significant
**Potential Effects:** Cimetidine inhibits the metabolism of propranolol, resulting in increased propranolol levels and effects.
**Recommendations:** Patients receiving these agents concurrently should be monitored for increased beta-blocking activity. The dose of either agent may need to be reduced, or alternative agents to cimetidine (famotidine, ranitidine) or propranolol (atenolol, pindolol) that do not interact may be considered.
**Summary:** Concurrent administration of cimetidine and propranolol have resulted in an increase in propranolol plasma concentrations. Resting pulse rates may be significantly lower when cimetidine is administered with propranolol.
**Related Drugs:** Cimetidine interacted similarly with metoprolol and labetalol. Because of conflicting results, it is difficult to determine whether an interaction would occur between cimetidine and other beta-blocking agents. Ranitidine has been shown to interact similarly to cimetidine; however, all data do not support this. Propranolol would not be expected to interact with famotidine.
**Mechanism:** Cimetidine reduces hepatic blood flow, decreasing the extraction rate of propranolol, and it may inhibit propranolol metabolism.
**Detailed Information:** See *EDI*, 11/19.00

## Propranolol-Cocaine

**Significance:** 2—moderately clinically significant
**Potential Effects:** Cocaine-associated coronary vasoconstriction may be potentiated by propranolol.
**Recommendations:** Concurrent use of propranolol and cocaine should probably be avoided.
**Summary:** Cocaine-induced coronary vasoconstriction is potentiated by propranolol.
**Related Drugs:** A similar interaction may occur between cocaine and other beta-adrenergic blocking agents.
**Mechanism:** Propranolol potentiates the effects of cocaine.
**Detailed Information:** See *EDI*, 11/20.50

## Propranolol-Desipramine

**Significance:** 3—minimally clinically significant
**Recommendations:** Since substantial clinical evidence is lacking with respect to specific interactions of desipramine with propranolol, no additional precautions are necessary when these drugs are given concurrently. However, precautions appropriate to the individual use of these drugs should be observed.
**Summary:** The use of propranolol in patients receiving desipramine requires caution until reports are fully substantiated.
**Related Drugs:** Other beta-blocking agents may interact with desipramine in a similar manner to propranolol.
**Mechanism:** Desipramine may antagonize propranolol in myocardial tissue and may counteract the bradycardia and decrease the inotropic effects produced by propranolol.
**Detailed Information:** See *EDI*, 11/21.00

## Propranolol-Diatrizoate

**Significance:** 3—minimally clinically significant

**Potential Effects:** Administration of these agents together may result in hypotension.

**Recommendations:** Further documentation of the incidence of adverse reactions to radiocontrast agents with concurrent beta-blocking drug therapy is necessary before the extent of such an interaction can be determined. In order to minimize the likelihood of such an interaction, one study recommended withdrawing the beta-blocking agent for two to three days before radiologic examination and administering an antihistamine two hours before examination. However, abruptly withdrawing beta-blocker therapy can be associated with the development of other adverse reactions. Until further information is available, practitioners should be aware of the possibility of hypotension development with concurrent radiocontrast agent and beta-blocker use.

**Summary:** A patient taking propranolol received sodium meglumine diatrizoate and experienced severe reactions characterized by progressive erythema of the upper extremities, hypotension, and tachycardia.

**Related Drugs:** Nadolol was documented to cause a similar interaction. The other beta-blocking agents may have the same ability to potentiate hypotensive reactions of diatrizoate. It is not known if other radiopaque agents would interact similarly with propranolol.

**Mechanism:** Iodinated contrast agents may cause histamine release and the development of hypotension or an anaphylactic reaction.

**Detailed Information:** See *EDI*, 11/22.10

## Propranolol-Epinephrine

**Significance:** 1—highly clinically significant

**Recommendations:** Sympathomimetic drugs with alpha agonist activity should be avoided if possible or used very cautiously in patients taking nonselective beta antagonists. This includes the use of local anesthetics with epinephrine. It has been recommended that the epinephrine dose not exceed 3 mg/kg every 30 minutes in these patients, with continuous blood pressure and pulse monitoring. If possible, a cardioselective beta$_1$-blocking agent (acebutolol, atenolol, and metoprolol) may be cautiously used in place of propranolol, beginning a few days before the patient is scheduled to receive the sympathomimetic drug.

**Summary:** Administration of epinephrine with propranolol may result in a considerable increase in systolic and diastolic blood pressure and a marked decrease in heart rate, potentiating a stroke.

**Related Drugs:** There are ample data indicating that epinephrine may interact with other beta-blockers; however, the data are conflicting. Epinephrine has been documented to interact with beta-blocking ophthalmic preparations as well.

**Mechanism:** Concurrent administration of propranolol and epinephrine results in blocking of the beta agonist activity of epinephrine while the alpha adrenergic effects are unopposed.

**Detailed Information:** See *EDI*, 11/23.00

## Propranolol-Ergotamine

**Significance:** 3—minimally clinically significant

**Recommendations:** In certain patients receiving concomitant propranolol and ergot alkaloids, the dose of the ergot alkaloid may need to be adjusted downward.

**Summary:** There are data to show that administration of propranolol may necessitate an adjustment downward of the ergot alkaloids. Peripheral vasoconstriction and migraine headache have been reported when propranolol was added to the regimen.

**Related Drugs:** A similar interaction is not expected to occur between the $beta_1$ cardioselective beta-blocking agents, if the mechanism involves the blocking of the vasodilatory effect of $beta_2$-adrenergic receptors in the vessels. The other noncardioselective beta-blocking agents may interact similarly with ergotamine. The other ergot alkaloids may interact with propranolol.

**Mechanism:** Vasodilation is blocked by the noncardioselective beta-adrenergic blocking agents, allowing the ergot alkaloid to produce a maximum vasoconstriction.

**Detailed Information:** See *EDI*, 11/25.00

## Propranolol-Flecainide

**Significance:** 3—minimally clinically significant

**Potential Effects:** Use of these agents together may result in an increase in plasma levels of both drugs and an additive effect on cardiac function.

**Recommendations:** Use of these agents together need not routinely be avoided. However, the patient's cardiac status should be monitored.

**Summary:** There are data to show that coadministration of these agents may result in an increase in plasma levels of both drugs and an additive effect on cardiac function.

**Related Drugs:** A similar interaction may occur between flecainide and other beta-blocking agents. It is not known whether an interaction would occur between propranolol and the other class IC antiarrhythmic agents.

**Mechanism:** The mechanism of this interaction is unknown.

**Detailed Information:** See *EDI*, 11/26.10

## Propranolol-Fluoxetine

**Significance:** 2—moderately clinically significant

**Potential Effects:** Increased cardiac effects of propranolol may be seen following the addition of fluoxetine.

**Recommendations:** Patients receiving concurrent selective serotonin reuptake inhibitors and beta-blockers should be monitored closely for increased pharmacologic action of beta-blockers. The beta-blocker dosage may need to be decreased.

**Summary:** Increased cardiac effects of propranolol have been seen following the addition of fluoxetine.

**Related Drugs:** Similar interactions have been reported between fluoxetine and metoprolol, sertraline and propranolol, and fluvoxamine and both metoprolol and propranolol. Although documentation is lacking, based on the proposed mechanism fluoxetine would be expected to interact with the other beta-adrenergic blockers which undergo hepatic metabolism and a similar reaction would be expected to occur between paroxetine and the hepatically metabolized beta-blockers.

**Mechanism:** It was postulated that fluoxetine may increase the duration of action of 5-HT in the atrium, thus impairing atrioventricular conduction, and that fluoxetine may inhibit the metabolism of metoprolol and other lipophilic beta-blockers which undergo extensive first-pass metabolism by the cytochrome P450 enzyme. Sertraline and the other selective serotonin reuptake inhibitors may worsen coronary artery disease by causing vasoconstriction in affected coronary arteries.

**Detailed Information:** See *EDI*, 11/26.50

## Propranolol-Furosemide

**Significance:** 2—moderately clinically significant

**Recommendations:** The concurrent use of these agents need not be avoided. However, patients should be closely monitored, and a corresponding dosage adjustment of either agent should be made if necessary.

**Summary:** The concurrent administration of furosemide and propranolol results in higher blood levels of propranolol, and this increase can be accompanied by a simultaneous increase in beta-adrenergic blockade.

**Related Drugs:** Documentation is lacking regarding an interaction between furosemide and other beta-blocking agents. A similar interaction is expected to occur between propranolol and the other loop diuretics.

**Mechanism:** A furosemide-induced reduction in extracellular fluid volume may be responsible for this mechanism.

**Detailed Information:** See *EDI*, 11/27.00

## Propranolol-Hydralazine

**Significance:** 3—minimally clinically significant

**Recommendations:** The clinical significance of the increased propranolol bioavailability has not been determined in long-term administration studies. Some patients may develop symptoms of propranolol toxicity (e.g., bradycardia, bronchospasm). If such symptoms appear, plasma propranolol should be monitored, and decreasing the propranolol dosage may be indicated.

**Summary:** Concurrent administration of hydralazine and propranolol significantly increases the bioavailability of propranolol and may enhance the antihypertensive effect of hydralazine.

**Related Drugs:** Hydralazine resulted in similar plasma concentration increases with metoprolol, but not with nadolol or acebutolol. Labetalol may interact with hydralazine similarly to propranolol. Beta-blocking agents that do not undergo significant first-pass metabolism would not interact with hydralazine. There are no drugs related to hydralazine.

**Mechanism:** Hydralazine may enhance the systemic availability of propranolol by alteration of first-pass clearance.

**Detailed Information:** See *EDI*, 11/29.00

## Propranolol-Indomethacin

**Significance:** 2—moderately clinically significant

**Potential Effects:** Indomethacin may reduce the hypotensive effects of propranolol.

**Recommendations:** Patients' blood pressure should be closely monitored when these agents are used together. The dose of propranolol may need to be increased or the indomethacin discontinued.

**Summary:** Indomethacin therapy may reduce the hypotensive effects of propranolol.

**Related Drugs:** A similar interaction is expected to occur between indomethacin and other beta-blocking agents. Oral and ophthalmic indomethacin did not affect the ability of ophthalmic timolol to lower intraocular pressure. Since NSAIAs inhibit prostaglandin synthesis to some extent, a similar interaction is expected to occur with propranolol.

**Mechanism:** Indomethacin inhibits the prostaglandin responsible for vasodilation, resulting in an increase in blood pressure.

**Detailed Information:** See *EDI*, 11/31.00

## Propranolol-Misoprostol

**Significance:** 3—minimally clinically significant

**Potential Effects:** Misoprostol may increase propranolol levels.

**Recommendations:** No special precautions appear necessary at the present time, since the existence and clinical significance of a misoprostol-propranolol interaction has not been established.

**Summary:** The addition of misoprostol to propranolol therapy may result in an increase in the maximum plasma propranolol concentration.

**Related Drugs:** No additional information is available concerning an interaction between misoprostol and other beta adrenergic blocking agents; therefore, it is not known whether a reaction would be expected to occur. There are no drugs related to misoprostol.

**Mechanism:** This interaction may result from changes in hepatic blood flow or reduced gastric acid secretion.

**Detailed Information:** See *EDI,* 11/32.05

## Propranolol-Pravastatin

**Significance:** 3—minimally clinically significant

**Potential Effects:** Propranolol may decrease the bioavailability of pravastatin.

**Recommendations:** Although the patient should be monitored during concurrent propranolol and pravastatin administration, the clinical significance of the decrease in pravastatin concentration is likely to be small.

**Summary:** The coadministration of propranolol with pravastatin has been shown to decrease the pravastatin total mean serum concentration-time curve.

**Related Drugs:** A similar interaction is expected to occur between propranolol and other HMG-CoA reductase inhibitors. The other beta-adrenergic blocking agents that are primarily hepatically metabolized may interact. It is not known whether an interaction would occur between pravastatin and other beta-adrenergic blocking agents that are not hepatically metabolized.

**Mechanism:** Beta-adrenergic blocking agents decrease hepatic blood flow, increasing first-pass clearance of drugs having high extraction ratios.

**Detailed Information:** See *EDI,* 11/32.50

## Propranolol-Quinidine

**Significance:** 3—minimally clinically significant

**Potential Effects:** Propranolol may reduce the clearance of quinidine. Concurrent therapy may possibly result in orthostatic hypotension. However, these agents may have a beneficial effect when used together for arrhythmias.

**Recommendations:** Concurrent administration of these agents may be therapeutically beneficial in certain patients. However, patients should be monitored for quinidine levels and orthostatic hypotension.

**Summary:** There are data to show that administration of propranolol may reduce the clearance of quinidine and result in orthostatic hypotension.

**Related Drugs:** It would be expected that other beta-adrenergic blockers would exert the same beneficial effect with quinidine. It is not known if propranolol would interact with the quinine.

**Mechanism:** The mechanism of the decreased clearance of quinidine by propranolol is not known.

**Detailed Information:** See *EDI,* 11/33.00

Beta-Adrenergic Blocker

## Propranolol-Thyroid

**Significance:** 2—moderately clinically significant

**Recommendations:** Although a specific drug interaction has not been determined, it is prudent to be aware of a possible interaction while treating a patient with a thyroid abnormality. Therefore, when using a thyroid drug concurrently with propranolol or metoprolol, the dose of the beta-blocking agent may need to be increased. Alternatively, a noninteracting beta-blocking agent may be used.

**Summary:** Several studies indicate that patients taking a thyroid drug may show a decreased bioavailability of propranolol; however, other studies show conflicting results.

**Related Drugs:** Metoprolol undergoes extensive first-pass metabolism and is altered in the hyperthyroid state. Those beta-blocking agents that do not undergo significant first-pass metabolism do not appear to be affected by hyperthyroidism. A similar interaction may be expected between propranolol and other thyroid drugs.

**Mechanism:** The decreased bioavailability of propranolol and metoprolol results from an increase in presystemic clearance related to the extent of first-pass metabolism. In the hypothyroid state, the interaction may be produced by a decrease in presystemic clearance.

**Detailed Information:** See *EDI*, 11/35.00

## Propranolol-Tobacco

**Significance:** 2—moderately clinically significant

**Potential Effects:** Smoking decreased the levels of propranolol.

**Recommendations:** If a patient stabilized on propranolol changes smoking habits, the dose of propranolol may need to be adjusted.

**Summary:** Smoking has resulted in reduced steady-state serum propranolol concentrations and increased propranolol clearance.

**Related Drugs:** The other beta-blocking agents dependent on hepatic metabolism may interact similarly with tobacco. The beta-blocking agents that are not dependent on hepatic metabolism may not interact with tobacco.

**Mechanism:** Tobacco is known to induce hepatic microsomal enzymes, and propranolol is eliminated by hepatic clearance.

**Detailed Information:** See *EDI*, 11/37.00

## Timolol, Ophthalmic-Acetazolamide

**Significance:** 3—minimally clinically significant

**Potential Effects:** The use of the agents together in patients with chronic obstructive pulmonary disease (COPD) may result in acidosis.

**Recommendations:** The concurrent administration of acetazolamide and ophthalmic timolol, especially in patients with COPD, should be done with caution. If acidosis occurs, one or both agents may need to be discontinued. The use of ophthalmic betaxolol, a cardioselective agent, may be considered as an alternative to ophthalmic timolol.

**Summary:** There are data to show that coadministration of these agents in patients with COPD may result in acidosis.

**Related Drugs:** A similar interaction may occur between acetazolamide and other oral and ophthalmic noncardioselective beta blocking agents. A similar interaction may occur between ophthalmic timolol and other carbonic anhydrase inhibitors.

**Mechanism:** Acetazolamide produces metabolic acidosis by blocking the renal excretion of hydrogen ions.

**Detailed Information:** See *EDI*, 11/38.10

## Timolol, Ophthalmic-Prednisone

**Significance:** 2—moderately clinically significant

**Potential Effects:** The use of these agents together may cause an increase in the serum potassium level.

**Recommendations:** Monitor the patient's serum potassium level when these agents are used together. The ophthalmic timolol may need to be discontinued.

**Summary:** There are data to show that coadministration of these agents may cause an increase in serum potassium levels.

**Related Drugs:** A similar interaction may occur between prednisone and other beta blocking agents as well as the other ophthalmic beta blocking agents. A similar interaction is expected to occur between ophthalmic timolol and other corticosteroids.

**Mechanism:** Therapy with beta-blocking agents can cause small increases in potassium levels by suppression of renin and aldosterone release and by preventing $beta_2$-receptor mediated hepatic and skeletal muscle potassium uptake.

**Detailed Information:** See *EDI*, 11/39.00

# Chapter Twelve

# Cardiac Glycoside Drug Interactions

## Digitalis-Calcium Chloride (intravenous)

**Significance:** 2—moderately clinically significant

**Recommendations:** If intravenous administration of calcium is necessary in patients receiving digitalis therapy, it is recommended that this procedure be accomplished slowly and with caution. If cardiac toxicity does develop from intravenous calcium administration to a digitalized patient, supportive measures without additional antiarrhythmics may be sufficient, based on studies of massive digitalis intoxication. Calcium chelation with ethylenediaminetetraacetic acid (EDTA) may produce only transient improvement while adding its own toxicity; therefore, it has been considered unsatisfactory in treating digitalis toxicity in general.

**Summary:** Effects of digitalis glycosides on the heart are increased by extracellular concentrations of ionic calcium. Intravenous administration of calcium salts during digitalis therapy may result in altered cardiac electrophysiologic activity.

**Related Drugs:** The other digitalis glycosides may interact in a similar manner. Multiple forms of calcium compounds are available for parenteral administration and may interact in a similar manner with the digitalis glycosides.

**Mechanism:** Elevated extracellular concentrations of $Ca^{+2}$ facilitate inward calcium fluxes and modify transmembrane potentials and stronger contractions of cardiac muscle.

**Detailed Information:** See *EDI*, 12/1.00

## Digitalis-Phenytoin

**Significance:** 2—moderately clinically significant

**Recommendations:** With appropriate safeguards, phenytoin appears to be a useful adjunct to management of digitalis-induced supraventricular arrhythmias. It must be borne in mind that certain individuals may not respond, or may experience a worsening in cardiac function, after therapeutic doses of phenytoin. Long-term antiarrhythmic treatment with phenytoin may increase the elimination of digitalis, so use of an alternate antiarrhythmic drug may be advantageous. If phenytoin is deleted from combination therapy with digitalis, appropriate adjustment of the cardiac glycoside dosage may be necessary.

**Summary:** The administration of phenytoin to a patient experiencing supraventricular cardiotoxicity from digitalis has been utilized as a positive interaction with beneficial results.

**Related Drugs:** The other digitalis glycosides may interact in a similar manner with phenytoin. A similar interaction is expected to occur with other hydantoin anticonvulsants and digitalis.

**Mechanism:** Phenytoin antagonizes supraventricular arrhythmias induced by digitalis overdosage through a pharmacodynamic interaction on the membranes of myocardial pacemaker cells.

**Detailed Information:** See *EDI*, 12/3.00

## Digitalis-Reserpine

**Significance:** 3—minimally clinically significant

**Recommendations:** It may be wise to consider the many alternatives to reserpine for controlling hypertension in patients using digitalis glycosides. If reserpine is necessary in a digitalized individual, it can be successfully used, but careful observation of the patient is in order. If atrial fibrillation pre-exists, the potential for this adverse drug interaction appears to be greatly enhanced.

**Summary:** The clinical literature documents an interaction between cardiac glycosides and reserpine characterized by enhanced cardiotoxicity.

**Related Drugs:** A similar interaction is expected to occur with other digitalis glycosides and reserpine. Other rauwolfia alkaloids may interact with digitalis.
**Mechanism:** Direct or indirect effects of these two drugs may actually underlie this interaction.
**Detailed Information:** See *EDI,* 12/5.00

## Digitoxin-Aminoglutethimide

**Significance:** 3—minimally clinically significant
**Potential Effects:** Aminoglutethimide may increase the clearance of digitoxin, leading to decreased digitoxin levels.
**Recommendations:** Although concurrent use of these agents need not be avoided, digitoxin levels should be monitored and the dosage increased if necessary.
**Summary:** There are data to show that administration of aminoglutethimide may increase the clearance of digitoxin, leading to decreased digitoxin levels.
**Related Drugs:** Digitalis may interact in a similar manner with aminoglutethimide. The other digitalis glycosides would not be expected to interact with aminoglutethimide. A similar interaction may occur between glutethimide and digitoxin.
**Mechanism:** Aminoglutethimide increases the metabolism of digitoxin.
**Detailed Information:** See *EDI,* 12/6.10

## Digitoxin-Cholestyramine

**Significance:** 2—moderately clinically significant
**Potential Effects:** Cholestyramine may bind to digitoxin in the gastrointestinal tract, decreasing absorption and increasing elimination.
**Recommendations:** Monitor digitalis levels when these agents are used together. Separating administration by 1.5 hours or using digoxin capsules may avoid this interaction. Cholestyramine may be useful in treating digoxin toxicity.
**Summary:** Concurrent administration of cholestyramine and digitoxin can decrease the gastrointestinal absorption of digitoxin and result in reduced bioavailability.
**Related Drugs:** Administration of cholestyramine and digoxin resulted in reduced digoxin bioavailability. Based on the proposed mechanism, cholestyramine may interact with other digitalis glycosides. A similar interaction is expected to occur between colestipol and other digitalis glycosides.
**Mechanism:** Cholestyramine has been reported to bind digitoxin in the gastrointestinal tract, inhibiting absorption and enterohepatic circulation and resulting in reduced reabsorption and increased fecal excretion of digitoxin.
**Detailed Information:** See *EDI,* 12/7.00

## Digitoxin-Phenobarbital

**Significance:** 2—moderately clinically significant
**Recommendations:** When phenobarbital or another barbiturate is added to the regimen of a patient receiving digitoxin, careful monitoring for underdigitalization should be performed. It may be necessary to increase the digitoxin dose in some patients. Conversely, patients receiving combined therapy should be monitored carefully for digitalis toxicity if the barbiturate is withdrawn from the regimen.
**Summary:** Phenobarbital may decrease plasma digitoxin levels and shorten the digitoxin half-life.
**Related Drugs:** Digitalis leaf may interact in a similar manner with phenobarbital. Other barbiturates would interact with cardiac glycosides in a similar manner.

## Cardiac Glycoside

**Mechanism:** Phenobarbital may increase the metabolism of digitoxin to digoxin through hepatic microsomal enzymes.
**Detailed Information:** See *EDI*, 12/9.00

### Digitoxin-Phenylbutazone

**Significance:** 3—minimally clinically significant
**Recommendations:** Patients should be closely monitored during concurrent therapy, and the dose of digitoxin may need to be increased.
**Summary:** Phenylbutazone reduced serum digitoxin levels.
**Related Drugs:** A similar interaction is expected to occur between digitoxin and oxyphenbutazone and between phenylbutazone and other digitalis glycosides.
**Mechanism:** Phenylbutazone may increase the hepatic metabolism of digitoxin.
**Detailed Information:** See *EDI*, 12/11.00

### Digitoxin-Rifampin

**Significance:** 1—highly clinically significant
**Recommendations:** Patients should be monitored for underdigitalization during concurrent therapy with rifampin. It would be expected that the dosage of the glycoside will need to be increased within the first week of cotherapy.
**Summary:** Serum digitoxin concentrations can be significantly reduced with concurrent use of rifampin.
**Related Drugs:** Rifampin has caused subtherapeutic digoxin serum concentrations. A similar interaction is expected to occur with rifampin and other digitalis glycosides. There are no drugs related to rifampin.
**Mechanism:** Rifampin increases the metabolism of digitoxin.
**Detailed Information:** See *EDI*, 12/13.00

### Digoxin-Acarbose

**Significance:** 3—minimally clinically significant
**Potential Effects:** Concurrent administration of digoxin and acarbose may result in subtherapeutic levels of digoxin.
**Recommendations:** Serum digoxin levels should be monitored in patients receiving concurrent therapy with digoxin and acarbose. The dosage of digoxin may need to be adjusted or acarbose may need to be discontinued.
**Summary:** Concurrent administration of digoxin and acarbose resulted in subtherapeutic levels of digoxin as low as 0.48 ng/ml (therapeutic range: 0.8–2.1 ng/ml).
**Related Drugs:** A similar reaction would be expected to occur between acarbose and the other digitalis glycosides. There are no drugs related to acarbose.
**Mechanism:** The exact mechanism is unknown. An acarbose-induced change in gastrointestinal transit may alter the absorption of digoxin or acarbose may adsorb digoxin molecules. Alternatively, acarbose may inhibit the hydrolysis of digoxin prior to absorption, resulting in alterations in the digoxin laboratory analysis, since less genin, a digoxin hydrolysate, would be available to cross-react in the assay.
**Detailed Information:** See *EDI*, 12/15.00

### Digoxin-Aluminum Hydroxide, Magnesium Hydroxide, Magnesium Trisilicate

**Significance:** 2—moderately clinically significant

**Potential Effects:** Simultaneous administration of aluminum- or magnesium-containing antacids may decrease the gastrointestinal absorption of digoxin.

**Recommendations:** Oral digoxin tablets should not be given simultaneously with certain antacids (e.g., aluminum/magnesium hydroxide and magnesium trisilicate). When both digoxin and antacids are indicated, antacid preparations containing magnesium trisilicate, magnesium hydroxide, and aluminum hydroxide should be administered at least one to two hours before or after the digoxin. Serum digoxin levels and the clinical status of the patient should be monitored carefully for signs of underdigitalization. The use of digoxin with concurrent sucralfate should be monitored for decreased effects of digoxin. The sucralfate may have to be discontinued.

**Summary:** Administration of antacids containing magnesium trisilicate, magnesium hydroxide, and aluminum hydroxide may significantly decrease the gastrointestinal absorption of digoxin.

**Related Drugs:** The other digitalis glycosides may interact with antacids to a variable degree. The extent to which other magnesium- or aluminum-containing antacids affect digoxin absorption is not known. Sucralfate was shown to decrease digoxin area-under-curve.

**Mechanism:** The adsorptive capacity of antacids may be responsible for decreased digoxin absorption. Liquid antacids coat digoxin tablets and may interfere with dissolution or disintegration. Digoxin may bind to sucralfate, decreasing the extent of absorption.

**Detailed Information:** See *EDI*, 12/17.00

## Digoxin-Aminosalicylic Acid

**Significance:** 3—minimally clinically significant

**Recommendations:** Patients' digoxin serum levels should be monitored during concomitant use of these agents. An increased digoxin dose may be necessary, or separating the administration of the two drugs by as much time as possible may be beneficial.

**Summary:** Concurrent administration of digoxin and aminosalicylic acid resulted in a reduced digoxin area-under-curve.

**Related Drugs:** A similar interaction may occur between aminosalicylic acid and other digitalis glycosides. There are no drugs related to aminosalicylic acid.

**Mechanism:** Decreased gastrointestinal absorption of digoxin is believed to be the mechanism in this interaction.

**Detailed Information:** See *EDI*, 12/19.00

## Digoxin-Amiodarone

**Significance:** 1—highly clinically significant

**Potential Effects:** Amiodarone causes an increase in digoxin levels, which may result in digoxin toxicity.

**Recommendations:** Monitor patients for signs of digoxin toxicity and increased digoxin levels. The dose of digoxin may need to be decreased.

**Summary:** Several studies and case reports have shown that the concurrent administration of digoxin and amiodarone results in significant increases in digoxin serum levels, digoxin toxicity and side effects.

**Related Drugs:** A similar interaction may occur between amiodarone and other digitalis glycosides. There are no drugs related to amiodarone.

**Mechanism:** Amiodarone decreases renal and nonrenal clearance of digoxin, probably by a decrease in renal tubular secretion, or amiodarone may displace digoxin from its tissue binding sites.

**Detailed Information:** See *EDI*, 12/20.01

Cardiac Glycoside

## Digoxin-Captopril
**Significance:** 2—moderately clinically significant
**Potential Effects:** Captopril may cause an increase in digoxin levels.
**Recommendations:** Monitor patients for increased digoxin levels when these agents are used together.
**Summary:** There are data to show that administration of captopril may cause an increase in digoxin levels; however, studies have also shown that digoxin levels may slightly decrease.
**Related Drugs:** A similar interaction may occur between deslanoside and captopril, if the mechanism involves a reduced renal clearance of digoxin. A similar interaction may occur between digoxin and other ACE inhibitors.
**Mechanism:** Captopril increases digoxin levels by reducing digoxin's renal clearance.
**Detailed Information:** See *EDI*, 12/20.03

## Digoxin-Charcoal
**Significance:** 3—minimally clinically significant
**Recommendations:** Activated charcoal appears to be effective in the treatment of an acute digoxin overdose, especially in doses of 50 to 100 G, and one report suggests that it may also be effective in some cases of more chronic intoxications. However, if charcoal is not being used in this situation, it may be advisable to separate the administration of these agents by as much time as possible.
**Summary:** Activated charcoal has been shown to reduce the absorption and lower serum levels of digoxin.
**Related Drugs:** It may be expected that charcoal will reduce the absorption of the other digitalis glycosides.
**Mechanism:** Activated charcoal adsorbs digoxin, limiting its gastrointestinal absorption.
**Detailed Information:** See *EDI*, 12/20.10

## Digoxin-Cimetidine
**Significance:** 3—minimally clinically significant
**Recommendations:** Until further studies are done, the concurrent use of these agents need not be avoided. However, because of digoxin's low therapeutic index, serum digoxin levels should be monitored. An increased digoxin dose may be necessary.
**Summary:** There are data to show that cimetidine administration may decrease digoxin levels; however, all data do not support this interaction.
**Related Drugs:** The other digitalis glycosides may interact similarly with cimetidine. Documentation is lacking regarding a similar interaction between digoxin and other $H_2$-receptor antagonists.
**Mechanism:** Cimetidine may increase gastric pH, resulting in a decrease in digoxin absorption.
**Detailed Information:** See *EDI*, 12/20.30

## Digoxin-Cyclophosphamide, Prednisone, Procarbazine, Vincristine
**Significance:** 2—moderately clinically significant
**Potential Effects:** Use of these agents together may result in a decrease in digoxin levels.
**Recommendations:** Monitor digoxin levels in patients taking these agents together. Digitoxin or digoxin capsules may be an alternative to digoxin tablets.
**Summary:** There are data to show that administration of these agents with digoxin may lead to a decrease in digoxin levels.

**Related Drugs:** Digoxin has been shown to interact with other combination cytotoxic therapies; however, the data are conflicting. Because of conflicting results, it is difficult to determine if an interaction would occur with other digitalis glycosides.
**Mechanism:** Combination cytotoxic agents may reduce gastrointestinal absorption of digoxin, possibly resulting from impairment of the intestinal mucosal membrane by the cytotoxic drugs.
**Detailed Information:** See *EDI*, 12/21.00

## Digoxin-Cyclosporine

**Significance:** 2—moderately clinically significant
**Potential Effects:** Cyclosporine may increase digoxin levels, resulting in toxicity.
**Recommendations:** Monitor digoxin levels and cardiac status closely during concomitant therapy with cyclosporine.
**Summary:** There are data to show that administration of cyclosporine can increase digoxin levels, potentiating toxicity; however, the data are conflicting.
**Related Drugs:** It is not known if an interaction would occur between cyclosporine and other digitalis glycosides. There are no drugs related to cyclosporine.
**Mechanism:** Decreased digoxin clearance may be a result of a cyclosporine-induced reduction in renal blood flow.
**Detailed Information:** See *EDI*, 12/22.10

## Digoxin-Diazepam

**Significance:** 2—moderately clinically significant
**Potential Effects:** Concurrent digoxin and diazepam may result in an increase in digoxin half-life and a decrease in digoxin urinary excretion.
**Recommendations:** Patients should be monitored for an increase in digoxin levels, and a lower dose of digoxin may be necessary.
**Summary:** There are data to show that administration of diazepam may increase digoxin levels.
**Related Drugs:** A similar interaction is expected to occur between digoxin and deslanoside if the interaction results from a renal mechanism. Other benzodiazepines have been documented to interact with digoxin; however, the data are conflicting.
**Mechanism:** The mechanism of this interaction is unknown.
**Detailed Information:** See *EDI*, 12/23.00

## Digoxin-Disopyramide

**Significance:** 3—minimally clinically significant
**Recommendations:** Until further studies are done, the concurrent use of these agents need not be avoided, and no special precautions appear necessary.
**Summary:** The concurrent use of disopyramide does not significantly affect serum digoxin levels.
**Related Drugs:** It is not known whether an interaction would occur between disopyramide and other digitalis glycosides. There are no drugs related to disopyramide.
**Mechanism:** The mechanism of this interaction is unknown.
**Detailed Information:** See *EDI*, 12/25.00

## Digoxin-Erythromycin Base

**Significance:** 1—highly clinically significant
**Potential Effects:** The addition of erythromycin to a stable digoxin regimen may result in increased digoxin serum levels and toxicity.

## Cardiac Glycoside

**Recommendations:** Digoxin serum concentrations should be monitored when initiating or discontinuing concurrent erythromycin therapy. Patients who are receiving erythromycin and being digitalized should be closely monitored for overdigitalization.

**Summary:** The addition of erythromycin to the therapy of patients maintained on digoxin resulted in increased serum digoxin levels by as much as 104% and digoxin toxicity.

**Related Drugs:** One patient with a stable digoxin regimen experienced a 270% increase in digoxin serum levels after starting clarithromycin. Other erythromycin salts and macrolide antibiotics would be expected to undergo a similar interaction with digoxin. It is not known if an interaction would occur between erythromycin and the other digitalis glycosides.

**Mechanism:** Approximately 10% of the patients who receive digoxin convert a substantial portion of it to digoxin reduction products. These metabolites are not taken up as well by cardiac muscle and have less cardiac activity and some are more rapidly excreted in the urine. These products are formed predominantly by the bacteria in the gastrointestinal tract. The antibiotic, by destroying the bacteria, decreases digoxin metabolism, which would account for the increased digoxin serum concentrations.

**Detailed Information:** See *EDI*, 12/27.00

## Digoxin-Esmolol

**Significance:** 3—minimally clinically significant

**Potential Effects:** Concurrent administration of oral digoxin and a beta-blocking agent may result in an increase in the mean digoxin area-under-curve (AUC).

**Recommendations:** Concurrent use of these agents need not be avoided. However, digoxin levels should be monitored closely during concomitant beta-blocker therapy, especially at the initiation or discontinuation of beta-blocker therapy.

**Summary:** Concurrent administration of oral digoxin and esmolol resulted in an increase in the mean digoxin AUC. Other pharmacologic parameters were not affected. The clinical significance was not determined.

**Related Drugs:** Studies have shown conflicting results with carvedilol, nadolol, atenolol, propranolol, and sotalol; therefore it would be difficult to determine if an interaction would occur between digoxin and other beta-blocking agents. It is also not known if an interaction would occur between esmolol and the other digitalis glycosides.

**Mechanism:** The mechanism whereby esmolol increased the digoxin AUC is not known; however, it is unlikely that esmolol altered the clearance of digoxin. It has been suggested that the oral bioavailability of digoxin may have been increased as a result of intestinal vasodilation.

**Detailed Information:** See *EDI*, 12/28.01

## Digoxin-Fluoxetine

**Significance:** 2—moderately clinically significant

**Potential Effects:** The addition of fluoxetine to the therapy of a patient stabilized on digoxin may result in increased digoxin levels and digoxin toxic effects.

**Recommendations:** If fluoxetine is added to or discontinued from the therapy of a patient maintained on digoxin, the patient should be carefully monitored for serum digoxin level changes and toxicity. The digoxin dosage may need to be adjusted or an alternative to fluoxetine may need to be contemplated.

**Summary:** The addition of fluoxetine to the therapy of a patient stabilized on digoxin resulted in increased digoxin levels (from 1.4 nmol/L to 4.2 nmol/L) and digoxin toxic effects.

**Related Drugs:** In separate studies, sertraline, paroxetine, and fluvoxamine had no significant effects on digoxin pharmacokinetics. Based on structural and pharmacologic similarity, an interaction may be expected to occur between digoxin and citalopram, although this interaction is not expected to be of clinical significance. It is not known whether a similar interaction would be expected to occur between fluoxetine and the other digitalis glycosides.

**Mechanism:** The mechanism of this interaction is not known.

**Detailed Information:** See *EDI*, 12/28.50

## Digoxin-Furosemide

**Significance:** 2—moderately clinically significant

**Potential Effects:** Concurrent administration of these agents may result in increased digoxin effect and toxicity resulting from hypokalemia.

**Recommendations:** Monitor the patient's potassium level and cardiac status with concurrent administration of these agents.

**Summary:** Concurrent administration of digoxin and furosemide resulted in cardiac arrhythmias.

**Related Drugs:** Digitalis and digitoxin have also been reported to interact with diuretics. Deslanoside may be expected to interact similarly based on pharmacologic similarity. All potassium-depleting diuretics, including thiazides, other loop diuretics, the mercurial diuretic mersalyl, and thiazide-related diuretics may be expected to interact with digoxin similarly. Amphotericin B, although structurally and pharmacologically unrelated to the potassium-sparing diuretics, has caused hypokalemia, which can predispose patients to digoxin toxicity.

**Mechanism:** Digoxin acts on excitable tissues of the myocardium to inhibit sodium/potassium dependent ATPase. In hypokalemia there is less extracellular potassium available to exchange for intracellular sodium through remaining sodium pump activity, and membranes become even more depolarized. Thus, furosemide and other diuretics enhance the electrophysiologic effects of digoxin primarily by disturbing the normal potassium gradient across cell membranes.

**Detailed Information:** See *EDI*, 12/29.00

## Digoxin-Ginseng

**Significance:** 3—minimally clinically significant

**Potential Effects:** Concomitant ginseng and digoxin administration may lead to increased digoxin serum levels.

**Recommendations:** Patients should be carefully monitored for apparent changes in digoxin serum levels and possible toxicity with concurrent use of these agents. The dose of digoxin may need to be adjusted.

**Summary:** Elevated digoxin serum levels have occurred with concomitant digoxin and Siberian ginseng administration. No digoxin or digitoxin contamination was found in the ginseng capsules.

**Related Drugs:** It is not known whether a similar interaction would be expected to occur between ginseng and the other digitalis glycosides.

**Mechanism:** Siberian ginseng contains eleutherosides, which are chemically related to cardiac glycosides such as digoxin. Since no digoxin toxicity has been reported, it is unlikely that these compounds are converted to digoxin *in vivo* or that the elimination of digoxin is impaired. It is possible that the serum assay may have measured another compound, perhaps an eleutheroside or its derivative. Further studies are needed.

**Detailed Information:** See *EDI*, 12/30.05

## Digoxin-Guar Gum

**Significance:** 3—minimally clinically significant

**Potential Effects:** The concurrent use of digoxin and guar gum may result in decreased peak serum concentrations and decreased area under the curve (AUC) of digoxin. However, there was little change in digoxin bioavailability when compared to a control.

**Recommendations:** The concurrent administration of digoxin and guar gum only minimally reduced the amount of digoxin absorbed in a single dose study. Separating the dosing of digoxin by two to four hours from that of guar gum may help reduce the potential for decreased absorption. The patient receiving both digoxin and guar gum concurrently should be monitored for decreased digoxin levels as well as a possible decrease in efficacy.

**Summary:** Concurrent use of digoxin and guar gum resulted in decreased peak serum concentrations and AUC of digoxin when compared to the control. However, there was little difference in digoxin bioavailability when compared to the control

**Related Drugs:** A similar interaction may be expected between guar gum and the other digitalis glycosides. There are no agents related to guar gum. Other common names for guar gum include guar flour and jaguar gum.

**Mechanism:** It has been suggested that the serum digoxin concentration may be decreased due to the binding of bile acids by guar gum.

**Detailed Information:** See *EDI*, 12/30.07

## Digoxin-Heparin

**Significance:** 3—minimally clinically significant

**Recommendations:** Until further clinical studies are done, the concurrent use of these agents need not be avoided. However, caution should be used in patients receiving high dose heparin therapy, and digoxin levels should be monitored frequently.

**Summary:** The concomitant use of these agents should be used with caution.

**Related Drugs:** It is not known if heparin would interact with other digitalis glycosides.

**Mechanism:** Heparin releases free fatty acids, and these strongly bind to serum albumin and may remove digoxin from the albumin sites.

**Detailed Information:** See *EDI*, 12/30.10

## Digoxin-Hydroxychloroquine

**Significance:** 2—moderately clinically significant

**Recommendations:** Patients should be closely monitored for signs of digoxin toxicity during concurrent use of these agents, and the dose of digoxin may need to be reduced.

**Summary:** There are data to show that administration of hydroxychloroquine may increase serum digoxin levels.

**Related Drugs:** A similar interaction is expected to occur between the other digitalis glycosides and other aminoquinolines.

**Mechanism:** The mechanism of this interaction is unknown; however, hydroxychloroquine is related to quinidine, and the interaction between digoxin and quinidine is well documented (see Digoxin-Quinidine, page 287).

**Detailed Information:** See *EDI*, 12/31.00

## Cardiac Glycoside

### Digoxin-Hypericum
**Significance:** 3—minimally clinically significant
**Potential Effects:** The concurrent use of digoxin and St. John's wort (*Hypericum perforatum L.*) resulted in a decrease in the digoxin concentrations.
**Recommendations:** Patients maintained on digoxin should be monitored for changes in digoxin serum levels if St. John's wort is added to or discontinued from concurrent therapy. Digoxin toxicity may result if St. John's wort is discontinued from concurrent therapy with digoxin.
**Summary:** Concurrent use of digoxin and St. John's wort resulted in a decrease in digoxin concentrations.
**Related Drugs:** A similar interaction may occur between hypericum and the other digitalis glycosides.
**Mechanism:** St. John's wort has many constituents, with hypericin generally considered to be the active ingredient. *In vitro*, the extract induces cytochrome $P450_{3A4}$ and cytochrome $P450_{1A2}$; however, oxidative metabolism plays a minor role in digoxin elimination. Several flavonoids in St. John's wort are substrates or modulators of P-glycoprotein. Digoxin pharmacokinetics may be influenced by an induction of P-glycoprotein after multiple-dose administration of hypericum extract. This mediates the efflux function, which transports digoxin into the intestinal lumen.
**Detailed Information:** See *EDI*, 12/32.00

### Digoxin-Ibuprofen
**Significance:** 2—moderately clinically significant
**Potential Effects:** Ibuprofen may increase digoxin levels when added to therapy. One study reported an initial change in digoxin levels, but no change in digoxin levels after 28 days of cotherapy.
**Recommendations:** Monitor digoxin levels during concurrent therapy. The dose of digoxin may need to be decreased.
**Summary:** Ibuprofen may increase serum digoxin levels; however, there was no significant difference in digoxin levels after 28 days of concomitant therapy.
**Related Drugs:** A similar interaction is expected to occur between deslanoside and digitalis or digitoxin, if the mechanism involves a decreased renal excretion. Because of conflicting reports, it is difficult to determine if an interaction would occur between digoxin and the other NSAIAs.
**Mechanism:** NSAIAs are known to depress kidney function, and there may be a decreased digoxin renal excretion.
**Detailed Information:** See *EDI*, 12/33.00

### Digoxin-Itraconazole
**Significance:** 2—moderately clinically significant
**Potential Effects:** The addition of itraconazole to the therapy of a patient maintained on digoxin may result in increased digoxin serum levels.
**Recommendations:** Digoxin serum levels should be carefully monitored if itraconazole is added to, or withdrawn from, concurrent therapy. The dose of digoxin may need to be adjusted, and as much as a 75% decrease in digoxin dose may be needed with concurrent itraconazole. Ketoconazole may be a suitable alternative, but further controlled clinical studies are needed.
**Summary:** There are data to show that itraconazole may increase digoxin serum levels in digoxin maintained patients.

## Cardiac Glycoside

**Related Drugs:** An interaction may occur between itraconazole and other digitalis glycosides. Because of conflicting data, it is not known if an interaction would occur between digoxin and other imidazole antifungal agents.
**Mechanism:** The mechanism of the interaction is unknown.
**Detailed Information:** See *EDI,* 12/34.50

### Digoxin-Kaolin
**Significance:** 2—moderately clinically significant
**Recommendations:** A steady-state study indicates that the interaction is not of major clinical significance, although other studies report a significant decrease in digoxin bioavailability. Administering the kaolin-pectin suspension at least two hours after digoxin appears to avoid the interaction. If the agents must be administered simultaneously, then digoxin as the soft gelatin capsule or the elixir is recommended. The patient receiving both digoxin and kaolin-pectin suspension concurrently should be observed for signs and symptoms of underdigitalization.
**Summary:** Concurrent administration of kaolin-pectin suspension and digoxin tablets resulted in a significant reduction in digoxin bioavailability.
**Related Drugs:** A similar interaction is expected to occur between kaolin-pectin and other digitalis glycosides. Digoxin has been shown to be decreased by concurrent diphenoxylate and atropine.
**Mechanism:** Kaolin may prevent the gastrointestinal absorption of digoxin by adsorption of digoxin, or kaolin may alter the gastrointestinal motility.
**Detailed Information:** See *EDI,* 12/35.00

### Digoxin-Kyushin
**Significance:** 3—minimally clinically significant
**Potential Effects:** The concurrent administration of digoxin and kyushin may result in inaccurate measurements of digoxin levels.
**Recommendations:** Digoxin levels should be carefully evaluated in patients receiving concurrent therapy with digoxin and kyushin.
**Summary:** Concurrent administration of digoxin and kyushin resulted in inaccurate measurements of digoxin levels; although digoxin monitoring revealed a level of 2.5 ng/ml, the patient had no symptoms of digoxin toxicity.
**Related Drugs:** Kyushin is composed mainly of chan-su. Chan-su is the dried venom of the Cantor Chinese toad, *Bufo bufo gargarizans,* which is primarily composed of bufalin and cinobufaginal. Bufalin (a major component of chan-su, and the largest constituent of kyushin), resulted in positive interference when digitoxin was measured by fluorescence polarization assays. An interaction may occur between kyushin and the other digitalis glycosides.
**Mechanism:** The major effective component of kyushin is chan-su, which contains cardiotonic steroids with chemical structures similar to digoxin. Bufalin has been shown to be one of these cardiotonic compounds.
**Detailed Information:** See *EDI,* 12/35.70

### Digoxin-Methyldopa
**Significance:** 3—minimally clinically significant
**Recommendations:** Patients receiving methyldopa and digoxin concurrently should be observed carefully for symptomatic bradycardia. If sinus bradycardia occurs during concomitant therapy, hydralazine has been shown to be a beneficial alternative to methyldopa.

## Cardiac Glycoside

**Summary:** There are data to show that methyldopa administration may sometimes cause symptomatic bradycardia in patients on digoxin.

**Related Drugs:** A similar interaction is expected to occur between methyldopa and other digitalis glycosides. There are no drugs related to methyldopa.

**Mechanism:** Digoxin could augment the sympatholytic action of methyldopa.

**Detailed Information:** See *EDI*, 12/36.10

### Digoxin-Metoclopramide

**Significance:** 2—moderately clinically significant

**Recommendations:** Metoclopramide will influence digoxin absorption less from fast-dissolving digoxin tablets, digoxin capsules, or liquid preparations than from slow-dissolving tablets. Thus, slow-dissolving preparations may underdigitalize patients currently receiving metoclopramide. Digoxin serum concentrations should therefore be monitored when these agents are used concomitantly.

**Summary:** Metoclopramide was shown to increase serum digoxin concentrations; however, the pharmacokinetic changes will depend on the formulation of digoxin used.

**Related Drugs:** A similar interaction is expected to occur with other digitalis glycosides and metoclopramide. There are no drugs related to metoclopramide.

**Mechanism:** Peristalsis caused by metoclopramide may reduce the time digoxin is at the absorption site, causing less drug to be absorbed.

**Detailed Information:** See *EDI*, 12/37.00

### Digoxin-Mexiletine

**Significance:** 4—not clinically significant

**Potential Effects:** Mexiletine does not affect digoxin levels.

**Recommendations:** The concurrent administration of digoxin and mexiletine need not be avoided. Because of the lack of interaction, mexiletine may be considered as an alternative antiarrhythmic agent to other agents that have been shown to interact with digoxin (e.g., quinidine), although further study is needed to support this statement.

**Summary:** Mexiletine was shown to have no significant effect on serum digoxin levels.

**Related Drugs:** It is not known if an interaction would occur between digoxin and lidocaine or tocainide, or between mexiletine and the other digitalis glycosides.

**Mechanism:** Mexiletine does not appear to affect the serum levels of digoxin.

**Detailed Information:** See *EDI*, 12/38.10

### Digoxin-Moricizine

**Significance:** 4—not clinically significant

**Potential Effects:** Moricizine does not appear to alter digoxin levels.

**Recommendations:** Concurrent administration need not be avoided. Moricizine may be an alternative agent to those antiarrhythmics that interact with digoxin during concurrent digoxin therapy.

**Summary:** An interaction does not appear to occur between digoxin and moricizine.

**Related Drugs:** There are no reports demonstrating an interaction between moricizine and other digitalis glycosides. There are no drugs related to moricizine.

**Mechanism:** Moricizine does not appear to affect the serum levels of digoxin.

**Detailed Information:** See *EDI*, 12/38.30

## Digoxin-Neomycin

**Significance:** 2—moderately clinically significant

**Recommendations:** The interaction was seen with neomycin dosages from 1.0 to 3.0 G with tablets or solutions of both digoxin and neomycin, or when neomycin was given three or six hours before digoxin. Therefore, if neomycin is added to, or withdrawn from, concurrent digoxin therapy, patients must be monitored for changing digoxin serum concentrations and dosage adjustments should be made. Patients receiving neomycin who are being digitalized should be closely monitored for underdigitalization.

**Summary:** Concurrent administration of neomycin sulfate has been shown to depress serum digoxin concentrations.

**Related Drugs:** A similar interaction is expected to occur between neomycin and other digitalis glycosides or between digoxin and other available oral aminoglycosides.

**Mechanism:** Neomycin may cause a precipitation of digoxin, or neomycin may change the intestinal membrane permeability.

**Detailed Information:** See *EDI*, 12/39.00

## Digoxin-Penicillamine

**Significance:** 2—moderately clinically significant

**Recommendations:** Patients should be monitored for decreased digoxin levels. The dose of digoxin may need to be increased.

**Summary:** Concurrent use of digoxin and penicillamine results in significantly reduced serum digoxin levels.

**Related Drugs:** There is no documentation regarding a similar interaction between penicillamine and other digitalis glycosides. There are no drugs related to penicillamine.

**Mechanism:** The exact mechanism is not known.

**Detailed Information:** See *EDI*, 12/41.00

## Digoxin-Prazosin

**Significance:** 2—moderately clinically significant

**Potential Effects:** Prazosin may increase digoxin levels.

**Recommendations:** Patients maintained on digoxin should be monitored closely if prazosin is added to, or withdrawn from, cotherapy. The dose of digoxin may need to be adjusted.

**Summary:** There are data to show that prazosin administration may increase digoxin levels.

**Related Drugs:** It is not known if a similar interaction would occur between prazosin and other digitalis glycosides or between digoxin and other alpha-1-adrenergic blocking agents.

**Mechanism:** Prazosin may cause an increase in oral absorption, reduce tubular secretion, reduce hepatic clearance or alter the protein binding of digoxin.

**Detailed Information:** See *EDI*, 12/42.10

## Digoxin-Propafenone

**Significance:** 2—moderately clinically significant

**Potential Effects:** Propafenone may cause an increase in digoxin levels.

**Recommendations:** Concurrent use of digoxin and propafenone should be approached with caution. Digoxin levels should be monitored and the dose of digoxin may need to be adjusted.

**Summary:** Concurrent use of propafenone may increase digoxin serum levels.

**Related Drugs:** Flecainide has been shown to interact with digoxin; however, the data are conflicting. It is not known if propafenone would interact with other digitalis glycosides or if an interaction would occur between digoxin and indecainide.

**Mechanism:** Reduced renal elimination of digoxin may partially explain the serum digoxin concentration increase during concurrent propafenone administration.
**Detailed Information:** See *EDI*, 12/42.30

## Digoxin-Propantheline

**Significance:** 1—highly clinically significant
**Recommendations:** The problem presented by a patient who requires propantheline and digoxin can be circumvented by the selection of quickly absorbed digoxin preparations—either rapidly solubilized tablets or liquid digoxin. The soft gelatin capsule form of digoxin might also be considered because of its rapid dissolution. Should digitalized patients experience symptoms indicative of digitalis glycoside intoxication with the use of propantheline or similar drugs, it may be from excessive absorption of digoxin from a slowly disintegrating tablet. Changing to a rapidly absorbed preparation will give predictable blood levels.
**Summary:** Absorption of digoxin may be significantly increased by concomitant administration of propantheline.
**Related Drugs:** Undocumented risk may be anticipated with all the anticholinergics. All slow-dissolving digitalis glycoside preparations may be expected to interact similarly.
**Mechanism:** Medication in a slow-dissolving tablet will be more extensively absorbed if the time spent in the intestine is increased. Propantheline prolongs intestinal emptying time, facilitating more complete absorption.
**Detailed Information:** See *EDI*, 12/43.00

## Digoxin-Psyllium

**Significance:** 3—minimally clinically significant
**Recommendations:** Although information is limited, the interaction seems to produce some degree of reduced digoxin absorption. If long-term psyllium and digoxin cotherapy is undertaken, patients should be monitored for decreasing digoxin serum concentrations. A two-hour interval between dosage with these drugs may prevent any problem.
**Summary:** Coadministration of psyllium hydrophilic mucilloid has been shown to reduce the bioavailability of digoxin.
**Related Drugs:** There appear to be no reports that any of the digitalis glycosides interact similarly with other bulk producing laxatives.
**Mechanism:** Possible physical binding of digoxin to psyllium or other absorptive hindrance may explain this interaction.
**Detailed Information:** See *EDI*, 12/45.00

## Digoxin-Quinidine

**Significance:** 1—highly clinically significant
**Potential Effects:** Quinidine will cause an increase in digoxin levels.
**Recommendations:** Monitor digoxin levels closely when quinidine is added to, or withdrawn from, therapy. Some reports recommend reducing the digoxin dose by 30% to 50% when quinidine is added to therapy. Digoxin toxicity may be enhanced by concomitant quinidine, even at therapeutic serum digoxin levels.
**Summary:** It is well documented that quinidine alters digoxin pharmacokinetics, causing an approximately twofold increase in plasma digoxin concentration.
**Related Drugs:** Conflicting results make it difficult to determine whether a similar interaction would occur between quinidine and other digitalis glycosides. Quinine was found to increase plasma digoxin concentration.

## Cardiac Glycoside

**Mechanism:** Reduction in digoxin renal clearance and displacement from tissue digoxin binding sites, leading to a reduced volume of distribution, appear to be the predominant mechanisms involved in this interaction.
**Detailed Information:** See *EDI*, 12/47.00

### Digoxin-Spironolactone
**Significance:** 2—moderately clinically significant
**Recommendations:** Concurrent administration of spironolactone and digoxin should be closely monitored, and potassium and digoxin concentrations should be measured frequently to assess the potential for toxicity. Also, the patient should be monitored for changes in therapeutic effects.
**Summary:** Simultaneous administration of spironolactone and digoxin has been shown to decrease volume of distribution, plasma clearance, and renal clearance and increase plasma digoxin concentrations. Potassium levels have also been shown to fluctuate.
**Related Drugs:** Because of conflicting data, whether spironolactone increases or reduces the therapeutic action of digitoxin cannot be documented. Conflicting reports make it difficult to predict whether an interaction would occur between spironolactone and other digitalis glycosides.
**Mechanism:** Increases in steady-state digoxin concentrations associated with spironolactone have been attributed to reduced renal tubular digoxin clearance caused by competitive blocking by spironolactone.
**Detailed Information:** See *EDI*, 12/50.10

### Digoxin-Succinylcholine
**Significance:** 2—moderately clinically significant
**Recommendations:** Succinylcholine should be used with caution in patients receiving digoxin or other digitalis glycosides.
**Summary:** There have been reports of cardiac arrhythmias occurring after the administration of succinylcholine to patients stabilized on digoxin.
**Related Drugs:** Administration of digoxin and pancuronium has led to sinus tachycardia and atrial flutter. The other digitalis glycosides may also be expected to interact with succinylcholine.
**Mechanism:** This interaction may be due to a loss of intracellular potassium, sympathetic postganglionic stimulation, or a direct effect on the myocardium by succinylcholine.
**Detailed Information:** See *EDI*, 12/51.00

### Digoxin-Sulfasalazine
**Significance:** 2—moderately clinically significant
**Recommendations:** Careful monitoring of digoxin serum levels is recommended to detect subtherapeutic levels when digoxin is taken concurrently with sulfasalazine. Increasing the digoxin dosage or switching to the elixir form did not increase digoxin levels, nor did separating the times of administration, results suggesting that sulfasalazine may need to be discontinued. In an acute situation, parenteral digoxin may be indicated. No literature is available at this time regarding the interaction of sulfasalazine and the soft gelatin capsule form of digoxin.
**Summary:** Sulfasalazine has been shown to reduce the serum levels of digoxin.
**Related Drugs:** No documentation is available indicating sulfasalazine interacts similarly with other digitalis glycosides. There appears to be no evidence that other sulfonamides interact with digoxin.
**Mechanism:** The mechanism of this interaction is unknown.
**Detailed Information:** See *EDI*, 12/53.00

## Cardiac Glycoside

### Digoxin-Tetracycline
**Significance:** 1—highly clinically significant
**Recommendations:** Digoxin serum concentrations should be monitored when initiating or discontinuing concurrent tetracycline therapy. Patients who are receiving tetracycline and being digitalized should be closely monitored for overdigitalization.
**Summary:** There are data to show that tetracycline administration may increase steady-state serum digoxin concentrations.
**Related Drugs:** A similar interaction is expected to occur with the tetracycline derivatives and digoxin. There is no documentation that tetracycline undergoes a similar reaction with the other digitalis glycosides.
**Mechanism:** Antibiotics destroy bacteria and decrease digoxin metabolism, which would account for the increased digoxin serum concentrations.
**Detailed Information:** See *EDI*, 12/55.00

### Digoxin-Thyroid
**Significance:** 2—moderately clinically significant
**Recommendations:** Patients stabilized on digoxin should be monitored closely when concurrent thyroid therapy is initiated to avoid a decrease in the therapeutic effect of the digoxin. Conversely, increased digoxin sensitivity may result from withdrawal of thyroid preparations in patients maintained on the digitalis glycoside.
**Summary:** The therapeutic efficacy of digoxin may be decreased in patients with hyperthyroidism or in patients being treated with thyroid hormones.
**Related Drugs:** Digitoxin has been shown to be similarly affected by hyperthyroidism. The other digitalis glycosides may interact in a similar manner. The interaction with thyroid hormones may occur primarily with liothyronine, but all other thyroid preparations may be expected to interact.
**Mechanism:** Hyperthyroidism results in lower serum levels of digoxin and other digitalis glycosides.
**Detailed Information:** See *EDI*, 12/57.00

### Digoxin-Tolbutamide
**Significance:** 3—minimally clinically significant
**Potential Effects:** Tolbutamide may cause an increase in digoxin levels, leading to digoxin toxicity.
**Recommendations:** Concurrent administration of digoxin and tolbutamide should be done with caution, and digoxin levels should be closely monitored. Glyburide may be used instead of tolbutamide.
**Summary:** There are data to show that administration of tolbutamide may cause an increase in digoxin levels, leading to digoxin toxicity and increased adverse effects.
**Related Drugs:** Glyburide was shown to not significantly interact with digoxin. Because of conflicting results, it is difficult to determine if an interaction would occur between digoxin and other sulfonylurea hypoglycemic agents. It is not known if tolbutamide would interact with other digitalis glycosides.
**Mechanism:** The mechanism of this interaction is not known.
**Detailed Information:** See *EDI*, 12/58.01

### Digoxin-Trazodone
**Significance:** 3—minimally clinically significant
**Potential Effects:** The addition of trazodone to the therapy of a patient stabilized on digoxin may result in increased digoxin serum levels and toxicity.

**Recommendations:** Patients receiving these drugs concurrently should be carefully monitored for digoxin toxicity. Because conclusive documentation for this interaction is lacking, the incidence and clinical significance of the concurrent administration of these agents has not been determined.

**Summary:** The addition of trazodone to the therapy of a patient stabilized on digoxin resulted in increased digoxin serum levels from 0.8 ng/ml to 2.8 ng/ml (therapeutic range: 1.2–1.7 ng/ml) and digoxin toxicity.

**Related Drugs:** Concurrent nefazodone and digoxin has also resulted in increased digoxin levels, but without clinically significant changes in vital signs. It is not known whether an interaction would occur between either trazodone or nefazodone and the other digitalis glycosides. Trazodone and nefazodone are chemically and pharmacologically unrelated to the tricyclic and tetracyclic antidepressant agents.

**Mechanism:** The mechanism of this interaction is not known.

**Detailed Information:** See *EDI*, 12/58.10

## Digoxin-Trimethoprim

**Significance:** 3—minimally clinically significant

**Potential Effects:** Trimethoprim may cause an increase in digoxin levels.

**Recommendations:** If these agents are used together, digoxin levels should be monitored.

**Summary:** There are data to show that trimethoprim administration may cause an increase in digoxin levels.

**Related Drugs:** The other digitalis glycosides eliminated largely through renal mechanisms would be expected to interact similarly with trimethoprim. Other digitalis glycosides metabolized in the liver would not be expected to interact with trimethoprim. There are no drugs related to trimethoprim.

**Mechanism:** Trimethoprim may decrease the renal tubular secretion of digoxin.

**Detailed Information:** See *EDI*, 12/58.30

## Digoxin-Verapamil

**Significance:** 1—highly clinically significant

**Potential Effects:** Verapamil can significantly increase digoxin levels. Both the therapeutic and toxic effects of digoxin have been increased.

**Recommendations:** Monitor the patient's cardiac status and digoxin levels when these agents are used together. The dosage of digoxin may need to be decreased.

**Summary:** Serum digoxin concentrations are increased with concurrent verapamil therapy.

**Related Drugs:** Nifedipine, nicardipine, isradipine and bepridil have been documented to interact with digoxin; however, the data are conflicting. It is not known if verapamil or other calcium channel blocking agents would interact with other digitalis glycosides.

**Mechanism:** Verapamil impairs the renal and extrarenal clearance of digoxin. The reduction in renal clearance may result from inhibition of tubular secretion.

**Detailed Information:** See *EDI*, 12/59.00

# Chapter Thirteen

# Diuretic Drug Interactions

## Acetazolamide-Cyclosporine
**Significance:** 2—moderately clinically significant
**Potential Effects:** Acetazolamide may increase cyclosporine levels.
**Recommendations:** Acetazolamide should be used with caution in patients maintained on cyclosporine. Patients undergoing cotherapy should be monitored for an increase in cyclosporine levels and for nephrotoxicity. The dose of one or both agents may need to be adjusted.
**Summary:** There are data to show that acetazolamide administration may increase cyclosporine levels.
**Related Drugs:** Documentation is lacking regarding a similar interaction between cyclosporine and other carbonic anhydrase inhibitors. There are no drugs related to cyclosporine.
**Mechanism:** This interaction may be due to the alteration of cyclosporine entry into red blood cells or an increase in absorption of cyclosporine.
**Detailed Information:** See *EDI*, 13/0.05

## Bendroflumethiazide-Aminoglutethimide
**Significance:** 3—minimally clinically significant
**Potential Effects:** The concurrent use of these agents may result in hyponatremia.
**Recommendations:** Patients taking these agents together should have serum sodium monitored. Fludrocortisone may need to be added or the bendroflumethiazide discontinued if hyponatremia occurs.
**Summary:** There are data to show that coadministration of these agents may result in reversible hyponatremia.
**Related Drugs:** A similar interaction may occur between aminoglutethimide and other thiazide diuretics and thiazide-related diuretics.
**Mechanism:** A synergistic effect may occur with concurrent diuretic therapy and aminoglutethimide, resulting in hyponatremia.
**Detailed Information:** See *EDI*, 13/0.10

## Bendroflumethiazide-Indomethacin
**Significance:** 2—moderately clinically significant
**Potential Effects:** Indomethacin may decrease the hypotensive effects of bendroflumethiazide.
**Recommendations:** Patients' blood pressure should be closely monitored during concurrent therapy of these agents. The dose of bendroflumethiazide may need to be increased.
**Summary:** Indomethacin has been shown to reduce the hypotensive effects of concurrent bendroflumethiazide.
**Related Drugs:** Hydrochlorothiazide and indomethacin were shown to exhibit a similar interaction; however, the data are conflicting. Indomethacin may blunt the antihypertensive effect of chlorthalidone. Because of conflicting results, it is difficult to determine whether an interaction would occur between indomethacin and other thiazide diuretics or other thiazide-related diuretics and between bendroflumethiazide and other NSAIAs.
**Mechanism:** Indomethacin may inhibit prostaglandin synthesis responsible for vasodilation, causing an increase in blood pressure. Indomethacin has been shown to acutely reduce sodium and water excretion.
**Detailed Information:** See *EDI*, 13/1.00

## Chlorothiazide-Calcium Carbonate

**Significance:** 2—moderately clinically significant

**Potential Effects:** Concurrent use of these agents may result in hypercalcemia, metabolic alkalosis, and renal failure.

**Recommendations:** Use these agents together with caution. If milk-alkali syndrome develops, the calcium carbonate and chlorothiazide should be discontinued and electrolyte and fluid abnormalities corrected.

**Summary:** There are data to show that coadministration of these agents may result in milk-alkali syndrome, characterized by hypercalcemia, metabolic alkalosis, and renal failure.

**Related Drugs:** An interaction may occur with the other thiazide diuretics and calcium carbonate. It is not known if a similar interaction would occur between chlorothiazide and other calcium salts.

**Mechanism:** Many factors contribute to the development of milk-alkali syndrome: the blockage of renal excretory capacity, bicarbonate reabsorption, increased calcium intake, volume depletion and decreased glomerular filtration rate.

**Detailed Information:** See *EDI*, 13/2.10

## Chlorothiazide-Colestipol

**Significance:** 3—minimally clinically significant

**Recommendations:** If concurrent use of colestipol and chlorothiazide is necessary, it may be advisable to separate their administration by as much time as possible. However, patients should still be closely monitored since an increased dose of the thiazide diuretic may be necessary.

**Summary:** Chlorothiazide and colestipol resulted in a significant reduction in the excretion of chlorothiazide.

**Related Drugs:** A similar interaction was documented with cholestyramine. A similar interaction is expected to occur between chlorothiazide and cholestyramine. Similar results may be expected between colestipol and other thiazide diuretics and thiazide-related diuretics.

**Mechanism:** Colestipol and cholestyramine have been shown to bind chlorothiazide and hydrochlorothiazide.

**Detailed Information:** See *EDI*, 13/3.00

## Chlorothiazide-Metoclopramide

**Significance:** 3—minimally clinically significant

**Recommendations:** Although the bioavailability of chlorothiazide, when administered as a solution, is decreased by metoclopramide, it was not determined if the pharmacologic activity of chlorothiazide decreased as well. Based on this limited information, the concurrent use of these agents need not be avoided, and it seems that no special precautions are necessary.

**Summary:** Metoclopramide has been documented to reduce the recovery of chlorothiazide.

**Related Drugs:** The other thiazide diuretics and thiazide-related diuretics may undergo a similar interaction with metoclopramide. There are no drugs related to metoclopramide.

**Mechanism:** Metoclopramide causes thiazides to have less time for dissolution and/or shorter contact time with the intestinal membrane.

**Detailed Information:** See *EDI*, 13/4.10

Diuretic

## Chlorothiazide-Probenecid

**Significance:** 3—minimally clinically significant

**Potential Effects:** Probenecid may increase the diuretic effect of chlorothiazine.

**Recommendations:** If serum uric acid concentrations become elevated, an increase in the dose of probenecid should be considered.

**Summary:** Probenecid may increase the diuretic effect of chlorothiazide. Chlorothiazide has the potential to elevate serum uric acid concentrations and diminish the uricosuric effect of probenecid.

**Related Drugs:** Bendroflumethiazide, hydrochlorothiazide, methyclothiazide, chlorthalidone, diazoxide, triamterene, indapamide, trichlormethiazide, cyclopenthiazide, and quinethazone cause serum uric acid elevation and may be expected to antagonize the uricosuric effect of probenecid. Probenecid has been shown to increase the activity of metolazone. Other thiazide diuretics may be expected to interact similarly, although no documentation on such interactions exists. Loop diuretics exhibit a similar reaction.

**Mechanism:** Probenecid blocks the secretion of chlorothiazide at the proximal renal tubule, resulting in enhancement, through prolongation, of the diuretic effect of chlorothiazide. Hyperuricemia from the thiazide diuretics is attributed to either competitive inhibition of uric acid secretion within the kidney or to indirect enhancement of renal reabsorption of uric acid through redistribution of blood flow.

**Detailed Information:** See *EDI*, 13/5.00

## Chlorothiazide-Propantheline

**Significance:** 3—minimally clinically significant

**Recommendations:** Although the bioavailability of chlorothiazide, when administered as a solution, is increased by propantheline, it was not determined if the pharmacologic activity of chlorothiazide increased as well. Based on this limited information, the concurrent use of these agents need not be avoided, and no special precautions are necessary.

**Summary:** Propantheline was shown to double the bioavailability of chlorothiazide.

**Related Drugs:** Hydrochlorothiazide bioavailability was increased with propantheline. The other thiazide diuretics and the thiazide-related diuretics may undergo a similar interaction. The other anticholinergics may be expected to enhance the bioavailability of chlorothiazide.

**Mechanism:** Propantheline delays gastric emptying rate and motility, allowing more time for thiazide dissolution and greater contact time with the intestinal membrane.

**Detailed Information:** See *EDI*, 13/6.10

## Ethacrynic Acid-Cisplatin

**Significance:** 2—moderately clinically significant

**Recommendations:** Although this interaction is based on animal studies only, the ototoxicity of each agent is well documented. Therefore, it is important to monitor eighth cranial nerve function during and after concurrent therapy. The use of lower doses of ethacrynic acid may also avoid, or lessen, the potential for an interaction.

**Summary:** The concurrent use of ethacrynic acid and cisplatin has been shown to produce prolonged and permanent ototoxic effects in animals.

**Related Drugs:** There are no drugs related to cisplatin. A similar interaction is expected to occur between cisplatin and other loop diuretics.

**Mechanism:** The mechanism appears to be related to the synergistic toxicity of each agent.
**Detailed Information:** See *EDI*, 13/7.00

## Furosemide-Aspirin

**Significance:** 3—minimally clinically significant
**Recommendations:** During concurrent administration of these agents, the dose of furosemide may need to be adjusted if the diuretic effect decreases. However, whether this interaction occurs in all patients or only those with renal insufficiency remains to be determined.
**Summary:** There are data to show that coadministration of these agents suppresses hemodynamic effects of furosemide and reduces the diuretic effect. Signs of renal insufficiency were abolished when furosemide was added.
**Related Drugs:** Because of conflicting results, it is difficult to determine whether a similar interaction would occur between the other loop diuretics and other salicylates.
**Mechanism:** It has been suggested that aspirin and furosemide have opposing effects on renal prostaglandin synthesis.
**Detailed Information:** See *EDI*, 13/9.00

## Furosemide-Charcoal

**Significance:** 2—moderately clinically significant
**Potential Effects:** Concurrent furosemide and charcoal administration may decrease the absorption and diuretic effect of furosemide.
**Recommendations:** If charcoal and furosemide must be given concurrently, it is recommended that furosemide be administered two to three hours prior to charcoal to minimize the effect of charcoal.
**Summary:** Charcoal reduced the absorption and diuretic effect of furosemide.
**Related Drugs:** An interaction may occur between charcoal and other loop diuretics because of the high adsorptive capacity of activated charcoal.
**Mechanism:** The high adsorptive capacity of activated charcoal results in reduced absorption of drugs from the gastrointestinal tract.
**Detailed Information:** See *EDI*, 13/10.50

## Furosemide-Chloral Hydrate

**Significance:** 3—minimally clinically significant
**Recommendations:** In patients with acute coronary disease, the concurrent use of these agents may need to be avoided. However, since this interaction does not occur in all patients, concomitant administration should at least be used with caution. If the interaction does occur, the discontinuation of chloral hydrate has been shown to lead to a reversal of the symptoms. Alternatively, the use of flurazepam or another benzodiazepine may be considered as a nocturnal sedative.
**Summary:** Furosemide and chloral hydrate have resulted in uneasiness, diaphoresis, hot flashes, and blood pressure changes, including hypertension.
**Related Drugs:** A similar interaction is expected to occur between the loop diuretics and tricoflos.
**Mechanism:** Furosemide may displace a metabolite of chloral hydrate from plasma protein binding sites, which displaces thyroxine. This can result in a hypermetabolic state.
**Detailed Information:** See *EDI*, 13/11.00

Diuretic

## Furosemide-Cholestyramine

**Significance:** 2—moderately clinically significant

**Potential Effects:** The concurrent use of cholestyramine and furosemide may result in decreased furosemide bioavailability and diuretic effect.

**Recommendations:** The administration of furosemide and cholestyramine should be separated by two to three hours to help avoid a decrease in furosemide bioavailability and diuretic effect.

**Summary:** The absorption and diuretic effect of furosemide were decreased by concurrent cholestyramine.

**Related Drugs:** Colestipol has resulted in a decrease in furosemide bioavailability. An interaction may occur between other anionic exchange resins and other loop diuretics.

**Mechanism:** Furosemide is adsorbed to cholestyramine, an anionic exchange resin, because of the acidic nature of the furosemide molecule.

**Detailed Information:** See *EDI*, 13/12.10

## Furosemide-Ginseng

**Significance:** 3—minimally clinically significant

**Potential Effects:** The addition of a ginseng preparation to the therapy of a patient maintained on furosemide may result in decreased furosemide effects.

**Recommendations:** Caution is advised with concurrent use of these agents. The patient's renal status should be carefully monitored. Ginseng may need to be discontinued.

**Summary:** Addition of a ginseng preparation to the therapy of a patient maintained on furosemide resulted in hospitalization for edema and hypertension.

**Related Drugs:** An interaction may occur between ginseng and the other loop diuretics. There are no agents related to ginseng. There are several different species of the genus Panax that include ginseng in their names. These include Korean ginseng, Sanchi ginseng, American ginseng, Chikusetsu ginseng, Himalayan ginseng, and Dwarf ginseng. Another species is called Zhuzishen.

**Mechanism:** Long-term use of germanium, a component of many ginseng preparations, has been associated with chronic renal failure. This nephrotoxicity may be related to vacuolar degeneration in the distal tubular epithelium with intracellular deposition of lipofuscin granules deposited in the thick ascending loop of Henle.

**Detailed Information:** See *EDI*, 13/12.60

## Furosemide-Indomethacin

**Significance:** 3—minimally clinically significant

**Potential Effects:** Indomethacin may decrease the effects of furosemide, possibly by inhibition of prostaglandin synthesis.

**Recommendations:** If a decrease in furosemide's diuretic or natriuretic effects occurs with indomethacin cotherapy, indomethacin may need to be discontinued.

**Summary:** Indomethacin has been shown to decrease the diuretic and natriuretic effects and to block the acute audiologic effect and the rise in plasma renin activity associated with furosemide therapy. Furosemide has been reported to reduce indomethacin plasma concentrations; however, not all data support this.

**Related Drugs:** Indomethacin has reportedly produced a similar attenuation of the effects of ethacrynic acid and bumetanide. Furosemide has been shown to interact with many NSAIAs, and a similar interaction is expected to occur with the NSAIAs and furosemide.

# Diuretic

**Mechanism:** Indomethacin inhibits prostaglandin synthesis and decreases sodium diuresis, and this may vary with the individual NSAIA used.
**Detailed Information:** See *EDI,* 13/13.00

## Furosemide-Phenytoin

**Significance:** 3—minimally clinically significant
**Recommendations:** Patients should be monitored for a decreased effect of furosemide when phenytoin (and/or phenobarbital) is administered concurrently. The dose of furosemide may need to be increased.
**Summary:** There are data to show that phenytoin may significantly delay the diuretic response, and the dose of furosemide may need to be increased.
**Related Drugs:** It is difficult to relate whether or not other hydantoin anticonvulsants or other barbiturates would interact in a similar manner with other loop diuretics.
**Mechanism:** This interaction may be due to the decrease in absorption of furosemide or the increase in the reabsorption of sodium in the renal tubules.
**Detailed Information:** See *EDI,* 13/14.10

## Furosemide-Probenecid

**Significance:** 3—minimally clinically significant
**Potential Effects:** Concomitant furosemide and probenecid may increase furosemide serum levels and its diuretic effect.
**Recommendations:** Since probenecid may enhance the actions of furosemide, doses may need to be decreased in patients. Also, since furosemide has the potential to increase uric acid levels, probenecid doses may need to be increased.
**Summary:** Studies show concomitant use of furosemide and probenecid may increase furosemide serum levels and its diuretic effect. Furosemide may also elevate serum uric acid concentrations which may diminish the uricosuric effects of probenecid.
**Related Drugs:** Probenecid blocks the secretion of bumetanide and torsemide at the proximal renal tubule. This reduces both drugs' effects. Bumetanide, torsemide, and ethacrynic acid may also increase uric acid levels, antagonizing the effect of probenecid. Thiazide diuretics exhibit a similar reaction with probenecid.
**Mechanism:** Probenecid blocks the secretion of furosemide at the proximal renal tubule, resulting in enhancement, through prolongation, of the diuretic effect of furosemide. Another possible mechanism includes the displacement of furosemide from plasma protein binding sites by probenecid, resulting in the increased glomerular filtration of unbound furosemide. Hyperuricemia from the loop diuretics may be due to enhanced reabsorption of uric acid through redistribution of blood flow or competitive inhibition of uric acid secretion in the kidney.
**Detailed Information:** See *EDI,* 13/14.50

## Hydrochlorothiazide-Fenfluramine

**Significance:** 3—minimally clinically significant
**Recommendations:** Because of the combined anorectic and hypotensive effects of fenfluramine, it may be useful in combination with a thiazide diuretic in the hypertensive obese patient. Caution should be used when prescribing fenfluramine and a thiazide diuretic in a normotensive patient because of the possibility of hypotension.

## Diuretic

**Summary:** Fenfluramine with hydrochlorothiazide has been shown to reduce blood pressure in patients previously unresponsive to hydrochlorothiazide.

**Related Drugs:** A similar interaction is expected to occur between fenfluramine and other thiazide diuretics and thiazide-related diuretics as well as between hydrochlorothiazide and other anorexiants.

**Mechanism:** The mechanism of action of fenfluramine in lowering plasma norepinephrine levels and in enhancing the hypotensive effects of hydrochlorothiazide is not clear.

**Detailed Information:** See *EDI*, 13/15.00

### Hydrochlorothiazide, Triamterene-Amantadine

**Significance:** 3—minimally clinically significant

**Recommendations:** The concurrent use of these agents should be approached with caution. If symptoms of amantadine toxicity occur, the dose of amantadine may need to be decreased.

**Summary:** There are data to show that one or both agents of the combination drug (hydrochlorothiazide and triamterene) reduced the clearance and produced higher plasma levels and toxic effects of amantadine.

**Related Drugs:** Because it is not known which agent was responsible for the interaction, it is not known how other thiazide-related diuretics or other potassium-sparing diuretics would interact with amantadine. There are no drugs related to amantadine.

**Mechanism:** It has been postulated that one or both of the components of the combination diuretic reduces the tubular secretion of amantadine.

**Detailed Information:** See *EDI*, 13/17.00

### Spironolactone-Aspirin

**Significance:** 3—minimally clinically significant

**Recommendations:** The concurrent usage of spironolactone and aspirin need not be avoided, unless additional study establishes a clinically significant effect.

**Summary:** Concurrent usage of aspirin and spironolactone showed a decrease in the natriuretic effect of spironolactone.

**Related Drugs:** Further studies are needed to determine any possible effects caused by other salicylates. There is a lack of documentation regarding a similar interaction between aspirin and other potassium-sparing diuretics.

**Mechanism:** The mechanism of this interaction is controversial and unclear. Aspirin may block the renal tubular secretion of the active metabolite of spironolactone.

**Detailed Information:** See *EDI*, 13/19.00

### Spironolactone-Captopril

**Significance:** 3—minimally clinically significant

**Potential Effects:** The concurrent use of these agents may cause an increase in potassium levels.

**Recommendations:** Monitor potassium levels when using these agents together. The dose of either may need to be decreased or discontinued.

**Summary:** There are data to show that coadministration of these agents may cause an increase in potassium levels; the clinical signs may or may not be present.

**Related Drugs:** Captopril may interact similarly with other potassium-sparing diuretics. Enalapril has been shown to increase potassium levels.

**Mechanism:** Captopril causes potassium retention, and administration of these agents results in an additive interaction, increasing serum potassium concentrations.
**Detailed Information:** See *EDI,* 13/20.10

## Spironolactone-Potassium Chloride

**Significance:** 1—highly clinically significant
**Summary:** In the presence of a potassium-sparing diuretic, an added source of potassium can result in serious symptoms of hyperkalemia, which may lead to cardiac failure and arrest.
**Related Drugs:** Other potassium-sparing diuretics may interact in a similar manner with all absorbable forms of potassium.
**Mechanism:** Spironolactone produces retention of potassium ions, and a potassium supplement will increase the accumulation of potassium.
**Detailed Information:** See *EDI,* 13/21.00

## Triamterene-Cimetidine

**Significance:** 3—minimally clinically significant
**Potential Effects:** Cimetidine decreases the clearance of triamterene.
**Recommendations:** The use of these agents together need not to be avoided; however, if they are used together, the effects of triamterene should be monitored.
**Summary:** There are data to show that cimetidine administration will decrease the clearance of triamterene.
**Related Drugs:** The pharmacokinetics of other potassium-sparing diuretics differ from that of triamterene; therefore, it is not known if a similar interaction would occur with cimetidine. It is not known to what extent an interaction would occur between triamterene and the other $H_2$-receptor antagonists.
**Mechanism:** Cimetidine has reduced hepatic hydroxylation, reduced renal tubular secretion and reduced the absorption of triamterene.
**Detailed Information:** See *EDI,* 13/22.10

## Triamterene-Indomethacin

**Significance:** 2—moderately clinically significant
**Potential Effects:** The concurrent use of triamterene and indomethacin may lead to reversible acute renal failure.
**Recommendations:** The concurrent use of these agents requires caution. If renal function deteriorates during concomitant therapy, one or both agents may need to be discontinued.
**Summary:** A study and four case reports showed the concurrent use of triamterene and indomethacin may lead to reversible acute renal failure.
**Related Drugs:** Similar interactions have been reported with triamterene and ibuprofen, diclofenac, and fluribrofen. Reports cite the development of acute renal failure with amiloride and indomethacin or ibuprofen. Sulindac, prioxicam and naproxen have been reported not to interact with amiloride. Both indomethacin and diflunisal decreased the diuretic effect of spironolactone, and diflunisal decreased creatinine clearance.
**Mechanism:** Prostaglandin inhibition by nonsteroidal anti-inflammatory agents may unmask triamterene or amiloride toxicity and contribute to the pathogenesis of the renal failure observed.
**Detailed Information:** See *EDI,* 13/23.00

Diuretic

## Trichlormethiazide-Diazoxide

**Significance:** 3—minimally clinically significant

**Recommendations:** Patients should be monitored for blood glucose changes, and dosage adjustments should be made in one or both agents as indicated. The combination may be beneficial in elevating blood glucose in refractory patients or lowering blood pressure, since both agents share those pharmacologic activities.

**Summary:** Trichlormethiazide and diazoxide alone have been shown to produce hyperglycemia.

**Related Drugs:** Hyperglycemia has been reported when diazoxide is given with hydrochlorothiazide or bendroflumethiazide. Because of conflicting reports, it is not possible to determine whether hyperglycemia will occur when diazoxide is administered with other thiazide diuretics or thiazide-related diuretics.

**Mechanism:** Diazoxide and thiazide diuretics act synergistically to inhibit insulin secretion from the pancreas. Diuretics have been reported to precipitate latent diabetes or increase blood glucose levels.

**Detailed Information:** See *EDI*, 13/25.00

# Chapter Fourteen

# Hypoglycemic Drug Interactions

## Chlorpropamide-Alcohol, Ethyl

**Significance:** 1—highly clinically significant

**Potential Effects:** Alcohol consumed while receiving chlorpropamide may result in hypoglycemia. A disulfiram-like reaction may also occur.

**Recommendations:** Although abstinence from alcohol would be ideal for patients receiving antidiabetic therapy, practical management will more often involve recommending reduced alcohol intake and cautioning the patient regarding potential effects of alcohol while taking antidiabetic agents.

**Summary:** The combination of alcohol and antidiabetic agents can result in mild flushing to severe hypoglycemic reactions. A disulfiram-type reaction to alcohol has been produced by chlorpropamide.

**Related Drugs:** Ample documentation exists of an interaction between tolbutamide and alcohol. A similar interaction is expected to occur between alcohol and other first generation sulfonylureas. Glipizide and glyburide have been reported to have a very low incidence of disulfiram-like reactions with concurrent alcohol.

**Mechanism:** Alcohol, by means of its intrinsic hypoglycemic activity, can induce hypoglycemia and interfere with gluconeogenesis in the liver.

**Detailed Information:** See *EDI,* 14/1.00

## Chlorpropamide-Allopurinol

**Significance:** 3—minimally clinically significant

**Recommendations:** Because of the extremely limited evidence of this drug interaction, the clinical significance must be considered minimal. It would be prudent to monitor patients on oral hypoglycemic agents for increases in pharmacologic effect or serum half-life if allopurinol is administered concurrently.

**Summary:** The half-life of chlorpropamide may be increased by concurrent administration of allopurinol.

**Related Drugs:** A similar interaction is expected to occur with other sulfonylurea hypoglycemic drugs and allopurinol. Glyburide and glipizide may not interact to the same extent as the other sulfonylureas. There are no drugs related to allopurinol.

**Mechanism:** The suggested mechanism between chlorpropamide and allopurinol is a competition for renal tubular secretion.

**Detailed Information:** See *EDI,* 14/3.00

## Chlorpropamide-Aspirin

**Significance:** 2—moderately clinically significant

**Recommendations:** An individual receiving both chlorpropamide and aspirin may need to have the chlorpropamide dose adjusted downward. The patient should be carefully monitored. Blood or urinary glucose levels will facilitate proper management of such patients. Upon discontinuation of aspirin administration, the requirement for chlorpropamide will increase. It may be beneficial to consider switching to insulin or dietary control in patients requiring aspirin therapy, particularly those who exhibit poor response with the oral hypoglycemic drug. Cases of hypoglycemia can be treated by traditional methods or by the use of glucose plus diazoxide.

**Summary:** There is an increased risk of chlorpropamide toxicity with concurrent aspirin administration, and use of these agents may result in severe hypoglycemia.

**Related Drugs:** Insulin response to tolbutamide has been significantly augmented after aspirin. The other first generation sulfonylurea hypoglycemic agents may also interact with aspirin. Glyburide and glipizide may not interact to the same degree as other sulfonylureas. A similar interaction is expected to occur with other salicylates and chlorpropamide.

**Mechanism:** Sulfonylureas bind extensively to plasma protein where aspirin may cause a displacement and increased concentrations of free drug.

**Detailed Information:** See *EDI*, 14/5.00

## Chlorpropamide-Clofibrate

**Significance:** 2—moderately clinically significant

**Recommendations:** When clofibrate is added to the regimen of diabetic patients receiving chlorpropamide or other sulfonylureas, blood glucose levels should be monitored closely for hypoglycemia; it may be necessary to decrease the dose of the sulfonylurea in some patients. Conversely, when clofibrate is discontinued in patients receiving chlorpropamide concurrently, blood glucose levels should be monitored closely for deterioration in diabetic control.

**Summary:** The hypoglycemic activity of chlorpropamide may be enhanced by concurrent administration of clofibrate.

**Related Drugs:** Other sulfonylureas have demonstrated a similar interaction with clofibrate. Glyburide and glipizide may interact in a similar manner. Halofenate enhances the hypoglycemic effect of the sulfonylureas.

**Mechanism:** Clofibrate may increase half-life, decrease excretion, decrease insulin resistance, or displace chlorpropamide and other sulfonylureas from protein binding sites.

**Detailed Information:** See *EDI*, 14/7.00

## Chlorpropamide-Cortisone

**Significance:** 2—moderately clinically significant

**Recommendations:** Occurrence of glycosuria should not be an important factor in the decision to discontinue corticosteroid therapy or to initiate it in diabetic patients. However, patients on antidiabetic therapy should be monitored for decreased hypoglycemic action while on concurrent glucocorticoid treatment. To maintain diabetic control during high dose or long-term corticosteroid treatment, increased dosage of chlorpropamide may be required.

**Summary:** The intrinsic hyperglycemic activity of cortisone may decrease the hypoglycemic effects of concurrently administered chlorpropamide.

**Related Drugs:** Prolonged treatment with glucocorticoids has been found to elevate plasma glucagon. Other sulfonylurea hypoglycemics and other corticosteroids may be expected to interact similarly.

**Mechanism:** Chlorpropamide and other sulfonylureas acutely increase sensitivity to glucose, and chlorpropamide may inhibit gluconeogenesis and augment insulin-mediated suppression of hepatic glucose release.

**Detailed Information:** See *EDI*, 14/9.00

## Chlorpropamide-Hydrochlorothiazide

**Significance:** 2—moderately clinically significant

**Recommendations:** Diabetic patients controlled by diet with oral hypoglycemic agents or by insulin should be monitored closely for hyperglycemia before and after thiazide or thiazide-like diuretics are initiated. Also, patients who have been maintained on such combination therapy should be observed for symptoms of hypoglycemia when the diuretic is withdrawn from the regimen. Since the development of hypokalemia may be responsible for the pathogenesis of the interaction, therapy should be directed toward preventing abnormal potassium loss. Additionally, the dose of the hypoglycemic drug may be increased, or insulin therapy may be substituted in sufficient dosage to control the diabetic state.

**Summary:** Diabetic patients regulated by chlorpropamide may exhibit impaired diabetic control when hydrochlorothiazide is added to the drug regimen.

**Related Drugs:** This drug interaction may occur with other sulfonylurea hypoglycemics. All thiazide diuretics have the potential of producing hypokalemia, and there are ample data exhibiting interactions between chlorpropamide and agents related to hydrochlorothiazide.

**Mechanism:** Thiazides inhibit the release of insulin by the pancreas. Hypokalemia is believed to be a contributing factor in the pathogenesis of this interaction.

**Detailed Information:** See *EDI*, 14/11.00

## Chlorpropamide-Probenecid

**Significance:** 3—minimally clinically significant

**Recommendations:** No changes are necessary during combined therapy; however, patients should be observed for excessive hypoglycemic effects. Neither chlorpropamide nor probenecid should be used in patients with impaired renal function.

**Summary:** Probenecid was reported to increase the half-life of chlorpropamide.

**Related Drugs:** Probenecid was reported to prolong the half-life of tolbutamide. It is not known whether other sulfonylurea hypoglycemic agents would interact with probenecid in a similar manner.

**Mechanism:** Probenecid inhibits the renal excretion of chlorpropamide.

**Detailed Information:** See *EDI*, 14/13.00

## Chlorpropamide-Sucralfate

**Significance:** 4—not clinically significant

**Potential Effects:** Sucralfate does not affect the absorption of chlorpropamide.

**Recommendations:** Although multiple dose studies are needed, the concurrent use of these agents need not be avoided. Sucralfate may be an alternative to cimetidine, which has been shown to interact with glipizide and tolbutamide (see Glipizide-Cimetidine, page 305).

**Summary:** There are data to show sucralfate does not affect the absorption of chlorpropamide.

**Related Drugs:** It is not known if a similar lack of interaction would occur between sucralfate and other sulfonylureas. There are no drugs related to sucralfate.

**Mechanism:** Sucralfate does not appear to affect the pharmacokinetics of chlorpropamide.

**Detailed Information:** See *EDI*, 14/14.10

## Glipizide-Charcoal

**Significance:** 2—moderately clinically significant

**Potential Effects:** Charcoal adsorbs glipizide, resulting in decreased absorption.

**Recommendations:** Separating administration times may not avoid this interaction because of glipizide enterohepatic recirculation. Charcoal may be useful in glipizide overdose treatment.

## Hypoglycemic

**Summary:** Concurrent administration of glipizide and charcoal results in a decrease in glipizide absorption.

**Related Drugs:** A similar interaction would be expected to occur between charcoal and other sulfonylureas.

**Mechanism:** Glipizide is adsorbed onto the surface of activated charcoal.

**Detailed Information:** See *EDI*, 14/14.44

### Glipizide-Cholestyramine

**Significance:** 2—moderately clinically significant

**Potential Effects:** Cholestyramine may bind to glipizide, resulting in decreased absorption of glipizide.

**Recommendations:** Monitor patients for signs of decreased glipizide absorption with concurrent cholestyramine administration. Separation of administration may not avoid the interaction because of enterohepatic circulation of glipizide.

**Summary:** Concurrent glipizide and cholestyramine may result in decreased glipizide serum levels.

**Related Drugs:** It is not known whether an interaction would occur between cholestyramine and other sulfonylureas or between glipizide and colestipol.

**Mechanism:** Cholestyramine interferes with the absorption of acidic drugs, and glipizide may bind to cholestyramine, preventing absorption.

**Detailed Information:** See *EDI*, 14/14.45

### Glipizide-Cimetidine

**Significance:** 2—moderately clinically significant

**Recommendations:** Caution should be exercised when cimetidine or ranitidine is administered concurrently with glipizide. If a hypoglycemic response occurs, the dose of glipizide may need to be decreased. Although clinical studies are lacking, famotidine may be an alternative to cimetidine. Sucralfate, which was shown not to interact with chlorpropamide (see Chlorpropamide-Sucralfate, page 304), may also be an alternative to cimetidine for ulcer therapy when concurrent sulfonylurea therapy is required.

**Summary:** There are data to show that cimetidine increases the glipizide area-under-curve, suggesting that some patients are at risk of developing significant hypoglycemia.

**Related Drugs:** Tolbutamide and glyburide have been shown to interact similarly; however, all data do not support this. A similar interaction may occur between cimetidine and other sulfonylurea hypoglycemic agents. Ranitidine did not seem to significantly alter the pharmacokinetics of glipizide and glyburide. Documentation is lacking regarding an interaction between glipizide and other $H_2$-receptor antagonists.

**Mechanism:** It was suggested that cimetidine inhibits the hepatic metabolism of glipizide and tolbutamide, or there may be a reduction in hepatic blood flow.

**Detailed Information:** See *EDI*, 14/14.30

### Glipizide-Heparin

**Significance:** 3—minimally clinically significant

**Potential Effects:** Heparin may decrease the protein binding of glipizide or inhibit its metabolism/excretion, leading to an increased hypoglycemic effect.

**Recommendations:** Patients receiving concurrent administration of glipizide and heparin should be monitored for potential hypoglycemia. The dose of glipizide may need to be decreased, or the drug may need to be discontinued.

**Summary:** There are data to show that heparin may decrease the protein binding of glipizide or inhibit its metabolism and excretion, potentiating an increased hypoglycemic effect.

**Related Drugs:** Glyburide may interact with heparin similarly to glipizide. Because of differences in protein binding and activity of metabolites, it is not known if other sulfonylureas would interact with heparin. There are no drugs related to heparin.

**Mechanism:** Heparin may decrease the binding of glipizide, which is highly protein bound and may have inhibited the metabolism or excretion of glipizide.

**Detailed Information:** See *EDI*, 14/14.50

## Glyburide-Ciprofloxacin

**Significance:** 2—moderately clinically significant

**Potential Effects:** The effect of glyburide may be increased when ciprofloxacin is added to therapy.

**Recommendations:** Patients maintained on glyburide should be closely monitored for a change in blood glucose levels if ciprofloxacin is added to therapy. The dose of glyburide may need to be adjusted.

**Summary:** Glyburide's effect was increased when ciprofloxacin was added to therapy. Symptoms including slurred speech, confusion, diaphoresis, extreme hypoglycemia, and glyburide levels as high as 1,050 ng/ml have been reported.

**Related Drugs:** An interaction may occur between glyburide and other quinolone antibiotics that also inhibit the cytochrome $P450_{3A4}$ isozyme (e.g., norfloxacin). It is not known whether an interaction would occur between ciprofloxacin and the other sulfonylureas.

**Mechanism:** Ciprofloxacin may inhibit hepatic isoenzymes, elevating glyburide levels and causing hypoglycemia. Both ciprofloxacin and glyburide may decrease the activity of cytochrome $P450_{3A4}$ isoenzymes, and ciprofloxacin may cause an additive hypoglycemic effect due to blockade of adenosine triphosphate-sensitive $K^+$ channels; studies have shown that quinolones increase insulin release from rat pancreatic islet cells.

**Detailed Information:** See *EDI*, 14/14.43

## Glyburide-Gemfibrozil

**Significance:** 2—moderately clinically significant

**Potential Effects:** The effect of glyburide may be increased when gemfibrozil is added to therapy.

**Recommendations:** Patients maintained on glyburide should be closely monitored for a change in blood glucose levels if gemfibrozil is added to, or withdrawn from, therapy. The dose of glyburide may need to be adjusted. Gemfibrozil may be effective as an aid to glycemic control in some patients maintained on sulfonylureas.

**Summary:** The effect of glyburide may be increased when gemfibrozil is added to therapy.

**Related Drugs:** A similar interaction may occur between gemfibrozil and other sulfonylureas. There are no drugs related to gemfibrozil.

**Mechanism:** Gemfibrozil is strongly bound to plasma proteins, and glyburide may be displaced from its binding sites by gemfibrozil.

**Detailed Information:** See *EDI*, 14/14.46

## Glyburide-Rifampin

**Significance:** 3—minimally clinically significant

**Potential Effects:** Rifampin may increase the metabolism of glyburide, resulting in decreased levels.

**Recommendations:** Patients should be monitored for changes in blood glucose concentration if rifampin is added to, or withdrawn from, cotherapy.

**Summary:** Addition of rifampin to a stable glyburide regimen necessitated an increase in glyburide dosage to maintain blood glucose levels.

**Related Drugs:** An interaction may occur between rifampin and other sulfonylurea hypoglycemics. There are no drugs related to rifampin.

**Mechanism:** Rifampin may cause metabolic induction, which may result in an increase in the metabolism of glyburide.

**Detailed Information:** See *EDI*, 14/14.47

## Insulin-Aspirin

**Significance:** 3—minimally clinically significant

**Recommendations:** Patients should be monitored for a change in their blood glucose levels during concurrent use of these agents. If necessary, a lower dose of insulin may be administered.

**Summary:** The hypoglycemic activity of insulin may be potentiated by concurrent use of aspirin or other salicylates.

**Related Drugs:** A similar interaction may occur with other salicylates.

**Mechanism:** Aspirin may reduce plasma glucose, affect pancreatic islet cell function, change hepatic glucose production, inhibit intestinal glucose production, or increase peripheral glucose uptake and oxidation.

**Detailed Information:** See *EDI*, 14/15.00

## Insulin-Chlorpromazine

**Significance:** 3—minimally clinically significant

**Recommendations:** Patients receiving hypoglycemic therapy with insulin or sulfonylureas should be observed for loss of diabetic control if high doses of phenothiazines are added to their medication regimen.

**Summary:** Chlorpromazine may produce a dose- and duration-dependent increase in plasma glucose concentrations that may lead to loss of diabetic control in predisposed individuals.

**Related Drugs:** Other phenothiazines, thioxanthenes, butyrophenones, dihydroindolones, and dibenzoxazepines may interact with insulin in a similar manner. Because of the mechanism of this interaction, sulfonylurea hypoglycemic agents may also be affected.

**Mechanism:** This interaction is a result of the inhibition of insulin release from the pancreas.

**Detailed Information:** See *EDI*, 14/17.00

## Insulin-Clofibrate

**Significance:** 2—moderately clinically significant

**Recommendations:** It is important to monitor blood glucose levels during concurrent therapy with these agents. The dose of insulin may need to be adjusted.

**Summary:** Clofibrate has been shown to lower blood glucose levels in insulin-dependent diabetics.

**Related Drugs:** There are no drugs related to clofibrate. An interaction involving clofibrate and the oral sulfonylureas is discussed in another monograph (see Chlorpropamide-Clofibrate, page 303).

**Mechanism:** The mechanism of this interaction is unknown. Clofibrate may cause a change in tissue sensitivity to insulin and/or glucose.

**Detailed Information:** See *EDI*, 14/19.00

## Insulin-Diltiazem
**Significance:** 3—minimally clinically significant
**Potential Effects:** Diltiazem may increase insulin requirements.
**Recommendations:** Patients stabilized on insulin should be monitored for increases in insulin requirements if diltiazem therapy is initiated. The insulin dosage may need to be adjusted.
**Summary:** Insulin resistance was reported when diltiazem was administered to a patient. Diltiazem may increase insulin requirements.
**Related Drugs:** A similar interaction is expected to occur between insulin and other calcium channel blocking agents.
**Mechanism:** Calcium antagonists impair insulin-mediated glucose transport, and chelation of intracellular calcium can block insulin action in cells. Diltiazem may cause insulin resistance by its effect on intracellular calcium.
**Detailed Information:** See *EDI*, 14/20.10

## Insulin-Epinephrine
**Significance:** 3—minimally clinically significant
**Recommendations:** Patients stabilized on insulin should be monitored for possible increases in blood glucose levels with sympathomimetic administration. Since the parenteral administration of sympathomimetics usually occurs in emergency clinical situations, the elevation of blood glucose may not be of clinical importance. There is no evidence, however, that supports an interaction between epinephrine and exogenously administered insulin.
**Summary:** Epinephrine raises blood glucose levels and may increase insulin requirements.
**Related Drugs:** Other sympathomimetic agents may have the same hyperglycemic effect with insulin.
**Mechanism:** Epinephrine may act synergistically with glucagon to antagonize the effects of insulin.
**Detailed Information:** See *EDI*, 14/21.00

## Insulin-Fenfluramine
**Significance:** 2—moderately clinically significant
**Recommendations:** This interaction may be beneficial in certain diabetic patients, and this effect is most marked when fenfluramine is administered immediately before a meal. However, patients must be closely monitored when fenfluramine is added to, or withdrawn from, diabetic therapy.
**Summary:** The intrinsic hypoglycemic effect of fenfluramine may increase the effects of insulin and result in hypoglycemia when the agents are used concurrently.
**Related Drugs:** A similar interaction is expected to occur between insulin and other anorexiants. A similar interaction may be expected with other sulfonylureas.
**Mechanism:** Fenfluramine lowers blood sugar levels as a result of the increased uptake of glucose into skeletal muscle. This hypoglycemic effect is additive in combination with insulin.
**Detailed Information:** See *EDI*, 14/23.00

## Insulin-Fenugreek
**Significance:** 3—minimally clinically significant
**Potential Effects:** Fenugreek administration may result in a decrease in blood sugar levels in persons with non-insulin-dependent diabetes mellitus (NIDDM) (also called Type 2 Diabetes). This may necessitate a change in insulin dosage to avoid hypoglycemic episodes.

**Recommendations:** If a patient is maintained on a stable regimen of insulin or an oral antidiabetic agent, the dose may need to be adjusted if fenugreek is added to the regimen. The patient's blood sugar and clinical status should be carefully monitored.

**Summary:** Fenugreek administration resulted in a significant decrease in blood sugar levels in persons with NIDDM. This may necessitate a change in insulin dosage to avoid hypoglycemic episodes.

**Related Drugs:** The dosage of sulfonylureas or other antidiabetic agents may also need to be adjusted to avoid hypoglycemic symptoms and maintain glycemic control. Fenugreek (Trigonella foenum-graecum Leguminosae) is also called bockshornsame.

**Mechanism:** The mechanism of action of fenugreek's hypoglycemic effect is not known. In diabetic dogs, the addition of fenugreek resulted in a decrease in hyperglycemia and insulin dose. Feeding normal rats a fenugreek-supplemented diet for five weeks reduced the severity of the onset of experimental diabetes.

**Detailed Information:** See *EDI*, 14/24.00

## Insulin-Ginseng

**Significance:** 3—minimally clinically significant

**Potential Effects:** Ginseng administration may result in a decrease in blood sugar levels in persons with non-insulin-dependent diabetes mellitus (NIDDM) (also called Type 2 Diabetes). This may result in a loss of glycemic control.

**Recommendations:** If a patient is maintained on a stable regimen of insulin or an oral antidiabetic agent, the dose may need to be adjusted if ginseng is added to the regimen. The patient's blood sugar and clinical status should be carefully monitored.

**Summary:** Ginseng administration resulted in a decrease in blood sugar levels in persons with NIDDM. This may result in a loss of glycemic control.

**Related Drugs:** The dosage of sulfonylureas or other antidiabetic agents may need to be adjusted to avoid hypoglycemic symptoms and maintain glycemic control. Ginseng commonly refers to *Panax* q. L. or *Panax ginseng* C. A. Meyer (Korean ginseng). Other species of ginseng include Sanchi ginseng, Chikusetsu ginseng, Radix ginseng, Himalayan ginseng, Siberian ginseng, and Dwarf ginseng.

**Mechanism:** Studies in rats show inhibition of neuronal discharge frequency from the gastric compartment of the brainstem with American ginseng (*Panax* q.L.) and gastric secretion with Asian ginseng. This may slow the digestion of food, decreasing the rate of carbohydrate metabolism into portal hepatic circulation. Ginseng may also affect glucose transport mediated by nitric oxide. Asian ginseng increases both glucose transporter-2-protein in the livers of normal and hyperglycemic mice and glucose uptake into sheep erythrocytes in a dose-dependent manner. In alloxan diabetic mice, ginseng fractions increased blood insulin levels and glucose-stimulated insulin secretion and biosynthesis. This effect may be mediated by nitric oxide; nitric oxide stimulates glucose-dependent insulin secretion in rat islet cells.

**Detailed Information:** See *EDI*, 14/24.70

## Insulin-Guanethidine

**Significance:** 1—highly clinically significant

**Recommendations:** Diabetic patients should be closely observed when guanethidine is added to, or deleted from, the drug regimen. A decrease in insulin dose may be required when guanethidine is added, or an increase in insulin dose may be necessitated when guanethidine is withdrawn.

**Summary:** Long-term guanethidine therapy may improve glucose tolerance, necessitating a reduction in insulin dose.

**Related Drugs:** A similar interaction is expected to occur between insulin and other drugs related to guanethidine.

**Mechanism:** The exact mechanism is unknown. Long-term guanethidine depletes tissue catecholamines involved with raising blood sugar levels and may improve glucose tolerance.

**Detailed Information:** See *EDI*, 14/25.00

## Insulin-Isoniazid

**Significance:** 3—minimally clinically significant

**Recommendations:** Patients on concurrent therapy with antidiabetic agents and isoniazid should be monitored for possible increases in blood glucose levels. This may be of greater clinical significance in patients with hepatic dysfunction or in those who are slow acetylators of isoniazid.

**Summary:** Isoniazid antagonizes the hypoglycemic action of insulin by elevating blood sugar levels.

**Related Drugs:** Because of conflicting results, it is difficult to determine whether an interaction occurs between isoniazid and other sulfonylurea hypoglycemics. There are no drugs related to isoniazid.

**Mechanism:** By causing disturbances in carbohydrate metabolism, isoniazid may increase blood glucose levels and impair glucose tolerance.

**Detailed Information:** See *EDI*, 14/27.00

## Insulin-Oxytetracycline

**Significance:** 2—moderately clinically significant

**Recommendations:** Patients whose diabetes is controlled on insulin therapy who receive oxytetracycline should be monitored closely because of the possibility of hypoglycemia.

**Summary:** Several cases have been reported in which the administration of oxytetracycline to diabetic patients receiving insulin caused hypoglycemia, necessitating a decrease in insulin dosage.

**Related Drugs:** A similar interaction is expected to occur with other sulfonylurea hypoglycemics and oxytetracycline. A similar interaction is expected to occur with other tetracyclines.

**Mechanism:** Oxytetracycline exerts a hypoglycemic effect by increasing the half-life of insulin or by interfering with the action of epinephrine.

**Detailed Information:** See *EDI*, 14/29.00

## Insulin-Phenelzine

**Significance:** 2—moderately clinically significant

**Recommendations:** Concurrent MAO inhibitor therapy for depression in a diabetic patient will often require reduction in dosage of the hypoglycemic agent because of enhanced hypoglycemic effects. Since the extent of the reaction is highly unpredictable, any diabetic patients receiving MAO inhibitors should be monitored for possible excessive hypoglycemia.

**Summary:** Phenelzine can potentiate the action of insulin, resulting in an enhanced hypoglycemic state.

**Related Drugs:** It is well documented that agents that possess MAOI activity may interact similarly with insulin. A similar interaction is expected to occur with other sulfonylurea hypoglycemics.

## Insulin-Phenytoin

**Significance:** 3—minimally clinically significant

**Recommendations:** Diabetic patients receiving phenytoin should be closely monitored for elevation of serum glucose levels and symptoms of hyperglycemia. Dosage reduction of phenytoin may prevent or alleviate the symptoms, since some adverse reactions have occurred at high phenytoin dosages. Also, adjusting the sulfonylurea dose whenever phenytoin is added to, or withdrawn from, therapy may be advisable.

**Summary:** Phenytoin may inhibit endogenous insulin secretion, resulting in clinically significant symptoms of hyperglycemia

**Related Drugs:** The other hydantoin anticonvulsants may be expected to produce the same hyperglycemic effect as phenytoin. Oral sulfonylurea hypoglycemic agents may be affected by phenytoin.

**Mechanism:** Phenytoin can induce hyperglycemia through inhibition of endogenous insulin secretion.

**Detailed Information:** See *EDI*, 14/33.00

## Insulin-Propranolol

**Significance:** 1—highly clinically significant

**Potential Effects:** Propranolol can delay recovery from hypoglycemia as well as modify the normal cardiovascular response to hypoglycemia.

**Recommendations:** When use of a beta-blocking agent is indicated in a diabetic patient, particularly one prone to hypoglycemic attacks, one of the cardioselective agents (acebutolol, atenolol, or metoprolol), rather than propranolol, should be used, both to decrease the risk of a hypertensive response to hypoglycemia and to permit more rapid recovery from low blood glucose levels. The danger of unrecognized hypoglycemia in the insulin-dependent diabetic who is taking propranolol can be reduced if the patient is aware of the associated diaphoretic response.

**Summary:** Propranolol can delay recovery from hypoglycemia and mask hypoglycemic symptoms.

**Related Drugs:** The cardioselective beta-blocking agents do not seem to prolong the effect on insulin-induced hypoglycemia. A similar interaction is expected to occur between insulin and other noncardioselective beta-blocking agents. Effects of beta-adrenergic blockers on long-term sulfonylurea therapy have not been determined. Because of conflicting reports, it is difficult to determine whether an interaction would occur with other sulfonylurea hypoglycemics.

**Mechanism:** The mechanism is complicated and unclear, but it is known that propranolol does not affect plasma glucose or insulin concentrations or the rate or magnitude of the fall of plasma glucose.

**Detailed Information:** See *EDI*, 14/35.00

## Insulin-Thyroid

**Significance:** 2—moderately clinically significant

**Recommendations:** The management of patients on this combination requires attention to both diabetic control and thyroid function, especially at initiation of therapy.

**Summary:** The initiation of thyroid replacement therapy may cause an increase in insulin or oral hypoglycemic requirements. Insulin administration may affect thyroid hormone binding and disrupt thyroid function.

## Hypoglycemic

**Related Drugs:** There are no reports of an interaction between hypoglycemic therapy and thyroid replacement therapy. Based on the available evidence, it would seem that any thyroid hormone can interact with any hypoglycemic therapy.

**Mechanism:** Levothyroxine increases the rate of carbohydrate absorption from the gastrointestinal tract, and both liothyronine and thyroxine suppress insulin secretion from the pancreas.

**Detailed Information:** See *EDI*, 14/37.00

### Insulin-Tobacco

**Significance:** 3—minimally clinically significant

**Recommendations:** Because of conflicting results and limited data, it is difficult to determine if diabetic smokers will need a change in their insulin requirements. However, patients' blood glucose should be monitored regularly, and the insulin dose adjusted if necessary.

**Summary:** Insulin absorption may be decreased in patients who smoke tobacco.

**Related Drugs:** There are no drugs related to insulin.

**Mechanism:** The increased insulin requirement in diabetic smokers may be secondary to elevated catecholamine levels, or there may be a decreased absorption because of peripheral vasoconstriction.

**Detailed Information:** See *EDI*, 14/38.10

### Metformin-Iodinated Contrast Media

**Significance:** 1—highly clinically significant

**Potential Effects:** Concurrent metformin and iodinated contrast media administration may result in an increased risk of metformin-induced lactic acidosis levels.

**Recommendations:** Coadministration of parenteral iodinated contrast media and metformin is contraindicated. The manufacturer product information states, "Glucophage (metformin) should be withheld for at least 48 hours prior to, and 48 hours subsequent to, the procedure and reinstituted only after renal function has been re-evaluated and found to be normal."

**Summary:** Concurrent metformin and iodinated contrast media administration may result in an increased risk of metformin-induced lactic acidosis. Metformin does not react with the iodine, causing renal failure and lactic acidosis. If the parenteral administration of iodinated contrast media causes decreased renal function, metformin may accumulate and result in higher serum lactate levels, thus resulting in an increased risk of lactic acidosis.

**Related Drugs:** There are no drugs related to metformin.

**Mechanism:** Metformin does not undergo hepatic metabolism or biliary excretion and is excreted unchanged in the urine. Iodinated contrast media-induced renal failure may interfere with the renal elimination of metformin. Contrast materials may lead to acute renal failure, particularly in diabetic patients, and have been associated with lactic acidosis in patients receiving metformin. This association has been attributed to accumulation of high blood concentrations of metformin resulting from impairment of the renal clearance of metformin during acute renal failure.

**Detailed Information:** See *EDI*, 14/38.20

### Tolazamide-Doxepin

**Significance:** 3—minimally clinically significant

**Potential Effects:** Concurrent use of these agents may result in hypoglycemia.

**Recommendations:** Patients receiving doxepin and tolazamide concurrently should be monitored for low blood glucose levels. If hypoglycemia occurs, the patient should be appropriately treated with dextrose or glucagon, and the sulfonylurea may need to be discontinued or the dose decreased.

**Summary:** There are data to show that coadministration of these agents may result in hypoglycemia, necessitating a decreased tolazamide dosage.

**Related Drugs:** Documentation is lacking regarding a similar interaction between tolazamide and other tricyclic antidepressants or between doxepin and other sulfonylureas.

**Mechanism:** The mechanism of this interaction is not known.

**Detailed Information:** See *EDI,* 14/38.30

## Tolbutamide-Chloramphenicol

**Significance:** 2—moderately clinically significant

**Recommendations:** Reduction in the sulfonylurea dose may be necessary if concurrent chloramphenicol administration is indicated. Frequent monitoring of serum glucose levels may enable control during this time. Temporary use of insulin may be required if serum glucose levels cannot be controlled with the oral agent. Since some studies have shown higher serum tolbutamide levels in morning measurements than those later in the day, patients can be monitored for symptoms and cautioned accordingly.

**Summary:** Chloramphenicol and tolbutamide may cause prolonged hypoglycemic responses because of an increased tolbutamide half-life. Patients with renal insufficiency may be at greater risk for this interaction.

**Related Drugs:** Chlorpropamide half-life has been increased by chloramphenicol. Tolazamide, acetohexamide, glyburide and glipizide may be affected. There are no drugs related to chloramphenicol.

**Mechanism:** Interference with renal elimination has been proposed as a mechanism for the increased half-life and elevated serum levels of the sulfonylurea.

**Detailed Information:** See *EDI,* 14/39.00

## Tolbutamide-Diazoxide

**Significance:** 3—minimally clinically significant

**Recommendations:** Diabetic patients receiving diazoxide should be monitored for an increase in blood glucose levels. Should hyperglycemia occur, an appropriate adjustment in dosage of one or both drugs is necessary. Treatment with insulin should be considered in patients with severe hyperglycemia resulting from diazoxide administration.

**Summary:** Hyperglycemia has occurred in patients receiving diazoxide for treatment of severe hypertension, or after long-term administration in the treatment of hypoglycemia.

**Related Drugs:** The other sulfonylurea hypoglycemics may interact similarly with diazoxide. There are no drugs related to diazoxide.

**Mechanism:** Diazoxide has been shown to inhibit the release of insulin.

**Detailed Information:** See *EDI,* 14/41.00

## Tolbutamide-Dicumarol

**Significance:** 2—moderately clinically significant

**Recommendations:** If dicumarol and a sulfonylurea must be given concurrently, serum glucose concentrations should be closely monitored, and the sulfonylurea dose should be adjusted accordingly when dicumarol is added to, or withdrawn from, the drug reg-

imen. Also, it is prudent to closely monitor prothrombin times since the dose of dicumarol may need to be adjusted.
**Summary:** Dicumarol may significantly increase the serum half-life of tolbutamide and prolong prothrombin time.
**Related Drugs:** Dicumarol may interact with other sulfonylurea hypoglycemics. The other coumarin anticoagulants and the indandione derivatives do not interact with tolbutamide.
**Mechanism:** It has been suggested that dicumarol inhibits the hepatic metabolism of tolbutamide and chlorpropamide. Dicumarol may displace the sulfonylureas from their plasma protein binding sites.
**Detailed Information:** See *EDI*, 14/43.00

## Tolbutamide-Fluconazole

**Significance:** 3—minimally clinically significant
**Potential Effects:** Concomitant tolbutamide and fluconazole administration may result in increased tolbutamide levels and possible hypoglycemia symptoms.
**Recommendations:** Patients should be carefully monitored for changes in blood glucose levels and symptoms of hypoglycemia with concurrent administration of these agents. The dose of tolbutamide may need to be adjusted.
**Summary:** Concomitant administration of tolbutamide and fluconazole resulted in increased tolbutamide levels.
**Related Drugs:** An interaction would be expected to occur between fluconazole and other sulfonylureas and between tolbutamide and other imidazole antifungal agents.
**Mechanism:** Tolbutamide is metabolized by cytochrome P450 isozymes. Fluconazole has been shown to have an inhibitory effect on cytochrome P450 isozymes.
**Detailed Information:** See *EDI*, 14/44.05

## Tolbutamide-Methyldopa

**Significance:** 3—minimally clinically significant
**Recommendations:** Although the concurrent use of these agents need not be avoided, blood glucose levels should be monitored, and the dose of tolbutamide may need to be decreased.
**Summary:** The half-life of tolbutamide was found to be prolonged with coadministration of methyldopa.
**Related Drugs:** A similar interaction is expected to occur between methyldopa and other sulfonylureas. There are no drugs related to methyldopa.
**Mechanism:** Methyldopa may decrease the metabolism of tolbutamide by inhibiting the hepatic microsomal enzymes.
**Detailed Information:** See *EDI*, 14/44.10

## Tolbutamide-Phenylbutazone

**Significance:** 1—highly clinically significant
**Potential Effects:** Phenylbutazone displaces tolbutamide from its binding sites, resulting in enhanced hypoglycemia.
**Recommendations:** Because of the possibility that a severe, or even fatal, hypoglycemic reaction can result, use of this combination requires intense monitoring of serum glucose levels and probable dosage reduction of the sulfonylurea. If concurrent long-term therapy is necessary, agents other than phenylbutazone or oxyphenbutazone (e.g., sulindac) should be used whenever possible.
**Summary:** There are data to show that severe hypoglycemic reactions have occurred after phenylbutazone administration to patients on long-term tolbutamide therapy.

**Related Drugs:** Tolbutamide has been shown to interact with many NSAIAs; however, the data are conflicting. A similar interaction is expected to occur between tolbutamide and other NSAIAs.

**Mechanism:** Phenylbutazone may inhibit the excretion or delay the metabolism of tolbutamide or displace tolbutamide from plasma and tissue proteins.

**Detailed Information:** See *EDI*, 14/45.00

## Tolbutamide-Sulfamethizole

**Significance:** 2—moderately clinically significant

**Potential Effects:** Sulfamethizole may inhibit the metabolism of tolbutamide or displace it from protein binding sites, leading to enhanced hypoglycemic activity.

**Recommendations:** Concurrent use of these agents should be done with caution. Patients should be monitored for enhanced hypoglycemic effects. Glyburide or possible glipizide may be alternatives to tolbutamide.

**Summary:** Tolbutamide-treated patients have developed enhanced hypoglycemic effects after administration of sulfamethizole.

**Related Drugs:** There are contradictory reports regarding the effect of sulfisoxazole or sulfadiazine on serum glucose or serum tolbutamide. Because of conflicting results, it is difficult to determine whether an interaction would occur between tolbutamide and other sulfonamides. Glyburide and glipizide have been shown not to significantly interact.

**Mechanism:** Sulfamethizole may inhibit hepatic oxidation, carboxylation and the aromatic ring hydroxylating enzyme system of tolbutamide.

**Detailed Information:** See *EDI*, 14/47.00

# Chapter Fifteen

# Sedative-Hypnotic Drug Interactions

## Alcohol, Ethyl-Amitriptyline

**Significance:** 2—moderately clinically significant

**Recommendations:** The most hazardous of the possible interactions is the enhanced central nervous system depression by alcohol while the patient is on amitriptyline. Patients receiving amitriptyline should be informed that concurrent ingestion of alcohol may produce a greater than expected impairment of the ability to drive an automobile or operate dangerous machinery. The impairment in psychomotor skills caused by the combination of alcohol and amitriptyline may become less harmful with continued amitriptyline administration.

**Summary:** The effects of the concurrent use of amitriptyline and alcohol are unpredictable. Various studies have reported that amitriptyline can enhance, antagonize, or have no effect on CNS effects.

**Related Drugs:** Other tricyclic antidepressants and the tetracyclic antidepressants may interact similarly with alcohol.

**Mechanism:** Enhanced sedation seen with the combination of amitriptyline and alcohol may result from an additive effect.

**Detailed Information:** See *EDI,* 15/1.00

## Alcohol, Ethyl-Bromocriptine

**Significance:** 3—minimally clinically significant

**Recommendations:** If side effects of bromocriptine occur or become severe, patients should abstain from the use of alcohol. This interaction may be of benefit in alcoholic patients with severe alcohol withdrawal symptoms.

**Summary:** Alcohol may potentiate the side effects of bromocriptine.

**Related Drugs:** There are no drugs related to alcohol or bromocriptine.

**Mechanism:** Alcohol may enhance the sensitivity of the dopamine receptors, and bromocriptine is a dopamine receptor agonist.

**Detailed Information:** See *EDI,* 15/2.10

## Alcohol, Ethyl-Cimetidine

**Significance:** 3—minimally clinically significant

**Potential Effects:** Cimetidine may increase ethyl alcohol serum levels, leading to increased side effects.

**Recommendations:** Patients should be aware that alcohol blood levels may be increased during concurrent cimetidine, and an increased level of intoxication may result.

**Summary:** There are data to show that administration of cimetidine may increase alcohol levels, leading to increased side effects; however, it has been shown that cimetidine has no effect on alcohol blood levels when alcohol is administered intravenously.

**Related Drugs:** Ranitidine and famotidine, when given at recommended doses, do not affect alcohol metabolism. It is not known whether an interaction will occur between nizatidine and alcohol.

**Mechanism:** Alcohol absorption may be increased with concurrent cimetidine.

**Detailed Information:** See *EDI,* 15/3.00

## Alcohol, Ethyl-Diphenhydramine

**Significance:** 2—moderately clinically significant

**Recommendations:** Patients receiving diphenhydramine or other antihistamines should be advised that the concurrent use of alcohol may result in increased mental and motor impairment and may impair their ability to drive an automobile or operate dangerous equipment.

**Summary:** Concurrent administration of diphenhydramine and alcohol may result in a greater impairment of motor and mental performance.
**Related Drugs:** Evidence indicates that tripelennamine also interacts with alcohol. Other antihistamines may also interact with alcohol.
**Mechanism:** The mechanism is unknown.
**Detailed Information:** See *EDI,* 15/5.00

## Alcohol, Ethyl-Disulfiram

**Significance:** 1—highly clinically significant
**Recommendations:** Consumption of even small doses (e.g., 15 ml) of alcohol leads to this interaction; therefore, concomitant administration should be avoided. Patients have suffered this interaction from taking cough mixtures and using topical preparations such as aftershave lotions and antipsoriatic preparations that contained alcohol. However, the quantity of alcohol required to elicit the interaction varies with individuals. This reaction has also been reported in patients who came in contact with other organic solvents (e.g., paint, "mineral spirits") through inhalation; therefore, patients should be advised of this potential hazard as well.
**Summary:** Patients ingesting alcohol or using topical preparations that contain alcohol while taking disulfiram will experience throbbing in the head and neck, palpitations, tachycardia, hypotension, sweating, nausea, and vomiting.
**Related Drugs:** There are no drugs related to alcohol or disulfiram.
**Mechanism:** Disulfiram alters the intermediary metabolism of alcohol, causing an accumulation of acetaldehyde which is responsible for this unpleasant reaction.
**Detailed Information:** See *EDI,* 15/7.00

## Alcohol, Ethyl-Fluoxetine

**Significance:** 4—not clinically significant
**Potential Effects:** Concurrent use of these agents does not result in any alterations in the concentrations or effects of either agent.
**Recommendations:** Fluoxetine may be considered as an alternative antidepressant agent to the tricyclic or tetracyclic antidepressant agents in patients who consume alcohol. Also, fluoxetine may be beneficial in the treatment of alcoholism.
**Summary:** The concurrent use of these agents did not alter the plasma or blood concentrations of either drug. Psychomotor activity and subjective effects of alcohol were not affected.
**Related Drugs:** There are no drugs related to fluoxetine.
**Mechanism:** Please see summary.
**Detailed Information:** See *EDI,* 15/8.01

## Alcohol, Ethyl-Furazolidone

**Significance:** 2—moderately clinically significant
**Recommendations:** If disulfiram-like reactions (e.g., facial flushing, lightheadedness, tachycardia, dyspnea, nausea, vomiting) occur in a patient receiving furazolidone who ingests alcohol, the use of alcohol should be avoided.
**Summary:** The ingestion of alcohol in patients receiving furazolidone has been shown to result in acute alcohol intolerance similar to a disulfiram reaction.
**Related Drugs:** There is no evidence of alcohol interacting with nitrofurantoin.
**Mechanism:** The mechanism of this interaction is unknown.
**Detailed Information:** See *EDI,* 15/8.10

## Alcohol, Ethyl-Glutethimide

**Significance:** 2—moderately clinically significant

**Recommendations:** Concurrent ingestion of alcohol and glutethimide (or other central nervous system depressants previously mentioned) may result in an increased depressant activity. Patients should be warned of this possible enhancement of the depressant effects and also that this combination may produce a greater impairment of their ability to drive or operate hazardous machinery.

**Summary:** Concurrent ingestion of alcohol and glutethimide may result in a greater CNS depression than when either agent is taken alone.

**Related Drugs:** Methyprylon may interact with alcohol in a manner similar to that of glutethimide. Other drugs that possess CNS depressant activity, such as ethchlorvynol and methaqualone, may interact with alcohol.

**Mechanism:** The mechanism of this interaction is not documented. The CNS depressant effects result from synergism.

**Detailed Information:** See *EDI*, 15/9.00

## Alcohol, Ethyl-Ketoconazole

**Significance:** 3—minimally clinically significant

**Potential Effects:** The ingestion of alcohol with concurrent ketoconazole may result in a "sunburn-like" rash.

**Recommendations:** Patients should avoid alcohol if a rash develops when also taking ketoconazole.

**Summary:** A patient taking ketoconazole developed a "sunburn-like" rash that was confined to the face, upper chest, and back shortly after ingesting alcohol.

**Related Drugs:** There are no drugs related to ketoconazole.

**Mechanism:** Although the mechanism is unknown, ketoconazole is similar to metronidazole, and metronidazole has been shown to result in a disulfiram-like reaction with alcohol ingestion (see Alcohol, Ethyl-Metronidazole, below).

**Detailed Information:** See *EDI*, 15/10.10

## Alcohol, Ethyl-Metoclopramide

**Significance:** 3—minimally clinically significant

**Recommendations:** The clinical significance of the interaction is not completely documented. However, administration of these agents together led to an enhanced alcohol sedation, suggesting that concurrent use should be avoided.

**Summary:** Concurrent administration of metoclopramide and alcohol has significantly increased the rate of alcohol absorption and sedation.

**Related Drugs:** There are no drugs related to metoclopramide.

**Mechanism:** Metoclopramide hastens gastric emptying which results in a quicker absorption onset.

**Detailed Information:** See *EDI*, 15/11.00

## Alcohol, Ethyl-Metronidazole

**Significance:** 2—moderately clinically significant

**Potential Effects:** Metronidazole may inhibit the metabolism of alcohol, leading to an increase in acetaldehyde, which is responsible for the disulfiram-like reaction that may occur.

**Recommendations:** Patients receiving metronidazole should be advised of the potential for this interaction with alcohol ingestion.

**Summary:** Concurrent use of metronidazole with alcohol has been associated with a disulfiram-type reaction resulting in symptoms of hypotension, nausea, facial flushing, headache, and sweating.

## Sedative-Hypnotic

**Related Drugs:** There are no drugs related to metronidazole.
**Mechanism:** Metronidazole may produce an inhibition of aldehyde dehydrogenase, and the resultant accumulation of acetaldehyde is responsible for the disulfiram-like reaction.
**Detailed Information:** See *EDI*, 15/13.00

### Amobarbital-Tranylcypromine

**Significance:** 3—minimally clinically significant
**Recommendations:** Amobarbital, and possibly other barbiturates, should be used with caution in patients receiving tranylcypromine, other monoamine oxidase inhibitors, or other drugs that possess monoamine oxidase inhibitor activity, such as furazolidone or procarbazine. If concurrent administration is required, the dosage interval of the barbiturate may need to be lengthened because of the prolongation of CNS depression.
**Summary:** Pretreatment with tranylcypromine may prolong the CNS depressant effect of amobarbital.
**Related Drugs:** Other MAOIs may prolong the CNS depressant effects of other barbiturates.
**Mechanism:** MAOIs produce this effect by interference with the metabolism of barbiturates rather than through the effect on monoamine oxidase.
**Detailed Information:** See *EDI*, 15/15.00

### Chloral Hydrate-Alcohol, Ethyl

**Significance:** 2—moderately clinically significant
**Recommendations:** All patients taking chloral hydrate should be warned that the CNS depressant effects of both chloral hydrate and alcohol are increased by concurrent ingestion. Patients with cardiovascular disease who receive chloral hydrate long-term should be especially careful about ingesting alcohol in view of the tachycardia and hypotension that can result from the vasodilation reaction.
**Summary:** Concurrent ingestion of chloral hydrate and alcohol results in greater CNS depression than when either agent is taken alone.
**Related Drugs:** Based on the mechanism, triclofos and other products metabolized to yield trichloroethanol may be expected to interact with alcohol.
**Mechanism:** Enhanced CNS depression occurs because of an altered production of active metabolites of chloral hydrate and alcohol.
**Detailed Information:** See *EDI*, 15/17.00

### Chloral Hydrate-Furazolidone

**Significance:** 4—not clinically significant
**Recommendations:** Since the drug interaction between chloral hydrate and furazolidone is based on theoretic considerations and has not been documented in humans, the clinical significance of this drug interaction is unsubstantiated, and no special precautions are advised with concurrent use.
**Summary:** Furazolidone or its metabolite may inhibit the metabolism of chloral hydrate, enhancing the CNS depressant effect.
**Related Drugs:** Other MAOIs (e.g., procarbazine) may be expected to interact with chloral hydrate in a manner analogous to that of furazolidone.
**Mechanism:** Chloral hydrate could show exaggerated effects in the presence of monoamine oxidase inhibitors, primarily CNS depression.
**Detailed Information:** See *EDI*, 15/19.00

## Sedative-Hypnotic

### Chlormethiazole-Cimetidine

**Significance:** 3—minimally clinically significant

**Potential Effects:** Concurrent cimetidine and chlormethiazole may result in a decreased clearance of chlormethiazole.

**Recommendations:** Patients being administered concurrent cimetidine and chlormethiazole should be monitored for excess sedation and respiratory depression.

**Summary:** Cimetidine administration resulted in a decreased clearance of chlormethiazole, potentiating sedation and respiratory depression.

**Related Drugs:** Ranitidine did not appear to interact similarly to cimetidine. An interaction may not occur with famotidine and nizatadine since they do not inhibit mixed function oxidase activity.

**Mechanism:** The decrease in chlormethiazole is because of cimetidine's inhibition of hepatic mixed function oxidase activity.

**Detailed Information:** See *EDI*, 15/20.50

### Hexobarbital-Rifampin

**Significance:** 3—minimally clinically significant

**Recommendations:** A reduction in the effectiveness of hexobarbital may be expected with concurrent rifampin and may necessitate an increased hexobarbital dosage. Whether this occurs with other barbiturates is unknown at this time.

**Summary:** There are data to show that a reduction in the effectiveness of hexobarbital may occur with concurrent rifampin.

**Related Drugs:** Because of conflicting results, it is difficult to determine whether an interaction would occur between rifampin and the other barbiturates. There are no drugs related to rifampin.

**Mechanism:** Rifampin appears to significantly stimulate the metabolism of hexobarbital, reducing its effectiveness.

**Detailed Information:** See *EDI*, 15/21.00

### Meprobamate-Alcohol, Ethyl

**Significance:** 2—moderately clinically significant

**Recommendations:** Patients receiving meprobamate should be cautioned regarding the enhancement of the CNS depressant effects of this drug when alcohol is ingested concurrently, because more pronounced and possibly dangerous effects (impairment of driving ability) have been observed when meprobamate was administered to some patients on a long-term basis. If either drug is taken in large doses, these agents can enhance CNS depression, resulting in death. Habitual use of alcohol while taking meprobamate should likewise be avoided.

**Summary:** Acute alcohol intoxication in patients receiving meprobamate can lead to an additive or synergistic CNS depression as well as an increase in the half-life of meprobamate.

**Related Drugs:** Propanediol derivatives are related to meprobamate and may interact with alcohol.

**Mechanism:** The effects of this interaction may be described as enhanced CNS depression produced by two agents having sedative-hypnotic properties.

**Detailed Information:** See *EDI*, 15/23.00

### Meprobamate-Imipramine

**Significance:** 3—minimally clinically significant

**Recommendations:** Although one study suggested drowsiness and dizziness in humans were enhanced by the combination of meprobamate and a tricyclic antidepressant, it appears that this interaction is of minor clinical significance. However, patients should be aware that the combination of these drugs may result in enhanced drowsiness and dizziness.

**Summary:** Imipramine has been shown to enhance the CNS effect of meprobamate in animals.

**Related Drugs:** Propanediol derivatives are related to meprobamate and may interact with imipramine. Other tricyclic antidepressants and the tetracyclic antidepressants may also interact with meprobamate.

**Mechanism:** The enhanced sedative effects of meprobamate are mediated by hepatic microsomal enzyme inhibition rather than additive central depression.

**Detailed Information:** See *EDI*, 15/25.00

## Phenobarbital-Alcohol, Ethyl

**Significance:** 2—moderately clinically significant

**Recommendations:** The effects of this interaction are dose-related. Relatively moderate amounts of alcohol (90 to 120 ml of 100-proof whiskey ingested during one hour) may impair a patient's ability to drive or operate machinery, and this danger is increased when barbiturates are taken concurrently. Large amounts of alcohol (150 to 200 ml of 100-proof whiskey) should be avoided while the patient is receiving barbiturates. Although benzodiazepines also interact with alcohol, they may be preferred over barbiturates for treatment of alcohol withdrawal since they result in less respiratory depression and do not disturb sleep patterns.

**Summary:** Concurrent use of alcohol and barbiturates may result in enhanced CNS depressant effects.

**Related Drugs:** Pentobarbital has been shown to decrease half-life and action. Other barbiturates may interact with alcohol similarly to phenobarbital.

**Mechanism:** The CNS depression of this interaction is caused by a synergistic effect of phenobarbital and alcohol.

**Detailed Information:** See *EDI*, 15/27.00

## Phenobarbital-Charcoal

**Significance:** 3—minimally clinically significant

**Recommendations:** Activated charcoal may be an effective treatment in an acute phenobarbital overdose. It should be administered as soon as possible, and subsequent doses should be given to increase phenobarbital elimination. However, if charcoal is not used for phenobarbital overdose, the administration of these agents should be separated by as much time as possible.

**Summary:** Activated charcoal has been shown to reduce the absorption and increase the elimination of phenobarbital.

**Related Drugs:** Other barbiturates may also be adsorbed by activated charcoal. There are no drugs related to charcoal.

**Mechanism:** Activated charcoal adsorbs phenobarbital, limiting its absorption, and it may increase the nonrenal clearance of phenobarbital.

**Detailed Information:** See *EDI*, 15/28.10

## Phenobarbital-Chlorcyclizine

**Significance:** 3—minimally clinically significant

**Recommendations:** Patients receiving both antihistamines and barbiturates should be cautioned about the combined CNS depressant effects, particularly when driving or operating hazardous machinery. Patients should be reminded that antihistamines occur widely in nonprescription formulas, especially cough and cold remedies.

**Summary:** Concurrent administration of chlorcyclizine and phenobarbital may enhance CNS depression.
**Related Drugs:** Other antihistamines and other barbiturates may cause a similar additive depressant action.
**Mechanism:** The probable mechanism for this interaction is the additive synergistic CNS depressant effect of each agent.
**Detailed Information:** See *EDI,* 15/29.00

## Phenobarbital-Cimetidine

**Significance:** 3—minimally clinically significant
**Recommendations:** Although the concurrent use of these agents need not be avoided, the dose of cimetidine may need to be increased if lower cimetidine efficacy occurs.
**Summary:** There are data to show that coadministration of these agents may necessitate an increased cimetidine dosage secondary to decreased efficacy.
**Related Drugs:** A similar interaction may occur between cimetidine and other barbiturates. A similar interaction is expected to occur between phenobarbital and other $H_2$-receptor antagonists.
**Mechanism:** Phenobarbital may increase the hepatic metabolism of cimetidine through enzyme induction.
**Detailed Information:** See *EDI,* 15/30.10

## Phenobarbital-Cyclosporine

**Significance:** 2—moderately clinically significant
**Potential Effects:** Phenobarbital reduces cyclosporine serum levels by hepatic enzyme induction.
**Recommendations:** Monitor cyclosporine serum levels when these agents are used concurrently. The dose of cyclosporine may need to be adjusted if phenobarbital is added to, or withdrawn from, therapy.
**Summary:** Concurrent administration of phenobarbital and cyclosporine may decrease cyclosporine serum levels.
**Related Drugs:** Cyclosporine may interact similarly with other barbiturates. There are no drugs related to cyclosporine.
**Mechanism:** Phenobarbital, a known inducer of hepatic microsomal enzymes, enhances the metabolism of cyclosporine.
**Detailed Information:** See *EDI,* 15/30.30

## Phenobarbital-Dexamethasone

**Significance:** 2—moderately clinically significant
**Recommendations:** Current evidence reveals that if barbiturates, such as phenobarbital, are taken in high doses (120 mg/day or more) by patients dependent on steroid therapy, these patients should be observed for clinical evidence of decreased corticosteroid effectiveness. Alternative therapy should be considered in these patients, or a higher dose of the corticosteroid during concomitant therapy may be necessary. For treatment of anxiety and sedation, a benzodiazepine such as diazepam could be utilized. This agent has been shown not to significantly interact with steroids. Patients requiring physiologic replacement doses of steroids should be assessed for adrenal function and pharmacologic response to steroid treatment after initiation of barbiturate therapy. Barbiturates should be given with care to patients with borderline hypoadrenal function, whether of pituitary or adrenal origin.
**Summary:** Phenobarbital may act to decrease the systemic effects of corticosteroids such as dexamethasone.
**Related Drugs:** Other corticosteroids may interact with barbiturates. Other barbiturates have not been documented in the literature to interact with corticosteroids.

## Sedative-Hypnotic

**Mechanism:** Barbiturates can induce the activity of hepatic microsomes responsible for drug metabolism and have been shown to influence the metabolism of testosterone and cortisol.
**Detailed Information:** See *EDI,* 15/31.00

## Phenobarbital-Felbamate

**Significance:** 3—minimally clinically significant
**Potential Effects:** The addition of felbamate to the therapy of a patient maintained on phenobarbital may result in an increase in phenobarbital serum levels.
**Recommendations:** Monitor patients carefully for changes in phenobarbital serum levels when felbamate is added to or withdrawn from concurrent therapy. The dose of one or both agents may need to be adjusted.
**Summary:** In a single case report of a patient with a history of seizures who had been receiving sodium valproate, phenobarbital, and thioridazine for three months before institution of felbamate therapy, the phenobarbital serum level increased.
**Related Drugs:** It is not known whether an interaction would be expected to occur between felbamate and the other barbiturates or between meprobamate and phenobarbital.
**Mechanism:** Although the mechanism of this interaction is not known, it is postulated that felbamate may interfere with the metabolism of phenobarbital or that phenobarbital may induce felbamate clearance.
**Detailed Information:** See EDI, 15/32.50

## Phenobarbital-Oral Contraceptive Agents

**Significance:** 2—moderately clinically significant
**Recommendations:** Although the incidence of oral contraceptive failure is not known, a sign of developing failure is intermediate breakthrough bleeding or spotting. Two courses of action have been suggested. The first is to increase the ethinyl estradiol content of the oral contraceptive to 50 µg, or to 80 µg if bleeding persists. The second is to use a mechanical form of contraception. Patients receiving phenobarbital as an anticonvulsant should be monitored for changes in seizure control when oral contraceptive agents are added to, or withdrawn from, therapy.
**Summary:** Concurrent administration of phenobarbital may result in the failure of oral contraceptive agents.
**Related Drugs:** Phenobarbital treatment enhanced the metabolism of estrone, progesterone, estradiol, ethinyl estradiol, testosterone, and androsterone. Other barbiturates also induce hepatic enzymes and may interact similarly with oral contraceptive agents.
**Mechanism:** Phenobarbital is a potent inducer of microsomal enzyme systems, and hormonal steroids have their metabolism increased by this mechanism. Phenobarbital decreases the unbound serum concentration of the steroid. Fluid retention can cause changes in seizure frequency.
**Detailed Information:** See *EDI,* 15/33.00

## Phenobarbital-Pyridoxine

**Significance:** 3—minimally clinically significant
**Recommendations:** Although the concurrent use of these agents need not be avoided, serum phenobarbital levels should be monitored. If an increased frequency of seizures occurs in patients receiving phenobarbital and high doses of pyridoxine, the dose of phenobarbital may need to be increased. It is not known if a smaller dose of pyridoxine (e.g., a multivitamin preparation) would interact with phenobarbital.

**Summary:** The concurrent use of pyridoxine and phenobarbital may decrease phenobarbital plasma levels.

**Related Drugs:** A similar interaction may occur between pyridoxine and other barbiturates. An interaction would be expected to occur between pyridoxine and primidone. There are no drugs related to pyridoxine.

**Mechanism:** The reduced serum concentration of phenobarbital could result from increased activity of pyridoxal-phosphate dependent enzymes.

**Detailed Information:** See *EDI*, 15/35.00

## Zolpidem-Rifampin

**Significance:** 2—moderately clinically significant

**Potential Effects:** The concurrent administration of rifampin and zolpidem may result in decreased zolpidem effects.

**Recommendations:** Patients receiving concurrent therapy with rifampin and zolpidem should be monitored for decreased zolpidem effects.

**Summary:** The concurrent administration of rifampin and zolpidem resulted in decreased zolpidem serum concentrations and pharmacodynamic effects.

**Related Drugs:** Rifampin decreased zopiclone peak plasma concentration, half-life, and area-under-curve along with a significant reduction in zopiclone effects. If the other rifamycins (rifabutin, rifapentine) are also inducers of cytochrome $P450_{3A4}$, then a similar interaction may be expected to occur.

**Mechanism:** It was postulated that rifampin pretreatment decreased zolpidem and zopiclone metabolism by inducing cytochrome $P450_{3A4}$-mediated metabolism of these hypnotic agents.

**Detailed Information:** See *EDI*, 15/40.00

# Chapter Sixteen

# Vitamin/Nutrient/Food Drug Interactions

## Ascorbic Acid-Aspirin

**Significance:** 4—not clinically significant

**Recommendations:** Since there is no conclusive evidence that large doses of ascorbic acid will reduce the excretion of aspirin, or that aspirin causes a deficiency of ascorbic acid, the concurrent use of these agents need not be avoided.

**Summary:** There is no conclusive evidence that ascorbic acid reduces the excretion of aspirin, since ascorbic acid does not consistently acidify the urine.

**Related Drugs:** The administration of other salicylates, alone or in combination products, may produce a similar interaction. The ability of other NSAIAs to alter ascorbic acid leukocyte levels has not been sufficiently determined.

**Mechanism:** Aspirin has been reported to alter the uptake of ascorbic acid into the leukocytes. Aspirin may displace ascorbic acid from albumin binding sites. Ascorbic acid in large doses may cause a uricosuric effect.

**Detailed Information:** See *EDI*, 16/1.00

## Ascorbic Acid-Ethinyl Estradiol

**Significance:** 3—minimally clinically significant

**Recommendations:** Patients should be advised that starting and stopping ascorbic acid may lead to contraceptive failure. It has been suggested that the increase in plasma ethinyl estradiol during treatment with ascorbic acid might be of some benefit in permitting wider use of the very low dose ethinyl estradiol preparations.

**Summary:** There are data to show that coadministration of these agents may increase plasma ethinyl estradiol concentrations, and breakthrough bleeding has been documented with the withdrawal of ascorbic acid.

**Related Drugs:** The use of oral contraceptives may lower concurrent ascorbic acid levels in both leukocytes and platelets. A similar interaction may occur between ascorbic acid and other estrogenic substances. There are no drugs related to ascorbic acid.

**Mechanism:** This interaction may result from competition for sulfate, increasing the bioavailability and plasma concentrations of ethinyl estradiol. The breakthrough bleeding may be a withdrawal effect of the ascorbic acid, causing sudden falls in the ethinyl estradiol levels.

**Detailed Information:** See *EDI*, 16/3.00

## Cholecalciferol-Aluminum Hydroxide

**Significance:** 2—moderately clinically significant

**Potential Effects:** Concurrent administration of cholecalciferol (vitamin D3) and aluminum hydroxide may result in an increase in plasma aluminum levels, possibly leading to toxicity.

**Recommendations:** Patients taking concurrent aluminum hydroxide and cholecalciferol should be closely monitored for signs of aluminum toxicity. If possible, plasma aluminum concentrations should be monitored.

**Summary:** The concurrent administration of aluminum hydroxide and cholecalciferol resulted in elevated plasma aluminum concentrations.

**Related Drugs:** An interaction may occur between cholecalciferol and other aluminum salts. An interaction may occur between aluminum hydroxide and other vitamin D analogues.

**Mechanism:** The increase in plasma aluminum may be the result of increased intestinal absorption of aluminum and not tissue redistribution.

**Detailed Information:** See *EDI*, 16/4.50

## Cyanocobalamin-Omeprazole

**Significance:** 3—minimally clinically significant

**Potential Effects:** Concurrent cyanocobalamin and omeprazole resulted in a decrease in protein-bound cyanocobalamin absorption.

**Recommendations:** Cyanocobalamin levels should be monitored in patients maintained on long-term omeprazole therapy (it has been shown that cyanocobalamin malabsorption would not be detectable by the standard Schilling test). Because decreased cyanocobalamin levels can cause hematopoietic and irreversible neurologic and cognitive effects, it may be prudent to institute adjunctive cyanocobalamin supplementation.

**Summary:** The concurrent administration of cyanocobalamin and omeprazole resulted in a decrease in protein-bound cyanocobalamin absorption.

**Related Drugs:** There are no drugs related to omeprazole. Cimetidine and ranitidine were shown to cause a decrease in cyanocobalamin absorption. A similar interaction may occur between protein-bound cyanocobalamin and other $H_2$-receptor antagonists.

**Mechanism:** Decreased absorption of protein-bound cyanocobalamin may be a result of drug-induced achlorhydria. Cyanocobalamin absorption may be inhibited in patients following vagotomy and patients with achlorhydria. Protein-bound cyanocobalamin absorption may be increased by acidic drinks such as cranberry juice.

**Detailed Information:** See *EDI*, 16/4.70

## Ergocalciferol-Phenytoin

**Significance:** 2—moderately clinically significant

**Recommendations:** Patients receiving phenytoin with risk factors for the development of osteomalacia (e.g., inadequate dietary vitamin D intake, limited sunlight exposure, relative inactivity) should be monitored periodically for decreased serum calcium levels and evidence of bone demineralization. Adequate nutrition, with the ingestion of foods rich in vitamin D such as milk, fish, and eggs, and sufficient sunlight exposure are necessary for patients receiving phenytoin and other anticonvulsants. Ergocalciferol therapy, at an individualized dosage, may be required in certain high-risk patients to prevent development of osteomalacia and rickets, and in patients with evidence of impaired bone and mineral metabolism. Vitamin D may be given in a daily dose of 400-800 IU. If phenytoin-induced demineralization is identified, 2000 IU of vitamin D may be given daily.

**Summary:** Phenytoin may increase the metabolic inactivation of ergocalciferol and decrease the half-life of the vitamin in the body, potentiating hypocalcemia, osteomalacia or rickets.

**Related Drugs:** A similar interaction may occur with other hydantoin derivatives.

**Mechanism:** Phenytoin may cause an increase in hydroxylation and hepatic glucuronidation of cholecalciferol, decreasing serum calcium and increasing serum alkaline phosphatase levels.

**Detailed Information:** See *EDI*, 16/5.00

## Ferrous Sulfate-Allopurinol

**Significance:** 4—not clinically significant

**Recommendations:** Clinical studies do not support the existence of this interaction; therefore, no additional precautions are required when these drugs are given together.

**Summary:** Studies do not support an interaction between allopurinol and ferrous ion preparations.

**Related Drugs:** Other ferrous salts are not expected to interact with allopurinol. There are no drugs related to allopurinol.
**Mechanism:** Please refer to summary.
**Detailed Information:** See *EDI,* 16/7.00

## Ferrous Sulfate-Aluminum Hydroxide, Magnesium Carbonate, Magnesium Hydroxide

**Significance:** 3—minimally clinically significant
**Potential Effects:** The antacids may decrease the absorption of ferrous sulfate.
**Recommendations:** The administration of antacids and ferrous salts should be separated by several hours.
**Summary:** There are data to show that antacids may decrease the absorption of ferrous sulfate, reducing the hematologic response expected with ferrous sulfate iron therapy.
**Related Drugs:** A similar interaction may occur between ferrous sulfate and other antacids. There are data supporting an interaction; however, conflicting data are available.
**Mechanism:** The mechanism of this potential interaction is not fully known.
**Detailed Information:** See *EDI,* 16/9.00

## Ferrous Sulfate-Ascorbic Acid

**Significance:** 3—minimally clinically significant
**Recommendations:** Since the absorption of ferrous salts alone has been shown to be adequate in most humans, there is little justification for concurrent use of ascorbic acid in the treatment of uncomplicated iron deficiency states.
**Summary:** It has been reported that ferrous ion absorption is facilitated by concurrent administration of ascorbic acid.
**Related Drugs:** The absorption of other iron salts may also be enhanced in the presence of ascorbic acid.
**Mechanism:** Ascorbic acid is thought to increase the absorption of ferrous ion by its ability to lower pH, reducing the ferric ion to a more soluble ferrous ion.
**Detailed Information:** See *EDI,* 16/11.00

## Ferrous Sulfate-Cimetidine

**Significance:** 3—minimally clinically significant
**Recommendations:** If altered iron metabolism occurs because of impaired absorption during concurrent use of cimetidine and ferrous sulfate, it may be necessary to give iron parenterally.
**Summary:** There are data to show that coadministration of these agents may alter iron metabolism secondary to impaired absorption with concurrent use of cimetidine and ferrous sulfate.
**Related Drugs:** A similar interaction may occur with other iron salts. It is not known whether a similar interaction would occur between ferrous sulfate and other $H_2$-receptor antagonists.
**Mechanism:** The prolonged reduction of gastric acid secretion induced by high doses of cimetidine may decrease the gastrointestinal absorption of ferrous sulfate.
**Detailed Information:** See *EDI,* 16/12.01

## Ferrous Sulfate-Penicillamine

**Significance:** 2—moderately clinically significant
**Recommendations:** The concomitant administration of penicillamine and ferrous salts should be avoided. If both need to be administered, they should be separated by as much time as possible. One

report suggests the ferrous salt should be taken two hours after penicillamine. If patients stabilized on a combination of penicillamine and ferrous salts discontinue the ferrous salt, they should be observed for signs and symptoms of penicillamine toxicity and the penicillamine dose decreased if necessary.

**Summary:** Concomitant administration of ferrous sulfate with penicillamine has been shown to reduce the absorption of penicillamine.

**Related Drugs:** Ferrous fumarate has been shown to interact similarly to ferrous sulfate. Other ferrous salts may interact similarly. There are no drugs related to penicillamine.

**Mechanism:** It is proposed that the ferrous ion chelates to the penicillamine, reducing the absorption of penicillamine.

**Detailed Information:** See *EDI*, 16/12.10

## Folic Acid-Sulfasalazine

**Significance:** 3—minimally clinically significant

**Recommendations:** In patients with inflammatory bowel disease who require sulfasalazine and folic acid, the administration of folic acid by the parenteral route may avoid this interaction.

**Summary:** There are data to show that sulfasalazine administration may reduce folate absorption in patients with inflammatory bowel disease.

**Related Drugs:** A similar interaction may occur between folic acid and other sulfonamides. There are no drugs related to folic acid.

**Mechanism:** It is not known how the use of sulfasalazine further decreases the absorption of folic acid.

**Detailed Information:** See *EDI*, 16/13.00

## Garlic-Saquinavir

**Significance:** 2—moderately clinically significant

**Potential Effects:** The addition of a garlic supplement to a saquinavir regimen resulted in a decrease in saquinavir mean trough, area-under-curve (AUC), and maximum concentration ($C_{max}$) values.

**Recommendations:** Patients taking saquinavir should avoid taking garlic supplements. Garlic from food sources is not likely to cause a problem; however, there may be some concern if patients are ingesting a very large quantity of garlic on a regular basis.

**Summary:** Addition of a garlic supplement to a saquinavir regimen resulted in a decrease in saquinavir mean trough, AUC, and $C_{max}$ values.

**Related Drugs:** A similar interaction may occur with other protease inhibitors.

**Mechanism:** Garlic may induce the cytochrome $P450_{3A4}$ isozyme; *p*-glycoproteins may also be involved.

**Detailed Information:** See *EDI*, 16/13.05

## Grapefruit Juice-Amiodarone

**Significance:** 2—moderately clinically significant

**Potential Effects:** Concurrent administration of grapefruit juice and amiodarone resulted in an increase in amiodarone serum levels and a decrease in levels of N-desethylamiodarone (N-DEA), the major active metabolite of amiodarone.

**Recommendations:** Caution is advised with the consumption of grapefruit juice and amiodarone administration. Experimental data have shown a correlation between N-DEA plasma concentrations and amiodarone antiarrhythmic properties. Because of the dramatic alteration of amiodarone metabolism by grapefruit juice, the concurrent administration of grapefruit juice and amiodarone should be avoided.

**Summary:** Concurrent administration of grapefruit juice and amiodarone resulted in an increase in amiodarone serum levels and a decrease in levels of N-DEA, the major active metabolite of amiodarone.

**Related Drugs:** It is not known whether grapefruit juice ingestion would cause an interaction with other class III antiarrhythmic agents (e.g., bretylium, dofetilide, ibutilide, and sotalol).

**Mechanism:** Grapefruit juice selectively down-regulates cytochrome P-450$_{3A4}$, which may mediate amiodarone metabolism to N-DEA, thereby increasing amiodarone serum levels.

**Detailed Information:** See *EDI*, 16/13.10

## Grapefruit Juice-Clomipramine

**Significance:** 2—moderately clinically significant

**Potential Effects:** The administration of grapefruit juice with clomipramine resulted in elevated levels of desmethylclomipramine and clomipramine and decreased the desmethylclomipramine/clomipramine ratio.

**Recommendations:** The routine administration of clomipramine with grapefruit juice should be approached with caution. While simultaneous administration may result in a decreased desmethylclomipramine/clomipramine ratio and clinical improvement in some patients, clomipramine and desmethylclomipramine levels should be closely monitored.

**Summary:** The administration of grapefruit juice with clomipramine resulted in elevated levels of desmethylclomipramine and clomipramine and a decrease in the desmethylclomipramine/clomipramine ratio in two patients. One patient experienced clinical improvement.

**Related Drugs:** Concurrent administration of carbamazepine with grapefruit juice increased the carbamazepine $C_{max}$, AUC, and minimum concentration. An interaction may occur between grapefruit juice and other tricyclic antidepressant agents, provided the metabolism of these agents involves the cytochrome P450$_{3A4}$ isoenzyme.

**Mechanism:** Furocoumarin derivatives found in grapefruit juice may selectively inhibit cytochrome P450$_{3A4}$ in the small intestine, preventing presystemic metabolism mediated by this isoenzyme; therefore, clomipramine and carbamazepine metabolism may be inhibited in some individuals.

**Detailed Information:** See *EDI*, 16/13.30

## Grapefruit Juice-Colchicine

**Significance:** 2—moderately clinically significant

**Potential Effects:** The addition of grapefruit juice to the diet of a patient maintained on colchicine resulted in colchicine intoxication.

**Recommendations:** Patients should be instructed not to consume large quantities of grapefruit juice during therapy with colchicine. If small quantities of grapefruit juice are consumed during concurrent colchicine therapy, patients should be advised to discontinue colchicine and consult their physician if gastrointestinal symptoms appear.

**Summary:** The addition of grapefruit juice to the diet of a patient maintained on colchicine resulted in colchicine intoxication.

**Related Drugs:** There are no drugs related to colchicine.

**Mechanism:** Colchicine is hepatically metabolized, mainly by cytochrome $P450_{3A4}$ isozymes. It has been determined that the flavonoids quercetin, kaempferol, and naringenin in grapefruit juice are potent inhibitors of cytochrome $P450_{3A4}$ metabolism. This interruption in the cytochrome metabolic pathway can cause increased colchicine levels and resultant toxicity.

**Detailed Information:** See *EDI*, 16/13.34

## Grapefruit Juice-Ethinyl Estradiol

**Significance:** 3—minimally clinically significant

**Potential Effects:** Grapefruit juice may increase serum concentration of exogenously administered ethinyl estradiol.

**Recommendations:** Patients ingesting grapefruit juice and concurrent ethinyl estradiol may have increased plasma ethinyl estradiol levels. Because of the large intersubject variation, this combination may be clinically significant in some patients and patients should be monitored.

**Summary:** Grapefruit juice increased the serum concentration of exogenously administered ethinyl estradiol in a randomized, crossover study.

**Related Drugs:** An interaction may occur between grapefruit juice and the other estrogenic substances (e.g., estropipate, mestranol, quinestrol), provided these agents are metabolized by the same process as ethinyl estradiol.

**Mechanism:** *In vitro* studies indicate that while cytochrome $P450_{3A4}$ is the major mediator for the 2-hydroxylation of ethinyl estradiol, cytochrome $P450_{2C}$ and cytochrome $P450_{2E}$ may also play a role. The flavonoids quercitin, kaempferol, and naringenin found in grapefruit juice are significant inhibitors of cytochrome $P450_{3A4}$. Therefore, it is postulated that naringin or naringenin (an aglycon of naringin) formed in the gut inhibits the 2-hydroxylation of ethinyl estradiol via cytochrome $P450_{3A4}$ mediation, thereby causing increases in pharmacokinetic parameters.

**Detailed Information:** See *EDI*, 16/13.40

## Grapefruit Juice-Quinidine

**Significance:** 3—minimally clinically significant

**Potential Effects:** Concurrent quinidine and grapefruit juice administration may result in changes in the rate-corrected QT interval ($QT_c$) and delayed quinidine absorption.

**Recommendations:** Patients maintained on quinidine should be monitored for changes in the $QT_c$ interval and delayed absorption of quinidine if grapefruit juice is given concurrently. Further study is needed to determine how these changes may affect clinically unstable patients or stabilized patients on long-term therapy.

**Summary:** The concurrent administration of quinidine with grapefruit juice delayed the absorption of quinidine and led to a delayed maximal effect on the $QT_c$.

**Related Drugs:** It is not known whether a similar interaction would occur between grapefruit juice and quinine, a stereoisomer of quinidine.

**Mechanism:** Grapefruit juice reduced the area-under-curve and maximum concentration of 3-hydroxyquinidine. This may suggest inhibition of gut wall metabolism by grapefruit juice during absorption of the drug from the gastrointestinal tract. The absorption of quinidine by grapefruit juice appears to be delayed only with concomitant administration because quinidine, a weak base, is likely to remain in the ionized form with concurrent grapefruit juice administration since grapefruit juice has a pH of approximately 4. Previous *in vitro* studies have suggested that, in grapefruit juice, the flavonoids quercetin, kaempferol, and naringenin, which are potent inhibitors of cytochrome P450 metabolism, may increase the bioavailability of quinidine by inhibition of cytochrome $P450_{3A4}$ isozymes.

**Detailed Information:** See *EDI*, 16/13.50

## Grapefruit Juice-Saquinavir

**Significance:** 2—moderately clinically significant

**Potential Effects:** The addition of grapefruit juice may increase the bioavailability of saquinavir.

**Recommendations:** Saquinavir blood levels should be carefully monitored if grapefruit juice is given concurrently. The dose of saquinavir may need to be adjusted. The normally low oral bioavailability of saquinavir can be increased twofold by grapefruit juice intake.

**Summary:** The addition of grapefruit juice increased the bioavailability of saquinavir. It was also noted that there was a large interindividual variability in saquinavir bioavailability.

**Related Drugs:** It is not known whether an interaction would occur between grapefruit juice and the other protease inhibitors.

**Mechanism:** It has been shown that saquinavir is metabolized by cytochrome $P450_{3A4}$ and that grapefruit juice selectively down-regulates $P450_{3A4}$ in the small intestine. It also has been shown that $P450_{3A4}$ is expressed in the small intestine and predominantly in the liver and gut. This prevents presystemic metabolism mediated by $P450_{3A4}$ in the small intestine.

**Detailed Information:** See *EDI*, 16/13.70

## Grapefruit Juice-Sertraline

**Significance:** 3—minimally clinically significant

**Potential Effects:** Grapefruit juice may increase the serum concentration of sertraline.

**Recommendations:** It has been demonstrated that grapefruit juice inhibits sertraline metabolism; however, the clinical significance is not known. Until further studies are done, it would be prudent to withhold grapefruit juice during sertraline therapy.

**Summary:** Grapefruit juice increased the mean trough serum concentration of sertraline.

**Related Drugs:** An interaction would be expected to occur between grapefruit juice and other selective serotonin inhibitors that are metabolized by a similar mechanism (citalopram, fluoxetine). It is not known whether an interaction would occur between grapefruit juice and the other selective serotonin reuptake inhibitors (fluvoxamine, paroxetine).

**Mechanism:** Grapefruit juice inhibits the formation of desmethylsertraline (sertraline's primary metabolite) in a dose-dependent manner. The flavonoids quercitin, kaempferol, and naringenin found in grapefruit juice are significant inhibitors of cytochrome $P450_{3A4}$ isozymes, which are responsible for the metabolism of sertraline.

**Detailed Information:** See *EDI*, 16/13.80

## Grapefruit Juice-Terfenadine

**Significance:** 2—moderately clinically significant

**Potential Effects:** The concurrent administration of terfenadine and grapefruit juice may result in increased terfenadine serum levels and associated cardiac changes.

**Recommendations:** Caution is advised for the consumption of grapefruit juice with terfenadine administration. An effect of QT prolongation can be demonstrated even with a two-hour separation in the administration of these two agents. Because of the variability of terfenadine pharmacokinetics and pharmacodynamics among individuals, further study is needed. Because of the absence of cardiac effects with increased serum levels of loratadine or fexofenadine, these agents could be considered as possible therapy alternatives to terfenadine.

**Summary:** Concurrent administration of grapefruit juice resulted in increased terfenadine levels by as much as fivefold and increases in the mean QT interval.

**Related Drugs:** It is not known whether a similar interaction would occur with grapefruit juice and the other nonsedating $H_1$ receptor antagonists. Two studies have shown no effect on electrocardiogram parameters when either loratadine or fexofenadine were given with grapefruit juice.

**Mechanism:** Naringenin, quercetin, and kaempferol, flavonoids found in grapefruit, are potent inhibitors of cytochrome P450 metabolism. Studies suggest that grapefruit juice inhibits cytochrome $P450_{3A}$ activity *in vitro* and that neither naringin nor naringenin is primarily responsible for this effect. Further studies are needed.

**Detailed Information:** See *EDI*, 16/14.00

## Niacin-Aspirin

**Significance:** 3—minimally clinically significant

**Potential Effects:** Niacin induces prostaglandin-mediated vascular dilatation of the skin which can be ameliorated by aspirin.

**Recommendations:** One aspirin taken 30 minutes before a scheduled niacin dose may be helpful in patients in whom flushing is bothersome. Alternatively, one morning dose of aspirin for fourteen days may suffice.

**Summary:** The administration of aspirin before niacin administration effectively reduces the flushing response, a common side effect of niacin.

**Related Drugs:** A similar interaction may occur with other salicylates if the mechanism is related to prostaglandin synthesis inhibition. There are no drugs related to niacin.

**Mechanism:** The flushing response seen with niacin administration may be related to prostaglandin liberation; if so, then aspirin would be expected to antagonize this effect of niacin.

**Detailed Information:** See *EDI*, 16/15.00

## Pyridoxine-Levodopa

**Significance:** 1—highly clinically significant

**Recommendations:** Patients receiving levodopa therapy should avoid products containing more than the pyridoxine dietary allowance (2 mg per day). Patients with conditions causing pyridoxine deficiency (diabetes mellitus, chronic alcoholism, malnutrition, and malignancy) may be exceptions to this recommendation. Also included as possible exceptions are patients requiring pyridoxine supplementation because of other drug therapy (those taking isoniazid, cycloserine, or penicillamine, and those with cystinuria or heavy metal poisoning). Concurrent use of carbidopa, a peripheral decarboxylase inhibitor, prevents the inhibitory effect of pyridoxine on levodopa and is recommended for use in patients receiving pyridoxine supplementation.

**Summary:** Pyridoxine may reduce or abolish the beneficial effects of levodopa in parkinsonism.

**Related Drugs:** There are no drugs related to pyridoxine and levodopa.

**Mechanism:** Pyridoxine may alter levodopa metabolism, increase transamination of levodopa or accelerate peripheral nonenzymatic conversion of levodopa to dopamine.

**Detailed Information:** See *EDI*, 16/17.00

## Vitamin A-Neomycin

**Significance:** 3—minimally clinically significant

**Recommendations:** It may be advisable to monitor patients on concurrent vitamin A and oral neomycin therapy for a decrease in vitamin A levels. An increased vitamin A dose may be necessary.

**Summary:** There are data to show that coadministration of these agents may potentiate a decrease in vitamin A levels, necessitating an increased vitamin A dose.

**Related Drugs:** Isotretinoin, which is chemically related to vitamin A, may also decrease levels with concurrent neomycin. A similar interaction is expected to occur between vitamin A and other oral aminoglycosides.

**Mechanism:** Neomycin is thought to interfere with activity of bile acids, reducing uptake of vitamin A, and neomycin may cause morphologic changes in the small intestine, interfering with vitamin A absorption.

**Detailed Information:** See *EDI,* 16/19.00

## Watercress-Chlorzoxazone

**Significance:** 3—minimally clinically significant

**Potential Effects:** The consumption of watercress increased the chlorzoxazone area-under-curve (AUC) and prolonged the chlorzoxazone elimination half-life.

**Recommendations:** Patients maintained on chlorzoxazone should be monitored for changes in chlorzoxazone serum levels if watercress ingestion is instituted or discontinued. In patients who regularly consume watercress, the dosage of chlorzoxazone may need to be adjusted downward.

**Summary:** Watercress increased the chlorzoxazone AUC and prolonged the chlorzoxazone elimination half-life.

**Related Drugs:** Chlorzoxazone is a centrally acting skeletal muscle relaxant not structurally related to the other skeletal muscle relaxants.

**Mechanism:** The 6-hydroxylation of chlorzoxazone may be mediated by the cytochrome $P450_{2E1}$ isozyme, which is inhibited by gluconasturtiin, a phenylethylisothiocyanate precursor found in watercress.

**Detailed Information:** See *EDI,* 16/22.00

# Chapter Seventeen

# Xanthine Drug Interactions

## Aminophylline-Halothane

**Significance:** 1—highly clinically significant

**Recommendations:** Although some believe there is a wide margin of safety associated with the concurrent use of these agents, caution should be observed since arrhythmias have been reported. It appears that the use of aminophylline after halothane anesthesia reduces the incidence of this interaction. Alternatively, the use of a noninteracting anesthetic agent such as enflurane may be considered.

**Summary:** The concurrent use of halothane and aminophylline may lead to cardiac arrhythmias.

**Related Drugs:** A similar interaction may occur between halothane and other theophylline derivatives. Enflurane anesthesia has been shown to not induce cardiac arrhythmias. Documentation is lacking regarding an interaction between aminophylline and other halogenated inhalation anesthetics.

**Mechanism:** The exact mechanism of this interaction is unknown. Halothane may potentiate the arrhythmogenic effects of aminophylline by the same metabolic pathway.

**Detailed Information:** See *EDI*, 17/1.00

## Aminophylline-Imipenem

**Significance:** 3—minimally clinically significant

**Potential Effects:** Concurrent administration of these agents may result in central nervous system (CNS) toxicity and seizures.

**Recommendations:** Patients should be carefully monitored for signs of CNS toxicity and seizures with concurrent administration of these agents.

**Summary:** The concomitant administration of aminophylline and imipenem may have resulted in seizures.

**Related Drugs:** Concurrent theophylline and imipenem therapy has also caused generalized seizures. It is not known whether an interaction would occur between aminophylline and the other carbapenem antibiotic agent, meropenem, or between imipenem and the other theophylline derivatives.

**Mechanism:** CNS toxicity is an adverse effect of theophylline. Theophylline-induced seizures are often not predictable because they are often not preceded by other signs of theophylline toxicity, they often occur in the presence of therapeutic theophylline concentrations (10–20 μg/ml), and they may occur during oral theophylline therapy. Imipenem has been associated with seizures in approximately 1% of patients during clinical trials. It is postulated that an interaction occurs between imipenem and theophylline based on the temporal relationship of seizures and on the absence of seizures during therapy with either imipenem or theophylline alone. Further studies are needed.

**Detailed Information:** See *EDI*, 17/1.05

## Aminophylline-Interferon

**Significance:** 2—moderately clinically significant

**Potential Effects:** Interferon inhibits the metabolism of theophylline (from aminophylline), leading to increased theophylline levels.

**Recommendations:** Patients receiving aminophylline should be monitored for increased theophylline levels when interferon is administered concurrently. The dose of aminophylline may need to be decreased.

**Summary:** There are data to show that coadministration of these agents may lead to increased theophylline levels.

**Related Drugs:** A similar interaction may occur between interferon and other theophylline derivatives that are hepatically metabolized. Dyphylline may not interact with interferon. There are no drugs related to interferon.

**Mechanism:** Interferon inhibited the metabolism of theophylline by decreasing the activity of the hepatic cytochrome P450 mixed oxidase enzyme system.
**Detailed Information:** See *EDI*, 17/2.01

## Aminophylline-Isoproterenol

**Significance:** 3—minimally clinically significant
**Potential Effects:** Data show that isoproterenol may decrease theophylline levels.
**Recommendations:** In patients maintained on theophylline and in whom isoproterenol is initiated, serum theophylline concentrations should be monitored. While decreased levels of theophylline have been reported, dosing modifications may not be necessary.
**Summary:** Data show that isoproterenol may decrease serum theophylline concentrations.
**Related Drugs:** Interactions between isoproterenol and other theophylline derivatives have not been reported. Dyphylline may not interact if the mechanism involves altered hepatic metabolism of aminophylline. There are data available regarding an interaction between albuterol or terbutaline and aminophylline; however, data are conflicting. Documentation is lacking regarding an interaction between aminophylline and other direct-acting sympathomimetics.
**Mechanism:** The mechanism of the interaction is unknown.
**Detailed Information:** See *EDI*, 17/2.10

## Aminophylline-Ketamine

**Significance:** 3—minimally clinically significant
**Recommendations:** The concurrent use of these agents need not be avoided; however, caution should be used. The administration of succinylcholine was successful in resolving the interaction.
**Summary:** Aminophylline administration and ketamine given before surgery could precipitate convulsive seizures.
**Related Drugs:** There are no drugs related to ketamine. Documentation is lacking regarding a similar interaction with the other theophylline derivatives.
**Mechanism:** The mechanism of this interaction is unknown. However, neither drug significantly lowers seizure threshold.
**Detailed Information:** See *EDI*, 17/3.00

## Aminophylline-Levothyroxine

**Significance:** 3—minimally clinically significant
**Potential Effects:** Levothyroxine, by altering thyroid function, may increase theophylline clearance. This interaction may result from the correction of a disease state rather than a direct effect of levothyroxine on theophylline.
**Recommendations:** Patients' theophylline levels should be monitored while establishing a euthyroid state with thyroid replacement therapy. Similarly, patients receiving aminophylline should be monitored for a change in theophylline levels or signs of toxicity if they develop hypothyroidism. The dose of aminophylline may need to be adjusted.
**Summary:** Levothyroxine, by correcting thyroid function, may increase theophylline clearance.
**Related Drugs:** A similar interaction may occur between levothyroxine and other theophylline derivatives that are hepatically metabolized. Dyphylline may not interact with levothyroxine. The other thyroid hormones may interact similarly with aminophylline.
**Mechanism:** Thyroid function may alter the hepatic metabolism of some drugs via the microsomal mixed function oxidase system.
**Detailed Information:** See *EDI*, 17/4.10

## Aminophylline-Oral Contraceptive Agents
**Significance:** 3—minimally clinically significant
**Potential Effects:** Oral contraceptive agents may decrease aminophylline clearance, resulting in increased aminophylline levels.
**Recommendations:** Theophylline levels should be monitored when these agents are used together.
**Summary:** There are data to show that administration of oral contraceptive agents may decrease aminophylline clearance, resulting in increased aminophylline levels; however, all data do not support this.
**Related Drugs:** Theophylline has been shown to interact similarly with oral contraceptive agents. Dyphylline may not interact with oral contraceptive agents.
**Mechanism:** It has been suggested that oral contraceptive agents inhibit the metabolism of aminophylline.
**Detailed Information:** See *EDI*, 17/5.00

## Aminophylline-Tacrine
**Significance:** 2—moderately clinically significant
**Potential Effects:** Concurrent administration of tacrine and aminophylline may result in an increase in theophylline elimination half-life and mean plasma concentrations.
**Recommendations:** Patients receiving concurrent tacrine and aminophylline should be monitored for increases in theophylline concentration and possible associated toxicity. The theophylline dose may need to be adjusted.
**Summary:** The concurrent administration of tacrine and aminophylline may result in a significant increase in theophylline elimination half-life and mean plasma concentrations.
**Related Drugs:** A similar interaction may occur between tacrine and other theophylline derivatives that are hepatically metabolized. Caffeine would be expected to interact with tacrine; dyphylline would not. There are no drugs related to tacrine.
**Mechanism:** It has been postulated that tacrine inhibits theophylline clearance.
**Detailed Information:** See *EDI*, 17/6.50

## Aminophylline-Terbinafine
**Significance:** 2—moderately clinically significant
**Potential Effects:** The concurrent administration of terbinafine with aminophylline may lead to changes in theophylline pharmacokinetic parameters, which may predispose some patients to theophylline side effects and toxicity.
**Recommendations:** Theophylline serum levels, efficacy, and signs of toxicity should be monitored when terbinafine is added to or discontinued from therapy. Closer monitoring should be instituted in patients whose maintenance theophylline serum concentrations approach the upper limits of theophylline's therapeutic range. The dose of theophylline may need to be adjusted.
**Summary:** Administration of terbinafine with aminophylline resulted in changes in theophylline pharmacokinetic parameters, including an increase in theophylline AUC and half-life and a decrease in elimination rate constant and oral clearance of theophylline. There were no significant changes in theophylline maximum concentration ($C_{max}$) or time to $T_{max}$.
**Related Drugs:** A similar interaction has been noted with caffeine. If the mechanism involves inhibition of hepatic metabolism by terbinafine, dyphylline, which is not converted to theophylline or metabolized by the liver, would not be expected to interact. A similar interaction may occur between terbinafine and other theophylline derivatives.

# Xanthine

**Mechanism:** Although the mechanism of this interaction is not known, it has been postulated that terbinafine may disrupt the P450 reductase membranes, resulting in the inhibition of theophylline metabolism by the $P450_{1A2}$ isoenzyme.

**Detailed Information:** See *EDI*, 17/6.70

## Aminophylline-Thiabendazole

**Significance:** 2—moderately clinically significant

**Recommendations:** Theophylline levels should be closely monitored during concomitant use of these agents. The dose of aminophylline may need to be decreased, or another anthelmintic may be considered.

**Summary:** There are data to show that coadministration of these agents may cause an increase in aminophylline levels, causing nausea, lethargy, and general malaise.

**Related Drugs:** A similar interaction may occur between thiabendazole and other theophylline derivatives. Dyphylline would not be expected to interact similarly. There are no drugs related to thiabendazole.

**Mechanism:** Thiabendazole may inhibit the hepatic microsomal enzymes responsible for aminophylline's metabolism.

**Detailed Information:** See *EDI*, 17/7.00

## Caffeine-Adenosine

**Significance:** 3—minimally clinically significant

**Potential Effects:** Caffeine may inhibit the pharmacologic effects of adenosine.

**Recommendations:** The concurrent use of these two agents need not be avoided. In patients who regularly take in large amounts of caffeine, the dosage of adenosine may need to be reduced.

**Summary:** Caffeine has been reported to inhibit the pharmacologic effects of adenosine.

**Related Drugs:** Theophylline has been shown to interact with adenosine; however, data are conflicting. It is not known whether an interaction would occur between adenosine and other xanthine derivatives that are hepatically metabolized. There are no drugs related to adenosine.

**Mechanism:** The cardiovascular effects of caffeine and theophylline may result from the antagonism of exogenous adenosine.

**Detailed Information:** See *EDI*, 17/8.05

## Caffeine-Methoxsalen

**Significance:** 3—minimally clinically significant

**Potential Effects:** Methoxsalen may inhibit the metabolism of caffeine.

**Recommendations:** Concurrent use of these agents may need to be avoided. Also, it may be prudent to monitor patients receiving other xanthine derivatives (e.g., theophylline) with methoxsalen.

**Summary:** There are data to show that administration of methoxsalen will reduce the clearance of caffeine and increase its half-life. The potential for increased adverse effects of caffeine may exist in patients receiving methoxsalen.

**Related Drugs:** A similar interaction may occur between methoxsalen and other xanthine derivatives that are hepatically metabolized. Dyphylline would not be expected to interact with methoxsalen. A similar interaction may occur between caffeine and the other psoralen, trioxsalen.

**Mechanism:** Methoxsalen therapy may cause selective induction of hepatic metabolism, inhibiting metabolism of caffeine.

**Detailed Information:** See *EDI*, 17/8.10

## Caffeine-Oral Contraceptive Agents
**Significance:** 3—minimally clinically significant
**Recommendations:** The concurrent use of these agents need not be avoided. However, if central nervous system stimulation appears, the dose of caffeine may need to be decreased.
**Summary:** The total plasma clearance of a single dose of caffeine was reduced and its elimination half-life prolonged in women taking oral contraceptive agents.
**Related Drugs:** There are no drugs related to caffeine.
**Mechanism:** Oral contraceptive agents may inhibit the hepatic metabolism of caffeine.
**Detailed Information:** See *EDI*, 17/9.00

## Caffeine-Phenylpropanolamine
**Significance:** 3—minimally clinically significant
**Potential Effects:** Phenylpropanolamine may inhibit the metabolism of caffeine resulting in increased caffeine levels and side effects.
**Recommendations:** Monitor patients for increased side effects when these agents are administered concurrently. Caffeine-containing beverages may also interact with phenylpropanolamine.
**Summary:** Phenylpropanolamine may increase caffeine serum levels.
**Related Drugs:** A similar interaction may occur between phenylpropanolamine and other xanthine derivatives that are hepatically metabolized. It is not known whether an interaction would occur between phenylpropanolamine and dyphylline or between caffeine and other indirect-acting sympathomimetics.
**Mechanism:** The increased plasma levels of caffeine may be the result of inhibition of caffeine metabolism by phenylpropanolamine.
**Detailed Information:** See *EDI*, 17/10.50

## Dyphylline-Probenecid
**Significance:** 2—moderately clinically significant
**Recommendations:** If a patient is currently on dyphylline therapy and probenecid is added, the patient should be monitored for increased dyphylline levels (not detectable by theophylline assays); a decrease in the dosage of dyphylline may be necessary. This interaction may be of greater clinical importance in aminophylline-sensitive patients.
**Summary:** The concurrent administration of probenecid and dyphylline has been shown to increase the half-life, decrease the elimination rate constant and decrease the total body clearance of dyphylline.
**Related Drugs:** The same results may be expected when probenecid is used with theophylline and oxtriphylline. The concurrent use of sulfinpyrazone and theophylline has resulted in an increase in total plasma theophylline clearance.
**Mechanism:** Probenecid, which inhibits the renal transport of some compounds, may also inhibit the renal elimination of dyphylline.
**Detailed Information:** See *EDI*, 17/11.00

## Theophylline-Allopurinol
**Significance:** 2—moderately clinically significant
**Recommendations:** Large daily doses of allopurinol may decrease theophylline clearance when both drugs are used for longer than two weeks. Since increases in serum theophylline concentrations of 25% have been reported, some patients may require monitoring for signs of possible theophylline toxicity and may need lower doses during concurrent allopurinol therapy.

**Summary:** Allopurinol may decrease theophylline clearance and increase the risk of toxicity.
**Related Drugs:** A similar interaction may occur between allopurinol and other theophylline derivatives. Dyphylline is not expected to interact with allopurinol. There are no drugs related to allopurinol.
**Mechanism:** Allopurinol may inhibit the hepatic drug metabolizing enzymes.
**Detailed Information:** See *EDI*, 17/13.00

## Theophylline-Aluminum Hydroxide, Magnesium Hydroxide

**Significance:** 3—minimally clinically significant
**Potential Effects:** Some antacid preparations may increase theophylline absorption.
**Recommendations:** These agents may be given together; however, theophylline levels should be monitored when initiating therapy.
**Summary:** There are data to show that coadministration of some antacid preparations may increase theophylline absorption; however, all data do not support this interaction.
**Related Drugs:** There are data to show that other antacid products may interact with theophylline; however, data are conflicting. Because of conflicting results, it is not known if other theophylline derivatives would interact with an aluminum and magnesium hydroxide combination antacid.
**Mechanism:** Factors such as gastrointestinal fluid pH may influence the degradation and/or absorption of some slow release theophylline formulations.
**Detailed Information:** See *EDI*, 17/14.01

## Theophylline-Aminoglutethimide

**Significance:** 3—minimally clinically significant
**Recommendations:** Although concurrent use of these agents need not be avoided, theophylline levels should be monitored and the theophylline dosage increased if necessary.
**Summary:** There are data to show that aminoglutethimide administration increases theophylline clearance, possibly decreasing the pharmacologic effects of theophylline.
**Related Drugs:** A similar interaction may occur between aminoglutethimide and other theophylline derivatives. Dyphylline is not expected to interact with aminoglutethimide. A similar interaction may occur between glutethimide and theophylline.
**Mechanism:** Aminoglutethimide may increase the metabolism of theophylline.
**Detailed Information:** See *EDI*, 17/14.10

## Theophylline-Caffeine

**Significance:** 2—moderately clinically significant
**Potential Effects:** The addition of caffeine to a theophylline regimen may result in increased serum theophylline levels.
**Recommendations:** Patients receiving theophylline should be carefully monitored for changes in theophylline serum levels when changes in caffeine consumption occur.
**Summary:** Concurrent caffeine and theophylline may result in an increase in theophylline serum levels.
**Related Drugs:** It is not known whether an interaction would occur between caffeine and oxtriphylline. Dyphylline would not be expected to interact with caffeine, if the mechanism of this interaction results from an interference of theophylline hepatic metabolism.

**Mechanism:** Saturation of theophylline metabolism and/or competition between caffeine and theophylline may result in the delay of theophylline elimination.
**Detailed Information:** See *EDI,* 17/14.50

## Theophylline-Carbamazepine
**Significance:** 2—moderately clinically significant
**Potential Effects:** The concomitant use of these agents may result in increased or decreased theophylline levels as well as decreased carbamazepine levels. The patient's clinical condition may also worsen.
**Recommendations:** Patients should be monitored for changes in the levels of both theophylline and carbamazepine, and the dosage of each agent may need to be adjusted until therapeutic levels are maintained and efficacy is achieved.
**Summary:** Concurrent administration of theophylline and carbamazepine resulted in decreased levels of theophylline in one patient and increased carbamazepine levels in another.
**Related Drugs:** Concurrent administration of aminophylline has resulted in a decrease in carbamazepine levels and bioavailability. A similar interaction may be expected to occur between carbamazepine and oxtriphylline, which, like theophylline, is hepatically metabolized. Dyphylline is not converted to theophylline in vivo, is not metabolized by the liver, and is rapidly removed from the blood by glomerular filtration, active secretion, or both, and approximately 82% is excreted unchanged in the urine. If the mechanism of this interaction results from increased hepatic metabolism of theophylline, dyphylline would not be expected to interact with carbamazepine. No interaction has been seen between carbamazepine and caffeine. There are no drugs related to carbamazepine.
**Mechanism:** The mechanism of this interaction is not known. However, it has been suggested that the hepatic metabolism of theophylline is increased by carbamazepine, and theophylline increases the hepatic metabolism of carbamazepine. It is not known why theophylline levels were elevated in one study.
**Detailed Information:** See *EDI,* 17/15.00

## Theophylline-Cefaclor
**Significance:** 3—minimally clinically significant
**Potential Effects:** Cefaclor may increase theophylline levels.
**Recommendations:** Theophylline dosage may need to be decreased if toxicity or increased levels occur. Cefaclor may need to be discontinued.
**Summary:** The addition of cefaclor to a stabilized theophylline regimen has been shown to result in an increase in theophylline serum levels.
**Related Drugs:** It is not known whether an interaction would occur between theophylline and other cephalosporins or between cefaclor and other theophylline derivatives.
**Mechanism:** The mechanism of this interaction is not known. The presence of an acute viral illness has been associated with decreased hepatic cytochrome P450 activity and decreased theophylline clearance, but the patient was afebrile in this case report.
**Detailed Information:** See *EDI,* 17/16.10

## Theophylline-Charcoal
**Significance:** 1—highly clinically significant
**Potential Effects:** Charcoal adsorbs theophylline, reducing absorption and increasing clearance.

**Recommendations:** Charcoal should be administered as soon as possible to decrease theophylline absorption; however, continued administration will increase theophylline clearance. Sorbitol will increase the effectiveness of charcoal. If charcoal is not being used to treat a theophylline overdose, a higher dose of theophylline or separating the administration times is necessary.

**Summary:** Activated charcoal administration has been shown to decrease the absorption of oral theophylline.

**Related Drugs:** Other oral theophylline derivatives may also be adsorbed by activated charcoal.

**Mechanism:** Activated charcoal adsorbs oral theophylline, limiting its absorption from the gastrointestinal tract, and decreases enterohepatic recirculation, increasing theophylline clearance.

**Detailed Information:** See *EDI,* 17/17.00

## Theophylline-Cimetidine

**Significance:** 1—highly clinically significant

**Potential Effects:** Cimetidine can inhibit the metabolism of theophylline, resulting in increased theophylline levels.

**Recommendations:** If these agents are used together, theophylline serum levels should be closely monitored. Antacids, famotidine, or possibly ranitidine may be used as an alternative to cimetidine.

**Summary:** It is well documented that cimetidine impairs the elimination of theophylline, resulting in increased theophylline levels.

**Related Drugs:** Aminophylline, caffeine, pentoxifylline and oxtriphylline may also be involved in a similar interaction. Dyphylline is not expected to interact with cimetidine. Ranitidine and famotidine do not appear to significantly influence theophylline disposition.

**Mechanism:** Cimetidine inhibits the hepatic microsomal mono-oxygenase system, and this inhibition may cause cimetidine to bind to an enzyme system or to theophylline, forming a complex that interrupts metabolism.

**Detailed Information:** See *EDI,* 17/19.00

## Theophylline-Ciprofloxacin

**Significance:** 2—moderately clinically significant

**Potential Effects:** Ciprofloxacin or its metabolite may inhibit the hepatic metabolism of theophylline, resulting in increased theophylline levels.

**Recommendations:** Theophylline levels should be monitored when these agents are used concomitantly. The theophylline dose may need to be decreased or the ciprofloxacin discontinued. Norfloxacin may be substituted for ciprofloxacin; however, indications for the different quinolones may vary. Theophylline levels should still be monitored.

**Summary:** Several cases have been reported in which ciprofloxacin or its metabolite inhibited the hepatic metabolism of theophylline, resulting in increased theophylline levels and theophylline toxicity.

**Related Drugs:** Concurrent administration of aminophylline and ciprofloxacin has also been shown to affect theophylline levels, leading to theophylline toxicity. A similar interaction may be expected to occur between ciprofloxacin and the other theophylline derivative that is hepatically metabolized, oxtriphylline. Dyphylline, a theophylline derivative that is not converted to theophylline in vivo and is not metabolized by the liver, would not be expected to interact with ciprofloxacin. Norfloxacin and lomefloxacin have shown conflicting results when administered with theophylline. Enoxacin has increased theophylline levels in several studies, but conflicting data are available. Temafloxacin, nalidixic acid, fleroxacin, and ofloxacin have not been shown to interact with theophylline. Clinafloxacin interacted in a similar fashion as ciprofloxacin. The quinolone antibiotics have also been shown to affect caffeine pharmacokinetics similarly, although conflicting data are available. An interaction would not be expected to occur between theophylline and the other quinolone that is not hepatically metabolized, cinoxacin.

**Mechanism:** Ciprofloxacin may inhibit the hepatic metabolism of theophylline via the cytochrome P450 enzyme system, the site at which both agents are metabolized. The specific sites within the cytochrome P450 enzyme may be the $CYP_{1A2}$ and $CYP_{3A4}$ sites, and the interindividual variation in the expression of the $CYP_{1A2}$ site may be responsible for the interindividual response seen during concurrent administration of theophylline and ciprofloxacin. There is evidence that this interaction is not caused by the parent drug, ciprofloxacin, but by its 4-oxo metabolite.

**Detailed Information:** See *EDI*, 17/20.21

## Theophylline-Dipyridamole Injection

**Significance:** 2—moderately clinically significant

**Potential Effects:** The performance of a dipyridamole-thallium imaging test on patients receiving therapeutic doses of theophylline may result in false-negative results.

**Recommendations:** Patients scheduled for dipyridamole-thallium imaging tests should have a xanthine-free (including caffeine-containing products) period for at least 24 hours prior to their exam. It has been suggested that patients with congestive heart failure and decreased hepatic function may need a longer xanthine-free period prior to dipyridamole-thallium imaging tests because the metabolism of xanthine derivatives may be decreased in these patients. In patients with severe bronchospastic disease, theophylline may need to be substituted with other bronchodilators or an alternative diagnostic procedure may be indicated.

**Summary:** The performance of a dipyridamole-thallium imaging test on patients receiving therapeutic doses of theophylline resulted in false-negative results.

**Related Drugs:** A similar interaction has occurred with caffeine. Based on the proposed mechanism, a similar interaction may occur between dipyridamole and other theophylline derivatives.

**Mechanism:** The xanthine derivatives are adenosine receptor antagonists. It has been postulated that the concurrent administration of xanthines with dipyridamole may inhibit dipyridamole-induced increases in endogenous plasma adenosine levels, thus decreasing dipyridamole's vasodilator effects.

**Detailed Information:** See *EDI*, 17/20.26

## Theophylline-Disulfiram

**Significance:** 2—moderately clinically significant

**Potential Effects:** Disulfiram may inhibit the metabolism of theophylline, increasing its half-life and serum levels. The metabolism of caffeine may also be inhibited by disulfiram.

**Recommendations:** Patients receiving disulfiram and theophylline concurrently should be monitored for increased theophylline levels. The dose of theophylline may need to be decreased by as much as 50% depending on the dose of disulfiram. Caffeine should be avoided in patients receiving disulfiram.

**Summary:** There are data to show that disulfiram administration may inhibit the metabolism of theophylline, increasing its half-life and serum levels.

**Related Drugs:** A similar interaction may occur between disulfiram and other theophylline derivatives that are hepatically metabolized. Dyphylline is not expected to interact with disulfiram. There are no drugs related to disulfiram.

**Mechanism:** Disulfiram may inhibit the hepatic metabolism of theophylline by its inhibitory effect on the cytochrome P450 enzyme system.

**Detailed Information:** See *EDI,* 17/20.30

## Theophylline-Erythromycin

**Significance:** 1—highly clinically significant

**Potential Effects:** Erythromycin decreases the elimination of theophylline leading to increased theophylline levels. Theophylline may also decrease erythromycin levels.

**Recommendations:** Monitor theophylline levels when erythromycin is added to or withdrawn from therapy. Also, monitor erythromycin efficacy when these agents are used together.

**Summary:** Concurrent administration of theophylline and erythromycin has resulted in decreased theophylline clearance, increased theophylline levels, and decreased erythromycin levels in some subjects.

**Related Drugs:** Azithromycin has not interacted with theophylline; however, a male smoker had an 80% decrease in serum theophylline concentration after discontinuing azithromycin from concurrent therapy and a 33% decrease in theophylline dosage. Clarithromycin has been shown to elevate theophylline levels slightly. In separate studies, dithromycin showed no significant effect on theophylline pharmacokinetics and a decreased theophylline mean average steady-state concentration. No significant effect on theophylline concentrations by spiramycin has been documented. Concomitant administration of troleandomycin and theophylline decreased theophylline clearance by 50%. Several studies showed that the administration of aminophylline with erythromycin resulted in decreased theophylline clearance and increased theophylline half-life, blood levels, and toxicity. Several studies found no effect on theophylline kinetics during the concurrent administration of aminophylline and erythromycin, either as stearate or lactobionate. An infusion of aminophylline following erythromycin therapy for eight days resulted in a 30% decrease in erythromycin serum concentrations. Administering erythromycin stearate with oxtriphylline decreased theophylline clearance by 40% and increased theophylline half-life by 57%. Caffeine would be expected to interact with erythromycin. Dyphylline, which is not metabolized by the liver and is rapidly removed from the blood, would not be expected to interact with erythromycin.

**Mechanism:** The mechanism is not clearly established. Theophylline is metabolized to a significant degree, and erythromycin may block one or more of the metabolic pathways. Troleandomycin inhibits theophylline metabolism *in vitro*. Duration of erythromycin administration, smoking habits, patient age, and concomitant disease states may play a role in the interaction. It has been proposed that an interaction between erythromycin and 1-methyluric acid, a theophylline metabolite, is responsible for the decrease in erythromycin levels during concurrent therapy.

**Detailed Information:** See *EDI,* 17/21.00

## Theophylline-Fluvoxamine

**Significance:** 3—minimally clinically significant

**Potential Effects:** The addition of fluvoxamine to a theophylline regimen may result in increased theophylline serum levels and toxicity.

**Recommendations:** The addition or removal of fluvoxamine from the therapy of a patient maintained on theophylline may result in altered theophylline serum levels. The fluvoxamine may have to be discontinued or the theophylline dose adjusted.

**Summary:** Fluvoxamine administration may result in increased theophylline levels and toxicity.

**Related Drugs:** It is not known whether an interaction would occur between fluvoxamine and other theophylline derivatives or between theophylline and other serotonin reuptake inhibitors.

**Mechanism:** Competitive inhibition of hepatic microsomal enzymes by fluvoxamine may be a factor in the elevated theophylline concentrations.

**Detailed Information:** See *EDI*, 17/24.50

## Theophylline-Furosemide

**Significance:** 2—moderately clinically significant

**Potential Effects:** Furosemide may alter theophylline levels.

**Recommendations:** Monitor theophylline levels when administering these agents together. Separating the dosing of these agents by as much time as possible may avoid this interaction.

**Summary:** There are data to show that furosemide administration may cause theophylline levels to decrease.

**Related Drugs:** A similar interaction may occur between furosemide and other theophylline derivatives. Dyphylline is not expected to interact with furosemide. A similar interaction is expected to occur between theophylline and other loop diuretics.

**Mechanism:** Furosemide may decrease hepatic congestion, increasing theophylline clearance, or displace theophylline from serum proteins.

**Detailed Information:** See *EDI*, 17/25.00

## Theophylline-Hydrocortisone

**Significance:** 3—minimally clinically significant

**Potential Effects:** The concurrent administration of these agents may result in increased theophylline levels.

**Recommendations:** Theophylline levels should be monitored in patients receiving concurrent hydrocortisone. A lower dose of theophylline may be necessary.

**Summary:** There are data to show that hydrocortisone administration may result in increased theophylline levels; however, there are conflicting data.

**Related Drugs:** Methylprednisolone and dexamethasone were shown to have no significant effect on theophylline levels. Because of conflicting results, it is difficult to determine if theophylline would interact with other corticosteroids. A similar interaction is expected to occur between hydrocortisone and other theophylline derivatives. Dyphylline would not be expected to interact with hydrocortisone, whereas aminophylline and oxtriphylline would interact similarly.

**Mechanism:** The mechanism of this interaction is unknown.

**Detailed Information:** See *EDI*, 17/27.00

## Theophylline-Hypericum

**Significance:** 3—minimally clinically significant

**Potential Effects:** The addition of St. John's wort (*Hypericum perforatum* L.) to a stable theophylline regimen may require an increased theophylline dosage to maintain theophylline serum levels and therapeutic effect.

## Xanthine

**Recommendations:** Patients maintained on a theophylline regimen should be carefully monitored for changes in theophylline serum levels if St. John's wort is added to or removed from concurrent therapy.

**Summary:** The addition of 300 mg/day of St. John's wort to a stable theophylline regimen required an increased theophylline dosage to maintain theophylline serum levels and therapeutic effect.

**Related Drugs:** An interaction may occur between hypericum and other theophylline derivatives that are hepatically metabolized (aminophylline and oxtriphylline). Dyphylline, which is not converted to theophylline *in vivo*, is not metabolized by the liver, and is rapidly removed from the blood by glomerular filtration or active secretion, or both, would not be expected to interact with hypericum based on the proposed mechanism.

**Mechanism:** St. John's wort is referred to as hypericum. Hypericum extract has many constituents, with hypericin, a naphthodianthrone, considered to be the active ingredient. Hypericin resembles compounds known to induce cytochrome $P450_{1A}$ and glutathione-S-transferase enzymes. This induction appears to be mediated via a transcriptional enhancer sequence. Hypericum may have induced cytochrome $P450_{1A2}$-mediated theophylline clearance, resulting in decreased theophylline serum levels.

**Detailed Information:** See *EDI*, 17/28.30

## Theophylline-Influenza Virus Vaccine

**Significance:** 3—minimally clinically significant

**Potential Effects:** Influenza virus vaccine may decrease theophylline metabolism, resulting in increased levels.

**Recommendations:** Patients maintained on theophylline should be monitored closely for increased theophylline levels if influenza virus vaccine is administered.

**Summary:** There are data to show that administration of influenza virus vaccine may decrease theophylline metabolism, resulting in increased levels and potentiating increased adverse effects.

**Related Drugs:** Oxtriphylline has been shown to interact similarly, whereas aminophylline has not. Dyphylline is not expected to interact with influenza virus vaccine.

**Mechanism:** Influenza vaccine may decrease theophylline biotransformation because of a depression of the cytochrome P450 system.

**Detailed Information:** See *EDI*, 17/29.00

## Theophylline-Isoniazid

**Significance:** 3—minimally clinically significant

**Potential Effects:** Concomitant administration of these agents may result in an increase or decrease in theophylline clearance.

**Recommendations:** Concurrent use of these agents need not be avoided. However, until further clinical studies are done, theophylline levels should be routinely monitored since an adjustment in the dosage of theophylline may be necessary.

**Summary:** There are data to show that isoniazid administration may result in an increase or decrease in theophylline clearance.

**Related Drugs:** Isoniazid was shown to decrease the plasma clearance of theophylline and increase its serum concentrations. Because of conflicting results, it is difficult to determine if an interaction would occur between isoniazid and other theophylline derivatives. Dyphylline is not expected to interact with isoniazid. There are no drugs related to isoniazid.

**Mechanism:** Isoniazid may increase the hepatic metabolism of theophylline by enzyme induction or an unknown mechanism.

**Detailed Information:** See *EDI*, 17/30.10

## Theophylline-Ketoconazole

**Significance:** 3—minimally clinically significant

**Potential Effects:** Ketoconazole may decrease theophylline levels.

**Recommendations:** Theophylline levels should be monitored when ketoconazole is added to or withdrawn from therapy. The dose of theophylline may need to be increased.

**Summary:** Ketoconazole significantly reduced serum theophylline concentrations.

**Related Drugs:** Fluconazole has been reported to slightly decrease theophylline clearance. In contrast with oral theophylline, studies failed to show any effect of ketoconazole on theophylline levels following administration of intravenous aminophylline. Because of conflicting results, it is difficult to determine if an interaction would occur between ketoconazole and the other theophylline derivatives or between theophylline and the other imidazole antifungal agents.

**Mechanism:** The mechanism of this interaction is not known. It is possible that ketoconazole enhanced the metabolism of theophylline since it has been suggested that long-term ketoconazole administration may induce hepatic drug metabolism; however, this would be opposite its expected effect since ketoconazole has been shown to inhibit the hepatic metabolism of other agents.

**Detailed Information:** See *EDI*, 17/30.30

## Theophylline-Methimazole

**Significance:** 3—minimally clinically significant

**Potential Effects:** Methimazole, by affecting thyroid function, may decrease theophylline clearance. This interaction may be the result of a correction of a disease state rather than a direct effect of methimazole on theophylline.

**Recommendations:** Patients' theophylline levels should be monitored while establishing a euthyroid state with antithyroid replacement therapy. Similarly, patients receiving theophylline should be monitored for a change in theophylline levels if they develop hyperthyroidism. The dose of theophylline may need to be adjusted.

**Summary:** There are data to show that methimazole administration may decrease theophylline clearance. This interaction may be the result of a disease state correction rather than a direct effect on theophylline clearance.

**Related Drugs:** A similar interaction may occur between methimazole and other theophylline derivatives that are hepatically metabolized. Dyphylline is not expected to interact with methimazole. A similar interaction is expected to occur between theophylline and propylthiouracil.

**Mechanism:** Hyperthyroidism may increase the activity of the hepatic microsomal enzymes responsible for the metabolism of theophylline.

**Detailed Information:** See *EDI*, 17/30.50

## Theophylline-Mexiletine

**Significance:** 2—moderately clinically significant

**Potential Effects:** Concurrent use may result in increased theophylline serum levels.

**Recommendations:** These agents may be given concurrently, but theophylline levels should be monitored and the theophylline dose reduced if necessary.

**Summary:** There are data to show that mexiletine administration may cause an increase in theophylline levels, increasing theophylline side effects.

# Xanthine

**Related Drugs:** Mexiletine reduced the clearance of caffeine. A similar interaction may occur between mexiletine and other hepatically metabolized xanthines, if the mechanism involves inhibition of hepatic metabolism. It is not known if dyphylline would interact with mexiletine.

**Mechanism:** Impaired hepatic metabolism of theophylline by mexiletine may be an explanation.

**Detailed Information:** See *EDI*, 17/30.70

## Theophylline-Moricizine

**Significance:** 2—moderately clinically significant

**Potential Effects:** Theophylline serum levels may be decreased with concurrent moricizine.

**Recommendations:** Theophylline levels should be carefully monitored with concomitant moricizine administration. The dose of theophylline may need to be adjusted.

**Summary:** Theophylline clearance increased and half-life decreased with concurrent moricizine.

**Related Drugs:** It is not known whether an interaction would occur between moricizine and other theophylline derivatives or between theophylline and other class I antiarrhythmic agents.

**Mechanism:** Changes in theophylline clearance are most likely the result of enzyme induction by moricizine.

**Detailed Information:** See *EDI*, 17/30.85

## Theophylline-Omeprazole

**Significance:** 4—not clinically significant

**Potential Effects:** Omeprazole does not appear to interact with theophylline to a clinically significant extent.

**Recommendations:** No special precautions appear necessary with the concurrent use of these agents.

**Summary:** Omeprazole does not appear to interact with theophylline to a clinically significant extent. Although one study showed increased theophylline absorption when the two drugs were taken concurrently, theophylline serum level changes were not statistically significant.

**Related Drugs:** Studies on omeprazole's effect on caffeine metabolism are conflicting. The clinical significance of an increase in caffeine metabolism has not been determined. Lansoprazole and pantoprazole have not shown clinically significant effects on the pharmacokinetics of theophylline. Based on the mechanism of omeprazole metabolism, an interaction would not be expected to occur between omeprazole and the other theophylline derivatives.

**Mechanism:** Although omeprazole is metabolized in the liver by S-mephenytoin hydroxylase in the cytochrome P450 enzyme system, present studies indicate that this agent does not seem to compete with theophylline for metabolism. Omeprazole has been postulated to be an inducer of the cytochrome $P450_{1A2}$ isozyme system both in studies discussed above and in other *in vivo* and *in vitro* studies.

**Detailed Information:** See *EDI*, 17/30.90

## Theophylline-Phenobarbital

**Significance:** 2—moderately clinically significant

**Potential Effects:** Phenobarbital may induce the metabolism of theophylline, resulting in decreased theophylline levels.

**Recommendations:** Theophylline plasma levels should be closely monitored when a barbiturate is added to, or withdrawn from, theophylline therapy. The dose of theophylline may need to be adjusted.

**Summary:** The concurrent use of phenobarbital and theophylline may reduce theophylline serum levels.

**Related Drugs:** Secobarbital was shown to interact with theophylline. A similar interaction may occur between theophylline and other barbiturates. A similar interaction is expected to occur between phenobarbital and other theophylline derivatives. Dyphylline is not expected to interact with phenobarbital.

**Mechanism:** Phenobarbital induces the hepatic microsomal enzymes responsible for theophylline metabolism.

**Detailed Information:** See *EDI*, 17/31.00

## Theophylline-Phenytoin

**Significance:** 2—moderately clinically significant

**Recommendations:** It is important to monitor the levels of both phenytoin and theophylline during concurrent therapy. If necessary, the dose of theophylline or phenytoin may need to be increased.

**Summary:** There are data to show that coadministration may lead to a decrease in theophylline or in phenytoin levels.

**Related Drugs:** A similar interaction is expected to occur between theophylline and other hydantoin anticonvulsants. Dyphylline is not expected to interact with phenytoin.

**Mechanism:** Phenytoin may increase the metabolism of theophylline by inducing hepatic microsomal enzymes. Theophylline induces the metabolism of phenytoin or interferes with its absorption.

**Detailed Information:** See *EDI*, 17/33.00

## Theophylline-Propafenone

**Significance:** 2—moderately clinically significant

**Potential Effects:** The addition of propafenone to a theophylline regimen may result in increased theophylline serum concentration.

**Recommendations:** Theophylline levels should be carefully monitored if propafenone is added to, or withdrawn from, concurrent therapy. The dose of theophylline may need to be adjusted.

**Summary:** The addition of propafenone to the therapy of a patient maintained on theophylline resulted in increased theophylline serum concentrations.

**Related Drugs:** It is not known if a similar interaction would occur between theophylline and other class IC antiarrhythmic agents. A similar interaction is expected to occur between propafenone and other theophylline derivatives. Dyphylline is not expected to interact with propafenone.

**Mechanism:** An inhibition of theophylline hepatic metabolism may occur.

**Detailed Information:** See *EDI*, 17/34.50

## Theophylline-Propranolol

**Significance:** 2—moderately clinically significant

**Potential Effects:** Propranolol may cause an increase in theophylline serum levels.

**Recommendations:** Since propranolol may increase bronchial resistance, the patient's clinical status as well as theophylline serum levels should be monitored. The dose of theophylline may need to be adjusted.

**Summary:** There are data to show that propranolol administration may cause an increase in theophylline serum levels and reduce clearance.

**Related Drugs:** A similar interaction may occur between propranolol and other theophylline derivatives. Dyphylline is not expected to interact with propranolol. The noncardioselective beta blocking agents that are not extensively hepatically metabolized are expected to interact with theophylline to some degree.

**Mechanism:** Propranolol and theophylline may have some antagonistic effects that cause this interaction. Propranolol may interfere with the metabolism of theophylline by blocking cyclic AMP in the cytochrome system.

**Detailed Information:** See *EDI*, 17/35.00

## Theophylline-Pyrantel Pamoate

**Significance:** 2—moderately clinically significant

**Potential Effects:** Pyrantel pamoate may increase theophylline levels, resulting in toxicity.

**Recommendations:** The patient should be carefully monitored for changes in theophylline serum levels and for signs of theophylline toxicity when theophylline is administered concomitantly with pyrantel pamoate. The dose of theophylline may need to be adjusted.

**Summary:** There are data to show that pyrantel pamoate administration may increase theophylline levels, resulting in toxicity and increased adverse effects.

**Related Drugs:** A similar interaction may occur between pyrantel pamoate and other theophylline derivatives that are hepatically metabolized. Dyphylline is not expected to interact with pyrantel pamoate. There are no drugs related to pyrantel pamoate.

**Mechanism:** Pyrantel pamoate may inhibit theophylline clearance by inhibition of hepatic enzymes, or it may increase the rate of drug release, increasing the theophylline level.

**Detailed Information:** See *EDI*, 17/36.05

## Theophylline-Rifampin

**Significance:** 2—moderately clinically significant

**Recommendations:** Patients maintained on theophylline should have their serum concentrations monitored if rifampin is to be added to, or deleted from, their therapeutic regimen. While most patients may require only monitoring, appropriate dosage adjustments of up to 25% have been suggested.

**Summary:** Concurrent administration of rifampin and theophylline may result in a more rapid clearance of theophylline.

**Related Drugs:** Rifampin has been shown to reduce the aminophylline area-under-curve, increase the metabolic clearance and volume of distribution of aminophylline. Dyphylline is not expected to interact with rifampin. There are no drugs related to rifampin.

**Mechanism:** It is speculated that the increased activity of the hepatic cytochrome P450 enzymes by rifampin is involved in this interaction.

**Detailed Information:** See *EDI*, 17/36.10

## Theophylline-Sucralfate

**Significance:** 3—minimally clinically significant

**Potential Effects:** Sucralfate may decrease the absorption of theophylline. This interaction may be clinically significant with the sustained-release dosage form of theophylline.

**Recommendations:** Although further studies are necessary, theophylline levels should be monitored during concurrent sucralfate administration. The dose of theophylline may need to be adjusted.

**Summary:** There are data to show that sucralfate administration may decrease the absorption of theophylline; however, there are conflicting data.

**Related Drugs:** It is not known if sucralfate would affect the absorption of other theophylline derivatives.

**Mechanism:** Sustained-release theophylline products release drug over a prolonged period, allowing a greater opportunity for an interaction to occur. This may explain the differences in the interaction between sustained-release and immediate-release theophylline products and sucralfate.
**Detailed Information:** See *EDI*, 17/36.70

## Theophylline-Tacrolimus

**Significance:** 3—minimally clinically significant
**Potential Effects:** The addition of theophylline to a tacrolimus regimen may result in increased tacrolimus serum levels and serum creatinine.
**Recommendations:** If low-dose theophylline is used concurrently with tacrolimus in renal transplant patients, tacrolimus serum levels and renal function should be carefully monitored. The dosages of theophylline and/or tacrolimus may need to be adjusted.
**Summary:** Addition of theophylline to a tacrolimus regimen resulted in increased tacrolimus serum levels and serum creatinine in a kidney transplant patient.
**Related Drugs:** Single doses of aminophylline are used to increase urine flow during tacrolimus toxicity, with improved renal function and lower tacrolimus levels resulting. A similar interaction may occur between tacrolimus and oxtriphylline, multiple doses of aminophylline, and theophylline derivatives that are hepatically metabolized. Dyphylline, which is not converted to theophylline and is rapidly removed from the blood by glomerular filtration and/or active secretion, would not be expected to interact with tacrolimus. Sirolimus may interact with the other theophylline derivatives.
**Mechanism:** Theophylline may inhibit the cytochrome $P450_{3A4}$-mediated hepatic metabolism of tacrolimus. Data showing that single doses of aminophylline improved urine flow and decreased tacrolimus toxicity suggest that multiple aminophylline doses are needed to inhibit $P450_{3A4}$-mediated tacrolimus metabolism.
**Detailed Information:** See *EDI*, 17/36.80

## Theophylline-Tetracycline

**Significance:** 3—minimally clinically significant
**Potential Effects:** Tetracycline may increase theophylline levels. An increased incidence of gastrointestinal complaints may occur from concomitant administration.
**Recommendations:** These agents may be used together, but theophylline levels should routinely be monitored.
**Summary:** There are data to show that tetracycline administration may increase theophylline levels and potentiate increased theophylline side effects.
**Related Drugs:** Doxycycline has not been shown to significantly interact with theophylline. Because of conflicting results, it is difficult to determine if an interaction would occur between theophylline and other tetracyclines and between tetracycline and other theophylline derivatives.
**Mechanism:** The mechanism of this interaction is unknown. Gastrointestinal complaints may occur with both agents, and this interaction may be a summation response.
**Detailed Information:** See *EDI*, 17/37.00

## Theophylline-Ticlopidine

**Significance:** 2—moderately clinically significant
**Potential Effects:** Concurrent administration of theophylline and ticlopidine may result in increased theophylline levels.

**Recommendations:** Patients should be monitored for increased theophylline levels and signs of theophylline toxicity if ticlopidine is added to therapy.

**Summary:** Use of ticlopidine resulted in an increase in plasma concentration and half-life of theophylline and a decrease in total plasma clearance and the theophylline elimination rate constant.

**Related Drugs:** Although documentation is lacking, based on the possible mechanism of action and pharmacologic and structural similarity derivatives of theophylline may be expected to interact with ticlopidine in a similar fashion. If the mechanism involves competition for the N-demethylation metabolic process, dyphylline may not be expected to interact similarly with ticlopidine.

**Mechanism:** One possible mechanism for this interaction is the interference of theophylline hepatic metabolism by ticlopidine.

**Detailed Information:** See *EDI*, 17/38.00

## Theophylline-Tobacco

**Significance:** 1—highly clinically significant

**Potential Effects:** Tobacco use induces the metabolism of theophylline, leading to decreased levels.

**Recommendations:** Theophylline levels should be monitored if tobacco use is started or stopped.

**Summary:** There are data to show that tobacco use induces the metabolism of theophylline, leading to decreased levels and necessitating an increase in dosage.

**Related Drugs:** Aminophylline undergoes the same interaction. Dyphylline is not expected to interact with tobacco.

**Mechanism:** Smoking is thought to enhance theophylline metabolism by inducing hepatic microsomal enzymes.

**Detailed Information:** See *EDI*, 17/39.00

## Theophylline-Verapamil

**Significance:** 2—moderately clinically significant

**Potential Effects:** Verapamil may cause an increase in theophylline serum levels.

**Recommendations:** Monitor theophylline levels closely when these agents are used together. The dose of theophylline may need to be decreased.

**Summary:** Verapamil has been shown to cause a doubling of theophylline serum concentrations and clinical manifestations of theophylline toxicity.

**Related Drugs:** Nifedipine and diltiazem have been documented to interact similarly to verapamil; however, documentation is conflicting. A similar interaction is expected to occur between verapamil and other theophylline derivatives. Dyphylline is not expected to interact similarly with verapamil.

**Mechanism:** Theophylline clearance has been shown to be affected by substances that may compete with its metabolism, and theophylline and verapamil have a metabolic process in common.

**Detailed Information:** See *EDI*, 17/41.00

## Theophylline-Vidarabine

**Significance:** 3—minimally clinically significant

**Recommendations:** Although this interaction has not been clearly established, patients receiving theophylline and vidarabine should be monitored for increasing theophylline serum concentrations. The dose of theophylline may need to be decreased.

# Xanthine

**Summary:** There are data to show that vidarabine administration may potentiate an increase in serum theophylline levels.

**Related Drugs:** Oxtriphylline would be expected to interact similarly. Dyphylline would not be expected to interact with vidarabine. There are no drugs related to vidarabine.

**Mechanism:** The major metabolite of vidarabine may compete with theophylline, decreasing theophylline's metabolism and leading to increased serum concentrations.

**Detailed Information:** See *EDI*, 17/43.00

# Chapter Eighteen

# Miscellaneous Drug Interactions

## Miscellaneous

### Adenosine-Dipyridamole

**Significance:** 3—minimally clinically significant

**Potential Effects:** Dipyridamole may reduce the required dose of adenosine.

**Recommendations:** Patients maintained on intravenous adenosine should be monitored for increased adenosine effects if dipyridamole is added to cotherapy. The dose of intravenous adenosine may need to be reduced.

**Summary:** Dipyridamole has been shown to reduce the dose of adenosine necessary to achieve a therapeutic response. There are data to show that concurrent administration of these agents causes an increased reduction in heart rate.

**Related Drugs:** There are no drugs related to adenosine or dipyridamole.

**Mechanism:** Dipyridamole in high plasma concentrations may inhibit the uptake of adenosine by erythrocytes or platelets, or by other tissues, inhibiting metabolism of adenosine.

**Detailed Information:** See *EDI*, 18/0.03

### Alteplase-Nitroglycerin

**Significance:** 2—moderately clinically significant

**Potential Effects:** Thrombolytic effects of alteplase may be reduced by concurrent nitroglycerin administration.

**Recommendations:** Caution should be exercised when intravenous nitroglycerin and alteplase are administered concomitantly since nitroglycerin has been shown to decrease the thrombolytic activity of alteplase.

**Summary:** Decreased thrombolytic effect of alteplase (tissue plasminogen activator) may result with concomitant nitroglycerin administration, studies have shown.

**Related Drugs:** There is no documentation of an interaction between alteplase and other nitrate derivatives; however, because of the similarity in pharmacologic activity an interaction may be expected to occur.

**Mechanism:** Nitroglycerin given concomitantly with alteplase may decrease the thrombolytic effect of alteplase by decreasing the plasma alteplase antigen concentrations. It has been postulated that nitroglycerin may enhance hepatic blood flow, thereby facilitating the degradation of alteplase.

**Detailed Information:** See *EDI*, 18/0.04

### Aluminum Hydroxide-Citric Acid

**Significance:** 3—minimally clinically significant

**Potential Effects:** Citric acid may increase the absorption of aluminum.

**Recommendations:** Simultaneous administration of citric acid and aluminum hydroxide should be avoided since significant systemic absorption of aluminum may occur. This may be of additional concern in patients on long-term dialysis or with impaired renal function.

**Summary:** The systemic absorption of aluminum is enhanced by concomitant citric acid administration.

**Related Drugs:** An interaction may occur between citric acid or oral citrates and other aluminum salts.

**Mechanism:** Citric acid and aluminum hydroxide will increase serum levels of a nonionized aluminum-citrate complex which may pass the gastrointestinal barrier.

**Detailed Information:** See *EDI*, 18/0.05

## Miscellaneous

### Amphetamine-Ammonium Chloride

**Significance:** 3—minimally clinically significant

**Recommendations:** Since the urinary excretion of amphetamine can be increased by the concurrent administration of ammonium chloride, this interaction may be useful in cases of amphetamine toxicity or overdose. If this effect is not desired, the dose of amphetamine may need to be increased or the ammonium chloride discontinued.

**Summary:** There are data to show that concurrent ammonium chloride and amphetamine administration may increase the elimination of unchanged amphetamine in the urine, decreasing the pharmacologic effects of amphetamine.

**Related Drugs:** The other indirect-acting sympathomimetics may interact with ammonium chloride based on a similar metabolic fate. Other agents that acidify the urine may also interact with amphetamine.

**Mechanism:** The tubular reabsorption of amphetamine is decreased as the pH of the urine becomes more acidic following the administration of ammonium chloride.

**Detailed Information:** See *EDI*, 18/0.10

### Amphetamine-Sodium Bicarbonate

**Significance:** 3—minimally clinically significant

**Recommendations:** If increased pharmacologic or toxic effects of amphetamine are observed when sodium bicarbonate is administered concurrently, the dose of amphetamine may need to be decreased or the sodium bicarbonate discontinued.

**Summary:** Sodium bicarbonate was shown to increase the half-life and metabolism, and decrease the excretion, of amphetamine, potentially causing amphetamine toxicity.

**Related Drugs:** The other indirect-acting sympathomimetics may interact with sodium bicarbonate. Other agents that alkalinize the urine may interact with amphetamine.

**Mechanism:** As sodium bicarbonate makes the urine more basic, the tubular reabsorption of amphetamine is increased.

**Detailed Information:** See *EDI*, 18/0.30

### Cimetidine-Aluminum Hydroxide, Magnesium Hydroxide

**Significance:** 3—minimally clinically significant

**Potential Effects:** Concomitant antacid administration may decrease the absorption of cimetidine.

**Recommendations:** If the concomitant use of these agents is necessary, separate the administration of each by as much time as possible, or administer cimetidine with meals followed by the antacid one hour later.

**Summary:** There are data to show that aluminum hydroxide administration may decrease the absorption of cimetidine; however, data are conflicting.

**Related Drugs:** Because of conflicting results, it is difficult to determine if an interaction would occur between cimetidine and other antacids. There are data to show that antacids have no effect on ranitidine absorption; however, the data do vary. There are conflicting data regarding the concurrent use of famotidine.

**Mechanism:** Some component of the antacids may interfere with cimetidine absorption, or the total neutralizing capacity of the antacid may be responsible for the interaction.

**Detailed Information:** See *EDI*, 18/1.00

## Cimetidine-Metoclopramide

**Significance:** 3—minimally clinically significant

**Recommendations:** If metoclopramide is administered concurrently with cimetidine, the dose of cimetidine may need to be increased depending on the therapeutic outcome of the combination.

**Summary:** Metoclopramide and cimetidine administration has resulted in a decreased bioavailability of cimetidine.

**Related Drugs:** There are no drugs related to metoclopramide. There is a lack of documentation concerning a similar interaction between other $H_2$-receptor antagonists and metoclopramide.

**Mechanism:** Metoclopramide increases gastric emptying time, and this may decrease cimetidine absorption.

**Detailed Information:** See *EDI*, 18/3.00

## Cimetidine-Praziquantel

**Significance:** 3—minimally clinically significant

**Potential Effects:** The concurrent administration of praziquantel and cimetidine may result in increased praziquantel serum concentrations.

**Recommendations:** Praziquantel serum concentrations should be monitored if cimetidine is added to or removed from concurrent therapy. The concurrent use of cimetidine has been advocated as an adjunct to praziquantel therapy.

**Summary:** Concurrent administration of praziquantel and cimetidine has resulted in increased praziquantel serum concentrations, half-life, and AUC.

**Related Drugs:** Mebendazole serum concentrations increased when administered with cimetidine. Increased serum, bile, and cystic fluid levels of albendazole occurred when given with cimetidine. It is not known whether an interaction would occur between praziquantel and the other $H_2$ receptor antagonists.

**Mechanism:** Although the mechanism of this interaction is not known, cimetidine blocks praziquantel's metabolism in rats, increasing praziquantel bioavailability. Other cytochrome P450 inhibitors (ketoconazole and miconazole) increase the bioavailability of praziquantel.

**Detailed Information:** See *EDI*, 18/3.50

## Cimetidine-Propantheline

**Significance:** 3—minimally clinically significant

**Recommendations:** The concurrent use of these agents need not be avoided. However, if both drugs must be used concomitantly, it may be advisable to separate their administration by as much time as possible to avoid a possible interaction.

**Summary:** There are data to show that propantheline administration may alter cimetidine concentrations; however, these alterations are not very significant.

**Related Drugs:** A similar interaction may occur between cimetidine and other anticholinergics. Ranitidine was shown to act in contrast to cimetidine when administered with propantheline.

**Mechanism:** The reduced bioavailability of cimetidine when administered with propantheline may be a consequence of delayed gastric emptying or decreased intestinal motility.

**Detailed Information:** See *EDI*, 18/4.10

## Miscellaneous

### Clofibrate-Oral Contraceptive Agents
**Significance:** 3—minimally clinically significant
**Recommendations:** Until further studies are done, the concurrent administration of these agents need not be avoided. However, if the antihyperlipidemic effect of clofibrate decreases in the patient receiving concomitant oral contraceptive agents, the dose of clofibrate may need to be increased.
**Summary:** Clofibric acid (a form of clofibrate) clearance was found to be greater in those who were receiving oral contraceptive agents.
**Related Drugs:** There are no drugs related to clofibrate.
**Mechanism:** The oral contraceptive agents may induce the metabolism of clofibric acid.
**Detailed Information:** See *EDI*, 18/4.30

### Clomiphene-Cimetidine
**Significance:** 3—minimally clinically significant
**Potential Effects:** Cimetidine may decrease the ability of clomiphene to stimulate ovulation.
**Recommendations:** The dose of clomiphene may need to be increased in patients receiving cimetidine.
**Summary:** Cimetidine has been shown to reduce the ovulation-stimulatory effects of clomiphene during concurrent administration of these agents.
**Related Drugs:** There is no documentation that other $H_2$-receptor antagonists would interact similarly with clomiphene. There are no drugs related to clomiphene.
**Mechanism:** The mechanism of this interaction is not known.
**Detailed Information:** See *EDI*, 18/4.32

### Cyclosporine-Allopurinol
**Significance:** 2—moderately clinically significant
**Potential Effects:** The addition of allopurinol to a stable cyclosporine regimen may result in increased cyclosporine serum levels.
**Recommendations:** Patients should be closely monitored for changes in cyclosporine levels and renal status when allopurinol is added to therapy. The dose of cyclosporine may need to be decreased.
**Summary:** The addition of allopurinol to the therapy of a patient maintained on cyclosporine resulted in increased cyclosporine levels.
**Related Drugs:** It is unknown if tacrolimus and allopurinol would exhibit the same interaction.
**Mechanism:** The mechanism of this interaction is not known.
**Detailed Information:** See *EDI*, 18/4.38

### Cyclosporine-Azathioprine
**Significance:** 3—minimally clinically significant
**Potential Effects:** Azathioprine administration may decrease cyclosporine absorption and levels.
**Recommendations:** Cyclosporine levels should be monitored if azathioprine is added to, or withdrawn from, therapy. The dose of cyclosporine may need to be adjusted.
**Summary:** Azathioprine and concurrent cyclosporine may result in decreased cyclosporine plasma levels.
**Related Drugs:** There are no drugs related to cyclosporine or azathioprine.
**Mechanism:** Azathioprine is not metabolized by hepatic cytochrome P450, and azathioprine may interfere with cyclosporine absorption.
**Detailed Information:** See *EDI*, 18/4.41

## Miscellaneous

### Cyclosporine-Basiliximab

**Significance:** 2—moderately clinically significant

**Potential Effects:** Concurrent basiliximab and cyclosporine in pediatric patients may increase plasma levels of cyclosporine and decrease cyclosporine dose requirements.

**Recommendations:** Patients should be carefully monitored for possible graft rejection, changes in cyclosporine blood levels or toxic effects with concurrent basiliximab administration.

**Summary:** Two studies in pediatric patients reported that concurrent basiliximab and cyclosporine may increase plasma levels of cyclosporine and decrease cyclosporine dose requirements. Conversely, another study in pediatric patients reported episodes of acute rejection.

**Related Drugs:** There are no immunosuppressive agents pharmacologically related to basiliximab or cyclosporine.

**Mechanism:** The mechanism is thought to involve the effect by basiliximab of an interleukin-2 receptor-induced alteration of cyclosporine metabolism. This is thought to involve cytochrome $P450_{3A4}$ isozymes. Others have mentioned that differences in cyclosporine monitoring and accelerated cyclosporine reduction may have played a role.

**Detailed Information:** See *EDI*, 18/0.60

### Cyclosporine-Carbamazepine

**Significance:** 2—moderately clinically significant

**Potential Effects:** Cyclosporine blood levels may be reduced by concurrent carbamazepine.

**Recommendations:** Cyclosporine blood levels should be monitored if carbamazepine is added to, or deleted from, concurrent therapy. Carbamazepine may need to be discontinued; sodium valproate may be an acceptable alternative therapy.

**Summary:** There are data to show that carbamazepine increased cyclosporine whole blood levels when the carbamazepine was discontinued.

**Related Drugs:** There are no drugs related to carbamazepine or cyclosporine.

**Mechanism:** The reduction in cyclosporine blood levels may be the result of the induction of hepatic cytochrome P450 by carbamazepine.

**Detailed Information:** See *EDI*, 18/4.42

### Cyclosporine-Cholestyramine

**Significance:** 4—not clinically significant

**Potential Effects:** Cholestyramine may reduce cyclosporine absorption, but this has not been documented.

**Recommendations:** Although no interaction was found, cyclosporine levels should be closely monitored during cholestyramine coadministration.

**Summary:** Cholestyramine administration may reduce cyclosporine absorption, but this has not been documented.

**Related Drugs:** Documentation is lacking regarding an interaction between cyclosporine and colestipol. There are no drugs related to cyclosporine.

**Mechanism:** The effect of cholestyramine on cyclosporine absorption is not known. Cholestyramine could interfere with the oral absorption of cyclosporine.

**Detailed Information:** See *EDI*, 18/0.70

Miscellaneous

## Cyclosporine-Hypericum

**Significance:** 2—moderately clinically significant

**Potential Effects:** The addition of St. John's wort (hypericum) to the regimen of a post-transplant patient maintained on cyclosporine may result in decreased cyclosporine blood levels and possible acute transplant rejection.

**Recommendations:** Patients maintained on cyclosporine therapy should be carefully monitored if hypericum is added to or discontinued from concurrent therapy. The dose of cyclosporine may need to be adjusted. If hypericum is added, cyclosporine blood levels may decrease and transplant rejection events may occur. If hypericum is discontinued, cyclosporine blood levels may be increased.

**Summary:** The addition of St. John's wort (*Hypericum perforatum L.*) to the regimen of two post-transplant patients maintained on cyclosporine resulted in decreased cyclosporine blood levels and acute transplant rejection.

**Related Drugs:** There are no drugs related to cyclosporine.

**Mechanism:** St. John's wort is also referred to as hypericum. Hypericum extract has many constituents, with hypericin, a naphthodianthrone, generally considered to be the active ingredient. The naphthodianthrones are known to induce the cytochrome P-450$_{3A}$ isoenzyme that metabolize cyclosporine. It has been suggested that St. John's wort induces intestinal P-glycoprotein drug transporters, which could also contribute to a decrease in cyclosporine oral bioavailability.

**Detailed Information:** See *EDI*, 18/4.44

## Cyclosporine-Methyltestosterone

**Significance:** 2—moderately clinically significant

**Potential Effects:** Cyclosporine levels may be increased by concurrent methyltestosterone use, and hepatic and renal dysfunction may occur even at low doses of cyclosporine.

**Recommendations:** Monitor hepatic and renal function and cyclosporine levels closely if these agents are given together. The dose of methyltestosterone may need to be decreased or the drug may need to be discontinued.

**Summary:** Administration of cyclosporine and methyltestosterone resulted in significant increases in blood levels of cyclosporine. Both severe renal and hepatic dysfunction were reported as a result of this interaction.

**Related Drugs:** Danazole, norethindrone, and oxymetholone have been reported to cause a similar interaction with cyclosporine. If the mechanism involves inhibition of hepatic metabolism of cyclosporine by methyltestosterone, then the other androgens may be expected to interact similarly based on a similar metabolic fate. There is no information on whether this interaction occurs with tacrolimus.

**Mechanism:** It has been suggested that methyltestosterone and other sex steroids may inhibit the hepatic microsomal enzymes responsible for the metabolism of cyclosporine. It has also been suggested that since cyclosporine is eliminated mainly through biliary excretion, reduced bile flow may result in increased cyclosporine levels with subsequent toxicity.

**Detailed Information:** See *EDI*, 18/4.43

## Cyclosporine-Metoclopramide

**Significance:** 2—moderately clinically significant

**Potential Effects:** Metoclopramide may increase the absorption of cyclosporine.

**Recommendations:** Monitor cyclosporine levels closely if the agents must be used together. Concurrent cyclosporine and metoclopramide should be avoided if possible.
**Summary:** There are data to show that metoclopramide may increase bioavailability, peak levels, area-under-curve and absorption, and decrease time to peak of cyclosporine.
**Related Drugs:** There are no drugs related to cyclosporine or metoclopramide.
**Mechanism:** By increasing gastric emptying rate, metoclopramide will increase the delivery of cyclosporine to its absorption site in the small intestine, resulting in increased absorption of cyclosporine.
**Detailed Information:** See *EDI*, 18/4.47

## Cyclosporine-Nafcillin

**Significance:** 2—moderately clinically significant
**Potential Effects:** Nafcillin may induce the metabolism of cyclosporine, leading to decreased levels.
**Recommendations:** Caution should be used when nafcillin therapy is instituted in a patient maintained on cyclosporine. Cyclosporine whole-blood levels may be reduced to subtherapeutic levels.
**Summary:** There are data to show that nafcillin may decrease cyclosporine blood levels.
**Related Drugs:** A similar interaction may occur between cyclosporine and other penicillins that are hepatically metabolized. It is not known whether an interaction would occur between cyclosporine and other penicillins. There are no drugs related to cyclosporine.
**Mechanism:** The enhanced hepatic clearance of cyclosporine may have resulted from cytochrome P450 enzyme induction.
**Detailed Information:** See *EDI*, 18/4.49

## Cyclosporine-Oral Contraceptive Agents

**Significance:** 3—minimally clinically significant
**Potential Effects:** The administration of oral contraceptive agents concurrently with cyclosporine may lead to an increase in cyclosporine levels and hepatotoxicity because of decreased elimination of cyclosporine.
**Recommendations:** Hepatic function should be monitored in patients receiving cyclosporine and oral contraceptive agents concurrently. The cyclosporine serum level and serum creatinine should also be monitored. The cyclosporine dose may need to be decreased.
**Summary:** The concurrent administration of cyclosporine and oral contraceptive agents may increase cyclosporine levels, potentiating the hepatotoxic effects.
**Related Drugs:** There are no drugs related to cyclosporine.
**Mechanism:** Oral contraceptive agents may decrease the elimination of cyclosporine, potentiating the hepatotoxic effect of cyclosporine.
**Detailed Information:** See *EDI*, 18/4.45

## Cyclosporine-Quinine

**Significance:** 2—moderately clinically significant
**Potential Effects:** Quinine may decrease cyclosporine levels by increasing its clearance.
**Recommendations:** The addition of quinine to a cyclosporine regimen should be approached with caution. Cyclosporine blood levels should be monitored, and quinine may have to be discontinued.
**Summary:** The addition of quinine to a cyclosporine regimen may reduce cyclosporine blood levels.

## Miscellaneous

**Related Drugs:** Quinidine is expected to interact with cyclosporine in a similar manner. There are no drugs related to cyclosporine.
**Mechanism:** Quinine could interfere with the bioavailability of cyclosporine or increase its clearance.
**Detailed Information:** See *EDI*, 18/4.48

### Dexamethasone-Aminoglutethimide

**Significance:** 2—moderately clinically significant
**Recommendations:** Patients receiving dexamethasone and aminoglutethimide should be observed and monitored for a decreased effect of dexamethasone. Increasing the dose of dexamethasone or substituting hydrocortisone appears to avoid the interaction.
**Summary:** Aminoglutethimide may cause an increased metabolism of dexamethasone and a reduction in its half-life and bioavailability. This may lead to a decrease in the therapeutic efficacy of dexamethasone.
**Related Drugs:** Because of conflicting results, it is difficult to determine if an interaction would occur between aminoglutethimide and other corticosteroids. A similar interaction may occur between glutethimide and dexamethasone.
**Mechanism:** Aminoglutethimide appears to induce the hepatic enzymes responsible for the metabolism of dexamethasone, reducing the bioavailability of dexamethasone.
**Detailed Information:** See *EDI*, 18/4.50

### Dexamethasone-Ephedrine

**Significance:** 3—minimally clinically significant
**Potential Effects:** Ephedrine may cause an increase in the clearance of dexamethasone.
**Recommendations:** If these agents are used together, the dose of dexamethasone may need to be increased.
**Summary:** There are data to show that ephedrine administration may decrease plasma half-life and increase the metabolic clearance of dexamethasone, decreasing its therapeutic effect.
**Related Drugs:** It is not known if an interaction would occur between dexamethasone and other indirect, direct or mixed acting sympathomimetics, if the mechanism involves increased liver perfusion or hepatic enzyme induction. A similar interaction may occur between ephedrine and other corticosteroids.
**Mechanism:** Ephedrine may increase the hepatic clearance of dexamethasone or induce hepatic microsomal enzymes.
**Detailed Information:** See *EDI*, 18/4.70

### Didanosine-Ganciclovir

**Significance:** 2—moderately clinically significant
**Potential Effects:** Concurrent didanosine and ganciclovir may increase didanosine serum levels.
**Recommendations:** The clinical significance of this interaction has not been determined.
**Summary:** In a study of 11 HIV patients, concurrent administration of didanosine and ganciclovir resulted in increased didanosine serum levels.
**Related Drugs:** It is not known if a similar interaction would occur between didanosine and the other antiviral agents pharmacologically related to ganciclovir (acyclovir, famciclovir, valacyclovir). It is also not known if the other antiretroviral agents will interact with ganciclovir.

**Mechanism:** It is postulated that ganciclovir may compete with didanosine for tubular secretion in the kidney with resultant increases in didanosine serum concentrations.
**Detailed Information:** See *EDI*, 18/4.90

## Dihydroergotamine-Nitroglycerin

**Significance:** 2—moderately clinically significant
**Recommendations:** Patients should be monitored for symptoms of ergotism (e.g., cold, pale, and numb feet and legs, muscle pain, headache, nausea, vomiting) when these agents are used concomitantly. The dosage of dihydroergotamine may need to be reduced in some patients.
**Summary:** There are data to show that nitroglycerin administration may cause the ergotism, secondary to an increased dihydroergotamine response, necessitating a decrease in dose.
**Related Drugs:** Ergoloid mesylates may interact with nitroglycerin in a similar manner. Other nitrates may interact similarly with the ergot alkaloids.
**Mechanism:** Nitroglycerin may decrease the first-pass metabolism of dihydroergotamine and increase its bioavailability.
**Detailed Information:** See *EDI*, 18/5.00

## Dobutamine-Cimetidine

**Significance:** 3—minimally clinically significant
**Potential Effects:** The effect of dobutamine may be exaggerated.
**Recommendations:** Patients maintained on cimetidine should be carefully monitored if dobutamine is administered, since the effect of dobutamine may be increased. The dose of dobutamine may need to be decreased to attain the expected effect.
**Summary:** Cimetidine has been shown to increase dobutamine response.
**Related Drugs:** It is not known whether an interaction would occur between cimetidine and other direct-acting sympathomimetics or between dobutamine and other $H_2$-receptor antagonists.
**Mechanism:** The exaggerated dobutamine response may be due to impaired dobutamine metabolism, resulting from cimetidine-induced inhibition of the hepatic mixed function oxidase system.
**Detailed Information:** See *EDI*, 18/6.50

## Ergonovine-Dopamine

**Significance:** 2—moderately clinically significant
**Recommendations:** Although limited documentation is available, it indicates that concurrent use of these agents should be avoided if possible. Hypertension that resulted from the use of these agents was successfully treated with chlorpromazine.
**Summary:** An isolated case report suggested that the vasoconstrictive properties of ergonovine and dopamine may be additive, leading to an increased incidence of gangrene.
**Related Drugs:** Other reports are lacking of similar interactions between other mixed acting sympathomimetic amines and other ergot alkaloids; however, an interaction may be expected to occur.
**Mechanism:** The interaction probably results from the synergistic peripheral vasoconstriction activity of both agents.
**Detailed Information:** See *EDI*, 18/7.00

## Miscellaneous

### Fat Emulsion, Intravenous-Cyclosporine
**Significance:** 2—moderately clinically significant
**Potential Effects:** The addition of intravenous fat emulsion to cyclosporine therapy may result in increased cyclosporine levels and toxicity.
**Recommendations:** Because of the changes in levels of serum lipoproteins that accompany the intravenous administration of fat emulsions, the use of these agents should be avoided in patients on cyclosporine therapy.
**Summary:** The addition of intravenous fat emulsion to patients maintained on cyclosporine may result in increased cyclosporine levels and toxicity.
**Related Drugs:** There are no drugs related to cyclosporine or fat emulsion.
**Mechanism:** Cyclosporine is lipophilic and it will bind to the components in the intravenous fat emulsion.
**Detailed Information:** See *EDI*, 18/8.20

### Foscarnet-Cyclosporine
**Significance:** 2—moderately clinically significant
**Potential Effects:** Concurrent use of cyclosporine and foscarnet may result in reversible acute renal failure.
**Recommendations:** Patients receiving concurrent therapy with cyclosporine and foscarnet should be monitored for a decrease in renal function. Foscarnet may need to be discontinued.
**Summary:** In two case reports, concurrent use of cyclosporine and foscarnet may have resulted in reversible acute renal failure without a significant increase in cyclosporine concentration.
**Related Drugs:** It is not known whether there is an interaction between foscarnet and tacrolimus.
**Mechanism:** It was proposed that the reversible acute renal failure may be due to additive or synergistic nephrotoxic effects of cyclosporine and foscarnet.
**Detailed Information:** See *EDI*, 18/8.40

### Glycopyrrolate-Ritodrine
**Significance:** 2—moderately clinically significant
**Potential Effects:** Ritodrine may potentiate the effect of glycopyrrolate on heart rate, possibly leading to severe tachycardia.
**Recommendations:** Caution should be exercised in patients who are receiving, or have recently received, ritodrine if glycopyrrolate is to be given.
**Summary:** There are data to show that ritodrine administration may potentiate the effect of glycopyrrolate on heart rate, possibly leading to severe tachycardia.
**Related Drugs:** The other anticholinergic agents may interact in a similar manner with ritodrine. Other sympathomimetic agents may potentiate the cardiovascular effect of glycopyrrolate.
**Mechanism:** Ritodrine has been implicated in tachyarrhythmias, and glycopyrrolate may increase heart rate because of its parasympatholytic effects.
**Detailed Information:** See *EDI*, 18/8.50

### Hydrocortisone-Cholestyramine
**Significance:** 3—minimally clinically significant
**Recommendations:** Patients should be observed for a change in their clinical response to the corticosteroid, and an increase in the dose may be necessary.

## Miscellaneous

**Summary:** Cholestyramine has been shown to cause a reduction in the hydrocortisone plasma concentration area-under-curve.
**Related Drugs:** Because of conflicting data, it would be difficult to determine if a similar interaction would occur between cholestyramine and other corticosteroids. Documentation is lacking regarding an interaction with colestipol.
**Mechanism:** Cholestyramine has been demonstrated to bind hydrocortisone and may also decrease and delay the absorption of hydrocortisone.
**Detailed Information:** See *EDI*, 18/9.00

## Indinavir-Carbamazepine

**Significance:** 2—moderately clinically significant
**Potential Effects:** The concurrent administration of indinavir and carbamazepine may result in higher than anticipated carbamazepine levels, decreased indinavir plasma concentrations, and antiretroviral therapy failure.
**Recommendations:** Concurrent use of carbamazepine and indinavir should be avoided. When alternate therapy is not possible, indinavir levels and antiretroviral response should be closely monitored. Carbamazepine levels should also be monitored.
**Summary:** Concurrent administration of indinavir and carbamazepine resulted in high carbamazepine levels, decreased indinavir plasma concentrations, and antiretroviral therapy failure.
**Related Drugs:** Based on the postulated mechanism, an interaction would be expected to occur between carbamazepine and the other protease inhibitors, as well as between indinavir or ritonavir with oxcarbazepine.
**Mechanism:** Although the mechanism of this interaction is not known, it has been postulated that carbamazepine may induce cytochrome $P450_{3A4}$, increasing the metabolism of indinavir, and that, in a single case study, ritonavir might have inhibited carbamazepine metabolism. This was based on *in vitro* data that reported a 100-fold stronger inhibitor effect for ritonavir on the cytochrome $P450_{3A4}$ subsystem than that noted for saquinavir. However, an interaction involving both of these protease inhibitors cannot be totally excluded.
**Detailed Information:** See *EDI*, 18/9.15

## Indinavir-Hypericum

**Significance:** 2—moderately clinically significant
**Potential Effects:** The addition of St. John's wort (hypericum) to a concurrent indinavir regimen may result in decreased indinavir serum levels. This could lead to the development of drug resistance and possible treatment failure.
**Recommendations:** Hypericum should be avoided in patients receiving indinavir as their sole protease inhibitor. Since other protease inhibitors are metabolized in a fashion similar to indinavir, in the absence of definitive data it would be prudent to also avoid concurrent hypericum with these agents.
**Summary:** The addition of St. John's wort (*Hypericum perforatum L.*) to a concurrent indinavir regimen resulted in decreased indinavir serum levels. This could lead to the development of drug resistance and possible treatment failure.
**Related Drugs:** An interaction would be expected to occur between hypericum and the other protease inhibitors that also inhibit the cytochrome $P450_{3A4}$ isoenzyme.

## Miscellaneous

**Mechanism:** St. John's wort is also referred to as hypericum. Hypericum extract has many constituents, with hypericin, a naphthodianthrone, considered to be the active ingredient. The naphthodianthrones induce the cytochrome $P450_{3A}$ isoenzyme. The protease inhibitors all inhibit and induce cytochrome $P450_{3A4}$. Ritonavir is one of the most potent inhibitors of this isoenzyme. It has been suggested that cytochrome $P450_{3A4}$ induction is the mechanism for the decrease in indinavir serum levels when given concurrently with hypericum.
**Detailed Information:** See *EDI*, 18/9.20

## Indinavir-Omeprazole

**Significance:** 3—minimally clinically significant
**Potential Effects:** The concurrent use of indinavir and omeprazole may have resulted in decreased indinavir levels in some patients.
**Recommendations:** Patients receiving concurrent therapy with indinavir and a proton pump inhibitor should be monitored for decreased indinavir levels and antiviral effects of indinavir. The dosage of indinavir may need to be adjusted or the proton pump inhibitor may need to be discontinued.
**Summary:** The concurrent use of indinavir and omeprazole resulted in decreased indinavir levels in some patients. It was also noted that there was a large interindividual variability in indinavir levels among the subjects in the retrospective review.
**Related Drugs:** Although documentation is lacking, a similar interaction would be expected between indinavir and the other proton pump inhibitors based on the proposed mechanism and pharmacologic similarity. It is not known whether omeprazole would interact with the other protease inhibitors.
**Mechanism:** An omeprazole-induced increase in gastric pH may have decreased the solubility, and therefore absorption, of indinavir and the omeprazole may have induced indinavir metabolism by the cytochrome $P450_{3A}$ isoenzyme. Omeprazole has been shown *in vitro* to be a mixed inducer of cytochrome $P450_{3A}$. Interpatient variability of indinavir levels may also be a factor.
**Detailed Information:** See *EDI*, 18/9.30

## Levodopa-Aluminum Hydroxide, Magnesium Hydroxide

**Significance:** 3—minimally clinically significant
**Recommendations:** The addition of an antacid containing aluminum hydroxide and magnesium hydroxide 30 minutes before levodopa therapy may allow the dosage of levodopa to be decreased in some patients, thus minimizing gastrointestinal side effects. Other patients refractory to levodopa therapy may benefit as well. If this interaction is not desired, separating the dosage of these agents by as much time as possible or decreasing the dose of levodopa may be necessary.
**Summary:** Antacids containing aluminum hydroxide and magnesium hydroxide may enhance the rate of absorption of levodopa.
**Related Drugs:** A similar interaction may occur between levodopa and other antacids. There are no drugs related to levodopa.
**Mechanism:** Antacids may increase gastric emptying time, decreasing levodopa's gastric metabolism and leading to increased levels in the central nervous system.
**Detailed Information:** See *EDI*, 18/10.10

## Miscellaneous

### Levodopa-Domperidone
**Significance:** 3—minimally clinically significant
**Potential Effects:** This agent also reduces the incidence of gastrointestinal side effects of levodopa and may enable a higher optimum levodopa dose. Domperidone results in increased levodopa plasma concentrations.
**Recommendations:** No precautions are necessary regarding the concurrent use of levodopa and domperidone.
**Summary:** There are data to show that domperidone administration can increase levodopa plasma concentrations.
**Related Drugs:** There are no drugs related to levodopa or domperidone.
**Mechanism:** The mechanism of this interaction is unknown.
**Detailed Information:** See *EDI*, 18/10.21

### Levodopa-Ferrous Sulfate
**Significance:** 2—moderately clinically significant
**Potential Effects:** Ferrous sulfate may chelate with levodopa, leading to decreased levodopa levels.
**Recommendations:** Patients should be monitored closely if ferrous sulfate is added to, or withdrawn from, concomitant therapy with levodopa. The dose of levodopa may need to be adjusted.
**Summary:** There are data to show that ferrous sulfate administration may chelate with levodopa, reducing levodopa bioavailability and levels.
**Related Drugs:** An interaction would be expected to occur between levodopa and other oral ferrous salts. There are no drugs related to levodopa.
**Mechanism:** This mechanism is similar to the one that causes a decrease in the absorption of methyldopa with concurrent ferrous sulfate (see Methyldopa-Ferrous Sulfate, page 173). Ferrous sulfate may decrease levodopa absorption by chelation.
**Detailed Information:** See *EDI*, 18/10.25

### Levodopa, Benserazide-Orphenadrine
**Significance:** 3—minimally clinically significant
**Potential Effects:** Concurrent levodopa/benserazide and orphenadrine may result in erratic absorption of levodopa, resulting in impaired motor responses.
**Recommendations:** Therapeutic response to levodopa/benserazide should be carefully evaluated and monitored with concurrent orphenadrine therapy for parkinsonism.
**Summary:** A study showed that administering orphenadrine with levodopa/benserazide results in variable levodopa absorption and therapeutic response.
**Related Drugs:** There is no information on whether orphenadrine interacts with carbidopa/levodopa.
**Mechanism:** The proposed mechanism may be related to anticholinergic effects on gastric motility leading to erratic absorption; however, the exact mechanism is unknown.
**Detailed Information:** See *EDI*, 18/10.27

### Levodopa-Papaverine
**Significance:** 3—minimally clinically significant
**Potential Effects:** Papaverine may block the effects of levodopa, causing a worsening of parkinsonism.
**Recommendations:** Patients should be monitored for worsening of the symptoms of Parkinson's disease when papaverine is added to levodopa therapy. The dose of levodopa may need to be increased.

## Miscellaneous

**Summary:** There are data to show that concurrent papaverine and levodopa therapy will result in the antagonism of levodopa's pharmacologic effect.

**Related Drugs:** A similar interaction is expected to occur between levodopa and ethaverine. There are no drugs related to levodopa.

**Mechanism:** The antagonism in this interaction may be due to papaverine blocking the dopamine receptors in the striatum.

**Detailed Information:** See *EDI*, 18/10.30

### Levodopa-Trihexyphenidyl

**Significance:** 4—not clinically significant

**Potential Effects:** Trihexyphenidyl may decrease levodopa levels; however, this has not been demonstrated in humans.

**Recommendations:** No precautions need be made for patients receiving concurrent levodopa and trihexyphenidyl. Patients maintained on levodopa may need to be monitored if trihexyphenidyl is added to, or withdrawn from, therapy. The dose of levodopa may need to be adjusted.

**Summary:** The effectiveness of levodopa may be decreased by the addition of trihexyphenidyl; however, this has not been demonstrated in humans.

**Related Drugs:** It is not known if an interaction would occur between levodopa and other anticholinergic agents. There are no drugs related to levodopa.

**Mechanism:** When gastric emptying is prolonged, the metabolism of levodopa by gastric mucosa may be increased, and this may decrease the plasma levodopa levels.

**Detailed Information:** See *EDI*, 18/10.50

### Levothyroxine-Calcium Carbonate

**Significance:** 3—minimally clinically significant

**Potential Effects:** Simultaneous ingestion of calcium carbonate formulations and sodium levothyroxine may result in increased serum thyroid stimulating hormone levels and reduced levothyroxine efficacy.

**Recommendations:** If concurrent use of the agents is necessary, separating the administration by at least four hours should maintain levothyroxine efficacy.

**Summary:** Simultaneous ingestion of calcium carbonate formulations and sodium levothyroxine reduced levothyroxine efficacy. However, conflicting data are available.

**Related Drugs:** Based on structural and pharmacologic similarity and the proposed mechanism, an interaction may be expected to occur between levothyroxine and the other orally administered calcium compounds and between the other orally administered calcium compounds and other thyroid preparations.

**Mechanism:** It is thought that calcium carbonate might form insoluble chelates with levothyroxine. This would lead to decreased levothyroxine bioavailability. The formation of insoluble complexes has been shown to occur between levothyroxine and ferrous sulfate.

**Detailed Information:** See *EDI*, 18/10.70

### Levothyroxine-Ferrous Sulfate

**Significance:** 3—minimally clinically significant

**Potential Effects:** Concurrent ferrous sulfate and levothyroxine may result in a reduction in levothyroxine efficacy.

**Recommendations:** If concurrent therapy with these two agents is necessary, it may be possible to reduce the extent of the iron-levothyroxine interaction by separating the administration times of the medications by two or more hours. Routine thyroid function monitoring should also be undertaken.

**Summary:** There are data to show that ferrous sulfate may cause a reduction in levothyroxine efficacy.

**Related Drugs:** An interaction may occur between levothyroxine and other orally administered iron compounds and between ferrous sulfate and other thyroid drugs.

**Mechanism:** The formation of an insoluble ferric-levothyroxine complex may reduce the absorption of levothyroxine.

**Detailed Information:** See *EDI,* 18/11.05

## Levothyroxine-Lovastatin

**Significance:** 3—minimally clinically significant

**Potential Effects:** The addition of lovastatin to, or withdrawal from, levothyroxine therapy may result in a change in serum thyroxine levels.

**Recommendations:** A patient maintained on levothyroxine should be carefully monitored for changes in serum thyroxine levels if lovastatin is added to, or deleted from, cotherapy.

**Summary:** There are data to show that increases in the serum thyroxine levels have been documented when lovastatin is given concomitantly with levothyroxine.

**Related Drugs:** All thyroid compounds structurally similar to levothyroxine may interact with lovastatin. A similar interaction would be expected to occur between levothyroxine and the other HMG-CoA reductase inhibitors, although documentation is lacking.

**Mechanism:** A synergism may occur between lovastatin and levothyroxine, causing myolysis mediated by the thyrotoxic state.

**Detailed Information:** See *EDI,* 18/11.00

## Levothyroxine-Sucralfate

**Significance:** 3—minimally clinically significant

**Potential Effects:** Administration of sucralfate and levothyroxine at the same time may decrease the absorption of levothyroxine.

**Recommendations:** Patients receiving concurrent levothyroxine and sucralfate should be monitored for decreased response to thyroid hormone replacement therapy. Adjustment of levothyroxine dosage, separating the administration of these agents by several hours, or alternative therapy for sucralfate may need to be considered.

**Summary:** Three case reports and a follow-up study describe concurrent levothyroxine and sucralfate administration that resulted in decreased levothyroxine absorption. However, other reports in the literature dispute these findings.

**Related Drugs:** An aluminum hydroxide-containing antacid caused elevated levels of thyroid stimulating hormone (TSH) in a patient stabilized for five years on levothyroxine. Discontinuation returned TSH levels to normal, but two individual rechallenges with the antacid produced similar results. An interaction would be expected to occur between levothyroxine and other aluminum-containing compounds.

**Mechanism:** The exact mechanism for this interaction is unknown. One possible mechanism is the interference of either intraluminal or transintestinal transport of the levothyroxine by sucralfate. Another possible mechanism is the binding of levothyroxine to sucralfate or aluminum. Sucralfate has been shown to bind levothyroxine *in vitro,* and other studies have reported that aluminum hydroxide has a considerable nonspecific absorptive capacity for levothyroxine.

**Detailed Information:** See *EDI,* 18/11.20

## Miscellaneous

### Lovastatin-Cyclosporine

**Significance:** 2—moderately clinically significant

**Potential Effects:** Concurrent use of these agents may result in myolysis.

**Recommendations:** Concurrent use of lovastatin and cyclosporine should be approached with caution. If possible, lovastatin levels should be monitored and patients should be instructed to report any unexplained muscle pain, tenderness, or weakness. Pravastatin appears to have the lowest propensity to cause myopathy in cyclosporine-treated patients and can be safely used in these patients provided it is administered in moderated doses and with careful monitoring of liver and renal functions, and provided that there is a synergistic immunosuppressive effect with concurrent pravastatin and cyclosporine. Pravastatin or fluvastatin may be alternatives to lovastatin.

**Summary:** Concurrent administration of lovastatin and cyclosporine has resulted in myolysis.

**Related Drugs:** Patients receiving concurrent cyclosporine and simvastatin have required hospitalization due to significantly decreased cyclosporine clearance and increased lactate dehydrogenase levels (indicative of tissue injury) following the addition of cyclosporine to a simvastatin regimen. Conversely, no significant alteration in cyclosporine levels and no rhabdomyolysis were seen in other studies. Increases in the mean simvastatin AUC and simvastatin maximum concentration ($C_{max}$) were observed in patients receiving concurrent cyclosporine and simvastatin. Three cases of rhabdomyolysis occurred during concurrent administration of simvastatin and cyclosporine in cardiac transplant patients. No changes in cyclosporine pharmacokinetics have occurred with concurrent pravastatin; however, concurrent cyclosporine administration resulted in approximately a five-fold to seven-fold increase in pravastatin AUC values. No rhabdomyolysis occurred in 40 cardiac transplant recipients receiving pravastatin and cyclosporine during a one-year post-transplant follow-up period. Fluvastatin was judged to be safe and effective with concurrent cyclosporine.

**Mechanism:** Although lovastatin may cause myolysis and increased creatinine kinase when administered alone, cyclosporine may increase lovastatin levels, thereby increasing the incidence of myolysis. Lovastatin and cyclosporine are both substrates of cytochrome $P450_{3A}$ isoenzymes. Since both are hepatically metabolized, there may be a reduced clearance or decreased first-pass extraction of lovastatin. Because it is unlikely that cytochrome isozymes significantly contribute to pravastatin elimination, it can be speculated that cyclosporine interacts with pravastatin transport processes.

**Detailed Information:** See *EDI*, 18/12.01

### Lovastatin-Diltiazem

**Significance:** 2—moderately clinically significant

**Potential Effects:** The concurrent administration of lovastatin and diltiazem may result in elevated levels of lovastatin.

**Recommendations:** Patients receiving concurrent therapy with lovastatin and diltiazem should be carefully monitored for increased lovastatin serum levels and possible adverse reactions. A reduction of the dose of lovastatin may need to be considered.

**Summary:** Pretreatment with diltiazem resulted in increases in the lovastatin AUC and maximum concentration ($C_{max}$) by 2.6-fold and 3.3-fold, respectively.

**Related Drugs:** Pretreatment with verapamil has caused an increase in the AUC and Cmax of simvastatin and simvastatin acid with a 2.1-

fold variation in the AUC of verapamil. There was a significant positive correlation between the AUC of verapamil and the ratio of simvastatin Cmax in the verapamil phase to the simvastatin $C_{max}$ value in the placebo phase. Pretreatment with diltiazem had no effect on pravastatin pharmacokinetics. An interaction might occur between lovastatin and calcium channel blocking agents that inhibit cytochrome $P450_{3A4}$ isoenzymes. It is not known whether an interaction would occur between lovastatin and the other calcium channel blocking agents; however, an interaction may occur between diltiazem and other HMG-CoA reductase inhibitors whose metabolism is mediated by cytochrome $P450_{3A4}$ isoenzymes.

**Mechanism:** Although the mechanism of this interaction is not known, it may occur as a result of diltiazem inhibition of cytochrome $P450_{3A4}$-mediated lovastatin metabolism.

**Detailed Information:** See *EDI*, 18/12.02

## Lovastatin-Erythromycin

**Significance:** 1—highly clinically significant

**Potential Effects:** Concurrent administration of lovastatin and erythromycin may result in increased lovastatin levels and rhabdomyolysis.

**Recommendations:** Extreme caution should be exercised when administering these two agents concurrently. If alternative antimicrobials or temporary discontinuation of lovastatin is not possible, patients should be instructed to report any unexplained muscle pain, tenderness, or weakness.

**Summary:** Concurrent administration of lovastatin and erythromycin may result in increased lovastatin levels to as high as 97.6 ng equivalent/ml (normal: approximately 12.2 ng equivalent/ml) and rhabdomyolysis.

**Related Drugs:** Similar interactions have been reported between lovastatin and clarithromycin and between atorvastatin and erythromycin. *In vitro*, the metabolism of cerivastatin was inhibited in the presence of troleandomycin. Since pravastatin is not metabolized by the cytochrome $P450_{3A}$ system, it would not be expected to interact with the macrolide antibiotics. An interaction would be expected between atorvastatin, lovastatin, simvastatin, or cerivastatin and the other macrolide antibiotics as well as between the macrolides and the other HMG-CoA reductase inhibitors.

**Mechanism:** Atorvastatin, cerivastatin, lovastatin, and simvastatin are metabolized by the cytochrome $P450_{3A}$ isoenzyme system. Erythromycin may affect the metabolism of these agents either by competitive or noncompetitive inhibition.

**Detailed Information:** See *EDI*, 18/12.05

## Lovastatin-Gemfibrozil

**Significance:** 2—moderately clinically significant

**Potential Effects:** Concurrent use of these agents may result in myolysis.

**Recommendations:** Concurrent use of lovastatin and gemfibrozil should be approached with caution. Patients should be instructed to report any unexplained muscle pain, tenderness, weakness, or discolored urine. Alternative therapy may need to be considered.

**Summary:** Concurrent use of lovastatin and gemfibrozil may result in rhabdomyolysis and acute renal failure.

**Related Drugs:** Subjects receiving combined therapy with pravastatin and gemfibrozil had creatine kinase elevations and musculoskeletal symptoms; severe myopathies did not occur. Rhabdomyolosis has been related to the concurrent use of gemfibrozil and atorvastatin, simvastatin, and pravastatin. No interaction has been seen between gemfibrozil and fluvastatin. An interaction would be expected to occur between gemfibrozil and cerivastatin or between lovastatin and the other fibric acid derivatives.

**Mechanism:** Although lovastatin administration alone has been reported to cause myolysis and increased creatine kinase, gemfibrozil may increase the incidence by an unknown mechanism.

**Detailed Information:** See *EDI*, 18/12.03

## Lovastatin-Grapefruit Juice

**Significance:** 1—highly clinically significant

**Potential Effects:** The concurrent administration of lovastatin and grapefruit juice may result in increased serum concentrations of lovastatin and its active metabolite.

**Recommendations:** The administration of grapefruit juice during therapy with lovastatin should be avoided.

**Summary:** Concurrent administration of lovastatin and grapefruit juice resulted in greatly increased serum concentrations of lovastatin and lovastatin acid, its active metabolite.

**Related Drugs:** Based on the postulated mechanism and pharmacologic similarity, an interaction may be expected to occur between grapefruit juice and the HMG-CoA reductase inhibitors simvastatin, atorvastatin, and cerivastatin provided the metabolism of these agents involves cytochrome $P450_{3A4}$ inhibition. It is not known whether an interaction would occur between grapefruit juice and pravastatin or fluvastatin.

**Mechanism:** The mechanism probably involves bioflavonoids present in grapefruit juice. Grapefruit juice selectively down-regulates cytochrome $P450_{3A4}$ in the small intestine, where this isoenzyme is extensively expressed. This prevents presystemic metabolism mediated by cytochrome $P450_{3A4}$. Even though the hydrolysis of lovastatin to lovastatin acid is not mediated by cytochrome $P450_{3A4}$, the concentration of lovastatin acid increases with the level of lovastatin. Cytochrome $P450_{3A4}$ also plays an important role in the metabolism of the HMG-CoA reductase inhibitors simvastatin and atorvastatin. However, other enzymes are mainly responsible for the metabolism of pravastatin and fluvastatin. It has been demonstrated that the metabolic pathways involved in cerivastatin first-pass metabolism are insensitive to those cytochrome P450 isozymes induced by cimetidine (2C8-10, 2D6, 3A3); however, other investigators have found that cytochrome P450 isoenzymes play a major role in cerivastatin metabolism.

**Detailed Information:** See *EDI*, 18/12.04

## Lovastatin-Nicotinic Acid

**Significance:** 2—moderately clinically significant

**Potential Effects:** Concurrent use of these agents may result in myolysis.

**Recommendations:** If concurrent therapy of these agents is required, patients should be monitored for signs of myolysis.

**Summary:** The concurrent use of these agents may result in an increased incidence of myolysis.

**Related Drugs:** There are no drugs related to lovastatin or nicotinic acid.

**Mechanism:** Lovastatin has been reported to cause myolysis and increased creatine kinase; however, the mechanism of this interaction is not known.

**Detailed Information:** See *EDI*, 18/12.07

## Magnesium Hydroxide-Sodium Polystyrene Sulfonate

**Significance:** 2—moderately clinically significant

**Recommendations:** The concurrent use of magnesium hydroxide-containing antacids and sodium polystyrene sulfonate should be avoided, if possible, in patients with renal disease. However, if the combined use of these agents is necessary, separate their administration by several hours.

**Summary:** It has been documented in two patients with renal disease that metabolic alkalosis occurred in one patient and metabolic acidosis was reversed in the other after concurrent administration of sodium polystyrene sulfonate and an antacid containing magnesium hydroxide.

**Related Drugs:** The concurrent use of other combination antacids and sodium polystyrene sulfonate has been documented to result in a rapid alkalinization of the blood. There are no drugs related to sodium polystyrene sulfonate.

**Mechanism:** In the presence of sodium polystyrene sulfonate, the magnesium chloride interacts and bicarbonate is secreted in the small bowel and reabsorbed, leading to metabolic alkalosis.

**Detailed Information:** See *EDI,* 18/12.10

## Medroxyprogesterone-Aminoglutethimide

**Significance:** 3—minimally clinically significant

**Recommendations:** Patients receiving these agents concurrently should be monitored for a decrease in the therapeutic efficacy of medroxyprogesterone. A high dose of medroxyprogesterone may be necessary.

**Summary:** There are data to show that aminoglutethimide may decrease the therapeutic efficacy of medroxyprogesterone; however, there are conflicting data.

**Related Drugs:** An interaction may occur between aminoglutethimide and other progestins. A similar interaction is expected to occur between medroxyprogesterone and glutethimide.

**Mechanism:** Aminoglutethimide may induce the hepatic enzymes responsible for medroxyprogesterone metabolism.

**Detailed Information:** See *EDI,* 18/12.30

## Metoclopramide-Atropine

**Significance:** 3—minimally clinically significant

**Recommendations:** Since these agents antagonize the pharmacologic effect of one another, their concurrent use should be avoided. If the two drugs are to be used, metoclopramide should precede atropine by two hours.

**Summary:** These agents are antagonists. When metoclopramide was given first, atropine reversed metoclopramide. When atropine was given first, metoclopramide reversed the atropine-induced depression of sphincter pressure.

**Related Drugs:** A similar interaction is expected to occur between metoclopramide and other anticholinergics. There are no drugs related to metoclopramide.

**Mechanism:** It is postulated that metoclopramide may lead to an increase in lower esophageal sphincter pressure, which may be antagonized or potentiated by effects on cholinergic receptors.

**Detailed Information:** See *EDI,* 18/13.00

## Metoclopramide-Levodopa

**Significance:** 3—minimally clinically significant

**Recommendations:** The evidence suggests that a competitive antagonism is possible with the coadministration of these two agents. Therefore, patients should be monitored for such an interaction, with an appropriate adjustment made in the dosage of levodopa if necessary.

**Summary:** There is evidence that the concurrent use of levodopa will reverse some of the pharmacologic activities of metoclopramide.

**Related Drugs:** There are no drugs related to metoclopramide or levodopa.

**Mechanism:** Metoclopramide is a dopaminergic antagonist and levodopa, the precursor of dopamine, apparently antagonizes by inhibiting the action of metoclopramide.

**Detailed Information:** See *EDI*, 18/15.00

## Metronidazole-Cyclosporine

**Significance:** 3—minimally clinically significant

**Potential Effects:** The addition of metronidazole to the therapy of a patient maintained on cyclosporine may increase cyclosporine whole blood levels.

**Recommendations:** Patients' renal function and cyclosporine trough concentrations should be carefully monitored during concurrent cyclosporine and metronidazole therapy. The dosage of cyclosporine may need to be adjusted during and following the completion of metronidazole therapy.

**Summary:** The addition of metronidazole to the therapy of two patients maintained on cyclosporine resulted in increased cyclosporine whole blood levels.

**Related Drugs:** There are no drugs related to cyclosporine or metronidazole.

**Mechanism:** Metronidazole may inhibit the hepatic metabolism of cyclosporine by the cytochrome $P450_{3A4}$ isoenzyme.

**Detailed Information:** See *EDI*, 18/15.40

## Metyrapone-Phenytoin

**Significance:** 3—minimally clinically significant

**Potential Effects:** The addition of oral metyrapone may elicit a subnormal response resulting from decreased metyrapone blood levels in subjects maintained on phenytoin.

**Recommendations:** Invalid results for the metapyrone test may occur in patients maintained on phenytoin. Doubling the metyrapone dose has produced valid results.

**Summary:** The addition of oral metyrapone elicited a subnormal response resulting from decreased metyrapone blood levels in subjects maintained on phenytoin.

**Related Drugs:** Although no documentation exists for a similar interaction between metyrapone and the other hydantoin anticonvulsants, one would be expected based on structural and pharmacologic similarity. There are no drugs related to metyrapone.

**Mechanism:** It is postulated that phenytoin induced hepatic enzymes, resulting in an increased metyrapone metabolism.

**Detailed Information:** See *EDI*, 18/15.50

## Misoprostol-Aluminum Hydroxide, Magnesium Hydroxide

**Significance:** 3—minimally clinically significant

**Potential Effects:** The antacid may decrease the bioavailability of misoprostol.

**Recommendations:** The concurrent use of misoprostol and an aluminum/magnesium hydroxide antacid should be approached with caution. The efficacy of misoprostol may be decreased.

**Summary:** There are data to show that administration of misoprostol

## Miscellaneous

with an aluminum-magnesium hydroxide antacid will result in the reduced bioavailability of misoprostol.

**Related Drugs:** It is not known whether an interaction would occur between misoprostol and other antacids that contain aluminum or magnesium. There are no drugs related to misoprostol.

**Mechanism:** This interaction is believed to result from the decreased bioavailability of misoprostol.

**Detailed Information:** See *EDI*, 18/16.03

## Mycophenolate-Cyclosporine

**Significance:** 3—minimally clinically significant

**Potential Effects:** Discontinuation of cyclosporine from an immunosuppressive therapy regimen that also included mycophenolate mofetil and prednisone may result in significantly elevated mycophenolic acid trough levels.

**Recommendations:** Patients maintained on concomitant mycophenolate mofetil and cyclosporine should be monitored for side effects if cyclosporine is discontinued.

**Summary:** Discontinuation of cyclosporine from an immunosuppressive therapy regimen that also included mycophenolate mofetil and prednisone resulted in significantly elevated mycophenolic acid trough levels.

**Related Drugs:** There are no drugs related to mycophenolate or cyclosporine.

**Mechanism:** It has been postulated that cyclosporine might decrease the amount of glucuronidase producing bacteria in the gut, resulting in less deglucuronidation of the mycophenolic acid glucuronide. The discontinuation of cyclosporine might result in restoration of the normal bacterial flora of the gut, leading to increased deglucuronidation and an increased amount of mycophenolic acid available for reabsorption.

**Detailed Information:** See *EDI*, 18/16.04

## Nizatidine-Charcoal

**Significance:** 3—minimally clinically significant

**Potential Effects:** Charcoal adsorbs nizatidine, reducing its absorption.

**Recommendations:** Separate administration time as much as possible, unless the charcoal is being used to treat nizatidine overdose.

**Summary:** There are data to show that charcoal adsorbs nizatidine and reduces its absorption.

**Related Drugs:** There is no documentation of an interaction between charcoal and other $H_2$-receptor antagonists. There are no drugs related to charcoal.

**Mechanism:** Charcoal adsorbs nizatidine in the gastrointestinal tract, preventing the absorption of nizatidine.

**Detailed Information:** See *EDI*, 18/16.05

## Octreotide-Cyclosporine

**Significance:** 2—moderately clinically significant

**Potential Effects:** The concurrent administration of octreotide and cyclosporine resulted in a decrease in cyclosporine levels, which may lead to graft rejection episodes.

**Recommendations:** The concurrent administration of octreotide and cyclosporine should be approached with caution. Cyclosporine levels should be closely monitored in patients receiving concurrent therapy with octreotide and cyclosporine. The dosage of cyclosporine may need to be adjusted if octreotide is added to or

## Miscellaneous

discontinued from cyclosporine therapy. Octreotide may need to be discontinued. Supplementation with intravenous cyclosporine may not increase cyclosporine levels in all patients.

**Summary:** Concurrent administration of octreotide and cyclosporine resulted in a decrease in cyclosporine levels, which led to graft rejection episodes.

**Related Drugs:** There are no drugs related to either cyclosporine or octreotide.

**Mechanism:** The exact mechanism is not known. Octreotide may delay or inhibit the intestinal absorption of cyclosporine or may interfere with the enterohepatic circulation of cyclosporine.

**Detailed Information:** See *EDI*, 18/16.06

## Omeprazole-Clarithromycin

**Significance:** 3—minimally clinically significant

**Potential Effects:** The concurrent use of omeprazole and clarithromycin may result in increased serum levels for both agents.

**Recommendations:** The concurrent use of these agents may be advantageous, leading to increased tissue levels of the antibiotic. This combination may be especially effective against Helicobacter pylori infection.

**Summary:** Concurrent administration of omeprazole and clarithromycin resulted in increased serum levels for both agents.

**Related Drugs:** Lansoprazole has also been reported to interact with clarithromycin, causing glossitis, stomatitis, and/or black tongue. Although there is no documentation regarding an interaction between omeprazole and the other macrolide antibiotics that form inactive cytochrome P450 metabolite complexes to some extent (erythromycin, troleandomycin, josamycin), if the mechanism involves inhibition of the cytochrome $P450_{3A}$ isozyme, then an interaction would be expected to occur that may result in increased levels of one or both interacting agents. The macrolides that form inactive cytochrome P450 metabolite complexes (spiramycin, dirithromycin, azithromycin) would not be expected to affect the serum level of omeprazole based on the postulated mechanism, but it is not known whether omeprazole would affect the macrolide serum level. An interaction would be expected to occur between clarithromycin and the other proton pump inhibitor, pantoprazole.

**Mechanism:** It has been postulated that clarithromycin inhibits the cytochrome $P450_{3A}$ isozyme, that this isozyme makes a significant contribution to the metabolism of omeprazole *in vivo*, and that clarithromycin may have an inhibitory effect on omeprazole metabolism.

**Detailed Information:** See *EDI*, 18/16.07

## Omeprazole-Cyclosporine

**Significance:** 2—moderately clinically significant

**Potential Effects:** Omeprazole may inhibit cyclosporine metabolism, resulting in increased levels.

**Recommendations:** When omeprazole is added to, or withdrawn from, a cyclosporine regimen, the patient should be carefully monitored for changes in cyclosporine levels. The dose of cyclosporine may need to be adjusted.

**Summary:** There are data to show that omeprazole will inhibit cyclosporine metabolism and increase its levels.

**Related Drugs:** There are no drugs related to cyclosporine or omeprazole.

**Mechanism:** These agents may compete for the cytochrome P450 system, which may result in an inhibition of cyclosporine metabolism.

**Detailed Information:** See *EDI*, 18/16.08

## Miscellaneous

### Oxybutynin-Clomipramine

**Significance:** 3—minimally clinically significant

**Potential Effects:** The addition of oxybutynin to the regimen of a patient maintained on clomipramine and fluvoxamine may result in a decrease in clomipramine blood levels.

**Recommendations:** Clomipramine levels and depressive symptoms should be carefully monitored in patients maintained on clomipramine if oxybutynin is added to or discontinued from concurrent therapy. The dose of clomipramine may need to be adjusted or an alternative agent to oxybutynin may need to be considered.

**Summary:** The addition of oxybutynin to the regimen of a patient maintained on clomipramine and fluoxetine resulted in a decrease in clomipramine blood levels in a single case report.

**Related Drugs:** It is not known whether an interaction would occur between oxybutynin and other tricyclic antidepressant agents or between clomipramine and other anticholinergic agents.

**Mechanism:** Oxybutynin may have induced the metabolism of clomipramine through induction of the cytochrome $P450_{3A}$ isozyme system.

**Detailed Information:** See *EDI*, 18/16.09

### Penicillamine-Aluminum Hydroxide, Magnesium Hydroxide

**Significance:** 3—minimally clinically significant

**Recommendations:** The concomitant administration of penicillamine with an aluminum hydroxide-magnesium hydroxide antacid should be avoided. Although documentation is lacking, if both preparations need to be administered, separate administration by as much time as possible.

**Summary:** There are data to show that administration of a combination antacid product containing aluminum hydroxide and magnesium hydroxide with penicillamine will reduce penicillamine bioavailability and absorption.

**Related Drugs:** A similar interaction is expected to occur between penicillamine and other antacids if the mechanism involves chelation of penicillamine.

**Mechanism:** Aluminum and magnesium ions are thought to chelate penicillamine, limiting its absorption.

**Detailed Information:** See *EDI*, 18/16.10

### Penicillamine-Chloroquine

**Significance:** 3—minimally clinically significant

**Potential Effects:** Chloroquine may increase penicillamine levels.

**Recommendations:** Patients maintained on penicillamine therapy should be monitored for penicillamine toxicity if chloroquine is added to therapy. The dose of penicillamine may need to be reduced.

**Summary:** There are data to show that chloroquine administration will increase plasma penicillamine concentrations.

**Related Drugs:** It is not known whether an interaction would occur between penicillamine and other aminoquinolones. There are no drugs related to penicillamine.

**Mechanism:** The mechanism of this interaction is not known.

**Detailed Information:** See *EDI*, 18/16.27

Miscellaneous

### Penicillamine-Indomethacin

**Significance:** 3—minimally clinically significant
**Potential Effects:** Indomethacin may increase penicillamine levels.
**Recommendations:** Patients maintained on penicillamine therapy should be monitored for penicillamine toxicity if indomethacin is added to therapy. The dose of penicillamine may need to be reduced.
**Summary:** There are data to show that indomethacin administration will increase plasma penicillamine concentrations.
**Related Drugs:** It is not known whether an interaction would occur between penicillamine and other NSAIAs. There are no drugs related to penicillamine.
**Mechanism:** The mechanism of this interaction is not known.
**Detailed Information:** See *EDI*, 18/16.25

### Prednisolone-Cyclosporine

**Significance:** 2—moderately clinically significant
**Potential Effects:** The concurrent use of these agents may result in increased levels of either agent.
**Recommendations:** If increased levels of prednisolone (e.g., cushingoid symptoms) or cyclosporine (e.g., nephrotoxicity) occur, the dose of one or both agents may need to be decreased.
**Summary:** There are data to show that coadministration of these agents may result in increased levels of either agent.
**Related Drugs:** Prednisolone has been shown to decrease cyclosporine levels. Methylprednisolone has been shown to increase cyclosporine levels. The concurrent use of cyclosporine and other corticosteroids may result in increased levels of either agent. However, which drug would be affected is difficult to determine.
**Mechanism:** Prednisolone may decrease cyclosporine clearance by a hepatotoxic effect, cyclosporine may reduce the hepatic cytochrome P450 needed for prednisolone metabolism, or there may be a competitive inhibition of these agents.
**Detailed Information:** See *EDI*, 18/16.30

### Prednisolone-Glycyrrhiza

**Significance:** 3—minimally clinically significant
**Potential Effects:** The concurrent administration of prednisolone with compounds containing glycyrrhiza may result in increased, decreased, or no changes in prednisolone levels.
**Recommendations:** The dosage of corticosteroids may need to be adjusted in patients concurrently taking glycyrrhiza-containing compounds. Glycyrrhiza may need to be discontinued.
**Summary:** Concurrent administration of prednisolone with compounds containing glycyrrhiza either resulted in increased, decreased, or no changes in prednisolone levels.
**Related Drugs:** An interaction may occur between glycyrrhiza and other corticosteroids. There are no agents related to glycyrrhiza. Glycyrrhiza is commonly known as licorice.
**Mechanism:** Glycyrrhizic acid, the active form of glycyrrhizin, has been shown to inhibit 11-beta-hydroxysteroid dehydrogenase, the enzyme that catalyzes the oxidation of the 11-beta-hydroxycorticosteroids to their inactive metabolites.
**Detailed Information:** See *EDI*, 18/16.40

### Prednisolone-Oral Contraceptive Agents

**Significance:** 2—moderately clinically significant
**Potential Effects:** Oral contraceptive agents may decrease the clearance of prednisolone.

**Recommendations:** Patients taking these agents together should be monitored for increased corticosteroid effects. The dose of prednisolone may need to be reduced.
**Summary:** There are data to show that oral contraceptive agents may inhibit the elimination of oral or intravenous prednisolone.
**Related Drugs:** A similar interaction is expected to occur between oral contraceptive agents and other corticosteroids.
**Mechanism:** Oral contraceptives may inhibit the hepatic metabolism of prednisolone and other corticosteroids. Oral contraceptives may also decrease endogenous cortisol clearance, competitively inhibiting prednisolone metabolism.
**Detailed Information:** See *EDI*, 18/17.00

## Prednisone-Aluminum Hydroxide

**Significance:** 3—minimally clinically significant
**Recommendations:** Patients should be observed for a change in their clinical response to the corticosteroid. The dose of the corticosteroid may need to be increased.
**Summary:** Study results conflict as to whether administration of prednisone and an aluminum hydroxide antacid preparation may decrease the oral bioavailability of prednisone.
**Related Drugs:** An antacid preparation containing aluminum and magnesium hydroxide interacted similarly. A similar interaction is expected to occur between other corticosteroids and other antacid preparations.
**Mechanism:** Antacid preparations may physically adsorb prednisone.
**Detailed Information:** See *EDI*, 18/19.00

## Probucol-Cyclosporine

**Significance:** 2—moderately clinically significant
**Potential Effects:** Concurrent cyclosporine and probucol may result in a decrease in cyclosporine levels.
**Recommendations:** Patients on cyclosporine therapy in whom probucol therapy is added or discontinued should be monitored for changes in cyclosporine levels. The dosage of cyclosporine may need to be adjusted.
**Summary:** In two studies, concurrent administration of cyclosporine and probucol resulted in a decrease in cyclosporine levels.
**Related Drugs:** It is not known if there is an interaction between probucol and tacrolimus.
**Mechanism:** It is speculated that probucol may have inhibited the absorption of cyclosporine by increasing the excretion of bile acid in the feces, or it may have altered the disposition of cyclosporine by altering lipid concentrations.
**Detailed Information:** See *EDI*, 18/20.00

## Pyridostigmine-Methylprednisolone

**Significance:** 3—minimally clinically significant
**Recommendations:** If severe muscle weakness occurs during concurrent use of these agents, ventilatory assistance should be provided. It may also be necessary to discontinue the corticosteroid.
**Summary:** The concurrent administration of methylprednisolone and pyridostigmine may decrease muscle strength, possibly necessitating mechanical ventilation.
**Related Drugs:** Neostigmine administration resulted in the same interaction. Documentation is lacking regarding an interaction between other anticholinesterases and other corticosteroids.
**Mechanism:** The mechanism of this interaction is unknown.
**Detailed Information:** See *EDI*, 18/21.00

Miscellaneous

## Ranitidine-Sucralfate

**Significance:** 3—minimally clinically significant

**Potential Effects:** Ranitidine may bind to sucralfate, resulting in decreased absorption of ranitidine.

**Recommendations:** Until further multiple dose studies are done, the concurrent administration of these agents need not be avoided. It may be best to separate the administration of these agents by as much time as possible.

**Summary:** There are data to show that ranitidine may bind to sucralfate, resulting in decreased absorption of ranitidine; however, there are some conflicting data.

**Related Drugs:** Because of conflicting results, it is difficult to determine if an interaction would occur between sucralfate and other $H_2$-receptor antagonists. There are no drugs related to sucralfate.

**Mechanism:** The mechanism of the potential interaction between ranitidine and sucralfate is not known. Ranitidine may bind to the sucralfate paste in the gastrointestinal fluids.

**Detailed Information:** See *EDI*, 18/22.10

## Ritonavir-Desipramine

**Significance:** 2—moderately clinically significant

**Potential Effects:** The concurrent administration of ritonavir and desipramine may result in increased desipramine plasma levels.

**Recommendations:** In subjects maintained on ritonavir for whom antidepressant therapy is indicated, or if ritonavir is added to the therapy of a patient maintained on desipramine, the patient should be closely monitored for elevated plasma desipramine levels and side effects. The dose of desipramine may need to be adjusted.

**Summary:** Concurrent administration of ritonavir and desipramine resulted in increased desipramine plasma levels, probably because ritonavir inhibited the transformation of desipramine to hydroxydesipramine.

**Related Drugs:** Indinavir, nelfinavir, and saquinavir also appear to inhibit the transformation of desipramine to hydroxydesipramine, but to a lesser extent. An interaction may also occur between tricyclic antidepressant agents that are metabolized by cytochrome $P450_{2D6}$ or $P450_{3A4}$ and protease inhibitors that inhibit cytochrome $P450_{2D6}$ or amprenavir, which inhibits cytochrome $P450_{3A4}$. It is not known whether an interaction would occur between the other protease inhibitors and tricyclic antidepressant agents that have not been shown to inhibit cytochrome $P450_{2D6}$ (amoxapine, doxepin, protriptyline, trimipramine).

**Mechanism:** Ritonavir may have inhibited the metabolism of desipramine; both are metabolized by cytochrome $P450_{2D6}$ isozymes. Ritonavir is also a potent inhibitor of cytochrome $P450_{3A4}$. Virtually all tricyclic antidepressant agents are metabolized in part by one or both of these isozymes, though not all to the same degree.

**Detailed Information:** See *EDI*, 18/22.15

## Selegiline-Oral Contraceptive Agents

**Significance:** 3—moderately clinically significant

**Potential Effects:** The concomitant use of selegiline and oral contraceptive agents may result in marked increases in selegiline area under the curve (AUC) and selegiline serum concentration.

**Recommendations:** Patients who take selegiline and oral contraceptives concurrently should be monitored for elevation of selegiline levels and signs of selegiline toxicity.

**Summary:** Concomitant use of selegiline and oral contraceptive agents resulted in marked increases in selegiline AUC and serum concentrations.
**Related Drugs:** It is not known whether an interaction would occur between oral contraceptive agents and other monoamine oxidase inhibitors.
**Mechanism:** It was postulated that the interaction between selegiline and oral contraceptive agents is due to the inhibition of N-demethylation of selegiline to desmethylselegiline.
**Detailed Information:** See *EDI*, 18/22.17

## Simvastatin-Nefazodone

**Significance:** 3—minimally clinically significant
**Potential Effects:** Concurrent administration of simvastatin and nefazodone may result in rhabdomyolysis and myositis.
**Recommendations:** Concurrent use of simvastatin and nefazodone should be approached with caution. Patients should be monitored for signs of myositis and rhabdomyolysis. One or both agents may need to be discontinued.
**Summary:** Concurrent administration of simvastatin and nefazodone may have resulted in rhabdomyolysis and myositis.
**Related Drugs:** Although documentation is lacking, based on the proposed mechanism a similar interaction would be expected to occur between nefazodone and the other HMG-CoA reductase inhibitors. There are no drugs related to nefazodone.
**Mechanism:** Nefazodone is an inhibitor of the cytochrome $P450_{3A4}$ isoenzyme system. Simvastatin is thought to be metabolized by the $P450_{3A4}$ isoenzyme. It is postulated that nefazodone inhibits the metabolism of simvastatin.
**Detailed Information:** See *EDI*, 18/22.20

## Tacrine-Hormonal Contraceptive Agents

**Significance:** 3—minimally clinically significant
**Potential Effects:** Hormone replacement therapy with estradiol and levonorgestrel may increase tacrine plasma concentrations.
**Recommendations:** Tacrine plasma concentrations should be carefully monitored during concurrent estrogen/progestogen therapy. The dose of tacrine may need to be adjusted.
**Summary:** Hormone replacement therapy with estradiol and levonorgestrel significantly increased tacrine plasma concentrations.
**Related Drugs:** A similar interaction may occur between tacrine and the other estrogen/progestogen hormonal contraceptive agents based on the postulated mechanism. There are no drugs related to tacrine.
**Mechanism:** Concurrent tacrine and estradiol/levonorgestrel significantly increased tacrine plasma concentration, but no similar effect was observed on the concentrations of 1-hydroxytacrine, the major metabolite of tacrine. The mechanism of this interaction may involve a cytochrome $P450_{1A2}$-mediated reduction of tacrine 1-hydroxylation.
**Detailed Information:** See *EDI*, 18/22.25

## Tacrolimus-Erythromycin

**Significance:** 2—moderately clinically significant
**Potential Effects:** Concurrent use of tacrolimus and erythromycin may result in increased tacrolimus plasma levels.
**Recommendations:** Concurrent tacrolimus and erythromycin may result in increased tacrolimus plasma levels with possible associated central nervous system toxicity or nephrotoxicity. Tacrolimus

plasma levels should be carefully monitored. The dose of tacrolimus may need to be adjusted, and consideration should be given to an alternative for erythromycin.

**Summary:** There are data to show that concurrent tacrolimus and erythromycin may result in increased tacrolimus plasma levels.

**Related Drugs:** An interaction would be expected to occur between tacrolimus and other macrolide antibiotics that form inactive cytochrome P450 metabolite complexes. Azithromycin and spiramycin would not be expected to interact with tacrolimus.

**Mechanism:** This interaction may result from inhibition of hepatic cytochrome P450 metabolism.

**Detailed Information:** See *EDI,* 18/22.70

## Tacrolimus-Fluconazole

**Significance:** 2—moderately clinically significant

**Potential Effects:** The concurrent administration of tacrolimus and fluconazole may result in elevated levels of tacrolimus, which may lead to the development of nephrotoxicity.

**Recommendations:** Patients maintained on tacrolimus should be carefully monitored for increased tacrolimus levels and possible associated nephrotoxicity if fluconazole is added to therapy. The dose of tacrolimus may need to be adjusted if fluconazole is added to or discontinued from therapy with tacrolimus.

**Summary:** Concurrent administration of tacrolimus and fluconazole resulted in elevated levels of tacrolimus, which may lead to the development of nephrotoxicity.

**Related Drugs:** Tacrolimus concentrations decreased after coadministration with clotrimazole, itraconazole, or ketoconazole. An interaction between tacrolimus and other systemic imidazole antifungal agents may occur. Tacrolimus is a macrolide immunosuppressant agent that differs pharmacologically from the macrolide antibiotic agents; however, an interaction may occur between the systemic imidazole antifungal agents and sirolimus.

**Mechanism:** The intestinal metabolism of tacrolimus may be reduced in the presence of fluconazole, causing an alteration in the kinetics of tacrolimus. Ketoconazole inhibits the small intestine metabolism of tacrolimus; fluconazole may inhibit the hepatic $P450_{3A}$ enzymes responsible for tacrolimus metabolism. Sirolimus is also metabolized by cytochrome $P450_{3A4}$ isoenzymes in the wall of the intestine and the liver.

**Detailed Information:** See *EDI,* 18/22.30

## Tacrolimus-Metronidazole

**Significance:** 3—minimally clinically significant

**Potential Effects:** The addition of metronidazole may increase tacrolimus plasma levels.

**Recommendations:** Patients' renal function and tacrolimus plasma levels should be monitored during concurrent therapy of tacrolimus and metronidazole. The dose of tacrolimus may need to be decreased during concurrent use.

**Summary:** The addition of metronidazole has resulted in an increase in tacrolimus plasma levels.

**Related Drugs:** Tacrolimus is a macrolide immunosuppressant agent that differs pharmacologically from the macrolide antibiotic agents. A similar interaction might occur between metronidazole and other macrolide immunosuppressant agent (sirolimus). There are no drugs related to metronidazole.

**Mechanism:** Metronidazole may inhibit the hepatic metabolism of tacrolimus, which is extensively metabolized by the cytochrome $P450_{3A}$ enzyme system. Metronidazole has been shown to be a weak inhibitor of cytochrome $P450_{3A4}$ *in vitro*.
**Detailed Information:** See *EDI*, 18/22.74

## Tacrolimus-Nefazodone

**Significance:** 2—moderately clinically significant
**Potential Effects:** The concurrent administration of nefazodone and tacrolimus may result in increased levels and adverse effects of tacrolimus.
**Recommendations:** In patients maintained on tacrolimus, tacrolimus levels and signs of adverse effects should be monitored closely when nefazodone therapy is initiated. The dosage of tacrolimus may need to be adjusted or nefazodone may need to be discontinued. Tacrolimus levels may need to be adjusted if nefazodone is discontinued from concurrent therapy.
**Summary:** The concurrent administration of nefazodone and tacrolimus resulted in increased levels and adverse effects of tacrolimus.
**Related Drugs:** Although documentation is lacking, based on the postulated mechanism an interaction may be expected to occur between tacrolimus and trazodone, an antidepressant agent that inhibits serotonin uptake and is chemically and pharmacologically unrelated to the tricyclic and tetracyclic antidepressant agents. There are no drugs related to tacrolimus.
**Mechanism:** It has been postulated that nefazodone inhibits the metabolism of tacrolimus. *In vitro* studies have indicated that tacrolimus is metabolized at the cytochrome $P450_{3A4}$ isozyme in both the human small intestine and liver. *In vitro* studies have shown that nefazodone inhibits the $P450_{3A4}$ isozyme.
**Detailed Information:** See *EDI*, 18/22.77

## Tacrolimus-Nifedipine

**Significance:** 3—minimally clinically significant
**Potential Effects:** Concurrent administration of nifedipine and tacrolimus may result in increased tacrolimus levels requiring decreased tacrolimus dosages.
**Recommendations:** Tacrolimus blood levels should be carefully monitored in patients receiving concurrent nifedipine therapy, especially when nifedipine is initiated or discontinued. The dosage of tacrolimus may need to be adjusted.
**Summary:** Concurrent administration of nifedipine and tacrolimus resulted in increased tacrolimus levels by as much as 55%, requiring decreased tacrolimus dosages.
**Related Drugs:** An *in vitro* study in human liver microsomes found verapamil to be a competitive inhibitor of tacrolimus metabolism. Conflicting data are available on the effect of diltiazem. A similar interaction may be expected to occur between tacrolimus and the other calcium channel blockers. There are no agents related to tacrolimus.
**Mechanism:** Tacrolimus is metabolized by cytochrome $P450_{3A4}$ in the small intestine and liver. *In vivo* studies using isolated human liver and intestinal microsomes with high cytochrome $P450_{3A4}$ content have found nifedipine to be a competitive inhibitor of tacrolimus metabolism. Elevated concentrations of tacrolimus have been associated with an increased incidence of nephrotoxicity, neurotoxicity, and diabetogenicity.
**Detailed Information:** See *EDI*, 18/22.80

## Miscellaneous

### Tacrolimus-Rifampin

**Significance:** 2—moderately clinically significant

**Potential Effects:** The concurrent administration of tacrolimus and rifampin may result in decreased levels of tacrolimus and the need to adjust the dosage of tacrolimus.

**Recommendations:** The concurrent administration of rifampin with tacrolimus should be approached with caution. If concurrent therapy is warranted, tacrolimus levels should be carefully monitored. The dosage of tacrolimus may need to be adjusted when rifampin is initiated or discontinued.

**Summary:** Concurrent administration of tacrolimus and rifampin resulted in decreased levels of tacrolimus and the need to adjust the tacrolimus dosage.

**Related Drugs:** A similar interaction may occur between tacrolimus and the other rifamycins, and between rifamycins and sirolimus. There are no agents related to tacrolimus.

**Mechanism:** Rifampin may have induced the metabolism of tacrolimus at the cytochrome $P450_{3A4}$ isozyme. Rifampin, rifapentine, and rifabutin induce the $P450_{3A}$ isozyme, although rifampin and rifapentine are more potent inducers than rifabutin. Induction by rifapentine has been shown to occur within four days of the first dose and return to baseline 14 days after discontinuation of rifapentine.

**Detailed Information:** See *EDI*, 18/22.85

### Thyroid-Cholestyramine

**Significance:** 2—moderately clinically significant

**Recommendations:** Thyroxine and cholestyramine should be administered as far apart as possible (optimally four to six hours). When these drugs are used concurrently, the patient should be observed for symptoms of hypothyroidism (e.g., weakness, fatigue, cold intolerance, and dry, puffy skin). If possible, before cholestyramine is added to the drug regimen of a patient maintained on a thyroid preparation, baseline thyroid status should be determined. Periodic evaluation of thyroid status should be performed to detect changes in thyroid response.

**Summary:** Cholestyramine has been shown to cause a clinically significant decrease in the absorption of thyroid hormones.

**Related Drugs:** All thyroid compounds are expected to interact with cholestyramine. Colestipol may bind thyroid.

**Mechanism:** Cholestyramine forms strong ionic bonds with thyroid in the gastrointestinal tract, decreasing its absorption.

**Detailed Information:** See *EDI*, 18/23.00

### Trazodone-Nefazodone

**Significance:** 3—minimally clinically significant

**Potential Effects:** The addition of trazodone to a regimen including nefazodone may result in serotonin syndrome.

**Recommendations:** In subjects who are maintained on nefazodone, the addition of trazodone as a hypnotic or for other uses should be avoided or approached with caution. Patients receiving concurrent therapy should be carefully monitored during the first few days of combination therapy.

**Summary:** The addition of trazodone to a regimen including nefazodone resulted in an episode of serotonin syndrome in a single case report.

**Related Drugs:** It is not known whether an interaction would occur between trazodone and the other non-selective serotonin reuptake inhibitor (venlafaxine). Trazodone is an antidepressant agent chemically unrelated to the tricyclic, tetracyclic, and other antidepressant agents.

# Miscellaneous

**Mechanism:** The mechanism of this interaction is not known. Potential causes of the symptoms the patient experienced, including a transient ischemic attack or an allergic reaction, were ruled out. It was determined that serotonin hyperstimulation was the cause of the symptoms.

**Detailed Information:** See *EDI*, 18/23.80

## Zidovudine-Atovaquone

**Significance:** 3—minimally clinically significant

**Potential Effects:** Concurrent administration of zidovudine and atovaquone may result in an increase in zidovudine serum levels.

**Recommendations:** The increase reported in zidovudine area-under-curve (AUC) by itself may not be clinically significant. However, this interaction may be clinically significant in those patients who are also receiving agents that may produce bone marrow toxicity. The dose of zidovudine may need to be decreased by one-third in those patients.

**Summary:** Concurrent administration of zidovudine and atovaquone resulted in increased zidovudine serum levels. Atovaquone pharmacokinetics were unaffected.

**Related Drugs:** It is not known whether an interaction would occur between atovaquone and the other reverse transcriptase inhibitors. There are no drugs related to atovaquone.

**Mechanism:** Atovaquone decreases the zidovudine-glucuronide AUC and the ratio of zidovudine-glucuronide AUC to zidovudine AUC. It is postulated that zidovudine glucuronidation is inhibited by atovaquone. It is also postulated that this elevated zidovudine concentration may allow a larger amount of the parent to be metabolized by the cytochrome P450 system. This would be important because formation of the 3'-amino-3'-deoxythymidine zidovudine metabolite is mediated by the cytochrome P450 system and has been shown to be five-fold to seven-fold more toxic to bone marrow cells than zidovudine.

**Detailed Information:** See *EDI*, 18/24.50

## Zidovudine-Ribavirin

**Significance:** 1—highly clinically significant

**Potential Effects:** The concurrent administration of zidovudine and ribavirin may decrease the effectiveness of zidovudine.

**Recommendations:** The manufacturer of zidovudine recommends that the concurrent use of zidovudine and ribavirin be avoided in HIV-infected patients.

**Summary:** The concurrent administration of zidovudine and ribavirin decreased the effectiveness of zidovudine.

**Related Drugs:** No significant change in didanosine AUC or $C_{max}$ has been noted during concurrent ribavirin administration, although a very slight increase in the elimination rate of didanosine has been seen. *In vitro*, ribavirin has caused a concentration-dependent increase in the anti-HIV activity of didanosine.

**Mechanism:** Zidovudine undergoes a series of phosphorylations to its active form, zidovudine triphosphate. Zidovudine triphosphate then competes with thymidine triphosphate for incorporation into the viral chain. Ribavirin increases the pool of thymidine triphosphate, which results in reduced activity of thymidine kinase. The rate limiting step in the formation of the active form of zidovudine is the conversion of zidovudine monophosphate to zidovudine diphosphate by thymidylate kinase, leading to a reduction in the phosphorylation of zidovudine. However, an *in vitro* extracellular study showed that ribavirin increased the anti-HIV activity of zidovudine triphosphate.

**Detailed Information:** See *EDI*, 18/24.90

## Zidovudine-Rifampin

**Significance:** 2—moderately clinically significant

**Potential Effects:** Concomitant zidovudine and rifampin may result in an increased clearance of zidovudine, which may lead to decreased effectiveness of antiretroviral therapy.

**Recommendations:** Zidovudine serum levels should be carefully monitored if rifampin is added to, or withdrawn from, concurrent therapy. The dose of zidovudine may need to be adjusted. This interaction may have clinical implications for optimal antiretroviral therapy.

**Summary:** There are data to show that concomitant zidovudine and rifampin may increase zidovudine clearance.

**Related Drugs:** Rifabutin was shown to interact similarly with zidovudine. There are no drugs related to zidovudine.

**Mechanism:** The interaction between rifampin or rifabutin and zidovudine may be caused by the induction of hepatic glucuronidation enzymes.

**Detailed Information:** See *EDI*, 18/25.00

## Undocumented Interaction

**Significance:** 1—highly clinically significant

**Potential Effects:** The concurrent use of these agents may result in a highly clinically significant drug interaction.

**Recommendations:** Concurrent use of these agents may be contraindicated or may require dosage adjustments and/or additional patient monitoring. Refer to the manufacturer's prescribing information for additional information on this interaction.

**Summary:** The concurrent use of these agents may result in a highly clinically significant drug interaction. These agents have been listed in the manufacturer's product information for one or both agents in connection with an associated drug interaction warning. The labeling may state that the concurrent use of these agents is contraindicated, should not be used, or should be avoided. The labeling may state that dosage adjustments and/or additional patient monitoring is required when these agents are concurrently administered. This information may be included in a "black box" warning, under the contraindications section, under the drug interaction section of the product information, or a combination of sections. There may be no published documentation. The inclusion of this information in the manufacturer's product information may be a result of (1) in-house, unpublished studies by the manufacturer; (2) theoretical interactions based on other agents that may have structural and/or pharmacologic similarities; (3) mandated class labeling that may or may not have any accompanying documentation or theoretical basis.

**Related Drugs:** Please refer to the manufacturer's prescribing information for information concerning related drug agents.

**Mechanism:** Please refer to the manufacturer's prescribing information for information on the mechanism by which this interaction occurs.

**Detailed Information:** See *EDI*, 18/901.00

# Appendices

## Appendix A

# RELATED DRUGS

For the purpose of uniformity and consistency, the following groups of drugs have been arranged based on pharmacologic and chemical relationships. This appendix contains a complete list of the agents in a specific related drug class. If any of these agents are specifically implicated in a monograph by documentation or the mechanism of action of the primary drug interaction, a statement discussing their involvement appears in the Related Drugs section of the monograph.

**Agents to Treat Shock**
  Dobutamine
  Dopamine
  Ephedrine
  Epinephrine
  Isoproterenol
  Mephentermine
  Metaraminol
  Methoxamine
  Norepinephrine
  Phenylephrine

**Aminoglycosides**
  Amikacin
  Gentamicin
  Kanamycin
  Neomycin
  Netilmicin
  Paromomycin
  Streptomycin
  Tobramycin

**Androgen Derivatives**
  *All Inclusive*
  Danazol
  Dromostanolone
  Ethylestrenol
  Fluoxymesterone
  Gestrinone
  Methandrostenolone
  Methyltestosterone
  Nandrolone
  Oxandrolone
  Oxymetholone
  Stanozolol
  Testolactone
  Testosterone

  *C-17 Alkylated*
  Danazol
  Ethylestrenol
  Fluoxymesterone
  Methandrostenolone
  Methyltestosterone
  Oxandrolone
  Oxymetholone
  Stanozolol

**Angiotensin Converting Enzyme Inhibitors**
  Benazepril
  Captopril
  Cilazapril
  Enalapril
  Enalaprilat
  Fosinopril
  Imidapril
  Lisinopril
  Moexipril
  Perindopril
  Quinapril
  Ramipril
  Trandolapril
  Trandolaprilat

**Angiotensin II Receptor Antagonists**
  Candesartan
  Eprosartan
  Irbesartan
  Losartan
  Telmisartan
  Valsartan

**Anorexiants**
  Amphetamine
  Benzphetamine
  Dexfenfluramine
  Dextroamphetamine
  Diethylpropion
  Fenfluramine
  Mazindol
  Phendimetrazine
  Phenmetrazine
  Phentermine
  Phenylpropanolamine

**Antacids**
  Aluminum Carbonate Gel, Basic
  Aluminum Hydroxide Gel
  Aluminum Phosphate Gel
  Calcium Carbonate
  Dihydroxyaluminum Aminoacetate
  Dihydroxyaluminum Sodium Carbonate
  Magaldrate
  Magnesium Hydroxide
  Magnesium Carbonate
  Magnesium Oxide
  Magnesium Trisilicate
  Sodium Bicarbonate

**Anthracycline Antineoplastics**
  Aclarubicin

# Appendix A

Daunorubicin
Doxorubicin
Epirubicin
Idarubicin
Valrubicin

## Antiadrenergic Agonists

*Centrally Acting*
Clondine
Guanabenz
Guanfacine
Lofexidine
Methyldopa
Methyldopate

## Antiarrhythmics, Class I

*(Subclass)*
Disopyramide (*A*)
Encainide (*C*)
Flecainide (*C*)
Indecainide (*C*)
Lidocaine (*B*)
Mexiletine (*B*)
Moricizine
Procainamide (*A*)
Propafenone (*C*)
Quinidine (*A*)
Tocainide (*B*)

## Antiarrhythmics, Class III

Amiodarone
Bretylium
Dofetilde
Ibutilide
Sotalol

## Anticholinergics

Anisotropine
Atropine
Belladonna
Benztropine
Biperiden
Clidinium
Dicyclomine
Emepronium
Ethopropazine
Glycopyrrolate
Hexocyclium
Hyoscyamine
Isopropamide
Mepenzolate
Methantheline
Methscopolamine
Oxybutynin
Oxyphencyclimine
Oxyphenonium
Procyclidine
Propantheline
Scopolamine
Tridihexethyl
Trihexyphenidyl

## Anticoagulants, Oral

*Coumarins*
Acenocoumarol
Coumarin
Dicumarol
Nicoumalone
Phenprocoumon
Warfarin

*Indandiones*
Anisindione
Phenindione

## Antihistamines

*Non-Sedating*
Astemizole
Desloratadine
Emedastine
Fexofenadine
Levocabastine
Loratadine
Mizolastine
Olopatadine
Terfenadine

*Sedating*
Azatadine
Azelastine
Bromodiphenhydramine
Brompheniramine
Buclizine
Carbinoxamine
Cetirizine
Chlorcyclizine
Chlorpheniramine
Clemastine
Cyclizine
Cyproheptadine
Dexchlorpheniramine
Dimethindine
Diphenhydramine
Diphenylpyraline
Hydroxyzine
Mebhydrolin
Meclizine
Mequitazine
Phenindamine
Pheniramine
Phenyltoloxamine
Pyrilamine
Tripelennamine
Triprolidine

## Antineoplastic Alkylating Agents

*Nitrogen Mustards*
Chlorambucil
Cyclophosphamide
Ifosfamide
Mechlorethamine
Melphalan
Treosulfan

## Appendix A

*Nitrosoureas*
- Busulfan
- Carmustine
- Lomustine
- Pipobroman
- Streptozocin
- Thiotepa
- Uracil Mustard

**Antineoplastic Antimetabolites**
- Cytarabine
- Floxuridine
- Fluorouracil
- Mercaptopurine
- Methotrexate
- Thioguanine

**Antiparkinsonism Anticholinergics**
- Belladonna
- Benztropine
- Biperiden
- Cycrimine
- Ethopropazine
- Orphenadrine
- Procyclidine
- Trihexyphenidyl

**Antipsychotics, Miscellaneous**
- Benperidol
- Chlorprothixene
- Clozapine
- Flupenthixol
- Haloperidol
- Loxapine
- Molindone
- Pimozide
- Reboxetine
- Risperidone
- Sertindole
- Thiothixene
- Trifluperidol

**Barbiturates**

*General*
- Amobarbital
- Aprobarbital
- Barbital
- Butabarbital
- Butalbital
- Butobarbitone
- Hexobarbital
- Mephobarbital
- Metharbital
- Pentobarbital
- Phenobarbital
- Primidone
- Secobarbital
- Talbutal

*Anesthesia*
- Methohexital
- Thiamylal
- Thiopental

**Benzodiazepines**
- Alprazolam
- Bromazepam
- Brotizolam
- Chlordiazepoxide
- Clobazam
- Clonazepam
- Clorazepate
- Diazepam
- Estazolam
- Flunitrazepam
- Flurazepam
- Halazepam
- Ketazolam
- Lorazepam
- Lormetazepam
- Medazepam
- Midazolam
- Nitrazepam
- Oxazepam
- Prazepam
- Quazepam
- Temazepam
- Triazolam

**Beta-Blocking Agents**

*Cardioselective ($\beta_1$)*
- Acebutolol
- Atenolol
- Betaxolol
- Bisoprolol
- Esmolol
- Metoprolol
- Nebivolol

*Noncardioselective ($\beta_1$ and $\beta_2$)*
- Carteolol
- Carvedilol
- Celiprolol
- Labetalol
- Levobunolol
- Nadolol
- Oxprenolol
- Penbutolol
- Pindolol
- Propranolol
- Sotalol
- Tertatolol
- Timolol

*Ophthalmic*
- Betaxolol
- Carteolol
- Levobunolol
- Metipranolol
- Timolol

# Appendix A

**Bisphosphonates**
  Alendronate
  Clodronate
  Etidronate
  Pamidronate
  Risedronate
  Tiludronate
  Zoledronic Acid

**Bulk Producing Laxatives**
  Hemicellulose
  Malt Extract
  Methylcellulose
  Psyllium

**Calcium Channel Blockers**
  Amlodipine
  Bepridil
  Diltiazem
  Felodipine
  Isradipine
  Lacidipine
  Lercanidipine
  Mibefradil
  Nicardipine
  Nifedipine
  Nilvadipine
  Nimodipine
  Nisoldipine
  Terodiline
  Verapamil

**Carbonic Anhydrase Inhibitors**
  Acetazolamide
  Brinzolamide, Ophthalmic
  Dichlorphenamide
  Dorzolamide, Ophthalmic
  Methazolamide

**Central Nervous System Depressants**
  Acetylcarbromal
  Alcohol, Ethyl
  Chloral Hydrate
  Ethchlorvynol
  Ethinamate
  Glutethimide
  Meprobamate
  Methyprylon
  Paraldehyde

**Cephalosporins**
  Cefaclor
  Cefadroxil
  Cefamandole
  Cefazaflur
  Cefazolin
  Cefdinir
  Cefepime
  Cefixime
  Cefmetazole
  Cefodizime
  Cefonicid
  Cefoperazone
  Ceforanide
  Cefotaxime
  Cefotetan
  Cefoxitin
  Cefpirome
  Cefpodoxime
  Cefprozil
  Cefsulodin
  Ceftazidime
  Ceftibutin
  Ceftizoxime
  Ceftriaxone
  Cefuroxime
  Cephalexin
  Cephaloglycin
  Cephalothin
  Cephapirin
  Cephradine
  Loracarbef
  Moxalactam

**Corticosteroids**
  Beclomethasone
  Betamethasone
  Budesonide
  Ciprocinonide
  Corticotropin
  Cortisone
  Cosyntropin
  Deflazacort
  Desoxycorticosterone
  Dexamethasone
  Diflucortolone
  Fludrocortisone
  Fluocinolone
  Fluocinonide
  Fluocortolone
  Flunisolide
  Fluticasone
  Hydrocortisone
  Loteprednol
  Methylprednisolone
  Paramethasone
  Prednicarbate
  Prednisolone
  Prednisone
  Procinonide
  Triamcinolone

**Digitalis Glycosides**
  Deslanoside
  Digitalis
  Digitoxin
  Digoxin

**Ergot Alkaloids**
  Bromocriptine
  Cabergoline
  Dihydroergotamine

# Appendix A

Ergoloid Mesylates
Ergonovine
Ergotamine
Methylergonovine
Methysergide
Pergolide

## Estrogenic Substances
Chlorotrianisene
Conjugated Estrogens
Diethylstilbestrol
Esterified Estrogens
Estradiol
Estriol
Estrone
Estropipate
Ethinyl Estradiol
Mestranol
Polyestradiol
Quinestrol

## Fibric Acid Derivatives
Bezafibrate
Cifrofibrate
Clofibrate
Fenofibrate
Gemfibrozil

## Gonadotropin-Releasing Hormones and Analogues
Chorionic Gonadotropin
Gonadorelin
Gonadotropin
Histrelin
Leuprolide
Nafarelin
Triptorelin

## $H_2$-Receptor Antagonists
Cimetidine
Famotidine
Nizatidine
Ranitidine

## HMG-CoA Reductase Inhibitors
Atorvastatin
Cerivastatin
Fluvastatin
Lovastatin
Pravastatin
Simvastatin

## Hydantoin Anticonvulsants
Ethotoin
Fosphenytoin
Mephenytoin
Phenytoin

## Hydroxytryptamine ($5HT_1$) Receptor Agonists
Almotriptan
Naratriptan
Sumatriptan
Rizatriptan
Zolmitriptan

## Imidazole Antifungal Agents
Butoconazole
Clotrimazole
Econazole
Fenticonazole
Fluconazole
Isoconazole
Itraconazole
Ketoconazole
Miconazole
Oxiconazole
Terconazole
Tioconazole

## Inhalation Anesthetic Agents
*General*
Cyclopropane
Ether
Nitrous Oxide
*Halogenated*
Desflurane
Enflurane
Halothane
Isoflurane
Methoxyflurane
Sevoflurane

## Local Anesthetics
Amethocaine
Benzocaine
Bupivacaine
Butacaine
Chloroprocaine
Dibucaine
Etidocaine
Lidocaine
Mepivacaine
Piperocaine
Prilocaine
Procaine
Propoxycaine
Ropivacaine
Tetracaine

## Loop Diuretics
Bumetanide
Ethacrynic Acid
Ethacrynate Sodium
Furosemide
Piretanide
Torsemide

## Low Molecular Weight Heparin and Heparinoids
Ardeparin
Certoparin
Dalteparin
Danaparoid

Enoxaparin
Tinzaparin

**Macrolide Antibiotics**
Azithromycin
Clarithromycin
Dirithromycin
Erythromycin
Josamycin
Spiramycin
Troleandomycin

**Monoamine Oxidase Inhibitors**
Furazolidone
Hypericum
Isocarboxazid
Moclobemide
Pargyline
Phenelzine
Procarbazine
Selegiline
Tranylcypromine

**Narcotics**
Alfentanil
Buprenorphine
Codeine
Dextromoramide
Dezocine
Diamorphine
Dihydrocodeine
Diphenoxylate
Diphenoxin
Ethoheptazine
Fentanyl
Hydrocodone
Hydromorphone
Levomethadyl
Levorphanol
Meperidine
Meptazinol
Methadone
Morphine
Nalbuphine
Oxycodone
Oxymorphone
Pentazocine
Phenoperidine
Propoxyphene
Remifentanil
Sufentanil
Tramadol

**Neuromuscular Blocking Agents**
*Depolarizing*
Succinylcholine
*Nondepolarizing*
Alcuronium
Atracurium
Cisatracurium
Doxacurium
Gallamine
Metocurine
Mivacurium
Pancuronium
Pipecuronium
Rapacuronium
Rocuronium
Tubocurarine
Vecuronium

**Nitrate Derivatives**
Amyl Nitrite
Erythrityl Tetranitrate
Isosorbide Dinitrate
Isosorbide Mononitrate
Nitroglycerin
Pentaerythritol Tetranitrate

**Non-Nucleoside Reverse Transcriptase Inhibitors (NNRTI's)**
Delavirdine
Efavirenz
Nevirapine

**Nonsteroidal Anti-inflammatory Agents**
Acemetacin
Bromfenac
Diclofenac
Etodolac
Feprazone
Felbinac
Fenbufen
Fenoprofen
Flurbiprofen
Ibuprofen
Indomethacin
Ketoprofen
Ketorolac
Meclofenamate
Mefenamic Acid
Meloxicam
Nabumetone
Naproxen
Nimesulide
Oxaprozin
Oxyphenbutazone
Phenylbutazone
Piroxicam
Sulindac
Suprofen
Tenoxicam
Tiaprofenic Acid
Tolfenamic Acid
Tolmetin

*Ophthalmic*
Diclofenac
Flurbiprofen
Indomethacin
Ketorolac
Oxyphenbutazone
Suprofen

## Appendix A

*Topical*
- Diclofenac
- Felbinac
- Ibuprofen
- Ketoprofen
- Naproxen
- Piroxicam

### Nucleoside Analogue Reverse Transcriptase Inhibitors
- Abacavir
- Didanosine
- Lamivudine
- Stavudine
- Zalcitabine
- Zidovudine

### Penicillins
- Amoxicillin
- Ampicillin
- Azlocillin
- Bacampicillin
- Benethamine Penicillin
- Carbenicillin
- Carfecillin
- Cloxacillin
- Cyclacillin
- Dicloxacillin
- Mecillinam
- Methicillin
- Mezlocillin
- Nafcillin
- Oxacillin
- Penicillin G
- Penicillin V
- Piperacillin
- Pivampicillin
- Pivmecillinam
- Temocillin
- Ticarcillin

### Phenothiazines
- Acetophenazine
- Carphenazine
- Chlorpromazine
- Flupenthixol
- Fluphenazine
- Mesoridazine
- Methdilazine
- Pericyazine
- Perphenazine
- Piperacetazine
- Pipotiazine
- Prochlorperazine
- Promazine
- Promethazine
- Propiomazine
- Thiethylperazine
- Thioproperazine
- Thioridazine
- Trifluoperazine
- Triflupromazine
- Trimeprazine
- Zuclopenthixol

### Polypeptide Antibiotics
- Bacitracin
- Capreomycin
- Colistimethate
- Colistin
- Polymyxin B

### Potassium-Sparing Diuretics
- Amiloride
- Potassium Canrenoate
- Spironolactone
- Triamterene

### Progestins
- Allylestrenol
- Desogestrel
- Dydrogesterone
- Gestodene
- Gestronol
- Hydroxyprogesterone
- Levonorgestrel
- Medroxyprogesterone
- Megestrol
- Norethindrone
- Norethynodrel
- Norgestimate
- Norgestrel
- Progesterone

### Propanediol Derivatives
- Carisoprodol
- Chlorphenesin
- Felbamate
- Mephenesin
- Meprobamate
- Methocarbamol

### Protease Inhibitors
- Amprenavir
- Indinavir
- Lopinavir
- Nelfinavir
- Ritonavir
- Saquinavir

### Proton Pump Inhibitors
- Esomeprazole
- Lansoprazole
- Omeprazole
- Pantoprazole
- Rabeprazole

### Quinolone Antibacterials
- Alatrofloxacin
- Cinoxacin
- Ciprofloxacin
- Clinafloxacin
- Enoxacin
- Fleroxacin
- Gatifloxacin

Grepafloxacin
Levofloxacin
Lomefloxacin
Moxifloxacin
Nalidixic Acid
Norfloxacin
Ofloxacin
Rosoxacin
Sparfloxacin
Temafloxacin
Trovafloxacin

*Ophthalmic*
Ciprofloxacin
Norfloxacin
Ofloxacin

## Rauwolfia Alkaloids
Alseroxylon
Deserpidine
Rauwolfia Serpentina
Rescinnamine
Reserpine

## Retinoic Acid Derivatives
Acitretin
Etretinate
Isotretinoin
Retinol (Vitamin A)
Tazarotene
Tretinoin

## Salicylates
Aloxiprin
Aspirin
Calcium Carbaspirin
Choline Salicylate
Diflunisal
Magnesium Salicylate
Salicylamide
Salsalate
Sodium Salicylate
Sodium Thiosalicylate

## Serotonin Reuptake Inhibitors
*Selective*
Citalopram
Fluoxetine
Fluvoxamine
Paroxetine
Sertraline

*Nonselective*
Nefazodone
Venlafaxine

## Sulfonamides
Sulfacytine
Sulfadiazine
Sulfadoxine
Sulfamerazine
Sulfamethazine
Sulfamethizole
Sulfamethoxazole
Sulfanilamide
Sulfapyridine
Sulfasalazine
Sulfisoxazole
Zonisamide

## Sulfonylureas
Acetohexamide
Chlorpropamide
Gliclazide
Glimepiride
Glipizide
Gliquidone
Glyburide
Tolazamide
Tolbutamide

## Sympathomimetics
(a = alpha agonist activity,
b = beta agonist activity)

*Direct Acting*
Albuterol - b
Bitolterol - b
Dobutamine - a, b
Eformoterol - b
Epinephrine - a, b
Ethylnorepinephrine - b
Fenterol - b
Formoterol - b
Isoetharine - b
Isoproterenol - b
Metaproterenol - b
Methoxamine - a
Midodrine - a
Norepinephrine - a, b
Pirbuterol - b
Procaterol - b
Rimiterol - b
Ritodrine - b
Salmeterol - b
Terbutaline - b

*Indirect Acting* (All have alpha
and beta agonist activity)
Amphetamine
Benzphetamine
Dexfenfluramine
Dextroamphetamine
Diethylpropion
Ephedrine
Etafedrine
Fenfluramine
Isometheptene
Mazindol
Mephentermine
Methamphetamine
Methylphenidate
Phendimetrazine
Phenmetrazine
Phentermine
Phenylpropanolamine
Prolintane

## Appendix A

Pseudoephedrine
Tyramine
*Mixed Acting*
Dopamine - a, b
Metaraminol - a, b
Phenylephrine - a, b

**Tetracyclines**
Chlortetracycline
Demeclocycline
Doxycycline
Methacycline
Minocycline
Oxytetracycline
Tetracycline

**Theophylline Derivatives**
Aminophylline
Dyphylline
Oxtriphylline
Theophylline

**Thiazide Diuretics**
Bendroflumethiazide
Benzthiazide
Chlorothiazide
Cyclopenthiazide
Cyclothiazide
Flumethiazide
Hydrochlorothiazide
Hydroflumethiazide
Methyclothiazide
Polythiazide
Trichlormethiazide
Xipamide

**Thiazide-Related Diuretics**
Chlorthalidone
Indapamide
Metolazone
Quinethazone

**Thyroid Drugs**
Dextrothyroxine
Levothyroxine
Liothyronine
Liotrix
Thyroglobulin
Thyroid
Thyrotropin

**Tricyclic Antidepressants**
Amitriptyline
Amoxapine
Butryptyline
Clomipramine
Desipramine
Dothiepin
Doxepin
Imipramine
Iprindole
Lofepramine
Nortriptyline
Opipramol
Protriptyline
Trimipramine

**Urinary Acidifiers**
Ammonium Biphosphate
Ammonium Chloride
Ascorbic Acid
Potassium Acid Phosphate
Sodium Acid Phosphate
Sodium Acid Pyrophosphate

**Urinary Alkalinizers**
Potassium Citrate
Sodium Acetate
Sodium Bicarbonate
Sodium Citrate
Sodium Lactate
Tromethamine

**Vitamin D Analogues**
Alfacalcidol
Calcifediol
Calcipotriene
Calcitriol
Cholecalciferol
Dihydrotachysterol
Ergocalciferol
Paricalcitol

# Appendix B

# CODE 1 INTERACTIONS

The following is an alphabetical listing of those drug-drug interactions that are classified in *Pocket Guide to EDI* as Code 1, or highly clinically significant, interactions. Receiving a Code 1 significance rating are interactions that are of great potential harm to the patient, that are predictable or frequent, and that are well documented. The page numbers of their respective monographs follow.

| | |
|---|---|
| Acetazolamide-Lithium Carbonate | 245 |
| Alcohol, Ethyl-Chlorpropamide | 302 |
| Alcohol, Ethyl-Disulfiram | 318 |
| Allopurinol-Dicumarol | 70 |
| Allopurinol-Mercaptopurine | 221 |
| Aluminum Hydroxide-Tetracycline | 211 |
| Aminophylline-Halothane | 337 |
| Amiodarone-Digoxin | 277 |
| Amiodarone-Quinidine | 62 |
| Amiodarone-Warfarin | 76 |
| Amphetamine-Furazolidone | 191 |
| Aspirin-Heparin | 72 |
| Aspirin-Methotrexate | 222 |
| Aspirin-Warfarin | 77 |
| Carbamazepine-Charcoal | 104 |
| Carbamazepine-Clozapine | 237 |
| Carbamazepine-Erythromycin | 105 |
| Carbenicillin-Gentamicin | 192 |
| Cephalothin-Gentamicin | 192 |
| Charcoal-Carbamazepine | 104 |
| Charcoal-Theophylline | 343 |
| Chlorothiazide-Lithium Carbonate | 247 |
| Chlorpromazine-Guanethidine | 169 |
| Chlorpropamide-Alcohol, Ethyl | 302 |
| Cimetidine-Fluorouracil | 220 |
| Cimetidine-Lidocaine | 54 |
| Cimetidine-Phenytoin | 117 |
| Cimetidine-Propranolol | 266 |
| Cimetidine-Theophylline | 344 |
| Cimetidine-Warfarin | 80 |
| Clofibrate-Warfarin | 81 |
| Clonidine-Propranolol | 167 |
| Clozapine-Carbamazepine | 237 |
| Cyclosporine-Diltiazem | 47 |
| Cyclosporine-Erythromycin | 190 |
| Cyclosporine-Ketoconazole | 199 |
| Cyclosporine-Rifampin | 209 |
| Desipramine-Guanethidine | 169 |
| Dicumarol-Allopurinol | 70 |
| Digitoxin-Rifampin | 276 |
| Digoxin-Amiodarone | 277 |
| Digoxin-Erythromycin Base | 279 |
| Digoxin-Propantheline | 287 |
| Digoxin-Quinidine | 287 |
| Digoxin-Tetracycline | 289 |
| Digoxin-Verapamil | 290 |
| Diltiazem-Cyclosporine | 47 |
| Disulfiram-Alcohol, Ethyl | 318 |

## Appendix B

Disulfiram-Phenytoin . . . . . . . . . . . . . . . . . . . . . . . . . . 120
Disulfiram-Warfarin . . . . . . . . . . . . . . . . . . . . . . . . . . . .82
Dopamine-Phenytoin . . . . . . . . . . . . . . . . . . . . . . . . . . 120
Epinephrine-Halothane . . . . . . . . . . . . . . . . . . . . . . . . . .28
Epinephrine-Propranolol . . . . . . . . . . . . . . . . . . . . . . . .267
Erythromycin-Carbamazepine . . . . . . . . . . . . . . . . . . . .105
Erythromycin-Cyclosporine . . . . . . . . . . . . . . . . . . . . . .190
Erythromycin-Lovastatin . . . . . . . . . . . . . . . . . . . . . . . .373
Erythromycin-Terfenadine . . . . . . . . . . . . . . . . . . . . . . .191
Erythromycin-Theophylline . . . . . . . . . . . . . . . . . . . . . .346
Erythromycin-Warfarin . . . . . . . . . . . . . . . . . . . . . . . . . .83
Erythromycin Base-Digoxin . . . . . . . . . . . . . . . . . . . . . .279
Ethacrynic Acid-Kanamycin . . . . . . . . . . . . . . . . . . . . . .198
Ether-Neomycin . . . . . . . . . . . . . . . . . . . . . . . . . . . . . . .27
Ferrous Sulfate-Tetracycline . . . . . . . . . . . . . . . . . . . . .212
Fluconazole-Phenytoin . . . . . . . . . . . . . . . . . . . . . . . . .121
Fluorouracil-Cimetidine . . . . . . . . . . . . . . . . . . . . . . . .220
Fluoxetine-Tranylcypromine . . . . . . . . . . . . . . . . . . . . .144
Furazolidone-Amphetamine . . . . . . . . . . . . . . . . . . . . .191
Gentamicin-Carbenicillin . . . . . . . . . . . . . . . . . . . . . . .192
Gentamicin-Cephalothin . . . . . . . . . . . . . . . . . . . . . . .192
Gentamicin-Tubocurarine . . . . . . . . . . . . . . . . . . . . . . . .41
Glucagon-Warfarin . . . . . . . . . . . . . . . . . . . . . . . . . . . .87
Glutethimide-Warfarin . . . . . . . . . . . . . . . . . . . . . . . . . .87
Grapefruit Juice-Lovastatin . . . . . . . . . . . . . . . . . . . . . .374
Guanethidine-Chlorpromazine . . . . . . . . . . . . . . . . . . .169
Guanethidine-Desipramine . . . . . . . . . . . . . . . . . . . . . .169
Guanethidine-Insulin . . . . . . . . . . . . . . . . . . . . . . . . . .309
Halothane-Aminophylline . . . . . . . . . . . . . . . . . . . . . . .337
Halothane-Epinephrine . . . . . . . . . . . . . . . . . . . . . . . . .28
Heparin-Aspirin . . . . . . . . . . . . . . . . . . . . . . . . . . . . . . .72
Insulin-Guanethidine . . . . . . . . . . . . . . . . . . . . . . . . . .309
Insulin-Propranolol . . . . . . . . . . . . . . . . . . . . . . . . . . .311
Iodinated Contrast Media-Metformin . . . . . . . . . . . . . . .312
Kanamycin-Ethacrynic Acid . . . . . . . . . . . . . . . . . . . . .198
Kaolin-Lincomycin . . . . . . . . . . . . . . . . . . . . . . . . . . . .202
Ketoconazole-Cyclosporine . . . . . . . . . . . . . . . . . . . . .199
Ketoconazole-Terfenadine . . . . . . . . . . . . . . . . . . . . . .201
Ketoconazole-Triazolam . . . . . . . . . . . . . . . . . . . . . . . .258
Leucovorin-Methotrexate . . . . . . . . . . . . . . . . . . . . . . .224
Levodopa-Phenelzine . . . . . . . . . . . . . . . . . . . . . . . . .157
Levodopa-Pyridoxine . . . . . . . . . . . . . . . . . . . . . . . . . .334
Lidocaine-Cimetidine . . . . . . . . . . . . . . . . . . . . . . . . . .54
Lincomycin-Kaolin . . . . . . . . . . . . . . . . . . . . . . . . . . . .202
Lithium Carbonate-Acetazolamide . . . . . . . . . . . . . . . .245
Lithium Carbonate-Chlorothiazide . . . . . . . . . . . . . . . .247
Lovastatin-Erythromycin . . . . . . . . . . . . . . . . . . . . . . .373
Lovastatin-Grapefruit Juice . . . . . . . . . . . . . . . . . . . . .374
Meperidine-Phenelzine . . . . . . . . . . . . . . . . . . . . . . . . .15
Mercaptopurine-Allopurinol . . . . . . . . . . . . . . . . . . . . .221
Metformin-Iodinated Contrast Media . . . . . . . . . . . . . .312
Methotrexate-Aspirin . . . . . . . . . . . . . . . . . . . . . . . . . .222
Methotrexate-Leucovorin . . . . . . . . . . . . . . . . . . . . . . .224
Methotrexate-Probenecid . . . . . . . . . . . . . . . . . . . . . .225
Methotrexate-Sulfamethoxazole, Trimethoprim . . . . . . .226
Methyltestosterone-Warfarin . . . . . . . . . . . . . . . . . . . . .91
Nalidixic Acid-Warfarin . . . . . . . . . . . . . . . . . . . . . . . . .93

| | |
|---|---|
| Neomycin-Ether | 27 |
| Oral Contraceptive Agents-Rifampin | 209 |
| Phenelzine-Levodopa | 157 |
| Phenelzine-Meperidine | 15 |
| Phenobarbital-Warfarin | 94 |
| Phenylbutazone-Tolbutamide | 314 |
| Phenylbutazone-Warfarin | 94 |
| Phenylpropanolamine-Tranylcypromine | 159 |
| Phenytoin-Cimetidine | 117 |
| Phenytoin-Disulfiram | 120 |
| Phenytoin-Dopamine | 120 |
| Phenytoin-Fluconazole | 121 |
| Phytonadione-Warfarin | 95 |
| Potassium Chloride-Spironolactone | 299 |
| Probenecid-Methotrexate | 225 |
| Propantheline-Digoxin | 287 |
| Propranolol-Cimetidine | 266 |
| Propranolol-Clonidine | 167 |
| Propranolol-Epinephrine | 267 |
| Propranolol-Insulin | 311 |
| Pyridoxine-Levodopa | 334 |
| Quinidine-Amiodarone | 62 |
| Quinidine-Digoxin | 287 |
| Quinidine-Verapamil | 65 |
| Ribavirin-Zidovudine | 387 |
| Rifampin-Cyclosporine | 209 |
| Rifampin-Digitoxin | 276 |
| Rifampin-Oral Contraceptive Agents | 209 |
| Rifampin-Warfarin | 97 |
| Spironolactone-Potassium Chloride | 299 |
| Sulfamethoxazole, Trimethoprim-Methotrexate | 226 |
| Sulfamethoxazole-Warfarin | 98 |
| Sulfinpyrazone-Warfarin | 98 |
| Terfenadine-Erythromycin | 191 |
| Terfenadine-Ketoconazole | 201 |
| Tetracycline-Aluminum Hydroxide | 211 |
| Tetracycline-Digoxin | 289 |
| Tetracycline-Ferrous Sulfate | 212 |
| Theophylline-Charcoal | 343 |
| Theophylline-Cimetidine | 344 |
| Theophylline-Erythromycin | 346 |
| Theophylline-Tobacco | 354 |
| Thyroid-Warfarin | 100 |
| Tobacco-Theophylline | 354 |
| Tolbutamide-Phenylbutazone | 314 |
| Tranylcypromine-Fluoxetine | 144 |
| Tranylcypromine-Phenylpropanolamine | 159 |
| Triazolam-Ketoconazole | 258 |
| Tubocurarine-Gentamicin | 41 |
| Undocumented Interaction | 388 |
| Verapamil-Digoxin | 290 |
| Verapamil-Quinidine | 65 |
| Warfarin-Amiodarone | 76 |
| Warfarin-Aspirin | 77 |
| Warfarin-Cimetidine | 80 |
| Warfarin-Clofibrate | 81 |
| Warfarin-Disulfiram | 82 |

## Appendix B

| | |
|---|---|
| Warfarin-Erythromycin | 83 |
| Warfarin-Glucagon | 87 |
| Warfarin-Glutethimide | 87 |
| Warfarin-Methyltestosterone | 91 |
| Warfarin-Nalidixic Acid | 93 |
| Warfarin-Phenobarbital | 94 |
| Warfarin-Phenylbutazone | 94 |
| Warfarin-Phytonadione | 95 |
| Warfarin-Rifampin | 97 |
| Warfarin-Sulfamethoxazole | 98 |
| Warfarin-Sulfinpyrazone | 98 |
| Warfarin-Thyroid | 100 |
| Zidovudine-Ribavirin | 387 |

# Index

# Index

The *Pocket Guide* index, an abbreviated version of the one found in *Evaluations of Drug Interactions*, includes all drugs mentioned in a monograph title and all other drugs involved in highly significant interactions. Drugs related to those mentioned in a monograph title that are involved in minimally significant interactions are not indexed.

Some of the index entries contain, in addition to page numbers, a boldface number. This refers to the significance code of a drug interaction. Significance codes are included for drugs mentioned in a monograph title, not for other drugs that may be mentioned in a monograph. In addition, numerous instances of significance code 1 (highly clinically significant) appear that refer to agents for which there are undocumented interactions (see Undocumented Interaction monograph, page 388). These agents (e.g., abciximab-dextran 70, acebutolol hydrochloride-arbutamine hydrochloride) have been listed in the manufacturer's product information for one or both agents in connection with an associated drug interaction warning, but no published studies exist on the interaction.

For an explanation of the significance coding, see *How to Use Pocket Guide to Evaluations of Drug Interactions*, page vii.

## A

abciximab,
 dextran 70 **1**, 388
acarbose,
 digoxin **3**, 276
 warfarin **3**, 75
acebutolol hydrochloride,
 arbutamine hydrochloride **1**, 388
 epinephrine, 267
 insulin, 311
acemetacin,
 ketorolac tromethamine **1**, 388
 ketorolac tromethamine, injectable **1**, 388
acenocoumarol,
 allopurinol, 70–71
 aloxiprin, 77
 aminoglutethimide, 87
 amiodarone hydrochloride, 76–77
 amobarbital, 94
 aprobarbital, 94
 aspirin, 77
 azapropazone dihydrate **1**, 388
 barbital, 94
 butabarbital sodium, 94
 butalbital, 94
 butobarbitone, 94
 calcium carbaspirin, 77
 cetirizine **3**, 70
 clarithromycin, 83
 clofibrate, 81
 danazol, 91
 dextrothyroxine sodium, 100
 diflunisal, 77
 disulfiram, 82–83
 erythromycin, 83
 erythromycin estolate, 83
 erythromycin ethylsuccinate, 83
 erythromycin gluceptate, 83
 erythromycin lactobionate, 83
 erythromycin stearate, 83
 ethylestrenol, 91
 feprazone, 94–95
 fluoxymesterone, 91
 gemfibrozil, 81
 glucagon, 87
 glucagon, recombinant, 87
 glutethimide, 87
 ivermectin **3**, 70
 levothyroxine sodium, 100
 liothyronine sodium, 100
 menadiol sodium diphosphate, vitamin K4, 95
 menadione, 95
 mephobarbital, 94
 methandrostenolone, 91
 metharbital, 94
 methohexital sodium, 94
 methyltestosterone, 91
 methyprylon, 87
 nalidixic acid, 93
 norfloxacin, 93
 oxandrolone, 91
 oxymetholone, 91
 oxyphenbutazone, 94–95
 pentobarbital sodium, 94
 phenobarbital, 94
 phenylbutazone, 94–95
 phytonadione, vitamin K1, 95
 primidone, 94
 rifabutin, 97
 rifampin, 97
 secobarbital, 94
 sodium salicylate, 77
 stanozolol, 91
 talbutal, 94
 thiamylal sodium, 94
 thiopental sodium, 94

# Index

thyroglobulin, 100
thyroid desiccated, 100
thyroid strong, 100
toremifene **1**, 388
acetaminophen,
  alcohol, ethyl–oral/injectable **3**, 2
  charcoal **3**, 2
  chloramphenicol **3**, 183
  hormonal contraceptive **3**, 2–3
  hormonal contraceptive, low–dose **3**, 2–3
  isoniazid **3**, 2
  lamotrigine **3**, 112
  phenobarbital **3**, 3
  phenytoin **2**, 3
  propranolol hydrochloride **3**, 3–4
  ranitidine hydrochloride, oral **3**, 4
  sulfinpyrazone **3**, 4
  terfenadine **2**, 5
  warfarin **3**, 76
  zidovudine **3**, 214
acetazolamide,
  aspirin **2**, 6–7
  cyclosporine **2**, 292
  lithium **1**, 245–246
  phenytoin **4**, 113–114
  primidone **3**, 130
  timolol maleate, ophthalmic **3**, 271
acetohexamide,
  alcohol, ethyl–oral/injectable, 302
  feprazone, 314–315
  oxyphenbutazone, 314–315
  phenylbutazone, 314–315
acetophenazine maleate,
  cabergoline **1**, 388
  cisapride **1**, 388
  grepafloxacin hydrochloride **1**, 388
  guanethidine, 169
  halofantrine hydrochloride **1**, 388
  pergolide mesylate **1**, 388
  pimozide **1**, 388
acetylcysteine,
  bacampicillin hydrochloride **3**, 181
acyclovir, oral,
  probenecid **3**, 180
  zidovudine **3**, 215
acyclovir sodium, injectable,
  lithium **3**, 246
adenosine, injectable,
  caffeine **3**, 340
  dipyridamole **3**, 357
albuterol sulfate,
  chloroform, 28
  enflurane, 28
  halothane, 28
  methoxyflurane, 28
  timolol maleate, oral, 267
alcohol, ethyl–oral/injectable,
  acetaminophen **3**, 2
  acetohexamide, 302
  amitriptyline hydrochloride **2**, 317
  aspirin **2**, 7
  bromocriptine mesylate **3**, 317
  calcium carbimide, 318
  cefoperazone sodium **2**, 181
  chloral hydrate **2**, 320
  chlorpromazine hydrochloride **2**, 232
  chlorpropamide **1**, 302
  cimetidine, oral **3**, 317
  diazepam **2**, 239
  diphenhydramine **2**, 317–318
  disopyramide phosphate **3**, 48
  disulfiram **1**, 318
  fluoxetine hydrochloride **4**, 318
  furazolidone **2**, 318
  gliclazide, 302
  glimepiride, 302
  glipizide, 302
  gliquidone, 302
  glutethimide **2**, 319
  glyburide, 302
  guanethidine **2**, 168
  ketoconazole, oral **3**, 319
  lithium **3**, 246
  meprobamate **2**, 321
  methotrexate **3**, 222
  metoclopramide hydrochloride **3**, 319
  metronidazole, oral/vaginal **2**, 319–320
  monosulfiram, 318
  nifedipine **3**, 58
  nitric oxide, inhalation **2**, 31
  phenobarbital **2**, 322
  phenytoin **2**, 114
  procainamide hydrochloride **3**, 59–60
  propoxyphene **2**, 22–23
  propranolol hydrochloride **3**, 263
  thiram, topical, 318
  tolazamide, 302
  tolbutamide, 302
  warfarin **3**, 76
alcuronium chloride,
  amikacin sulfate, 41
  bacitracin, 41
  colistin sulfate, 41
  demeclocycline hydrochloride, 41
  doxycycline hydrochloride, 41
  doxycycline hyclate, injectable, 41
  gentamicin sulfate, 41
  kanamycin sulfate, injectable, 41
  kanamycin sulfate, oral, 41
  lymecycline, 41
  methacycline hydrochloride, 41
  minocycline, injectable, 41
  minocycline hydrochloride, 41
  minocycline hydrochloride pellets, 41
  neomycin sulfate, injectable, 41
  neomycin sulfate, oral, 41

# Index

netilmicin, 41
oxytetracycline, 41
oxytetracycline, injectable, 41
paromomycin sulfate, 41
polymyxin B sulfate, 41
polymyxin B sulfate, vaccine use, 41
rolitetracycline, injectable, 41
streptomycin sulfate, 41
tetracycline, 41
tetracycline hydrochloride, injectable, 41
tobramycin, 41
aldesleukin, interleukin–2 human, dexamethasone **2**, 220–221
alendronate sodium, naproxen **2**, 20
alfacalcidol, paricalcitol **1**, 388
alfentanil hydrochloride,
erythromycin **2**, 5
fluconazole **3**, 5–6
isocarboxazid, 15
naltrexone hydrochloride **1**, 388
pargyline hydrochloride, 15
phenelzine sulfate, 15
selegiline hydrochloride, 15
tranylcypromine sulfate, 15
alfuzosin hydrochloride,
phenoxybenzamine hydrochloride **1**, 388
phentolamine **1**, 388
allergenic extracts,
propranolol hydrochloride **3**, 264
allopurinol,
acenocoumarol, 70–71
aluminum hydroxide **3**, 6
ampicillin sodium **3**, 180
anisindione, 70–71
azathioprine sodium, 221–222
captopril **3**, 163
chlorpropamide **3**, 302
coumarin, 70–71
cyclophosphamide **2**, 217
cyclosporine **2**, 360
dicumarol **1**, 70–71
ferrous sulfate **4**, 328–329
mercaptopurine **1**, 221–222
phenytoin **2**, 114
probenecid **3**, 6
theophylline **2**, 341–342
vidarabine **2**, 214
warfarin, 70–71
aloxiprin,
acenocoumarol, 77
anisindione, 77
coumarin, 77
dicumarol, 77
heparin, 72–73
ketorolac tromethamine **1**, 388
ketorolac tromethamine, injectable **1**, 388
methotrexate, 222
methotrexate sodium, injectable, 222
phenindione, 77
warfarin, 77
alprazolam,
fluoxetine hydrochloride **2**, 231
itraconazole, oral **1**, 388
kava **3**, 231
ketoconazole, oral **1**, 388
ritonavir **1**, 388
alteplase, recombinant,
nitroglycerin **2**, 357
altretamine,
pyridoxine hydrochloride **1**, 388
aluminum carbonate, basic,
demeclocycline hydrochloride, 211–212
doxycycline hydrochloride, 211–212
methacycline hydrochloride, 211–212
oxytetracycline, 211–212
tetracycline, 211–212
aluminum hydroxide,
allopurinol **3**, 6
aspirin **2**, 7
captopril **3**, 163
chlorpromazine hydrochloride **3**, 232–233
cholecalciferol, vitamin D3 **2**, 327
cimetidine, oral **3**, 358
ciprofloxacin hydrochloride **2**, 186
citric acid **3**, 357
clorazepate dipotassium **3**, 236
demeclocycline hydrochloride, 211–212
digoxin **2**, 276–277
doxycycline hydrochloride, 211–212
ethambutol hydrochloride **3**, 191
ferrous sulfate **3**, 329
indomethacin **3**, 13
isoniazid **3**, 195
ketoconazole, oral **2**, 198–199
levodopa **3**, 368
methacycline hydrochloride, 211–212
mexiletine hydrochloride **3**, 55
misoprostol **3**, 376–377
oxytetracycline, 211–212
penicillamine **3**, 379
phenytoin **3**, 114
prednisone **3**, 381
propranolol hydrochloride **3**, 264
tetracycline **1**, 211–212
theophylline **3**, 342
ticlopidine hydrochloride **3**, 74–75
valproic acid **3**, 132
vitamin D3, prenatal multivitamin use **2**, 327
aluminum oxide,

# Index

demeclocycline hydrochloride, 211–212
doxycycline hydrochloride, 211–212
methacycline hydrochloride, 211–212
oxytetracycline, 211–212
tetracycline, 211–212
aluminum phosphate,
  demeclocycline hydrochloride, 211–212
  doxycycline hydrochloride, 211–212
  methacycline hydrochloride, 211–212
  oxytetracycline, 211–212
  tetracycline, 211–212
amantadine hydrochloride,
  bupropion hydrochloride **3**, 138
  triamterene **3**, 298
amikacin sulfate,
  alcuronium chloride, 41
  amoxicillin, 192
  ampicillin sodium, 192
  atracurium besylate, 41
  azlocillin sodium, 192
  bacampicillin hydrochloride, 192
  benethamine penicillin, 192
  bumetanide, 198
  bumetanide, injectable, 198
  carbenicillin disodium, 192
  cefprozil, 192
  ceftibuten dihyrate, 192
  cefuroxime, 192
  cephalexin, 192
  cephalothin sodium, 192
  cloxacillin sodium, 192
  cyclacillin, 192
  dicloxacillin, 192
  doxacurium chloride, 41
  enflurane, 27
  ethacrynic acid, 198
  ethacrynic acid, injectable, 198
  ether, 27
  flucloxacillin, 192
  furosemide, 198
  furosemide, injectable, 198
  gallamine triethiodide, 41
  halothane, 27
  isoflurane, 27
  methicillin sodium, 192
  methoxyflurane, 27
  metocurine iodide, 41
  mezlocillin sodium, 192
  mivacurium chloride, 41
  moxalactam disodium, 192
  nafcillin sodium, 192
  nitrous oxide, 27
  oxacillin sodium, 192
  pancuronium bromide, 41
  penicillin G, 192
  penicillin G benzathine, 192
  penicillin G procaine, 192
  penicillin V, 192
  pipecuronium bromide, 41
  piperacillin sodium, 192
  piretanide, 198
  rapacuronium bromide, 41
  rocuronium bromide, 41
  succinylcholine chloride, 41
  temocillin sodium, 192
  ticarcillin disodium, 192
  torsemide, injectable, 198
  torsemide, oral, 198
  tubocurarine chloride, 41
  vecuronium bromide, 41
amiloride hydrochloride,
  dofetilide **2**, 388
  potassium, salt unspecified, 299
  potassium acetate, 299
  potassium bicarbonate, 299
  potassium biphosphate, 299
  potassium chloride, 299
  potassium citrate, 299
  potassium gluconate, 299
  potassium glycerophosphate, oral, 299
  potassium iodide, 299
  potassium iodide, prenatal multivitamin use, 299
  potassium perchlorate, 299
  potassium phosphate, 299
  potassium salicylate, 299
aminoglutethimide,
  acenocoumarol, 87
  anisindione, 87
  bendroflumethiazide **3**, 292
  coumarin, 87
  dexamethasone **2**, 364
  dicumarol, 87
  digitoxin **3**, 275
  medroxyprogesterone acetate **3**, 375
  propranolol hydrochloride **3**, 264
  theophylline **3**, 342
  warfarin, 87
aminophylline,
  cimetidine, oral, 344
  cimetidine hydrochloride, injectable, 344
  diazepam **3**, 239–240
  erythromycin, 346
  erythromycin estolate, 346
  erythromycin ethylsuccinate, 346
  erythromycin gluceptate, 346
  erythromycin lactobionate, 346
  erythromycin stearate, 346
  halothane **1**, 337
  hormonal contraceptive **3**, 339
  hormonal contraceptive, low–dose **3**, 339
  imipenem in combination with cilastatin **3**, 337
  interferon alfa–2a **2**, 337–338

# Index

isoproterenol **3**, 338
ketamine hydrochloride **3**, 338
levothyroxine sodium **3**, 338
pancuronium bromide **2**, 31
propofol **3**, 35
tacrine hydrochloride **2**, 339
terbinafine hydrochloride **2**, 339–340
thiabendazole **2**, 340
tobacco, 354
amiodarone hydrochloride,
  acenocoumarol, 76–77
  amprenavir **1**, 388
  anisindione, 76–77
  astemizole **1**, 388
  cholestyramine **3**, 46
  cisapride **1**, 388
  coumarin, 76–77
  cyclosporine **2**, 46
  deslanoside, 277
  dicumarol, 76–77
  digitalis, 277
  digitoxin, 277
  digoxin **1**, 277
  digoxin capsule, stabilized, 277
  diltiazem hydrochloride **2**, 46
  flecainide acetate **2**, 52
  grapefruit juice **2**, 330–331
  grepafloxacin hydrochloride **1**, 388
  halofantrine hydrochloride **1**, 388
  lidocaine hydrochloride, systemic **2**, 46–47
  metoprolol tartrate **2**, 262
  mizolastine **1**, 388
  moxifloxacin hydrochloride, oral **1**, 388
  phenytoin **2**, 115
  pimozide **1**, 388
  procainamide hydrochloride **2**, 60
  quinidine **1**, 62–63
  rifampin **2**, 208
  ritonavir **1**, 388
  sotalol hydrochloride **1**, 388
  sparfloxacin **1**, 388
  warfarin **1**, 76–77
amitriptyline hydrochloride,
  alcohol, ethyl-oral/injectable **2**, 317
  amprenavir **1**, 388
  arbutamine hydrochloride **1**, 388
  chlordiazepoxide **3**, 137
  cisapride **1**, 388
  disulfiram **3**, 137
  fluconazole **2**, 137–138
  grepafloxacin hydrochloride **1**, 388
  guanadrel sulfate, 169
  guanethidine, 169
  halofantrine hydrochloride **1**, 388
  methyldopa **3**, 173
  morphine **3**, 18
  pimozide **1**, 388
  thioridazine hydrochloride **1**, 388
  valproic acid **3**, 132
ammonium chloride,
  amphetamine **3**, 358
  flecainide acetate **2**, 52
  methadone hydrochloride **3**, 16
  mexiletine hydrochloride **3**, 56
amobarbital,
  acenocoumarol, 94
  anisindione, 94
  coumarin, 94
  dicumarol, 94
  tranylcypromine sulfate **3**, 320
  warfarin, 94
amoxapine,
  amprenavir **1**, 388
  arbutamine hydrochloride **1**, 388
  guanethidine, 169
amoxicillin,
  amikacin sulfate, 192
  gentamicin sulfate, 192
  netilmicin, 192
  tobramycin, 192
amphetamine,
  ammonium chloride **3**, 358
  chloroform, 28
  chlorpromazine hydrochloride **2**, 233
  enflurane, 28
  furazolidone **1**, 191–192
  halothane, 28
  isocarboxazid, 191–192
  methoxyflurane, 28
  pargyline hydrochloride, 191–192
  phenelzine sulfate, 191–192
  procarbazine hydrochloride, 191–192
  propoxyphene **3**, 23
  sodium bicarbonate **3**, 358
  tranylcypromine sulfate, 191–192
amphotericin B,
  cyclosporine **2**, 188
ampicillin sodium,
  allopurinol **3**, 180
  amikacin sulfate, 192
  atenolol **3**, 260
  gentamicin sulfate, 192
  hormonal contraceptive **2**, 180–181
  kanamycin sulfate, injectable, 192
  kanamycin sulfate, oral, 192
  khat **3**, 180
  neomycin sulfate, injectable, 192
  neomycin sulfate, oral, 192
  netilmicin, 192
  paromomycin sulfate, 192
  streptomycin sulfate, 192
  sulfasalazine **3**, 211
  tobramycin, 192
amprenavir,
  amiodarone hydrochloride **1**, 388
  amitriptyline hydrochloride **1**, 388
  amoxapine **1**, 388

# Index

astemizole **1**, 388
bepridil hydrochloride **1**, 388
cisapride **1**, 388
clomipramine hydrochloride **1**, 388
desipramine hydrochloride **1**, 388
dihydroergotamine mesylate **1**, 388
doxepin hydrochloride **1**, 388
doxepin hydrochloride, topical **1**, 388
ergotamine tartrate **1**, 388
imipramine **1**, 388
lidocaine hydrochloride, systemic **1**, 388
midazolam hydrochloride **1**, 388
nortriptyline hydrochloride **1**, 388
protriptyline hydrochloride **1**, 388
quinidine **1**, 388
rifampin **1**, 388
sildenafil citrate **1**, 388
terfenadine **1**, 388
triazolam **1**, 388
trimipramine maleate **1**, 388
amylase,
  miglitol **1**, 388
amyl nitrite,
  sildenafil citrate **1**, 388
anileridine,
  isocarboxazid, 15
  naltrexone hydrochloride **1**, 388
  pargyline hydrochloride, 15
  phenelzine sulfate, 15
  selegiline hydrochloride, 15
  tranylcypromine sulfate, 15
anisindione,
  allopurinol, 70–71
  aloxiprin, 77
  aminoglutethimide, 87
  amiodarone hydrochloride, 76–77
  amobarbital, 94
  aprobarbital, 94
  aspirin, 77
  azapropazone dihydrate **1**, 388
  butabarbital sodium, 94
  butalbital, 94
  butobarbitone, 94
  calcium carbaspirin, 77
  clofibrate, 81
  danazol, 91
  diflunisal, 77
  disulfiram, 82–83
  erythromycin, 83
  erythromycin estolate, 83
  erythromycin ethylsuccinate, 83
  erythromycin gluceptate, 83
  erythromycin lactobionate, 83
  erythromycin stearate, 83
  feprazone, 94–95
  glucagon, 87
  glucagon, recombinant, 87
  glutethimide, 87
  levothyroxine sodium, 100
  menadiol sodium diphosphate, vitamin K4, 95
  menadione, 95
  methyltestosterone, 91
  nalidixic acid, 93
  norfloxacin, 93
  oxymetholone, 91
  oxyphenbutazone, 94–95
  pentobarbital sodium, 94
  phenobarbital, 94
  phenylbutazone, 94–95
  phytonadione, vitamin K1, 95
  rifabutin, 97
  rifampin, 97
  secobarbital, 94
  sodium salicylate, 77
  thyroid desiccated, 100
  thyroid strong, 100
  toremifene **1**, 388
anisotropine methylbromide,
  digoxin, 287
apraclonidine hydrochloride,
  isocarboxazid **1**, 388
  moclobemide **1**, 388
  pargyline hydrochloride **1**, 388
  phenelzine sulfate **1**, 388
  tranylcypromine sulfate **1**, 388
aprobarbital,
  acenocoumarol, 94
  anisindione, 94
  coumarin, 94
  dicumarol, 94
  warfarin, 94
arbutamine hydrochloride,
  acebutolol hydrochloride **1**, 388
  amitriptyline hydrochloride **1**, 388
  amoxapine **1**, 388
  atenolol **1**, 388
  atropine **1**, 388
  betaxolol hydrochloride, ophthalmic **1**, 388
  betaxolol hydrochloride, oral **1**, 388
  bisoprolol fumarate **1**, 388
  carteolol hydrochloride **1**, 388
  carteolol hydrochloride, ophthalmic **1**, 388
  carvedilol **1**, 388
  chloroform, 28
  clomipramine hydrochloride **1**, 388
  desipramine hydrochloride **1**, 388
  digoxin **1**, 388
  doxepin hydrochloride **1**, 388
  enflurane, 28
  esmolol hydrochloride **1**, 388
  halothane, 28
  imipramine **1**, 388
  labetalol hydrochloride **1**, 388
  levobunolol hydrochloride, ophthalmic **1**, 388
  lidocaine hydrochloride,

# Index

    local–injectable **1**, 388
    lidocaine hydrochloride, systemic **1**, 388
    methoxyflurane, 28
    metipranolol hydrochloride, ophthalmic **1**, 388
    metoprolol tartrate **1**, 388
    nadolol **1**, 388
    nebivolol hydrochloride **1**, 388
    nortriptyline hydrochloride **1**, 388
    oxprenolol **1**, 388
    penbutolol sulfate **1**, 388
    pindolol **1**, 388
    propranolol hydrochloride **1**, 388
    protriptyline hydrochloride **1**, 388
    quinidine **1**, 388
    sotalol hydrochloride **1**, 388
    tertatolol hydrochloride **1**, 388
    timolol maleate, ophthalmic **1**, 388
    timolol maleate, oral **1**, 388
    trimipramine maleate **1**, 388
ardeparin sodium,
    sodium salicylate, 77
ascorbic acid, vitamin C,
    aspirin **4**, 327
    ethinyl estradiol **3**, 327
    ferrous sulfate **3**, 329
    warfarin **4**, 77
asparaginase, e. coli derived,
    methotrexate **1**, 388
    methotrexate sodium, injectable **1**, 388
aspirin,
    acenocoumarol, 77
    acetazolamide **2**, 6–7
    alcohol, ethyl–oral/injectable **2**, 7
    aluminum hydroxide **2**, 7
    anisindione, 77
    ascorbic acid, vitamin C **4**, 327
    captopril **2**, 164
    charcoal **3**, 8
    chlorpropamide **2**, 302–303
    coumarin, 77
    dicumarol, 77
    dipyridamole **3**, 8
    fluoxetine hydrochloride **3**, 141–142
    furosemide **3**, 295
    ginkgo biloba **3**, 8
    griseofulvin **3**, 9
    heparin **1**, 72–73
    hormonal contraceptive **3**, 10
    imipramine **3**, 146
    indomethacin **3**, 13
    insulin **3**, 307
    ketorolac tromethamine **1**, 388
    ketorolac tromethamine, injectable **1**, 388
    magnesium hydroxide **2**, 7
    methotrexate **1**, 222
    methotrexate sodium, injectable, 222
    methylprednisolone **2**, 9
    niacin, vitamin B3 **3**, 334
    nitroglycerin **3**, 9
    penicillin G **3**, 205
    phenytoin **4**, 115
    propranolol hydrochloride **3**, 264–265
    spironolactone **3**, 298
    sulfinpyrazone **2**, 24
    valproic acid **2**, 132–133
    warfarin **1**, 77
astemizole,
    amiodarone hydrochloride **1**, 388
    amprenavir **1**, 388
    bepridil hydrochloride **1**, 388
    cisapride **1**, 388
    clarithromycin, 191
    disopyramide phosphate **1**, 388
    efavirenz **1**, 388
    encainide hydrochloride **1**, 388
    erythromycin, 191
    erythromycin estolate, 191
    erythromycin ethylsuccinate, 191
    erythromycin gluceptate, 191
    erythromycin lactobionate, 191
    erythromycin stearate, 191
    flecainide acetate **1**, 388
    fluconazole **1**, 388
    fluoxetine hydrochloride **1**, 388
    fluvoxamine maleate **1**, 388
    grapefruit juice **1**, 388
    grepafloxacin hydrochloride **1**, 388
    halofantrine hydrochloride **1**, 388
    ibutilide fumarate **1**, 388
    indinavir sulfate **1**, 388
    itraconazole, oral **1**, 388
    ketoconazole, oral, 201–202
    metronidazole, injectable **1**, 388
    metronidazole, oral/vaginal **1**, 388
    mibefradil dihydrochloride **1**, 388
    miconazole nitrate **1**, 388
    nefazodone hydrochloride **1**, 388
    nelfinavir mesylate **1**, 388
    paroxetine hydrochloride **1**, 388
    procainamide hydrochloride **1**, 388
    propafenone hydrochloride **1**, 388
    quinidine **1**, 388
    quinine **1**, 388
    ritonavir **1**, 388
    saquinavir **1**, 388
    sertraline hydrochloride **1**, 388
    sotalol hydrochloride **1**, 388
    sparfloxacin **1**, 388
    spiramycin, 191
    sulfamethoxazole–trimethoprim **1**, 388
    terfenadine **1**, 388
    troleandomycin, 191
    zileuton **1**, 388
atenolol,
    ampicillin sodium **3**, 260

# Index

arbutamine hydrochloride **1**, 388
calcium carbonate, oral **3**, 260
clonidine hydrochloride, 167
clonidine hydrochloride,
 transdermal, 167
disopyramide phosphate **3**, 48
propantheline bromide **3**, 260
atorvastatin calcium,
 grapefruit juice, 374
 itraconazole, oral **1**, 388
atovaquone,
 zidovudine **2**, 387
atracurium besylate,
 amikacin sulfate, 41
 colistin sulfate, 41
 kanamycin sulfate, injectable, 41
 kanamycin sulfate, oral, 41
 neomycin sulfate, injectable, 41
 neomycin sulfate, oral, 41
 netilmicin, 41
 paromomycin sulfate, 41
 streptomycin sulfate, 41
 tranylcypromine sulfate **3**, 159
atropine,
 arbutamine hydrochloride **1**, 388
 digoxin, 287
 metoclopramide hydrochloride **3**, 375
 mexiletine hydrochloride **3**, 56
attapulgite,
 demeclocycline hydrochloride, 211–212
 doxycycline hydrochloride, 211–212
 kaolin, 211–212
 lymecycline, 211–212
 methacycline hydrochloride, 211–212
 minocycline hydrochloride, 211–212
 minocycline hydrochloride pellets, 211–212
 oxytetracycline, 211–212
 tetracycline, 211–212
ayahuasca,
 fluoxetine hydrochloride **2**, 142
azapropazone dihydrate,
 acenocoumarol **1**, 388
 anisindione **1**, 388
 dicumarol **1**, 388
 fosphenytoin sodium, injectable **1**, 388
 methotrexate **1**, 388
 methotrexate sodium, injectable **1**, 388
 phenytoin **1**, 388
 warfarin **1**, 388
azathioprine sodium,
 allopurinol, 221–222
 cyclosporine **3**, 360
 enalapril maleate **3**, 168
 pancuronium bromide **3**, 32
 warfarin **2**, 78

azithromycin,
 cyclosporine, 190
 lovastatin, 373
 mizolastine **1**, 388
 pimozide **1**, 388
 warfarin, 83
azlocillin sodium,
 amikacin sulfate, 192
 gentamicin sulfate, 192
 netilmicin, 192
 tobramycin, 192

# B

bacampicillin hydrochloride,
 acetylcysteine **3**, 181
 amikacin sulfate, 192
 gentamicin sulfate, 192
 netilmicin, 192
 tobramycin, 192
bacitracin,
 alcuronium chloride, 41
 doxacurium chloride, 41
 ether, 27
 gallamine triethiodide, 41
 methoxyflurane, 27
 metocurine iodide, 41
 mivacurium chloride, 41
 pancuronium bromide, 41
 pipecuronium bromide, 41
 rapacuronium bromide, 41
 rocuronium bromide, 41
 succinylcholine chloride, 41
 tubocurarine chloride, 41
 vecuronium bromide, 41
baclofen,
 ibuprofen **3**, 12–13
barbital,
 acenocoumarol, 94
 coumarin, 94
 dicumarol, 94
 phenindione, 94
 warfarin, 94
basiliximab,
 cyclosporine **2**, 361
belladonna,
 digoxin, 287
bellafoline,
 digoxin, 287
bendroflumethiazide,
 aminoglutethimide **3**, 292
 indomethacin **2**, 292
 lithium, 247
benethamine penicillin,
 amikacin sulfate, 192
 gentamicin sulfate, 192
 kanamycin sulfate, injectable, 192
 kanamycin sulfate, oral, 192
 neomycin sulfate, injectable, 192
 neomycin sulfate, oral, 192
 netilmicin, 192
 paromomycin sulfate, 192

# Index

streptomycin sulfate, 192
tobramycin, 192
benperidol,
  cabergoline **1**, 388
  pergolide mesylate **1**, 388
benserazide,
  orphenadrine citrate **3**, 369
benzphetamine hydrochloride,
  chloroform, 28
  enflurane, 28
  furazolidone, 191–192
  halothane, 28
  isocarboxazid, 191–192
  methoxyflurane, 28
  moclobemide, 159–160
  pargyline hydrochloride, 159–160
  phenelzine sulfate, 159–160
  procarbazine hydrochloride, 159–160
  tranylcypromine sulfate, 159–160
benzthiazide,
  lithium, 247
benztropine mesylate,
  chlorpromazine hydrochloride **2**, 234
  digoxin, 287
bepridil hydrochloride,
  amprenavir **1**, 388
  astemizole **1**, 388
  cisapride **1**, 388
  grepafloxacin hydrochloride **1**, 388
  ritonavir **1**, 388
  sparfloxacin **1**, 388
betaxolol hydrochloride, ophthalmic,
  arbutamine hydrochloride **1**, 388
betaxolol hydrochloride, oral,
  arbutamine hydrochloride **1**, 388
  epinephrine, 267
  insulin, 311
bethanidine sulphate,
  chlorpromazine hydrochloride, 169
  desipramine hydrochloride, 169
  mazindol **2**, 163
bexarotene,
  gemfibrozil **1**, 388
bezafibrate,
  coumarin, 81
  dicumarol, 81
  phenindione, 81
  warfarin, 81
biperiden,
  digoxin, 287
bismuth subsalicylate,
  demeclocycline hydrochloride, 211–212
  doxycycline hydrochloride, 211–212
  methacycline hydrochloride, 211–212
  oxytetracycline, 211–212
  tetracycline, 211–212
bisoprolol fumarate,
  arbutamine hydrochloride **1**, 388
  epinephrine, 267
  insulin, 311
bitolterol mesylate,
  chloroform, 28
  enflurane, 28
  halothane, 28
  methoxyflurane, 28
  metoprolol tartrate, 267
  timolol maleate, oral, 267
bleomycin sulfate,
  cisplatin **3**, 217
bretylium tosylate,
  grepafloxacin hydrochloride **1**, 388
  halofantrine hydrochloride **1**, 388
  moxifloxacin hydrochloride, oral **1**, 388
  pimozide **1**, 388
  sotalol hydrochloride **1**, 388
brimonidine tartrate, ophthalmic,
  furazolidone **1**, 388
  isocarboxazid **1**, 388
  moclobemide **1**, 388
  pargyline hydrochloride **1**, 388
  phenelzine sulfate **1**, 388
  procarbazine hydrochloride **1**, 388
  selegiline hydrochloride **1**, 388
  tranylcypromine sulfate **1**, 388
brinzolamide, ophthalmic,
  lithium, 245–246
bromocriptine mesylate,
  alcohol, ethyl–oral/injectable **3**, 317
  efavirenz **1**, 388
  indinavir sulfate **1**, 388
  rizatriptan benzoate **1**, 388
  saquinavir **1**, 388
  thioridazine hydrochloride **2**, 257
bumetanide,
  amikacin sulfate, 198
  gentamicin sulfate, 198
  kanamycin sulfate, injectable, 198
  kanamycin sulfate, oral, 198
  lithium, 247
  neomycin sulfate, injectable, 198
  neomycin sulfate, oral, 198
  netilmicin, 198
  probenecid **3**, 297
  streptomycin sulfate, 198
  tobramycin, 198
bumetanide, injectable,
  amikacin sulfate, 198
  gentamicin sulfate, 198
  kanamycin sulfate, injectable, 198
  kanamycin sulfate, oral, 198
  lithium, 247
  neomycin sulfate, injectable, 198
  neomycin sulfate, oral, 198
  netilmicin, 198
  streptomycin sulfate, 198
  tobramycin, 198
bupivacaine hydrochloride,

# Index

diazepam **3**, 26
ritodrine hydrochloride **2**, 26
buprenorphine hydrochloride,
  isocarboxazid, 15
  naltrexone hydrochloride **1**, 388
  pargyline hydrochloride, 15
  phenelzine sulfate, 15
  selegiline hydrochloride, 15
  tranylcypromine sulfate, 15
bupropion hydrochloride,
  amantadine hydrochloride **3**, 138
  carbamazepine **3**, 138–139
  furazolidone **1**, 388
  guanfacine hydrochloride **3**, 171–172
  imipramine **3**, 146
  isocarboxazid **1**, 388
  moclobemide **1**, 388
  pargyline hydrochloride **1**, 388
  phenelzine sulfate **1**, 388
  procarbazine hydrochloride **1**, 388
  ritonavir **1**, 388
  selegiline hydrochloride **1**, 388
  tranylcypromine sulfate **1**, 388
buspirone hydrochloride,
  cimetidine, oral **4**, 231–232
  erythromycin **3**, 139
  fluoxetine hydrochloride **3**, 139
  itraconazole, oral **3**, 197–198
  phenelzine sulfate **3**, 156
  rifampin **3**, 208
  ritonavir **3**, 232
butabarbital sodium,
  acenocoumarol, 94
  anisindione, 94
  coumarin, 94
  dicumarol, 94
  warfarin, 94
butalbital,
  acenocoumarol, 94
  anisindione, 94
  coumarin, 94
  dicumarol, 94
  warfarin, 94
butobarbitone,
  acenocoumarol, 94
  anisindione, 94
  coumarin, 94
  dicumarol, 94
  phenindione, 94
  warfarin, 94
butoconazole nitrate,
  cyclosporine, 199–200
  lovastatin **1**, 388
  mizolastine **1**, 388
  phenytoin, 121–122
  simvastatin **1**, 388
butorphanol tartrate,
  naltrexone hydrochloride **1**, 388
  pargyline hydrochloride, 15
  phenelzine sulfate, 15
  selegiline hydrochloride, 15
  tranylcypromine sulfate, 15
butriptyline hydrochloride,
  guanadrel sulfate, 169
  guanethidine, 169

## C

cabergoline,
  acetophenazine maleate **1**, 388
  benperidol **1**, 388
  chlorpromazine hydrochloride **1**, 388
  chlorprothixene **1**, 388
  efavirenz **1**, 388
  flupenthixol decanoate, injectable **1**, 388
  flupenthixol dihydrochloride, oral **1**, 388
  fluphenazine **1**, 388
  haloperidol **1**, 388
  indinavir sulfate **1**, 388
  mesoridazine besylate **1**, 388
  methdilazine **1**, 388
  pericyazine **1**, 388
  perphenazine **1**, 388
  prochlorperazine **1**, 388
  promazine hydrochloride **1**, 388
  promethazine **1**, 388
  propiomazine hydrochloride **1**, 388
  rizatriptan benzoate **1**, 388
  saquinavir **1**, 388
  sumatriptan succinate **1**, 388
  sumatriptan succinate, injectable **1**, 388
  sumatriptan succinate, oral **1**, 388
  thiethylperazine maleate **1**, 388
  thioridazine hydrochloride **1**, 388
  thiothixene **1**, 388
  trifluoperazine hydrochloride **1**, 388
  trifluperidol hydrochloride **1**, 388
  triflupromazine hydrochloride **1**, 388
  trimeprazine tartrate **1**, 388
caffeine,
  adenosine, injectable **3**, 340
  cimetidine, oral, 344
  cimetidine hydrochloride, injectable, 344
  clozapine **3**, 236–237
  erythromycin, 346
  erythromycin estolate, 346
  erythromycin ethylsuccinate, 346
  erythromycin gluceptate, 346
  erythromycin lactobionate, 346
  erythromycin stearate, 346
  hormonal contraceptive **3**, 341
  hormonal contraceptive, low-dose **3**, 341
  methoxsalen **3**, 340
  phenylpropanolamine **3**, 341

## Index

theophylline **2**, 342–343
calcifediol,
  paricalcitol **1**, 388
calcipotriene,
  paricalcitol **1**, 388
calcitriol,
  paricalcitol **1**, 388
calcium, oral salt unspecified,
  demeclocycline hydrochloride, 211–212
  doxycycline hydrochloride, 211–212
  methacycline hydrochloride, 211–212
  oxytetracycline, 211–212
  tetracycline, 211–212
calcium acetate,
  demeclocycline hydrochloride, 211–212
  doxycycline hydrochloride, 211–212
  methacycline hydrochloride, 211–212
  oxytetracycline, 211–212
  tetracycline, 211–212
calcium ascorbate,
  demeclocycline hydrochloride, 211–212
  doxycycline hydrochloride, 211–212
  methacycline hydrochloride, 211–212
  oxytetracycline, 211–212
  tetracycline, 211–212
calcium carbaspirin,
  acenocoumarol, 77
  anisindione, 77
  heparin, 72–73
  ketorolac tromethamine **1**, 388
  methotrexate, 222
  methotrexate sodium, injectable, 222
  phenindione, 77
  warfarin, 77
calcium carbimide,
  alcohol, ethyl–oral/injectable, 318
  warfarin, 82–83
calcium carbonate, oral,
  atenolol **3**, 260
  chlorothiazide **2**, 293
  demeclocycline hydrochloride, 211–212
  doxycycline hydrochloride, 211–212
  levothyroxine sodium **3**, 370
  methacycline hydrochloride, 211–212
  oxytetracycline, 211–212
  tetracycline, 211–212
calcium chloride, injectable,
  digitalis **2**, 274
calcium chloride, oral,
  demeclocycline hydrochloride, 211–212
  doxycycline hydrochloride, 211–212
  methacycline hydrochloride, 211–212
  oxytetracycline, 211–212
  tetracycline, 211–212
calcium citrate, oral,
  demeclocycline hydrochloride, 211–212
  doxycycline hydrochloride, 211–212
  methacycline hydrochloride, 211–212
  oxytetracycline, 211–212
  tetracycline, 211–212
calcium glubionate, oral,
  demeclocycline hydrochloride, 211–212
  doxycycline hydrochloride, 211–212
  methacycline hydrochloride, 211–212
  oxytetracycline, 211–212
  tetracycline, 211–212
calcium glucoheptonate,
  demeclocycline hydrochloride, 211–212
  doxycycline hydrochloride, 211–212
  methacycline hydrochloride, 211–212
  oxytetracycline, 211–212
  tetracycline, 211–212
calcium gluconate, oral,
  demeclocycline hydrochloride, 211–212
  doxycycline hydrochloride, 211–212
  methacycline hydrochloride, 211–212
  oxytetracycline, 211–212
  tetracycline, 211–212
  verapamil hydrochloride **2**, 66
calcium glycerophosphate, oral,
  demeclocycline hydrochloride, 211–212
  doxycycline hydrochloride, 211–212
  methacycline hydrochloride, 211–212
  oxytetracycline, 211–212
  tetracycline, 211–212
calcium iodate,
  demeclocycline hydrochloride, 211–212
  doxycycline hydrochloride, 211–212
  metformin hydrochloride **1**, 312
  methacycline hydrochloride, 211–212
  oxytetracycline, 211–212
  tetracycline, 211–212
calcium lactate, oral,
  demeclocycline hydrochloride, 211–212
  doxycycline hydrochloride, 211–212
  methacycline hydrochloride, 211–212
  oxytetracycline, 211–212

# Index

tetracycline, 211–212
calcium lactate gluconate,
  demeclocycline hydrochloride, 211–212
  doxycycline hydrochloride, 211–212
  methacycline hydrochloride, 211–212
  oxytetracycline, 211–212
  tetracycline, 211–212
calcium lactobionate, oral,
  demeclocycline hydrochloride, 211–212
  doxycycline hydrochloride, 211–212
  lymecycline, 211–212
  methacycline hydrochloride, 211–212
  minocycline hydrochloride, 211–212
  minocycline hydrochloride pellets, 211–212
  oxytetracycline, 211–212
  tetracycline, 211–212
calcium phosphate, oral,
  demeclocycline hydrochloride, 211–212
  doxycycline hydrochloride, 211–212
  methacycline hydrochloride, 211–212
  oxytetracycline, 211–212
  tetracycline, 211–212
captopril,
  allopurinol **3**, 163
  aluminum hydroxide **3**, 163
  aspirin **2**, 164
  chlorpromazine hydrochloride **2**, 164
  digoxin **2**, 278
  furosemide **2**, 164
  indomethacin **2**, 164–165
  magnesium carbonate **3**, 163
  magnesium hydroxide **3**, 163
  naloxone hydrochloride **3**, 165
  nitroprusside sodium **3**, 175–176
  potassium chloride **3**, 165
  probenecid **3**, 165–166
  spironolactone **3**, 298–299
carbamazepine,
  bupropion hydrochloride **3**, 138–139
  charcoal **1**, 104
  cimetidine, oral **2**, 104
  clarithromycin, 105
  clonazepam **3**, 110–111
  clozapine **2**, 237
  cyclosporine **2**, 361
  danazol **2**, 104
  desipramine hydrochloride **3**, 104–105
  doxycycline hydrochloride **2**, 189
  erythromycin **1**, 105
  erythromycin estolate, 105
  erythromycin ethylsuccinate, 105
  erythromycin gluceptate, 105
  erythromycin lactobionate, 105
  erythromycin stearate, 105
  ethosuximide **3**, 111
  felbamate **2**, 105
  haloperidol **2**, 243
  hormonal contraceptive **3**, 108
  hormonal contraceptive, low–dose **3**, 108
  hydrochlorothiazide **3**, 106
  indinavir sulfate **2**, 367
  isoniazid **2**, 106
  isotretinoin **3**, 106
  ketoconazole, oral **3**, 106–107
  lithium **2**, 246–247
  methylphenidate hydrochloride **3**, 107
  metoclopramide hydrochloride **3**, 107
  metronidazole, oral/vaginal **2**, 107–108
  niacinamide (nicotinamide) **3**, 108
  pancuronium bromide **3**, 32
  phenobarbital **3**, 108–109
  phenytoin **3**, 115
  propoxyphene **2**, 109
  terfenadine **3**, 109
  theophylline **2**, 343
  ticlopidine hydrochloride **2**, 109–110
  trazodone hydrochloride **3**, 110
  troleandomycin, 105
  valproic acid **2**, 133
  verapamil hydrochloride **2**, 110
  vincristine sulfate **2**, 229
carbenicillin disodium,
  amikacin sulfate, 192
  gentamicin sulfate **1**, 192
  heparin **2**, 73
  kanamycin sulfate, injectable, 192
  kanamycin sulfate, oral, 192
  neomycin sulfate, injectable, 192
  neomycin sulfate, oral, 192
  netilmicin, 192
  paromomycin sulfate, 192
  streptomycin sulfate, 192
  tobramycin, 192
carbonyl iron,
  doxycycline hydrochloride, 212
  lymecycline, 212
  methacycline hydrochloride, 212
  minocycline hydrochloride, 212
  minocycline hydrochloride pellets, 212
  oxytetracycline, 212
  tetracycline, 212
carfecillin,
  gentamicin sulfate, 192
carmustine,
  cimetidine, oral **2**, 217
  phenytoin **2**, 116

# Index

carteolol hydrochloride,
  arbutamine hydrochloride **1**, 388
  clonidine hydrochloride, 167
  clonidine hydrochloride,
    transdermal, 167
  epinephrine, 267
  insulin, 311
carteolol hydrochloride, ophthalmic,
  arbutamine hydrochloride **1**, 388
  clonidine hydrochloride, 167
  clonidine hydrochloride,
    transdermal, 167
carvedilol,
  arbutamine hydrochloride **1**, 388
  cimetidine, oral, 266
  cimetidine hydrochloride,
    injectable, 266
  clonidine hydrochloride, 167
  clonidine hydrochloride,
    transdermal, 167
  cyclosporine **3**, 260–261
  epinephrine, 267
  insulin, 311
cefaclor,
  gentamicin sulfate, 192
  theophylline **3**, 343
  tobramycin, 192
cefadroxil monohydrate,
  gentamicin sulfate, 192
  tobramycin, 192
cefamandole nafate,
  gentamicin sulfate, 192
  tobramycin, 192
  warfarin **2**, 78
cefazolin sodium,
  gentamicin sulfate, 192
  tobramycin, 192
cefdinir,
  gentamicin sulfate, 192
  tobramycin, 192
cefepime hydrochloride,
  gentamicin sulfate, 192
  tobramycin, 192
cefmetazole sodium,
  gentamicin sulfate, 192
  tobramycin, 192
cefonicid sodium,
  gentamicin sulfate, 192
  tobramycin, 192
cefoperazone sodium,
  alcohol, ethyl–oral/injectable **2**, 181
  gentamicin sulfate, 192
  tobramycin, 192
cefloranide,
  gentamicin sulfate, 192
  tobramycin, 192
cefotaxime sodium,
  cimetidine, oral **3**, 181–182
  gentamicin sulfate, 192
  tobramycin, 192
cefotetan disodium,
  gentamicin sulfate, 192
  tobramycin, 192
cefoxitin sodium,
  gentamicin sulfate, 192
  tobramycin, 192
cefpirome sulfate,
  gentamicin sulfate, 192
  tobramycin, 192
cefpodoxime proxetil,
  gentamicin sulfate, 192
  tobramycin, 192
cefprozil,
  amikacin sulfate, 192
  gentamicin sulfate, 192
  kanamycin sulfate, injectable, 192
  kanamycin sulfate, oral, 192
  neomycin sulfate, injectable, 192
  neomycin sulfate, oral, 192
  netilmicin, 192
  paromomycin sulfate, 192
  streptomycin sulfate, 192
  tobramycin, 192
ceftazidime,
  gentamicin sulfate, 192
  tobramycin, 192
ceftibuten dihyrate,
  amikacin sulfate, 192
  gentamicin sulfate, 192
  kanamycin sulfate, injectable, 192
  kanamycin sulfate, oral, 192
  neomycin sulfate, injectable, 192
  neomycin sulfate, oral, 192
  netilmicin, 192
  paromomycin sulfate, 192
  streptomycin sulfate, 192
  streptomycin sulfate, vaccine use,
    192
  tobramycin, 192
ceftizoxime sodium,
  gentamicin sulfate, 192
  tobramycin, 192
ceftriaxone sodium,
  gentamicin sulfate, 192
  tobramycin, 192
cefuroxime,
  amikacin sulfate, 192
  gentamicin sulfate, 192
  kanamycin sulfate, injectable, 192
  kanamycin sulfate, oral, 192
  neomycin sulfate, injectable, 192
  neomycin sulfate, oral, 192
  netilmicin, 192
  paromomycin sulfate, 192
  streptomycin sulfate, 192
  tobramycin, 192
celiprolol hydrochloride,
  clonidine hydrochloride, 167
  clonidine hydrochloride,
    transdermal, 167
  epinephrine, 267
  insulin, 311

cephalexin,
  amikacin sulfate, 192
  gentamicin sulfate, 192
  kanamycin sulfate, injectable, 192
  kanamycin sulfate, oral, 192
  neomycin sulfate, injectable, 192
  neomycin sulfate, oral, 192
  netilmicin, 192
  paromomycin sulfate, 192
  streptomycin sulfate, 192
  tobramycin, 192
cephalothin sodium,
  amikacin sulfate, 192
  colistimethate sodium **2**, 182
  gentamicin sulfate **1**, 192
  kanamycin sulfate, injectable, 192
  kanamycin sulfate, oral, 192
  neomycin sulfate, injectable, 192
  neomycin sulfate, oral, 192
  netilmicin, 192
  paromomycin sulfate, 192
  probenecid **2**, 182–183
  streptomycin sulfate, 192
  tobramycin, 192
cephapirin sodium,
  gentamicin sulfate, 192
  tobramycin, 192
cephradine,
  gentamicin sulfate, 192
  tobramycin, 192
cerivastatin,
  gemfibrozil **1**, 388
  grapefruit juice, 374
certoparin,
  sodium salicylate, 77
cetirizine,
  acenocoumarol **3**, 70
charcoal,
  acetaminophen **3**, 2
  aspirin **3**, 8
  carbamazepine **1**, 104
  digoxin **3**, 278
  disopyramide phosphate **2**, 48–49
  flecainide acetate **3**, 52–53
  furosemide **2**, 295
  glipizide **2**, 304–305
  miglitol **1**, 388
  nizatidine **3**, 377
  nortriptyline hydrochloride **3**, 151
  phenobarbital **3**, 322
  phenylbutazone **3**, 21
  phenytoin **2**, 116
  promazine hydrochloride **3**, 257
  propoxyphene **3**, 23
  theophylline **1**, 343–344
chloral hydrate,
  alcohol, ethyl–oral/injectable **2**, 320
  furazolidone **4**, 320
  furosemide **3**, 295
  warfarin **2**, 78–79
chloramphenicol,
  acetaminophen **3**, 183
  cyclophosphamide **2**, 218
  cyclosporine **3**, 183–184
  dicumarol **2**, 71
  penicillin G **4**, 205–206
  phenobarbital **3**, 184
  phenytoin **2**, 116
  rifampin **2**, 184
  tolbutamide **2**, 313
chlorcyclizine hydrochloride,
  phenobarbital **3**, 322–323
chlordiazepoxide,
  amitriptyline hydrochloride **3**, 137
  ketoconazole, oral **3**, 258
  warfarin **4**, 79
chlormethiazole,
  cimetidine, oral **3**, 321
chloroform,
  albuterol sulfate, 28
  amphetamine, 28
  arbutamine hydrochloride, 28
  benzphetamine hydrochloride, 28
  bitolterol mesylate, 28
  dexfenfluramine hydrochloride, 28
  dextroamphetamine, 28
  diethylpropion hydrochloride, 28
  dobutamine hydrochloride, 28
  dopamine hydrochloride, 28
  ephedrine, 28
  epinephrine, 28
  etafedrine hydrochloride, 28
  ethylnorepinephrine hydrochloride, 28
  fenfluramine hydrochloride, 28
  fenoterol hydrobromide, 28
  formoterol fumarate, inhl, 28
  isoetharine, 28
  isometheptene, 28
  isoproterenol, 28
  mazindol, 28
  mephentermine sulfate, 28
  metaproterenol sulfate, 28
  metaraminol bitartrate, 28
  methamphetamine hydrochloride, 28
  methoxamine hydrochloride, 28
  methylphenidate hydrochloride, 28
  norepinephrine bitartrate, 28
  phendimetrazine tartrate, 28
  phenmetrazine hydrochloride, 28
  phentermine hydrochloride, 28
  phenylephrine, 28
  phenylpropanolamine, 28
  pirbuterol acetate, 28
  procaterol hydrochloride, 28
  pseudoephedrine, 28
  rimiterol hydrobromide, 28
  salmeterol xinafoate, 28
  terbutaline sulfate, 28
chloroquine,
  cimetidine, oral **3**, 184

# Index

cyclosporine **2**, 184–185
kaolin **3**, 185
levothyroxine sodium **3**, 185
metronidazole, oral/vaginal **2**, 202–203
penicillamine **3**, 379
chlorothiazide,
  calcium carbonate, oral **2**, 293
  colestipol hydrochloride **3**, 293
  lithium **1**, 247
  metoclopramide hydrochloride **3**, 293
  probenecid **3**, 294
  propantheline bromide **3**, 294
chlorotrianisene,
  rifampin, 209
chlorpheniramine,
  phenytoin **2**, 117
  propranolol hydrochloride **4**, 265
chlorphenoxamine hydrochloride,
  digoxin, 287
  digoxin capsule, stabilized, 287
chlorpromazine hydrochloride,
  alcohol, ethyl–oral/injectable **2**, 232
  aluminum hydroxide **3**, 232–233
  amphetamine **2**, 233
  benztropine mesylate **2**, 234
  bethanidine sulphate, 169
  cabergoline **1**, 388
  captopril **2**, 164
  diazoxide, oral **2**, 234
  guanadrel sulfate, 169
  guanethidine **1**, 169
  insulin **3**, 307
  levodopa **3**, 234
  lithium **2**, 235
  magnesium hydroxide **3**, 232–233
  meperidine hydrochloride **2**, 15
  pergolide mesylate **1**, 388
  phenobarbital **3**, 235
  phenytoin **3**, 117
  piperazine **3**, 235
  propranolol hydrochloride **2**, 265
  tobacco **3**, 236
  valproic acid **3**, 133
chlorpropamide,
  alcohol, ethyl–oral/injectable **1**, 302
  allopurinol **3**, 302
  aspirin **2**, 302–303
  clofibrate **2**, 303
  cortisone acetate **2**, 303
  feprazone, 314–315
  hydrochlorothiazide **2**, 303–304
  oxyphenbutazone, 314–315
  phenylbutazone, 314–315
  probenecid **3**, 304
  sucralfate **4**, 304
chlorprothixene,
  cabergoline **1**, 388
  guanethidine, 169
  pergolide mesylate **1**, 388

chlortetracycline hydrochloride,
  penicillin G **2**, 206
chlorthalidone,
  lithium, 247
  warfarin **3**, 79
chlorzoxazone,
  isoniazid **3**, 195
  watercress **3**, 335
cholecalciferol, vitamin D3,
  aluminum hydroxide **2**, 327
  paricalcitol **1**, 388
cholestyramine,
  amiodarone hydrochloride **3**, 46
  cyclosporine **4**, 361
  digitoxin **2**, 275
  doxepin hydrochloride **3**, 141
  furosemide **2**, 296
  glipizide **2**, 305
  hydrocortisone, oral/systemic **3**, 366–367
  hydrocortisone acet, injectable **3**, 366–367
  hydrocortisone sodium phos **3**, 366–367
  hydrocortisone sodium succinate **3**, 366–367
  naproxen **3**, 20
  propranolol hydrochloride **3**, 265–266
  spironolactone **2**, 178
  thyroid strong **2**, 386
  warfarin **2**, 79–80
choline salicylate,
  methotrexate, 222
  methotrexate sodium, injectable, 222
cilostazol,
  grapefruit juice **1**, 388
cimetidine, oral,
  alcohol, ethyl–oral/injectable **3**, 317
  aluminum hydroxide **3**, 358
  aminophylline, 344
  buspirone hydrochloride **4**, 231–232
  caffeine, 344
  carbamazepine **2**, 104
  carmustine **2**, 217
  carvedilol, 266
  cefotaxime sodium **3**, 181–182
  chlormethiazole **3**, 321
  chloroquine **3**, 184
  cisapride **1**, 388
  clomiphene citrate **3**, 360
  clozapine **2**, 237–238
  diazepam **2**, 240
  digoxin **3**, 278
  dobutamine hydrochloride **3**, 365
  dofetilide **1**, 388
  erythromycin stearate **3**, 189–190
  ethotoin, 117–118
  ferrous sulfate **3**, 329

# Index

flecainide acetate **2**, 53
fluorouracil **3**, 220
fosphenytoin sodium, injectable, 117–118
glipizide **2**, 305
imipramine **2**, 147
indomethacin **3**, 13
ketoconazole, oral **2**, 199
labetalol hydrochloride, 266
lidocaine hydrochloride, local–injectable, 54
lidocaine hydrochloride, systemic **1**, 54
magnesium hydroxide **3**, 358
mephenytoin, 117–118
metoclopramide hydrochloride **3**, 359
metoprolol tartrate, 266
metronidazole, injectable **3**, 203
moricizine hydrochloride **3**, 57–58
morphine **2**, 18–19
nebivolol hydrochloride, 266
nifedipine **2**, 58
oxtriphylline, 344
paroxetine hydrochloride **3**, 154
pentoxifylline, 344
phenindione, 80
phenobarbital **3**, 323
phenytoin **1**, 117–118
praziquantel **3**, 359
procainamide hydrochloride **2**, 60
propantheline bromide **3**, 359
propranolol hydrochloride **1**, 266
quinidine **2**, 63
succinylcholine chloride **2**, 35–36
tetracycline **3**, 212
theophylline **1**, 344
triamterene **3**, 299
valproic acid **3**, 131
venlafaxine hydrochloride **3**, 161
warfarin **1**, 80
cimetidine hydrochloride, injectable,
 aminophylline, 344
 caffeine, 344
 carvedilol, 266
 cisapride **1**, 388
 dofetilide **1**, 388
 ethotoin, 117–118
 fosphenytoin sodium, injectable, 117–118
 labetalol hydrochloride, 266
 lidocaine hydrochloride, local–injectable, 54
 lidocaine hydrochloride, systemic, 54
 mephenytoin, 117–118
 metoprolol tartrate, 266
 nebivolol hydrochloride, 266
 oxtriphylline, 344
 pentoxifylline, 344
 phenindione, 80
 phenytoin, 117–118
 praziquantel **3**, 359
 propranolol hydrochloride, 266
 theophylline, 344
 warfarin, 80
cinoxacin,
 warfarin, 93
ciprofibrate,
 phenindione, 81
ciprofloxacin hydrochloride,
 aluminum hydroxide **2**, 186
 cyclosporine **2**, 186–187
 enteral nutrition **3**, 187–188
 ferrous sulfate **2**, 187
 glyburide **2**, 306
 magnesium hydroxide **2**, 186
 phenytoin **2**, 118
 theophylline **2**, 344–345
 warfarin, 93
ciprofloxacin hydrochloride, injectable,
 glyburide **2**, 306
 phenytoin **2**, 118
 warfarin, 93
cisapride,
 acetophenazine maleate **1**, 388
 amiodarone hydrochloride **1**, 388
 amitriptyline hydrochloride **1**, 388
 amprenavir **1**, 388
 astemizole **1**, 388
 bepridil hydrochloride **1**, 388
 cimetidine, oral **1**, 388
 cimetidine hydrochloride, injectable **1**, 388
 clarithromycin **1**, 388
 desipramine hydrochloride **1**, 388
 diltiazem hydrochloride **2**, 47
 disopyramide phosphate **1**, 388
 doxepin hydrochloride **1**, 388
 efavirenz **1**, 388
 erythromycin **1**, 388
 erythromycin estolate **1**, 388
 erythromycin ethylsuccinate **1**, 388
 erythromycin gluceptate **1**, 388
 erythromycin lactobionate **1**, 388
 erythromycin stearate **1**, 388
 fluconazole **1**, 388
 fluvoxamine maleate **1**, 388
 grapefruit juice **1**, 388
 grepafloxacin hydrochloride **1**, 388
 imipramine **1**, 388
 indinavir sulfate **1**, 388
 itraconazole, oral **1**, 388
 ketoconazole, oral **1**, 388
 mesoridazine besylate **1**, 388
 methdilazine **1**, 388
 mibefradil dihydrochloride **1**, 388
 miconazole nitrate **1**, 388
 mirtazapine **1**, 388
 nefazodone hydrochloride **1**, 388
 nelfinavir mesylate **1**, 388

# Index

pericyazine **1**, 388
piperacetazine **1**, 388
procainamide hydrochloride **1**, 388
promazine hydrochloride **1**, 388
promethazine **1**, 388
propiomazine hydrochloride **1**, 388
quinidine **1**, 388
ritonavir **1**, 388
saquinavir **1**, 388
sotalol hydrochloride **1**, 388
sparfloxacin **1**, 388
sulfamethoxazole–trimethoprim **1**, 388
terfenadine **1**, 388
terodiline hydrochloride **1**, 388
thiethylperazine maleate **1**, 388
thioproperazine mesylate **1**, 388
thioridazine hydrochloride **1**, 388
triflupromazine hydrochloride **1**, 388
trimeprazine tartrate **1**, 388
trimipramine maleate **1**, 388
troleandomycin **1**, 388
warfarin **2**, 80
cisplatin,
　bleomycin sulfate **3**, 217
　ethacrynic acid **2**, 294–295
　lithium **3**, 247
　methotrexate **2**, 222–223
　paclitaxel **2**, 227–228
citalopram hydrobromide,
　isocarboxazid **1**, 144–145
　moclobemide, 144–145
　pargyline hydrochloride **1**, 144–145
　phenelzine sulfate **1**, 144–145
　selegiline hydrochloride **1**, 144–145
　tranylcypromine sulfate **1**, 144–145
citric acid,
　aluminum hydroxide **3**, 357
clarithromycin,
　acenocoumarol, 83
　astemizole, 191
　carbamazepine, 105
　cisapride **1**, 388
　cyclosporine, 190
　digoxin, 279–280
　fluoxetine hydrochloride **3**, 143
　lovastatin, 373
　mizolastine **1**, 388
　omeprazole **3**, 378
　phenytoin **3**, 118
　pimozide **1**, 388
　simvastatin, 373
　terfenadine, 191
　theophylline, 346
　warfarin, 83
clidinium bromide,
　digoxin, 287
clindamycin,
　enflurane, 27
　ether, 27
　halothane, 27
　methoxyflurane, 27
　nitrous oxide, 27
　pancuronium bromide **2**, 32
clindamycin phosphate, injectable,
　enflurane, 27
　ether, 27
　halothane, 27
　methoxyflurane, 27
　nitrous oxide, 27
　pancuronium bromide **2**, 32
clofibrate,
　acenocoumarol, 81
　anisindione, 81
　chlorpropamide **2**, 303
　coumarin, 81
　dicumarol, 81
　hormonal contraceptive, low–dose **3**, 360
　insulin **2**, 307
　probenecid **3**, 22
　rifampin **3**, 208
　warfarin **1**, 81
clomiphene citrate,
　cimetidine, oral **3**, 360
clomipramine hydrochloride,
　amprenavir **1**, 388
　arbutamine hydrochloride **1**, 388
　grapefruit juice **2**, 331
　guanethidine, 169
　halofantrine hydrochloride **1**, 388
　oxybutynin chloride **3**, 379
　s–adneosylmethionine **3**, 158
clonazepam,
　carbamazepine **3**, 110–111
　phenelzine sulfate **3**, 156–157
　primidone **4**, 111
　valproic acid **3**, 133–134
clonidine hydrochloride,
　atenolol, 167
　carteolol hydrochloride, 167
　carteolol hydrochloride, ophthalmic, 167
　carvedilol, 167
　celiprolol hydrochloride, 167
　cyclosporine **2**, 166
　fluphenazine **3**, 243
　metoprolol tartrate, 167
　mirtazapine **2**, 166
　nadolol, 167
　naloxone hydrochloride **3**, 167
　nebivolol hydrochloride, 167
　penbutolol sulfate, 167
　pindolol, 167
　propranolol hydrochloride **1**, 167
　rifampin **4**, 167
　tertatolol hydrochloride, 167
　timolol maleate, oral, 167
clonidine hydrochloride, transdermal,
　atenolol, 167
　carteolol hydrochloride, 167

# Index

carteolol hydrochloride,
  ophthalmic, 167
carvedilol, 167
celiprolol hydrochloride, 167
metoprolol tartrate, 167
nadolol, 167
nebivolol hydrochloride, 167
penbutolol sulfate, 167
pindolol, 167
propranolol hydrochloride, 167
tertatolol hydrochloride, 167
timolol maleate, oral, 167
clorazepate dipotassium,
  aluminum hydroxide **3**, 236
  influenza virus vaccine, split virion **3**, 236
  magnesium hydroxide **3**, 236
  ritonavir **1**, 388
clotrimazole,
  cyclosporine, 199–200
  fosphenytoin sodium, injectable, 121–122
  lovastatin **1**, 388
  mizolastine **1**, 388
  phenytoin, 121–122
  simvastatin **1**, 388
cloxacillin sodium,
  amikacin sulfate, 192
  gentamicin sulfate, 192
  netilmicin, 192
  tobramycin, 192
clozapine,
  caffeine **3**, 236–237
  carbamazepine **2**, 237
  cimetidine, oral **2**, 237–238
  erythromycin stearate **2**, 238
  fluvoxamine maleate **2**, 238
  rifampin **2**, 239
  ritonavir **1**, 388
cocaine hydrochloride,
  propranolol hydrochloride **2**, 266
codeine,
  isocarboxazid, 15
  naltrexone hydrochloride **1**, 388
  pargyline hydrochloride, 15
  phenelzine sulfate, 15
  quinidine **2**, 10
  selegiline hydrochloride, 15
  tranylcypromine sulfate, 15
colchicine,
  cyclosporine **2**, 10–11
  grapefruit juice **2**, 331–332
colestipol hydrochloride,
  chlorothiazide **3**, 293
colistimethate sodium,
  cephalothin sodium **2**, 182
colistin sulfate,
  alcuronium chloride, 41
  atracurium besylate, 41
  doxacurium chloride, 41
  enflurane, 27
  ether, 27
  gallamine triethiodide, 41
  halothane, 27
  methoxyflurane, 27
  metocurine iodide, 41
  mivacurium chloride, 41
  nitrous oxide, 27
  pancuronium bromide, 41
  pipecuronium bromide, 41
  rapacuronium bromide, 41
  rocuronium bromide, 41
  succinylcholine chloride, 41
  tubocurarine chloride, 41
  vecuronium bromide, 41
conjugated estrogens,
  rifampin, 209
corticotropin,
  dicumarol **2**, 71
cortisone acetate,
  chlorpropamide **2**, 303
coumarin,
  allopurinol, 70–71
  aloxiprin, 77
  aminoglutethimide, 87
  amiodarone hydrochloride, 76–77
  amobarbital, 94
  aprobarbital, 94
  aspirin, 77
  barbital, 94
  bezafibrate, 81
  butabarbital sodium, 94
  butalbital, 94
  butobarbitone, 94
  clofibrate, 81
  danazol, 91
  dicumarol, 100
  diflunisal, 77
  disulfiram, 82–83
  erythromycin, 83
  erythromycin estolate, 83
  erythromycin ethylsuccinate, 83
  erythromycin gluceptate, 83
  erythromycin lactobionate, 83
  erythromycin stearate, 83
  ethylestrenol, 91
  fenofibrate, micronized, 81
  feprazone, 94–95
  fluoxymesterone, 91
  gemfibrozil, 81
  glucagon, 87
  glucagon, recombinant, 87
  glutethimide, 87
  levothyroxine sodium, 100
  liothyronine sodium, 100
  menadiol sodium diphosphate, vitamin K4, 95
  menadione, 95
  mephobarbital, 94
  methandrostenolone, 91
  metharbital, 94
  methohexital sodium, 94

# Index

methyltestosterone, 91
methyprylon, 87
nalidixic acid, 93
norfloxacin, 93
oxandrolone, 91
oxymetholone, 91
oxyphenbutazone, 94–95
pentobarbital sodium, 94
phenobarbital, 94
phenylbutazone, 94–95
phytonadione, vitamin K1, 95
primidone, 94
rifabutin, 97
rifampin, 97
secobarbital, 94
sodium salicylate, 77
stanozolol, 91
talbutal, 94
thiamylal sodium, 94
thiopental sodium, 94
thyroglobulin, 100
thyroid desiccated, 100
thyroid strong, 100
cyanocobalamin, vitamin B12,
  omeprazole **3**, 328
cyclacillin,
  amikacin sulfate, 192
  gentamicin sulfate, 192
  netilmicin, 192
  tobramycin, 192
cyclobenzaprine hydrochloride,
  guanadrel sulfate, 169
  guanethidine, 169
cyclopenthiazide,
  lithium, 247
cyclophosphamide,
  allopurinol **2**, 217
  chloramphenicol **2**, 218
  digoxin **2**, 278–279
  hydrochlorothiazide **3**, 218
  indomethacin **3**, 218
  methotrexate **3**, 218–219
  prednisone **3**, 219
  succinylcholine chloride **2**, 36
  trastuzumab **1**, 388
cyclosporine,
  acetazolamide **2**, 292
  allopurinol **2**, 360
  amiodarone hydrochloride **2**, 46
  amphotericin B **2**, 188
  azathioprine sodium **3**, 360
  azithromycin, 190
  basiliximab **2**, 361
  butoconazole nitrate, 199–200
  carbamazepine **2**, 361
  carvedilol **3**, 260–261
  chloramphenicol **3**, 183–184
  chloroquine **2**, 184–185
  cholestyramine **4**, 361
  ciprofloxacin hydrochloride **2**,
    186–187
  clarithromycin, 190
  clonidine hydrochloride **2**, 166
  clotrimazole, 199–200
  colchicine **2**, 10–11
  diclofenac **2**, 11
  digoxin **2**, 279
  diltiazem hydrochloride **1**, 47–48
  dirithromycin, 190
  disopyramide phosphate **3**, 49
  erythromycin **1**, 190
  erythromycin estolate, 190
  erythromycin ethylsuccinate, 190
  erythromycin gluceptate, 190
  erythromycin lactobionate, 190
  erythromycin stearate, 190
  etoposide **2**, 219–220
  fat emulsion, intraveneous **2**, 366
  fenticonazole nitrate, 199–200
  fluconazole, 199–200
  fluoxetine hydrochloride **3**, 143
  foscarnet sodium **2**, 366
  griseofulvin **3**, 193–194
  hormonal contraceptive **3**, 363
  hormonal contraceptive, low–dose
    **3**, 363
  hypericum **2**, 362
  imipenem in combination with
    cilastatin **2**, 194–195
  itraconazole, 199–200
  itraconazole, oral, 199–200
  ketoconazole, oral **1**, 199–200
  lercanidipine hydrochloride, 47–48
  lovastatin **2**, 372
  melphalan **2**, 221
  methyltestosterone **2**, 362
  metoclopramide hydrochloride **2**,
    362–363
  metronidazole, injectable **3**, 376
  metronidazole, oral/vaginal **3**, 376
  miconazole nitrate, 199–200
  morphine **2**, 19
  mycophenolate mofetil **3**, 377
  nafcillin sodium **2**, 363
  nicardipine hydrochloride, 47–48
  nicardipine hydrochloride,
    injectable, 47–48
  nifedipine, 47–48
  nisoldipine, 47–48
  octreotide acetate **2**, 377–378
  omeprazole **2**, 378
  oxiconazole nitrate, 199–200
  pancuronium bromide **2**, 33
  phenobarbital **2**, 323
  phenytoin **2**, 119
  prednisolone **2**, 380
  probucol **2**, 381
  propafenone hydrochloride **2**,
    61–62
  quinine **2**, 363–364
  rifabutin, 209
  rifampin **1**, 209

# Index

sulfadiazine **2**, 210
terbinafine hydrochloride **2**, 211
terconazole, 199–200
ticlopidine hydrochloride **2**, 75
tioconazole, 199–200
trimethoprim **3**, 210
troleandomycin, 190
verapamil hydrochloride, 47–48
verapamil hydrochloride, sustained-release, 47–48
verapamil hydrochloride pellets, 47–48
warfarin **2**, 81
cyclothiazide,
 lithium, 247
cyproheptadine hydrochloride,
 fluoxetine hydrochloride **2**, 143–144
cytarabine,
 methotrexate **3**, 223
 methotrexate sodium, injectable **3**, 223

## D

dalteparin sodium,
 sodium salicylate, 77
danazol,
 acenocoumarol, 91
 anisindione, 91
 carbamazepine **2**, 104
 coumarin, 91
 dicumarol, 91
 phenindione, 91
 warfarin, 91
danshen,
 warfarin **2**, 81
dantrolene sodium,
 vecuronium bromide **3**, 43
 verapamil hydrochloride **2**, 66
dapsone,
 rifampin **3**, 188
 trimethoprim **3**, 188–189
daunorubicin citrate liposome,
 trastuzumab **1**, 388
daunorubicin hydrochloride,
 trastuzumab **1**, 388
deferiprone,
 lymecycline, 212
demeclocycline hydrochloride,
 alcuronium chloride, 41
 aluminum carbonate, basic, 211–212
 aluminum hydroxide, 211–212
 aluminum oxide, 211–212
 aluminum phosphate, 211–212
 attapulgite, 211–212
 bismuth subsalicylate, 211–212
 calcium, oral salt unspecified, 211–212
 calcium acetate, 211–212
 calcium ascorbate, 211–212
 calcium carbonate, oral, 211–212
 calcium chloride, oral, 211–212
 calcium citrate, oral, 211–212
 calcium glubionate, oral, 211–212
 calcium glucoheptonate, 211–212
 calcium gluconate, oral, 211–212
 calcium glycerophosphate, oral, 211–212
 calcium iodate, 211–212
 calcium lactate, oral, 211–212
 calcium lactate gluconate, 211–212
 calcium lactobionate, oral, 211–212
 calcium phosphate, oral, 211–212
 digoxin, 289
 digoxin capsule, stabilized, 289
 dihydroxyaluminum, 211–212
 doxacurium chloride, 41
 ferric ammonium citrate, 212
 ferrous citrate, 212
 ferrous fumarate, 212
 ferrous gluconate, 212
 ferrous glycine sulfate, 212
 ferrous hydroxide polymaltose, 212
 ferrous ions, salt unspecified, 212
 ferrous succinate, 212
 ferrous sulfate, 212
 gallamine triethiodide, 41
 iron peptonized, 212
 kaolin, 211–212
 magaldrate, 211–212
 magnesium carbonate, 211–212
 magnesium chloride, oral, 211–212
 magnesium hydroxide, 211–212
 magnesium oxide, 211–212
 magnesium salicylate, 211–212
 magnesium sulfate, 211–212
 magnesium trisilicate, 211–212
 metocurine iodide, 41
 mivacurium chloride, 41
 pancuronium bromide, 41
 pipecuronium bromide, 41
 rapacuronium bromide, 41
 rocuronium bromide, 41
 succinylcholine chloride, 41
 sucralfate, 211–212
 tubocurarine chloride, 41
 vecuronium bromide, 41
desflurane,
 epinephrine, 28
desipramine hydrochloride,
 amprenavir **1**, 388
 arbutamine hydrochloride **1**, 388
 bethanidine sulphate, 169
 carbamazepine **3**, 104–105
 cisapride **1**, 388
 grepafloxacin hydrochloride **1**, 388
 guanadrel sulfate, 169
 guanethidine **1**, 169
 halofantrine hydrochloride **1**, 388
 phenylbutazone **3**, 21
 pimozide **1**, 388

# Index

propranolol hydrochloride **3**, 266
quinidine **3**, 140
ritonavir **2**, 382
thioridazine hydrochloride **1**, 140
deslanoside,
  amiodarone hydrochloride, 277
  propantheline bromide, 287
  rifampin, 276
dexamethasone,
  aldesleukin, interleukin–2 human **2**, 220–221
  aminoglutethimide **2**, 364
  ephedrine **3**, 364
  phenobarbital **2**, 323–324
  phenytoin **2**, 119
dexbrompheniramine maleate,
  watercress **3**, 335
dexfenfluramine hydrochloride,
  chloroform, 28
  enflurane, 28
  furazolidone, 191–192
  halothane, 28
  isocarboxazid, 159–160
  methoxyflurane, 28
  metoprolol tartrate, 267
  moclobemide, 159–160
  nebivolol hydrochloride, 267
  pargyline hydrochloride, 159–160
  phenelzine sulfate, 159–160
  phentermine hydrochloride **1**, 388
  procarbazine hydrochloride, 159–160
  propranolol hydrochloride, 267
  selegiline hydrochloride, 159–160
  timolol maleate, ophthalmic, 267
  timolol maleate, oral, 267
  tranylcypromine sulfate, 159–160
  venlafaxine hydrochloride, 159–160
dexpanthenol,
  succinylcholine chloride **4**, 36
dextran 40,
  heparin **2**, 73
dextran 40, inert/interacting,
  heparin **2**, 73
dextran 70,
  abciximab **1**, 388
  heparin **2**, 73
dextroamphetamine,
  chloroform, 28
  enflurane, 28
  furazolidone, 191–192
  guanethidine **2**, 170
  halothane, 28
  isocarboxazid, 159–160
  methoxyflurane, 28
  moclobemide, 159–160
  pargyline hydrochloride, 159–160
  phenelzine sulfate, 159–160
  procarbazine hydrochloride, 159–160
  tranylcypromine sulfate, 159–160

dextromethorphan hbr,
  isocarboxazid, 15
  linezolid, 15
  moclobemide, 15
  pargyline hydrochloride, 15
  paroxetine hydrochloride **2**, 154–155
  phenelzine sulfate, 15
  selegiline hydrochloride, 15
  tranylcypromine sulfate, 15
dextromoramide,
  naltrexone hydrochloride **1**, 388
dextrothyroxine sodium,
  acenocoumarol, 100
  dicumarol, 100
  warfarin, 100
dezocine,
  naltrexone hydrochloride **1**, 388
  selegiline hydrochloride, 15
diamorphine hydrochloride,
  naltrexone hydrochloride **1**, 388
diatrizoate meglumine,
  metformin hydrochloride **1**, 312
diatrizoate sodium,
  metformin hydrochloride **1**, 312
  propranolol hydrochloride **3**, 267
diazepam,
  alcohol, ethyl–oral/injectable **2**, 239
  aminophylline **3**, 239–240
  bupivacaine hydrochloride **3**, 26
  cimetidine, oral **2**, 240
  digoxin **2**, 279
  disulfiram **3**, 240
  gallamine triethiodide **3**, 27–28
  hormonal contraceptive **3**, 242
  hormonal contraceptive, low–dose **3**, 242
  isoniazid **3**, 241
  ketamine hydrochloride **2**, 29
  levodopa **3**, 241
  lithium **3**, 247–248
  methadone hydrochloride **3**, 16–17
  omeprazole **3**, 241
  phenytoin **3**, 119–120
  propofol **3**, 35
  propranolol hydrochloride **3**, 242
  rifampin **3**, 242
  ritonavir **1**, 388
  tobacco **3**, 243
diazoxide, oral,
  chlorpromazine hydrochloride **2**, 234
  phenytoin **2**, 120
  tolbutamide **3**, 313
  trichlormethiazide **3**, 300
  warfarin **3**, 82
dicalcium phosphate,
  tetracycline, 211–212
dichlorphenamide,
  lithium, 245–246
diclofenac,

# Index

cyclosporine **2**, 11
ketorolac tromethamine **1**, 388
ketorolac tromethamine, injectable **1**, 388
dicloxacillin,
  amikacin sulfate, 192
  gentamicin sulfate, 192
  netilmicin, 192
  tobramycin, 192
dicumarol,
  allopurinol **1**, 70–71
  aloxiprin, 77
  aminoglutethimide, 87
  amiodarone hydrochloride, 76–77
  amobarbital, 94
  aprobarbital, 94
  aspirin, 77
  azapropazone dihydrate **1**, 388
  barbital, 94
  bezafibrate, 81
  butabarbital sodium, 94
  butalbital, 94
  butobarbitone, 94
  chloramphenicol **2**, 71
  clofibrate, 81
  corticotropin **2**, 71
  coumarin, 100
  danazol, 91
  dextrothyroxine sodium, 100
  diflunisal, 77
  disulfiram, 82–83
  erythromycin, 83
  erythromycin estolate, 83
  erythromycin ethylsuccinate, 83
  erythromycin gluceptate, 83
  erythromycin lactobionate, 83
  erythromycin stearate, 83
  ethylestrenol, 91
  fenofibrate, micronized, 81
  feprazone, 94–95
  fluoxymesterone, 91
  gemfibrozil, 81
  glucagon, 87
  glucagon, recombinant, 87
  glutethimide, 87
  hormonal contraceptive **2**, 72
  levothyroxine sodium, 100
  liothyronine sodium, 100
  menadiol sodium diphosphate, vitamin K4, 95
  menadione, 95
  mephobarbital, 94
  methandrostenolone, 91
  metharbital, 94
  methohexital sodium, 94
  methylphenidate hydrochloride **3**, 71–72
  methyltestosterone, 91
  methyprylon, 87
  nalidixic acid, 93
  norfloxacin, 93
  oxandrolone, 91
  oxymetholone, 91
  oxyphenbutazone, 94–95
  pentobarbital sodium, 94
  phenobarbital, 94
  phenylbutazone, 94–95
  phenytoin **2**, 72
  phytonadione, vitamin K1, 95
  primidone, 94
  rifabutin, 97
  rifampin, 97
  secobarbital, 94
  sodium salicylate, 77
  stanozolol, 91
  talbutal, 94
  thiamylal sodium, 94
  thiopental sodium, 94
  thyroglobulin, 100
  thyroid desiccated, 100
  thyroid strong, 100
  tolbutamide **2**, 313–314
  toremifene **1**, 388
dicyclomine hydrochloride,
  digoxin, 287
didanosine,
  ganciclovir **2**, 364–365
  itraconazole, oral **2**, 198
  methadone hydrochloride **3**, 17
diethylpropion hydrochloride,
  chloroform, 28
  enflurane, 28
  furazolidone, 191–192
  halothane, 28
  isocarboxazid, 159–160
  methoxyflurane, 28
  moclobemide, 159–160
  pargyline hydrochloride, 159–160
  phenelzine sulfate, 159–160
  procarbazine hydrochloride, 159–160
  tranylcypromine sulfate, 159–160
diethylstilbestrol,
  rifampin, 209
  succinylcholine chloride **2**, 36–37
difenoxin hydrochloride,
  isocarboxazid, 15
  naltrexone hydrochloride **1**, 388
  pargyline hydrochloride, 15
  phenelzine sulfate, 15
  selegiline hydrochloride, 15
  tranylcypromine sulfate, 15
diflunisal,
  acenocoumarol, 77
  anisindione, 77
  coumarin, 77
  dicumarol, 77
  methotrexate, 222
  methotrexate sodium, injectable, 222
  oxazepam **3**, 256
  warfarin, 77

# Index

digitalis,
 amiodarone hydrochloride, 277
 calcium chloride, injectable **2**, 274
 phenytoin **2**, 274
 propantheline bromide, 287
 reserpine **3**, 274–275
 rifampin, 276
digitoxin,
 aminoglutethimide **3**, 275
 amiodarone hydrochloride, 277
 cholestyramine **2**, 275
 diltiazem hydrochloride, 290
 phenobarbital **2**, 275–276
 phenylbutazone **3**, 276
 propantheline bromide, 287
 quinidine, 287–288
 rifabutin, 276
 rifampin **1**, 276
 verapamil hydrochloride, 290
 verapamil hydrochloride, sustained-release, 290
 verapamil hydrochloride pellets, 290
digoxin,
 acarbose **3**, 276
 aluminum hydroxide **2**, 276–277
 amiodarone hydrochloride **1**, 277
 anisotropine methylbromide, 287
 arbutamine hydrochloride **1**, 388
 atropine, 287
 belladonna, 287
 bellafoline, 287
 benztropine mesylate, 287
 biperiden, 287
 captopril **2**, 278
 charcoal **3**, 278
 chlorphenoxamine hydrochloride, 287
 cimetidine, oral **3**, 278
 clarithromycin, 279–280
 clidinium bromide, 287
 cyclophosphamide **2**, 278–279
 cyclosporine **2**, 279
 demeclocycline hydrochloride, 289
 diazepam **2**, 279
 dicyclomine hydrochloride, 287
 diltiazem hydrochloride, 290
 disopyramide phosphate **3**, 279
 doxycycline hydrochloride, 289
 doxycycline hyclate, injectable, 289
 erythromycin **1**, 279–280
 erythromycin estolate, 279–280
 erythromycin ethylsuccinate, 279–280
 erythromycin glucceptate, 279–280
 erythromycin lactobionate, 279–280
 erythromycin stearate, 279–280
 esmolol hydrochloride **3**, 280
 ethoheptazine citrate, 287
 furosemide **2**, 281

ginseng **3**, 281–282
glycopyrrolate, 287
guar gum **3**, 282
heparin **3**, 282
hexocyclium methylsulfate, 287
hydroxychloroquine sulfate **2**, 282
hyoscyamine, 287
hypericum **3**, 283
ibuprofen **2**, 283
isopropamide iodide, 287
itraconazole, oral **2**, 283–284
kaolin **2**, 284
kyushin **3**, 284
lymecycline, 289
magnesium hydroxide **2**, 276–277
magnesium trisilicate **2**, 276–277
mepenzolate bromide, 287
mesalamine, oral **3**, 277
methacycline hydrochloride, 289
methantheline bromide, 287
methscopolamine bromide, 287
methscopolamine nitrate, 287
methyldopa **3**, 284–285
metoclopramide hydrochloride **2**, 285
mexiletine hydrochloride **4**, 285
minocycline, injectable, 289
minocycline hydrochloride, 289
minocycline hydrochloride pellets, 289
moricizine hydrochloride **4**, 285
neomycin sulfate, oral **2**, 286
nifedipine, 290
oxybutynin chloride, 287
oxyphencyclimine hydrochloride, 287
oxytetracycline, 289
oxytetracycline, injectable, 289
penicillamine **2**, 286
pirenzepine dihydrochloride, 287
prazosin hydrochloride **2**, 286
prednisone **2**, 278–279
procarbazine hydrochloride **2**, 278–279
procyclidine hydrochloride, 287
propafenone hydrochloride **2**, 286–287
propantheline bromide **1**, 287
psyllium **3**, 287
quinidine **1**, 287–288
rifabutin, 276
rifampin, 276
rolitetracycline, injectable, 289
scopolamine, ophthalmic, 287
scopolamine, systemic, 287
spironolactone **2**, 288
succinylcholine chloride **2**, 288
sulfasalazine **2**, 288
tetracycline **1**, 289
tetracycline hydrochloride, injectable, 289

# Index

thyroid strong **2**, 289
tolbutamide **3**, 289
trazodone hydrochloride **3**, 289–290
tridihexethyl chloride, 287
trihexyphenidyl hydrochloride, 287
trimethoprim **3**, 290
verapamil hydrochloride **1**, 290
verapamil hydrochloride, sustained-release, 290
verapamil hydrochloride pellets, 290
vincristine sulfate **2**, 278–279
digoxin capsule, stabilized,
amiodarone hydrochloride, 277
chlorphenoxamine hydrochloride, 287
demeclocycline hydrochloride, 289
diltiazem hydrochloride, 290
doxycycline hydrochloride, 289
doxycycline hyclate, injectable, 289
erythromycin, 279–280
erythromycin estolate, 279–280
erythromycin ethylsuccinate, 279–280
erythromycin gluceptate, 279–280
erythromycin lactobionate, 279–280
erythromycin stearate, 279–280
fluoxetine hydrochloride **2**, 280–281
lymecycline, 289
methacycline hydrochloride, 289
minocycline, injectable, 289
minocycline hydrochloride, 289
nifedipine, 290
oxytetracycline, 289
oxytetracycline, injectable, 289
propafenone hydrochloride **2**, 286–287
quinidine, 287–288
rifampin, 276
rolitetracycline, injectable, 289
tetracycline, 289
tetracycline hydrochloride, injectable, 289
verapamil hydrochloride, 290
verapamil hydrochloride, sustained-release, 290
verapamil hydrochloride pellets, 290
dihydrocodeine bitartrate,
isocarboxazid, 15
naltrexone hydrochloride **1**, 388
pargyline hydrochloride, 15
phenelzine sulfate, 15
selegiline hydrochloride, 15
tranylcypromine sulfate, 15
dihydroergotamine mesylate,
amprenavir **1**, 388
efavirenz **1**, 388
indinavir sulfate **1**, 388
nitroglycerin **2**, 365
ritonavir **1**, 388
rizatriptan benzoate **1**, 388
saquinavir **1**, 388
sumatriptan, nasal **1**, 388
sumatriptan succinate **1**, 388
sumatriptan succinate, injectable **1**, 388
sumatriptan succinate, oral **1**, 388
zolmitriptan **1**, 388
dihydroergotamine mesylate, inhl,
efavirenz **1**, 388
indinavir sulfate **1**, 388
rizatriptan benzoate **1**, 388
saquinavir **1**, 388
sumatriptan succinate **1**, 388
sumatriptan succinate, injectable **1**, 388
sumatriptan succinate, oral **1**, 388
dihydrotachysterol,
paricalcitol **1**, 388
dihydroxyaluminum,
demeclocycline hydrochloride, 211–212
doxycycline hydrochloride, 211–212
methacycline hydrochloride, 211–212
oxytetracycline, 211–212
tetracycline, 211–212
diltiazem hydrochloride,
amiodarone hydrochloride **2**, 46
cisapride **2**, 47
cyclosporine **1**, 47–48
digitoxin, 290
digoxin, 290
digoxin capsule, stabilized, 290
insulin **3**, 308
lovastatin **2**, 372–373
quinidine, 65–66
diphenhydramine,
alcohol, ethyl-oral/injectable **2**, 317–318
temazepam **2**, 257
warfarin **4**, 82
diphenoxylate hydrochloride,
isocarboxazid, 15
naltrexone hydrochloride **1**, 388
pargyline hydrochloride, 15
phenelzine sulfate, 15
quinidine **3**, 63
selegiline hydrochloride, 15
tranylcypromine sulfate, 15
dipyridamole,
adenosine, injectable **3**, 357
aspirin **3**, 8
dipyridamole, injectable,
theophylline **2**, 345
dirithromycin,
cyclosporine, 190
mizolastine **1**, 388

# Index

pimozide **1**, 388
warfarin, 83
disodium hydrogen citrate,
  lithium, 245–246
disopyramide phosphate,
  alcohol, ethyl–oral/injectable **3**, 48
  astemizole **1**, 388
  atenolol **3**, 48
  charcoal **2**, 48–49
  cisapride **1**, 388
  cyclosporine **3**, 49
  digoxin **3**, 279
  erythromycin **2**, 49
  grepafloxacin hydrochloride **1**, 388
  halofantrine hydrochloride **1**, 388
  isosorbide dinitrate, sublingual **2**, 49–50
  mizolastine **1**, 388
  moxifloxacin hydrochloride, oral **1**, 388
  phenytoin **2**, 50
  pimozide **1**, 388
  quinidine **3**, 50
  rifampin **3**, 50–51
  sotalol hydrochloride **1**, 388
  sparfloxacin **1**, 388
  warfarin **3**, 82
disulfiram,
  acenocoumarol, 82–83
  alcohol, ethyl–oral/injectable **1**, 318
  amitriptyline hydrochloride **3**, 137
  anisindione, 82–83
  coumarin, 82–83
  diazepam **3**, 240
  dicumarol, 82–83
  ethotoin, 120
  fosphenytoin sodium, injectable, 120
  isoniazid **3**, 195
  mephenytoin, 120
  metronidazole, oral/vaginal **2**, 203
  perphenazine **3**, 256
  phenytoin **1**, 120
  theophylline **2**, 345–346
  warfarin **1**, 82–83
dobutamine hydrochloride,
  chloroform, 28
  cimetidine, oral **3**, 365
  enflurane, 28
  halothane, 28
  methoxyflurane, 28
  nebivolol hydrochloride, 267
  propranolol hydrochloride, 267
  timolol maleate, ophthalmic, 267
  timolol maleate, oral, 267
dofetilide,
  amiloride hydrochloride **2**, 388
  cimetidine, oral **1**, 388
  cimetidine hydrochloride, injectable **1**, 388
  ketoconazole, oral **1**, 388
  metformin hydrochloride **2**, 388
  sulfamethoxazole–trimethoprim **1**, 388
  thioridazine hydrochloride **1**, 388
  triamterene **2**, 388
  trimethoprim **1**, 388
  verapamil hydrochloride **1**, 388
  verapamil hydrochloride, sustained–release **1**, 388
  verapamil hydrochloride pellets **1**, 388
domperidone,
  levodopa **3**, 369
  levodopa, comb w/ carbidopa **3**, 369
donepezil hydrochloride,
  paroxetine hydrochloride **2**, 140–141
dong quai,
  warfarin **3**, 83
dopamine hydrochloride,
  chloroform, 28
  enflurane, 28
  ergonovine maleate **2**, 365
  fosphenytoin sodium, injectable, 120–121
  furazolidone, 159–160
  halothane, 28
  isocarboxazid, 159–160
  methoxyflurane, 28
  metoprolol tartrate, 267
  moclobemide, 159–160
  nebivolol hydrochloride, 267
  pargyline hydrochloride, 159–160
  phenelzine sulfate, 159–160
  phenytoin **1**, 120–121
  procarbazine hydrochloride, 159–160
  propranolol hydrochloride, 267
  timolol maleate, ophthalmic, 267
  timolol maleate, oral, 267
  tranylcypromine sulfate, 159–160
dorzolamide hydrochloride,
  lithium, 245–246
dothiepin hydrochloride,
  guanethidine, 169
doxacurium chloride,
  amikacin sulfate, 41
  bacitracin, 41
  colistin sulfate, 41
  demeclocycline hydrochloride, 41
  doxycycline hydrochloride, 41
  doxycycline hyclate, injectable, 41
  gentamicin sulfate, 41
  kanamycin sulfate, injectable, 41
  kanamycin sulfate, oral, 41
  lymecycline, 41
  methacycline hydrochloride, 41
  minocycline, injectable, 41
  minocycline hydrochloride, 41
  minocycline hydrochloride pellets,

# Index

41
neomycin sulfate, injectable, 41
neomycin sulfate, oral, 41
netilmicin, 41
oxytetracycline, 41
oxytetracycline, injectable, 41
paromomycin sulfate, 41
polymyxin B sulfate, 41
polymyxin B sulfate, vaccine use, 41
streptomycin sulfate, 41
tetracycline, 41
tobramycin, 41
doxepin hydrochloride,
  amprenavir **1**, 388
  arbutamine hydrochloride **1**, 388
  cholestyramine **3**, 141
  cisapride **1**, 388
  grepafloxacin hydrochloride **1**, 388
  guanadrel sulfate, 169
  guanethidine, 169
  halofantrine hydrochloride **1**, 388
  pimozide **1**, 388
  propoxyphene **3**, 141
  thioridazine hydrochloride **1**, 388
  tolazamide **2**, 312–313
doxepin hydrochloride, topical,
  amprenavir **1**, 388
  guanadrel sulfate, 169
  guanethidine, 169
doxorubicin hydrochloride,
  phenobarbital **3**, 219
  trastuzumab **1**, 388
doxorubicin hydrochloride liposome,
  trastuzumab **1**, 388
doxycycline hydrochloride,
  alcuronium chloride, 41
  aluminum carbonate, basic, 211–212
  aluminum hydroxide, 211–212
  aluminum oxide, 211–212
  aluminum phosphate, 211–212
  attapulgite, 211–212
  bismuth subsalicylate, 211–212
  calcium, oral salt unspecified, 211–212
  calcium acetate, 211–212
  calcium ascorbate, 211–212
  calcium carbonate, oral, 211–212
  calcium chloride, oral, 211–212
  calcium citrate, oral, 211–212
  calcium glubionate, oral, 211–212
  calcium glucoheptonate, 211–212
  calcium gluconate, oral, 211–212
  calcium glycerophosphate, oral, 211–212
  calcium iodate, 211–212
  calcium lactate, oral, 211–212
  calcium lactate gluconate, 211–212
  calcium lactobionate, oral, 211–212
  calcium phosphate, oral, 211–212
  carbamazepine **2**, 189
  carbonyl iron, 212
  digoxin, 289
  digoxin capsule, stabilized, 289
  dihydroxyaluminum, 211–212
  doxacurium chloride, 41
  ferric ammonium citrate, 212
  ferrous citrate, 212
  ferrous fumarate, 212
  ferrous gluconate, 212
  ferrous glycine sulfate, 212
  ferrous hydroxide polymaltose, 212
  ferrous ions, salt unspecified, 212
  ferrous succinate, 212
  ferrous sulfate, 212
  gallamine triethiodide, 41
  iron peptonized, 212
  kaolin, 211–212
  magaldrate, 211–212
  magnesium carbonate, 211–212
  magnesium chloride, oral, 211–212
  magnesium hydroxide, 211–212
  magnesium oxide, 211–212
  magnesium sulfate, 211–212
  magnesium trisilicate, 211–212
  metocurine iodide, 41
  mivacurium chloride, 41
  pancuronium bromide, 41
  phenobarbital **2**, 189
  phenytoin **2**, 189
  pipecuronium bromide, 41
  rapacuronium bromide, 41
  rocuronium bromide, 41
  succinylcholine chloride, 41
  sucralfate, 211–212
  tubocurarine chloride, 41
  vecuronium bromide, 41
doxycycline hyclate, injectable,
  alcuronium chloride, 41
  digoxin, 289
  digoxin capsule, stabilized, 289
  doxacurium chloride, 41
  gallamine triethiodide, 41
  metocurine iodide, 41
  mivacurium chloride, 41
  pancuronium bromide, 41
  pipecuronium bromide, 41
  rapacuronium bromide, 41
  rocuronium bromide, 41
  succinylcholine chloride, 41
  tubocurarine chloride, 41
  vecuronium bromide, 41
droperidol,
  guanethidine, 169
dyphylline,
  halothane, 337
  probenecid **2**, 341

# E

echothiophate iodide,
  succinylcholine chloride **2**, 37

# Index

econazole nitrate,
  lovastatin **1**, 388
  mizolastine **1**, 388
  phenytoin, 121–122
  simvastatin **1**, 388
efavirenz,
  astemizole **1**, 388
  bromocriptine mesylate **1**, 388
  cabergoline **1**, 388
  cisapride **1**, 388
  dihydroergotamine mesylate **1**, 388
  dihydroergotamine mesylate, inhl **1**, 388
  ergoloid mesylates **1**, 388
  ergonovine maleate **1**, 388
  ergotamine tartrate **1**, 388
  methylergonovine maleate **1**, 388
  methysergide maleate **1**, 388
  midazolam hydrochloride **1**, 388
  pergolide mesylate **1**, 388
  saquinavir **1**, 388
  terfenadine **1**, 388
  triazolam **1**, 388
enalapril maleate,
  azathioprine sodium **3**, 168
  lithium **2**, 248
  rifampin **3**, 168
encainide hydrochloride,
  astemizole **1**, 388
  grepafloxacin hydrochloride **1**, 388
  halofantrine hydrochloride **1**, 388
  pimozide **1**, 388
  ritonavir **1**, 388
enflurane,
  albuterol sulfate, 28
  amikacin sulfate, 27
  amphetamine, 28
  arbutamine hydrochloride, 28
  benzphetamine hydrochloride, 28
  bitolterol mesylate, 28
  clindamycin, 27
  clindamycin phosphate, injectable, 27
  colistin sulfate, 27
  dexfenfluramine hydrochloride, 28
  dextroamphetamine, 28
  diethylpropion hydrochloride, 28
  dobutamine hydrochloride, 28
  dopamine hydrochloride, 28
  ephedrine, 28
  epinephrine, 28
  etafedrine hydrochloride, 28
  ethylnorepinephrine hydrochloride, 28
  fenfluramine hydrochloride, 28
  fenoterol hydrobromide, 28
  formoterol fumarate, inhl, 28
  gentamicin sulfate, 27
  isoetharine, 28
  isometheptene, 28
  isoniazid **3**, 26
  isoproterenol, 28
  kanamycin sulfate, injectable, 27
  kanamycin sulfate, oral, 27
  mazindol, 28
  mephentermine sulfate, 28
  metaproterenol sulfate, 28
  metaraminol bitartrate, 28
  methamphetamine hydrochloride, 28
  methoxamine hydrochloride, 28
  methylphenidate hydrochloride, 28
  norepinephrine bitartrate, 28
  phendimetrazine tartrate, 28
  phenmetrazine hydrochloride, 28
  phentermine hydrochloride, 28
  phenylephrine, 28
  phenylpropanolamine, 28
  pirbuterol acetate, 28
  polymyxin B sulfate, 27
  polymyxin B sulfate, vaccine use, 27
  procaterol hydrochloride, 28
  pseudoephedrine, 28
  rimiterol hydrobromide, 28
  salmeterol xinafoate, 28
  streptomycin sulfate, 27
  terbutaline sulfate, 28
  tobramycin, 27
enoxacin,
  warfarin, 93
enoxaparin sodium,
  sodium salicylate, 77
entacapone,
  furazolidone **1**, 388
  hypericum **1**, 388
  isocarboxazid **1**, 388
  moclobemide **1**, 388
  pargyline hydrochloride **1**, 388
  phenelzine sulfate **1**, 388
  procarbazine hydrochloride **1**, 388
  tranylcypromine sulfate **1**, 388
enteral nutrition,
  ciprofloxacin hydrochloride **3**, 187–188
ephedrine,
  chloroform, 28
  dexamethasone **3**, 364
  enflurane, 28
  furazolidone, 191–192
  isocarboxazid, 159–160
  methoxyflurane, 28
  moclobemide, 159–160
  pargyline hydrochloride, 159–160
  phenelzine sulfate, 159–160
  procarbazine hydrochloride, 159–160
  reserpine **2**, 177
  tranylcypromine sulfate, 159–160
epinephrine,
  acebutolol hydrochloride, 267
  betaxolol hydrochloride, oral, 267

# Index

bisoprolol fumarate, 267
carteolol hydrochloride, 267
carvedilol, 267
celiprolol hydrochloride, 267
chloroform, 28
desflurane, 28
enflurane, 28
ether, 28
furazolidone, 191–192
halothane **1**, 28
imipramine **2**, 147
insulin **3**, 308
isoflurane, 28
isoproterenol, 28
methoxyflurane, 28
nadolol, 267
nebivolol hydrochloride, 267
norepinephrine bitartrate, 28
oxprenolol, 267
penbutolol sulfate, 267
pindolol, 267
propranolol hydrochloride **1**, 267
sevoflurane, 28
sotalol hydrochloride, 267
terbutaline sulfate, 28
tertatolol hydrochloride, 267
timolol maleate, ophthalmic, 267
timolol maleate, oral, 267
epirubicin hydrochloride,
  trastuzumab **1**, 388
eptifibatide,
  tirofiban hydrochloride **1**, 388
ergocalciferol, vitamin D2,
  paricalcitol **1**, 388
  phenytoin **2**, 328
ergoloid mesylates,
  efavirenz **1**, 388
  indinavir sulfate **1**, 388
  rizatriptan benzoate **1**, 388
  saquinavir **1**, 388
  sumatriptan, nasal **1**, 388
  sumatriptan succinate **1**, 388
  sumatriptan succinate, injectable **1**, 388
  sumatriptan succinate, oral **1**, 388
  zolmitriptan **1**, 388
ergonovine maleate,
  dopamine hydrochloride **2**, 365
  efavirenz **1**, 388
  indinavir sulfate **1**, 388
  rizatriptan benzoate **1**, 388
  saquinavir **1**, 388
  sumatriptan, nasal **1**, 388
  sumatriptan succinate **1**, 388
  sumatriptan succinate, injectable **1**, 388
  sumatriptan succinate, oral **1**, 388
  zolmitriptan **1**, 388
ergotamine tartrate,
  amprenavir **1**, 388
  efavirenz **1**, 388
  erythromycin **2**, 190–191
  indinavir sulfate **1**, 388
  propranolol hydrochloride **3**, 267–268
  ritonavir **1**, 388
  rizatriptan benzoate **1**, 388
  saquinavir **1**, 388
  sumatriptan, nasal **1**, 388
  sumatriptan succinate **1**, 388
  sumatriptan succinate, injectable **1**, 388
  sumatriptan succinate, oral **1**, 388
  zolmitriptan **1**, 388
erythrityl tetranitrate,
  sildenafil citrate **1**, 388
erythromycin,
  acenocoumarol, 83
  alfentanil hydrochloride **2**, 5
  aminophylline, 346
  anisindione, 83
  astemizole, 191
  buspirone hydrochloride **3**, 139
  caffeine, 346
  carbamazepine **1**, 105
  cisapride **1**, 388
  coumarin, 83
  cyclosporine **1**, 190
  dicumarol, 83
  digoxin **1**, 279–280
  digoxin capsule, stabilized, 279–280
  disopyramide phosphate **2**, 49
  ergotamine tartrate **2**, 190–191
  felodipine **3**, 51
  grepafloxacin hydrochloride **1**, 388
  lincomycin hydrochloride **3**, 202
  lovastatin **1**, 373
  midazolam hydrochloride **2**, 254–255
  mizolastine **1**, 388
  oxtriphylline, 346
  penicillin G **3**, 206
  pimozide **1**, 388
  simvastatin, 373
  tacrolimus **2**, 383–384
  terfenadine **2**, 191
  theophylline **1**, 346
  toremifene **1**, 388
  valproic acid **2**, 134
  vinblastine sulfate **3**, 228
  warfarin **1**, 83
erythromycin estolate,
  acenocoumarol, 83
  aminophylline, 346
  anisindione, 83
  astemizole, 191
  caffeine, 346
  carbamazepine, 105
  cisapride **1**, 388
  coumarin, 83
  cyclosporine, 190

# Index

dicumarol, 83
digoxin, 279–280
digoxin capsule, stabilized, 279–280
grepafloxacin hydrochloride **1**, 388
lovastatin, 373
mizolastine **1**, 388
oxtriphylline, 346
pimozide **1**, 388
simvastatin, 373
terfenadine, 191
theophylline, 346
toremifene **1**, 388
warfarin, 83
erythromycin ethylsuccinate,
acenocoumarol, 83
aminophylline, 346
anisindione, 83
astemizole, 191
caffeine, 346
carbamazepine, 105
cisapride **1**, 388
coumarin, 83
cyclosporine, 190
dicumarol, 83
digoxin, 279–280
digoxin capsule, stabilized, 279–280
grepafloxacin hydrochloride **1**, 388
lovastatin, 373
mizolastine **1**, 388
oxtriphylline, 346
pimozide **1**, 388
simvastatin, 373
terfenadine, 191
theophylline, 346
toremifene **1**, 388
valproic acid **2**, 134
warfarin, 83
erythromycin gluceptate,
acenocoumarol, 83
aminophylline, 346
anisindione, 83
astemizole, 191
caffeine, 346
carbamazepine, 105
cisapride **1**, 388
coumarin, 83
cyclosporine, 190
dicumarol, 83
digoxin, 279–280
digoxin capsule, stabilized, 279–280
grepafloxacin hydrochloride **1**, 388
lovastatin, 373
mizolastine **1**, 388
oxtriphylline, 346
pimozide **1**, 388
simvastatin, 373
terfenadine, 191
theophylline, 346
toremifene **1**, 388
warfarin, 83
erythromycin lactobionate,
acenocoumarol, 83
aminophylline, 346
anisindione, 83
astemizole, 191
caffeine, 346
carbamazepine, 105
cisapride **1**, 388
coumarin, 83
cyclosporine, 190
dicumarol, 83
digoxin, 279–280
digoxin capsule, stabilized, 279–280
grepafloxacin hydrochloride **1**, 388
lovastatin, 373
mizolastine **1**, 388
oxtriphylline, 346
pimozide **1**, 388
simvastatin, 373
terfenadine, 191
theophylline, 346
toremifene **1**, 388
warfarin, 83
erythromycin stearate,
acenocoumarol, 83
aminophylline, 346
anisindione, 83
astemizole, 191
caffeine, 346
carbamazepine, 105
cimetidine, oral **3**, 189–190
cisapride **1**, 388
clozapine **2**, 238
coumarin, 83
cyclosporine, 190
dicumarol, 83
digoxin, 279–280
digoxin capsule, stabilized, 279–280
grepafloxacin hydrochloride **1**, 388
lovastatin, 373
mizolastine **1**, 388
oxtriphylline, 346
pimozide **1**, 388
simvastatin, 373
terfenadine, 191
theophylline, 346
toremifene **1**, 388
warfarin, 83
esmolol hydrochloride,
arbutamine hydrochloride **1**, 388
digoxin **3**, 280
nitroprusside sodium **3**, 177–178
estazolam,
ritonavir **1**, 388
esterified estrogens,
rifampin, 209
estradiol,

# Index

rifabutin, 209
rifampin, 209
estradiol, transdermal,
  rifabutin, 209
  rifampin, 209
estriol,
  rifampin, 209
estrogen,
  rifampin, 209
estrone,
  rifampin, 209
estropipate,
  rifampin, 209
etafedrine hydrochloride,
  chloroform, 28
  enflurane, 28
  furazolidone, 191–192
  isocarboxazid, 159–160
  methoxyflurane, 28
  metoprolol tartrate, 267
  nebivolol hydrochloride, 267
  pargyline hydrochloride, 159–160
  phenelzine sulfate, 159–160
  procarbazine hydrochloride, 159–160
  propranolol hydrochloride, 267
  timolol maleate, ophthalmic, 267
  timolol maleate, oral, 267
  tranylcypromine sulfate, 159–160
ethacrynic acid,
  amikacin sulfate, 198
  cisplatin **2**, 294–295
  gentamicin sulfate, 198
  kanamycin sulfate, injectable, 198
  kanamycin sulfate, oral **1**, 198
  lithium, 247
  neomycin sulfate, injectable, 198
  neomycin sulfate, oral, 198
  netilmicin, 198
  streptomycin sulfate, 198
  tobramycin, 198
  warfarin **2**, 84
ethacrynic acid, injectable,
  amikacin sulfate, 198
  gentamicin sulfate, 198
  kanamycin sulfate, injectable, 198
  kanamycin sulfate, oral, 198
  lithium, 247
  neomycin sulfate, injectable, 198
  neomycin sulfate, oral, 198
  netilmicin, 198
  streptomycin sulfate, 198
  tobramycin, 198
ethambutol hydrochloride,
  aluminum hydroxide **3**, 191
ethchlorvynol,
  warfarin **2**, 84
ether,
  amikacin sulfate, 27
  bacitracin, 27
  clindamycin, 27
  clindamycin phosphate, injectable, 27
  colistin sulfate, 27
  epinephrine, 28
  gentamicin sulfate, 27
  isoproterenol, 28
  kanamycin sulfate, injectable, 27
  kanamycin sulfate, oral, 27
  neomycin sulfate, injectable, 27
  neomycin sulfate, oral **1**, 27
  norepinephrine bitartrate, 28
  oxytetracycline, 27
  oxytetracycline, injectable, 27
  polymyxin B sulfate, 27
  polymyxin B sulfate, vaccine use, 27
  rolitetracycline, injectable, 27
  streptomycin sulfate, 27
  terbutaline sulfate, 28
  tetracycline, 27
  tetracycline hydrochloride, injectable, 27
  tobramycin, 27
ethinyl estradiol,
  ascorbic acid, vitamin C **3**, 327
  grapefruit juice **3**, 332
  imipramine **3**, 147–148
  rifabutin, 209
  rifampin, 209
ethoheptazine citrate,
  digoxin, 287
  naltrexone hydrochloride **1**, 388
ethosuximide,
  carbamazepine **3**, 111
  isoniazid **3**, 111–112
  phenytoin **3**, 121
  valproic acid **3**, 112
ethotoin,
  cimetidine, oral, 117–118
  cimetidine hydrochloride, injectable, 117–118
  disulfiram, 120
  fluconazole, 121–122
  ranitidine hydrochloride, injectable, 117–118
  ranitidine hydrochloride, oral, 117–118
ethylestrenol,
  acenocoumarol, 91
  coumarin, 91
  dicumarol, 91
  warfarin, 91
ethylnorepinephrine hydrochloride,
  chloroform, 28
  enflurane, 28
  halothane, 28
  methoxyflurane, 28
  metoprolol tartrate, 267
  timolol maleate, oral, 267
etodolac,
  ketorolac tromethamine **1**, 388

# Index

ketorolac tromethamine, injectable **1**, 388
etomidate,
  verapamil hydrochloride **3**, 27
etoposide,
  cyclosporine **2**, 219–220
  mitomycin **3**, 227
  warfarin **3**, 84
etretinate,
  methotrexate **2**, 223
  warfarin **2**, 85

## F

fat emulsion, intraveneous,
  cyclosporine **2**, 366
felbamate,
  carbamazepine **2**, 105
  phenobarbital **3**, 324
  phenytoin **2**, 121
  valproic acid **2**, 134
  warfarin **2**, 85
felodipine,
  erythromycin **3**, 51
  itraconazole, oral **3**, 51–52
fenbufen,
  ketorolac tromethamine **1**, 388
  ketorolac tromethamine, injectable **1**, 388
fenfluramine hydrochloride,
  chloroform, 28
  enflurane, 28
  furazolidone, 191–192
  halothane, 28
  hydrochlorothiazide **3**, 297–298
  insulin **2**, 308
  isocarboxazid, 159–160
  methoxyflurane, 28
  moclobemide, 159–160
  pargyline hydrochloride, 159–160
  phenelzine sulfate, 159–160
  phentermine hydrochloride **1**, 388
  procarbazine hydrochloride, 159–160
  tranylcypromine sulfate, 159–160
fenofibrate, micronized,
  coumarin, 81
  dicumarol, 81
  phenindione, 81
  warfarin, 81
fenoprofen calcium,
  ketorolac tromethamine **1**, 388
  ketorolac tromethamine, injectable **1**, 388
  phenobarbital **3**, 11
fenoterol hydrobromide,
  chloroform, 28
  enflurane, 28
  halothane, 28
  methoxyflurane, 28
  metoprolol tartrate, 267
  timolol maleate, oral, 267

fentanyl citrate,
  naltrexone hydrochloride **1**, 388
  pargyline hydrochloride, 15
  phenelzine sulfate, 15
  propranolol hydrochloride **3**, 11–12
  selegiline hydrochloride, 15
  tranylcypromine sulfate, 15
fenticonazole nitrate,
  cyclosporine, 199–200
  fosphenytoin sodium, injectable, 121–122
  lovastatin **1**, 388
  mizolastine **1**, 388
  phenytoin, 121–122
  simvastatin **1**, 388
fenugreek,
  insulin **2**, 308–309
feprazone,
  acenocoumarol, 94–95
  acetohexamide, 314–315
  anisindione, 94–95
  chlorpropamide, 314–315
  coumarin, 94–95
  dicumarol, 94–95
  gliclazide, 314–315
  glimepiride, 314–315
  gliquidone, 314–315
  tolazamide, 314–315
  tolbutamide, 314–315
  warfarin, 94–95
ferric ammonium citrate,
  demeclocycline hydrochloride, 212
  doxycycline hydrochloride, 212
  lymecycline, 212
  methacycline hydrochloride, 212
  minocycline hydrochloride, 212
  minocycline hydrochloride pellets, 212
  oxytetracycline, 212
  tetracycline, 212
ferrous citrate,
  demeclocycline hydrochloride, 212
  doxycycline hydrochloride, 212
  lymecycline, 212
  methacycline hydrochloride, 212
  minocycline hydrochloride, 212
  minocycline hydrochloride pellets, 212
  oxytetracycline, 212
  tetracycline, 212
ferrous fumarate,
  demeclocycline hydrochloride, 212
  doxycycline hydrochloride, 212
  lymecycline, 212
  methacycline hydrochloride, 212
  minocycline hydrochloride, 212
  minocycline hydrochloride pellets, 212
  oxytetracycline, 212
  tetracycline, 212
ferrous gluconate,

## Index

demeclocycline hydrochloride, 212
doxycycline hydrochloride, 212
lymecycline, 212
methacycline hydrochloride, 212
minocycline hydrochloride, 212
minocycline hydrochloride pellets, 212
oxytetracycline, 212
tetracycline, 212

ferrous glycine sulfate,
  demeclocycline hydrochloride, 212
  doxycycline hydrochloride, 212
  lymecycline, 212
  methacycline hydrochloride, 212
  minocycline hydrochloride, 212
  minocycline hydrochloride pellets, 212
  oxytetracycline, 212
  tetracycline, 212

ferrous hydroxide polymaltose,
  demeclocycline hydrochloride, 212
  doxycycline hydrochloride, 212
  lymecycline, 212
  methacycline hydrochloride, 212
  minocycline hydrochloride, 212
  minocycline hydrochloride pellets, 212
  oxytetracycline, 212
  tetracycline, 212

ferrous ions, salt unspecified,
  demeclocycline hydrochloride, 212
  doxycycline hydrochloride, 212
  lymecycline, 212
  methacycline hydrochloride, 212
  minocycline hydrochloride, 212
  minocycline hydrochloride pellets, 212
  oxytetracycline, 212
  tetracycline, 212

ferrous succinate,
  demeclocycline hydrochloride, 212
  doxycycline hydrochloride, 212
  lymecycline, 212
  methacycline hydrochloride, 212
  minocycline hydrochloride, 212
  minocycline hydrochloride pellets, 212
  oxytetracycline, 212
  tetracycline, 212

ferrous sulfate,
  allopurinol **4**, 328–329
  aluminum hydroxide **3**, 329
  ascorbic acid, vitamin C **3**, 329
  cimetidine, oral **3**, 329
  ciprofloxacin hydrochloride **2**, 187
  demeclocycline hydrochloride, 212
  doxycycline hydrochloride, 212
  levodopa **2**, 369
  levothyroxine sodium **3**, 370–371
  lymecycline, 212
  magnesium carbonate **3**, 329
  magnesium hydroxide **3**, 329
  methacycline hydrochloride, 212
  methyldopa **2**, 173
  minocycline hydrochloride, 212
  minocycline hydrochloride pellets, 212
  oxytetracycline, 212
  penicillamine **2**, 329–330
  tetracycline **1**, 212

flecainide acetate,
  amiodarone hydrochloride **2**, 52
  ammonium chloride **2**, 52
  astemizole **1**, 388
  charcoal **3**, 52–53
  cimetidine, oral **2**, 53
  grepafloxacin hydrochloride **1**, 388
  halofantrine hydrochloride **1**, 388
  isoproterenol **2**, 53
  mizolastine **1**, 388
  pimozide **1**, 388
  propranolol hydrochloride **3**, 268
  quinine **3**, 53–54
  ritonavir **1**, 388
  sodium bicarbonate **2**, 54

flosequinan,
  warfarin, 93

flucloxacillin,
  amikacin sulfate, 192
  gentamicin sulfate, 192
  netilmicin, 192
  tobramycin, 192

fluconazole,
  alfentanil hydrochloride **3**, 5–6
  amitriptyline hydrochloride **2**, 137–138
  astemizole **1**, 388
  cisapride **1**, 388
  cyclosporine, 199–200
  ethotoin, 121–122
  fosphenytoin sodium, injectable, 121–122
  lovastatin **1**, 388
  mephenytoin, 121–122
  mizolastine **1**, 388
  phenytoin **1**, 121–122
  simvastatin **1**, 388
  tacrolimus **2**, 384
  terfenadine **1**, 388
  tolbutamide **3**, 314
  warfarin **2**, 85–86

flumethiazide,
  lithium, 247

fluorouracil,
  cimetidine, oral **3**, 220
  hydrochlorothiazide **3**, 218
  metronidazole, injectable **2**, 220
  metronidazole, oral/vaginal **2**, 220

fluoxetine hydrochloride,
  alcohol, ethyl–oral/injectable **4**, 318
  alprazolam **2**, 231
  aspirin **3**, 141–142

# Index

astemizole **1**, 388
ayahuasca **2**, 142
buspirone hydrochloride **3**, 139
clarithromycin **3**, 143
cyclosporine **3**, 143
cyproheptadine hydrochloride **2**, 143–144
digoxin capsule, stabilized **2**, 280–281
furazolidone, 144–145
haloperidol **3**, 243–244
isocarboxazid, 144–145
linezolid **1**, 388
lithium **2**, 248
marijuana **2**, 144
moclobemide, 144–145
nifedipine **3**, 58–59
nortriptyline hydrochloride **2**, 151–152
pargyline hydrochloride, 144–145
phenelzine sulfate, 144–145
phenytoin **2**, 122
pimozide **3**, 256–257
procarbazine hydrochloride, 144–145
propafenone hydrochloride **2**, 62
propranolol hydrochloride **2**, 268
selegiline hydrochloride, 144–145
thioridazine hydrochloride **1**, 388
tranylcypromine sulfate **1**, 144–145
trazodone hydrochloride **3**, 160
tryptophan **3**, 145
valproic acid **3**, 134–135
warfarin **3**, 86
fluoxymesterone,
acenocoumarol, 91
coumarin, 91
dicumarol, 91
warfarin, 91
flupenthixol decanoate, injectable,
cabergoline **1**, 388
guanethidine, 169
pergolide mesylate **1**, 388
flupenthixol dihydrochloride, oral,
cabergoline **1**, 388
guanethidine, 169
pergolide mesylate **1**, 388
fluphenazine,
cabergoline **1**, 388
clonidine hydrochloride **3**, 243
guanethidine, 169
pergolide mesylate **1**, 388
flurazepam hydrochloride,
ritonavir **1**, 388
flurbiprofen,
ketorolac tromethamine **1**, 388
ketorolac tromethamine, injectable **1**, 388
fluvoxamine maleate,
astemizole **1**, 388
cisapride **1**, 388

clozapine **2**, 238
furazolidone, 144–145
isocarboxazid, 144–145
melatonin **3**, 145
moclobemide, 144–145
olanzapine **3**, 255
pargyline hydrochloride, 144–145
phenelzine sulfate, 144–145
procarbazine hydrochloride, 144–145
selegiline hydrochloride, 144–145
tacrine hydrochloride **2**, 145–146
terfenadine **1**, 388
theophylline **3**, 347
thioridazine hydrochloride **1**, 388
tranylcypromine sulfate, 144–145
folic acid,
phenytoin **2**, 122
sulfasalazine **3**, 330
formoterol fumarate, inhl,
chloroform, 28
enflurane, 28
halothane, 28
methoxyflurane, 28
metoprolol tartrate, 267
timolol maleate, oral, 267
foscarnet sodium,
cyclosporine **2**, 366
fosphenytoin sodium, injectable,
azapropazone dihydrate **1**, 388
cimetidine, oral, 117–118
cimetidine hydrochloride, injectable, 117–118
clotrimazole, 121–122
disulfiram, 120
dopamine hydrochloride, 120–121
fenticonazole nitrate, 121–122
fluconazole, 121–122
isoconazole nitrate, 121–122
itraconazole, 121–122
itraconazole, oral, 121–122
ketoconazole, oral, 121–122
miconazole nitrate, 121–122
oxiconazole nitrate, 121–122
ranitidine hydrochloride, injectable, 117–118
ranitidine hydrochloride, oral, 117–118
terconazole, 121–122
thioridazine hydrochloride **1**, 388
tioconazole, 121–122
furazolidone,
alcohol, ethyl–oral/injectable **2**, 318
amphetamine **1**, 191–192
benzphetamine hydrochloride, 191–192
brimonidine tartrate, ophthalmic **1**, 388
bupropion hydrochloride **1**, 388
chloral hydrate **4**, 320
dexfenfluramine hydrochloride,

# Index

191–192
dextroamphetamine, 191–192
diethylpropion hydrochloride,
 191–192
dopamine hydrochloride, 159–160
entacapone **1**, 388
ephedrine, 191–192
epinephrine, 191–192
etafedrine hydrochloride, 191–192
fenfluramine hydrochloride, 191–192
fluoxetine hydrochloride, 144–145
fluvoxamine maleate, 144–145
indoramin **1**, 388
isometheptene, 159–160
levodopa, 157–158
mazindol, 191–192
meperidine hydrochloride, 15
mephentermine sulfate, 191–192
metaraminol bitartrate, 159–160
methamphetamine hydrochloride,
 191–192
methylphenidate hydrochloride,
 191–192
nalbuphine hydrochloride, 15
naphazoline hydrochloride,
 159–160
nefazodone hydrochloride **1**, 388
oxymetazoline hydrochloride,
 159–160
phendimetrazine tartrate, 191–192
phenmetrazine hydrochloride,
 191–192
phentermine hydrochloride,
 191–192
phenylephrine, 159–160
phenylpropanolamine, 191–192
pseudoephedrine, 191–192
rizatriptan benzoate **1**, 388
sertraline hydrochloride **1**, 388
sibutramine hydrochloride
 monohyd **1**, 388
sumatriptan, nasal **1**, 388
sumatriptan succinate **1**, 388
sumatriptan succinate, oral **1**, 388
tetrahydrozoline hydrochloride,
 159–160
tolcapone **1**, 388
venlafaxine hydrochloride, 144–145
xylometazoline hydrochloride,
 159–160
furosemide,
 amikacin sulfate, 198
 aspirin **3**, 295
 captopril **2**, 164
 charcoal **2**, 295
 chloral hydrate **3**, 295
 cholestyramine **2**, 296
 digoxin **2**, 281
 gentamicin sulfate, 198
 ginseng **3**, 296
 indomethacin **3**, 296–297
 kanamycin sulfate, injectable, 198
 kanamycin sulfate, oral, 198
 lithium, 247
 neomycin sulfate, injectable, 198
 neomycin sulfate, oral, 198
 netilmicin, 198
 pancuronium bromide **3**, 33
 phenytoin **3**, 297
 probenecid **3**, 297
 propranolol hydrochloride **2**, 269
 streptomycin sulfate, 198
 theophylline **2**, 347
 tobramycin, 198
furosemide, injectable,
 amikacin sulfate, 198
 gentamicin sulfate, 198
 kanamycin sulfate, injectable, 198
 kanamycin sulfate, oral, 198
 lithium, 247
 neomycin sulfate, injectable, 198
 neomycin sulfate, oral, 198
 netilmicin, 198
 streptomycin sulfate, 198
 tobramycin, 198

## G

gallamine triethiodide,
 amikacin sulfate, 41
 bacitracin, 41
 colistin sulfate, 41
 demeclocycline hydrochloride, 41
 diazepam **3**, 27–28
 doxycycline hydrochloride, 41
 doxycycline hyclate, injectable, 41
 gentamicin sulfate, 41
 kanamycin sulfate, injectable, 41
 kanamycin sulfate, oral, 41
 lymecycline, 41
 methacycline hydrochloride, 41
 minocycline, injectable, 41
 minocycline hydrochloride, 41
 minocycline hydrochloride pellets,
  41
 neomycin sulfate, injectable, 41
 neomycin sulfate, oral, 41
 netilmicin, 41
 oxytetracycline, 41
 oxytetracycline, injectable, 41
 paromomycin sulfate, 41
 polymyxin B sulfate, 41
 polymyxin B sulfate, vaccine use,
  41
 rolitetracycline, injectable, 41
 streptomycin sulfate, 41
 tetracycline, 41
 tetracycline hydrochloride,
  injectable, 41
 tobramycin, 41
ganciclovir,
 didanosine **2**, 364–365
garlic,

# Index

saquinavir **2**, 330
gemfibrozil,
  acenocoumarol, 81
  bexarotene **1**, 388
  cerivastatin **1**, 388
  coumarin, 81
  dicumarol, 81
  glyburide **2**, 306
  lovastatin **2**, 373–374
  phenindione, 81
  warfarin, 81
gentamicin sulfate,
  alcuronium chloride, 41
  amoxicillin, 192
  ampicillin sodium, 192
  azlocillin sodium, 192
  bacampicillin hydrochloride, 192
  benethamine penicillin, 192
  bumetanide, 198
  bumetanide, injectable, 198
  carbenicillin disodium **1**, 192
  carfecillin, 192
  cefaclor, 192
  cefadroxil monohydrate, 192
  cefamandole nafate, 192
  cefazolin sodium, 192
  cefdinir, 192
  cefepime hydrochloride, 192
  cefmetazole sodium, 192
  cefonicid sodium, 192
  cefoperazone sodium, 192
  ceforanide, 192
  cefotaxime sodium, 192
  cefotetan disodium, 192
  cefoxitin sodium, 192
  cefpirome sulfate, 192
  cefpodoxime proxetil, 192
  cefprozil, 192
  ceftazidime, 192
  ceftibuten dihyrate, 192
  ceftizoxime sodium, 192
  ceftriaxone sodium, 192
  cefuroxime, 192
  cephalexin, 192
  cephalothin sodium **1**, 192
  cephapirin sodium, 192
  cephradine, 192
  cloxacillin sodium, 192
  cyclacillin, 192
  dicloxacillin, 192
  doxacurium chloride, 41
  enflurane, 27
  ethacrynic acid, 198
  ethacrynic acid, injectable, 198
  ether, 27
  flucloxacillin, 192
  furosemide, 198
  furosemide, injectable, 198
  gallamine triethiodide, 41
  halothane, 27
  indomethacin **2**, 192–193
  isoflurane, 27
  mecillinam, 192
  methicillin sodium, 192
  methoxyflurane, 27
  metocurine iodide, 41
  mezlocillin sodium, 192
  mivacurium chloride, 41
  moxalactam disodium, 192
  nafcillin sodium, 192
  nitrous oxide, 27
  oxacillin sodium, 192
  pancuronium bromide, 41
  penicillin G, 192
  penicillin G benzathine, 192
  penicillin G procaine, 192
  penicillin V, 192
  pipecuronium bromide, 41
  piperacillin sodium, 192
  piretanide, 198
  polymyxin B sulfate **2**, 193
  rapacuronium bromide, 41
  rocuronium bromide, 41
  succinylcholine chloride, 41
  temocillin sodium, 192
  ticarcillin disodium, 192
  torsemide, injectable, 198
  torsemide, oral, 198
  tubocurarine chloride **1**, 41
  vancomycin hydrochloride **3**, 193
  vecuronium bromide, 41
ginkgo biloba,
  aspirin **3**, 8
  trazodone hydrochloride **3**, 161
  warfarin **3**, 86
ginseng,
  digoxin **3**, 281–282
  furosemide **3**, 296
  insulin **3**, 309
  phenelzine sulfate **3**, 157
  warfarin **3**, 87
gliclazide,
  alcohol, ethyl–oral/injectable, 302
  feprazone, 314–315
  oxyphenbutazone, 314–315
  phenylbutazone, 314–315
glimepiride,
  alcohol, ethyl–oral/injectable, 302
  feprazone, 314–315
  oxyphenbutazone, 314–315
  phenylbutazone, 314–315
glipizide,
  alcohol, ethyl–oral/injectable, 302
  charcoal **2**, 304–305
  cholestyramine **2**, 305
  cimetidine, oral **2**, 305
  heparin **3**, 305–306
gliquidone,
  alcohol, ethyl–oral/injectable, 302
  feprazone, 314–315
  oxyphenbutazone, 314–315
  phenylbutazone, 314–315

# Index

glucagon,
  acenocoumarol, 87
  anisindione, 87
  coumarin, 87
  dicumarol, 87
  warfarin **1**, 87
glucagon, recombinant,
  acenocoumarol, 87
  anisindione, 87
  coumarin, 87
  dicumarol, 87
  warfarin, 87
glutethimide,
  acenocoumarol, 87
  alcohol, ethyl–oral/injectable **2**, 319
  anisindione, 87
  coumarin, 87
  dicumarol, 87
  labetalol hydrochloride **3**, 261
  warfarin **1**, 87
glyburide,
  alcohol, ethyl–oral/injectable, 302
  ciprofloxacin hydrochloride **2**, 306
  ciprofloxacin hydrochloride, injectable **2**, 306
  gemfibrozil **2**, 306
  rifampin **3**, 306–307
glycopyrrolate,
  digoxin, 287
  ritodrine hydrochloride **2**, 366
glycyrrhiza, (licorice) inert,
  prednisolone **3**, 380
glycyrrhiza, (licorice) noninert,
  prednisolone **3**, 380
gold sodium thiomalate,
  naproxen **2**, 12
  tobacco **3**, 12
grapefruit juice,
  amiodarone hydrochloride **2**, 330–331
  astemizole **1**, 388
  atorvastatin calcium, 374
  cerivastatin, 374
  cilostazol **1**, 388
  cisapride **1**, 388
  clomipramine hydrochloride **2**, 331
  colchicine **2**, 331–332
  ethinyl estradiol **3**, 332
  lovastatin **1**, 374
  quinidine **3**, 332–333
  saquinavir **2**, 333
  sertraline hydrochloride **3**, 333
  simvastatin, 374
  tacrolimus **1**, 388
  terfenadine **2**, 333–334
grepafloxacin hydrochloride,
  acetophenazine maleate **1**, 388
  amiodarone hydrochloride **1**, 388
  amitriptyline hydrochloride **1**, 388
  astemizole **1**, 388
  bepridil hydrochloride **1**, 388
  bretylium tosylate **1**, 388
  cisapride **1**, 388
  desipramine hydrochloride **1**, 388
  disopyramide phosphate **1**, 388
  doxepin hydrochloride **1**, 388
  encainide hydrochloride **1**, 388
  erythromycin **1**, 388
  erythromycin estolate **1**, 388
  erythromycin ethylsuccinate **1**, 388
  erythromycin gluceptate **1**, 388
  erythromycin lactobionate **1**, 388
  erythromycin stearate **1**, 388
  flecainide acetate **1**, 388
  ibutilide fumarate **1**, 388
  imipramine **1**, 388
  lidocaine hydrochloride, local–injectable **1**, 388
  lidocaine hydrochloride, systemic **1**, 388
  mesoridazine besylate **1**, 388
  methdilazine **1**, 388
  mexiletine hydrochloride **1**, 388
  pentamidine isethionate **1**, 388
  pentamidine isethionate, inhalation **1**, 388
  pericyazine **1**, 388
  phenytoin **1**, 388
  piperacetazine **1**, 388
  procainamide hydrochloride **1**, 388
  promazine hydrochloride **1**, 388
  promethazine **1**, 388
  propafenone hydrochloride **1**, 388
  propiomazine hydrochloride **1**, 388
  quinidine **1**, 388
  sotalol hydrochloride **1**, 388
  sulfamethoxazole–trimethoprim **1**, 388
  terfenadine **1**, 388
  thiethylperazine maleate **1**, 388
  thioproperazine mesylate **1**, 388
  thioridazine hydrochloride **1**, 388
  triflupromazine hydrochloride **1**, 388
  trimeprazine tartrate **1**, 388
  trimipramine maleate **1**, 388
griseofulvin,
  aspirin **3**, 9
  cyclosporine **3**, 193–194
  hormonal contraceptive **2**, 194
  phenobarbital **3**, 194
  warfarin **2**, 88
guanadrel sulfate,
  amitriptyline hydrochloride, 169
  butriptyline hydrochloride, 169
  chlorpromazine hydrochloride, 169
  cyclobenzaprine hydrochloride, 169
  desipramine hydrochloride, 169
  doxepin hydrochloride, 169
  doxepin hydrochloride, topical, 169
  imipramine, 169
  maprotiline hydrochloride, 169
  nortriptyline hydrochloride, 169

## Index

opipramol, 169
protriptyline hydrochloride, 169
guanethidine,
  acetophenazine maleate, 169
  alcohol, ethyl oral/injectable **2**, 168
  amitriptyline hydrochloride, 169
  amoxapine, 169
  butriptyline hydrochloride, 169
  chlorpromazine hydrochloride **1**, 169
  chlorprothixene, 169
  clomipramine hydrochloride, 169
  cyclobenzaprine hydrochloride, 169
  desipramine hydrochloride **1**, 169
  dextroamphetamine **2**, 170
  dothiepin hydrochloride, 169
  doxepin hydrochloride, 169
  doxepin hydrochloride, topical, 169
  droperidol, 169
  flupenthixol decanoate, injectable, 169
  flupenthixol dihydrochloride, oral, 169
  fluphenazine, 169
  haloperidol, 169
  hydrochlorothiazide **2**, 170
  imipramine, 169
  insulin **2**, 309–310
  loxapine, 169
  maprotiline hydrochloride, 169
  mequitazine, 169
  mesoridazine besylate, 169
  methdilazine, 169
  methotrimeprazine, 169
  minoxidil **2**, 170–171
  nortriptyline hydrochloride, 169
  opipramol, 169
  oxypertine, 169
  pericyazine, 169
  perphenazine, 169
  phenelzine sulfate **2**, 171
  phenylephrine **2**, 171
  piperacetazine, 169
  prochlorperazine, 169
  promazine hydrochloride, 169
  promethazine, 169
  protriptyline hydrochloride, 169
  thiethylperazine maleate, 169
  thioproperazine mesylate, 169
  thioridazine hydrochloride, 169
  thiothixene, 169
  trifluoperazine hydrochloride, 169
  triflupromazine hydrochloride, 169
  trimeprazine tartrate, 169
  trimipramine maleate, 169
  zuclopenthixol, 169
guanfacine hydrochloride,
  bupropion hydrochloride **3**, 171–172
  phenobarbital **3**, 172
guar gum,

digoxin **3**, 282
penicillin V **3**, 207

## H

halofantrine hydrochloride,
  acetophenazine maleate **1**, 388
  amiodarone hydrochloride **1**, 388
  amitriptyline hydrochloride **1**, 388
  astemizole **1**, 388
  bretylium tosylate **1**, 388
  clomipramine hydrochloride **1**, 388
  desipramine hydrochloride **1**, 388
  disopyramide phosphate **1**, 388
  doxepin hydrochloride **1**, 388
  encainide hydrochloride **1**, 388
  flecainide acetate **1**, 388
  ibutilide fumarate **1**, 388
  imipramine **1**, 388
  indecainide hydrochloride **1**, 388
  mefloquine hydrochloride **1**, 388
  mesoridazine besylate **1**, 388
  methdilazine **1**, 388
  moricizine hydrochloride **1**, 388
  nortriptyline hydrochloride **1**, 388
  pericyazine **1**, 388
  perphenazine **1**, 388
  piperacetazine **1**, 388
  procainamide hydrochloride **1**, 388
  prochlorperazine **1**, 388
  promazine hydrochloride **1**, 388
  promethazine **1**, 388
  propafenone hydrochloride **1**, 388
  propiomazine hydrochloride **1**, 388
  protriptyline hydrochloride **1**, 388
  quinidine **1**, 388
  sotalol hydrochloride **1**, 388
  terfenadine **1**, 388
  thiethylperazine maleate **1**, 388
  thioproperazine mesylate **1**, 388
  thioridazine hydrochloride **1**, 388
  trifluoperazine hydrochloride **1**, 388
  triflupromazine hydrochloride **1**, 388
  trimeprazine tartrate **1**, 388
  trimipramine maleate **1**, 388
haloperidol,
  cabergoline **1**, 388
  carbamazepine **2**, 243
  fluoxetine hydrochloride **3**, 243–244
  guanethidine, 169
  itraconazole, oral **3**, 244
  lithium **2**, 248–249
  methyldopa **3**, 174
  pergolide mesylate **1**, 388
  phenindione **3**, 74
  rifampin **2**, 244–245
  tacrine hydrochloride **2**, 245
halothane,
  albuterol sulfate, 28

# Index

amikacin sulfate, 27
aminophylline **1**, 337
amphetamine, 28
arbutamine hydrochloride, 28
benzphetamine hydrochloride, 28
bitolterol mesylate, 28
clindamycin, 27
clindamycin phosphate, injectable, 27
colistin sulfate, 27
dexfenfluramine hydrochloride, 28
dextroamphetamine, 28
diethylpropion hydrochloride, 28
dobutamine hydrochloride, 28
dopamine hydrochloride, 28
dyphylline, 337
epinephrine **1**, 28
ethylnorepinephrine hydrochloride, 28
fenfluramine hydrochloride, 28
fenoterol hydrobromide, 28
formoterol fumarate, inhl, 28
gentamicin sulfate, 27
isoetharine, 28
isometheptene, 28
isoproterenol, 28
kanamycin sulfate, injectable, 27
kanamycin sulfate, oral, 27
ketamine hydrochloride **2**, 29
labetalol hydrochloride **2**, 261
mazindol, 28
mephentermine sulfate, 28
metaproterenol sulfate, 28
metaraminol bitartrate, 28
methamphetamine hydrochloride, 28
methoxamine hydrochloride, 28
methylphenidate hydrochloride, 28
neomycin sulfate, injectable, 27
neomycin sulfate, oral, 27
nifedipine **3**, 59
norepinephrine bitartrate, 28
oxtriphylline, 337
phendimetrazine tartrate, 28
phenmetrazine hydrochloride, 28
phentermine hydrochloride, 28
phenylephrine, 28
phenylpropanolamine, 28
phenytoin **3**, 28–29
pirbuterol acetate, 28
polymyxin B sulfate, 27
polymyxin B sulfate, vaccine use, 27
procaterol hydrochloride, 28
pseudoephedrine, 28
reserpine **3**, 177
rifampin **2**, 29
rimiterol hydrobromide, 28
salmeterol xinafoate, 28
streptomycin sulfate, 27
terbutaline sulfate, 28
theophylline, 337
tobramycin, 27
heparin,
  aloxiprin, 72–73
  aspirin **1**, 72–73
  calcium carbaspirin, 72–73
  carbenicillin disodium **2**, 73
  dextran 40, inert/interacting **2**, 73
  dextran 40 **2**, 73
  dextran 70 **2**, 73
  digoxin **3**, 282
  glipizide **3**, 305–306
  nitroglycerin **2**, 74
  sodium salicylate, 77
  tobacco **3**, 74
hexobarbital,
  rifampin **3**, 321
hexocyclium methylsulfate,
  digoxin, 287
hormonal contraceptive,
  acetaminophen **3**, 2–3
  aminophylline **3**, 339
  ampicillin sodium **2**, 180–181
  aspirin **3**, 10
  caffeine **3**, 341
  carbamazepine **3**, 108
  cyclosporine **3**, 363
  diazepam **3**, 242
  dicumarol **2**, 72
  griseofulvin **2**, 194
  hormonal contraceptive, low–dose **3**, 383
  hypericum **2**, 245
  metoprolol tartrate **3**, 262
  nevirapine **1**, 388
  phenobarbital **2**, 324
  phenytoin **3**, 123
  prednisolone **2**, 380–381
  rifabutin, 209
  rifampin **1**, 209
  selegiline hydrochloride **3**, 382–383
  tacrine hydrochloride **3**, 383
  tetracycline **2**, 212
  trimethoprim **3**, 210–211
  troleandomycin **2**, 214
hormonal contraceptive, low–dose,
  acetaminophen **3**, 2–3
  aminophylline **3**, 339
  caffeine **3**, 341
  carbamazepine **3**, 108
  clofibrate **3**, 360
  cyclosporine **3**, 363
  diazepam **3**, 242
  hormonal contraceptive **3**, 383
  hypericum **2**, 245
  nevirapine **1**, 388
  phenobarbital **2**, 324
  rifabutin, 209
  rifampin, 209
  selegiline hydrochloride **3**,

# Index

382–383
hydralazine hydrochloride,
  indomethacin **3**, 172
  propranolol hydrochloride **3**, 269
hydrochlorothiazide,
  carbamazepine **3**, 106
  chlorpropamide **2**, 303–304
  cyclophosphamide **3**, 218
  fenfluramine hydrochloride **3**, 297–298
  fluorouracil **3**, 218
  guanethidine **2**, 170
  lithium, 247
  methotrexate **3**, 218
hydrocodone bitartrate,
  isocarboxazid, 15
  naltrexone hydrochloride **1**, 388
  pargyline hydrochloride, 15
  phenelzine sulfate, 15
  selegiline hydrochloride, 15
  tranylcypromine sulfate, 15
hydrocortisone, oral/systemic,
  cholestyramine **3**, 366–367
  pancuronium bromide **3**, 33–34
  theophylline **3**, 347
hydrocortisone acet, injectable,
  cholestyramine **3**, 366–367
  pancuronium bromide **3**, 33–34
  theophylline **3**, 347
hydrocortisone sodium phos,
  cholestyramine **3**, 366–367
  pancuronium bromide **3**, 33–34
  theophylline **3**, 347
hydrocortisone sodium succinate,
  cholestyramine **3**, 366–367
  pancuronium bromide **3**, 33–34
  theophylline **3**, 347
hydroflumethiazide,
  lithium, 247
hydromorphone hydrochloride,
  isocarboxazid, 15
  naltrexone hydrochloride **1**, 388
  pargyline hydrochloride, 15
  phenelzine sulfate, 15
  selegiline hydrochloride, 15
  tranylcypromine sulfate, 15
hydroxychloroquine sulfate,
  digoxin **2**, 282
hyoscyamine,
  digoxin, 287
hypericum,
  cyclosporine **2**, 362
  digoxin **3**, 283
  entacapone **1**, 388
  hormonal contraceptive **2**, 245
  hormonal contraceptive, low-dose **2**, 245
  indinavir sulfate **2**, 367–368
  indoramin **1**, 388
  paroxetine hydrochloride **3**, 155
  rizatriptan benzoate **1**, 388
  sibutramine hydrochloride monohyd **1**, 388
  theophylline **3**, 347–348
  tolcapone **1**, 388

# I

ibuprofen,
  baclofen **3**, 12–13
  digoxin **2**, 283
  ketorolac tromethamine **1**, 388
  ketorolac tromethamine, injectable **1**, 388
  phenytoin **2**, 123
  warfarin **2**, 88
ibutilide fumarate,
  astemizole **1**, 388
  grepafloxacin hydrochloride **1**, 388
  halofantrine hydrochloride **1**, 388
  mizolastine **1**, 388
  moxifloxacin hydrochloride, oral **1**, 388
  pimozide **1**, 388
  sotalol hydrochloride **1**, 388
  sparfloxacin **1**, 388
idarubicin hydrochloride,
  trastuzumab **1**, 388
ifosfamide,
  warfarin **2**, 88–89
imipenem in combination with cilastatin,
  aminophylline **2**, 337
  cyclosporine **2**, 194–195
imipramine,
  amprenavir **1**, 388
  arbutamine hydrochloride **1**, 388
  aspirin **3**, 146
  bupropion hydrochloride **3**, 146
  cimetidine, oral **2**, 147
  cisapride **1**, 388
  epinephrine **2**, 147
  ethinyl estradiol **3**, 147–148
  grepafloxacin hydrochloride **1**, 388
  guanadrel sulfate, 169
  guanethidine, 169
  halofantrine hydrochloride **1**, 388
  levodopa **3**, 148
  liothyronine sodium **2**, 148
  lithium **3**, 148–149
  meprobamate **3**, 321–322
  methyltestosterone **3**, 149
  nitroglycerin, sublingual **2**, 149
  phenytoin **3**, 124
  pimozide **1**, 388
  reserpine **3**, 149
  thioridazine hydrochloride **1**, 388
  tobacco **3**, 150
  tranylcypromine sulfate **2**, 150
indapamide,
  lithium, 247
indecainide hydrochloride,
  halofantrine hydrochloride **1**, 388

# Index

pimozide **1**, 388
indinavir sulfate,
  astemizole **1**, 388
  bromocriptine mesylate **1**, 388
  cabergoline **1**, 388
  carbamazepine **2**, 367
  cisapride **1**, 388
  dihydroergotamine mesylate **1**, 388
  dihydroergotamine mesylate, inhl **1**, 388
  ergoloid mesylates **1**, 388
  ergonovine maleate **1**, 388
  ergotamine tartrate **1**, 388
  hypericum **2**, 367–368
  ketoconazole, oral **1**, 388
  methylergonovine maleate **1**, 388
  methysergide maleate **1**, 388
  midazolam hydrochloride **1**, 388
  nevirapine **1**, 388
  omeprazole **3**, 368
  pergolide mesylate **1**, 388
  rifampin **1**, 388
  rifapentine **1**, 388
  sildenafil citrate **1**, 388
  terfenadine **1**, 388
  triazolam **1**, 388
indomethacin,
  aluminum hydroxide **3**, 13
  aspirin **3**, 13
  bendroflumethiazide **2**, 292
  captopril **2**, 164–165
  cimetidine, oral **3**, 13
  cyclophosphamide **3**, 218
  furosemide **3**, 296–297
  gentamicin sulfate **2**, 192–193
  hydralazine hydrochloride **3**, 172
  ketorolac tromethamine **1**, 388
  ketorolac tromethamine, injectable **1**, 388
  lithium **2**, 249
  nitroglycerin **3**, 14
  penicillamine **3**, 380
  phenylpropanolamine **2**, 14
  prazosin hydrochloride **2**, 176
  probenecid **2**, 14
  propranolol hydrochloride **2**, 269
  triamterene **2**, 299
  warfarin **2**, 89
indomethacin sodium trihyd, injectable,
  ketorolac tromethamine **1**, 388
  ketorolac tromethamine, injectable **1**, 388
indoramin,
  furazolidone **1**, 388
  hypericum **1**, 388
  isocarboxazid **1**, 388
  moclobemide **1**, 388
  pargyline hydrochloride **1**, 388
  phenelzine sulfate **1**, 388
  procarbazine hydrochloride **1**, 388
  tranylcypromine sulfate **1**, 388
influenza virus vaccine, split virion,
  clorazepate dipotassium **3**, 236
  phenytoin **3**, 124
  theophylline **3**, 348
  warfarin **3**, 89
influenza virus vaccine, whole virion,
  theophylline **3**, 348
insulin,
  acebutolol hydrochloride, 311
  aspirin **3**, 307
  betaxolol hydrochloride, oral, 311
  bisoprolol fumarate, 311
  carteolol hydrochloride, 311
  carvedilol, 311
  celiprolol hydrochloride, 311
  chlorpromazine hydrochloride **3**, 307
  clofibrate **2**, 307
  diltiazem hydrochloride **3**, 308
  epinephrine **3**, 308
  fenfluramine hydrochloride **2**, 308
  fenugreek **2**, 308–309
  ginseng **3**, 309
  guanethidine **2**, 309–310
  isoniazid **3**, 177
  labetalol hydrochloride, 311
  nadolol, 311
  nebivolol hydrochloride, 311
  oxprenolol, 311
  oxytetracycline **2**, 310
  penbutolol sulfate, 311
  phenelzine sulfate **2**, 310–311
  phenytoin **3**, 311
  pindolol, 311
  propranolol hydrochloride **1**, 311
  sotalol hydrochloride, 311
  tertatolol hydrochloride, 311
  thyroid desiccated **3**, 311–312
  timolol maleate, ophthalmic, 311
  timolol maleate, oral, 311
  tobacco **3**, 312
interferon alfa-2a,
  aminophylline **2**, 337–338
  paroxetine hydrochloride **3**, 155–156
iocetamic acid,
  metformin hydrochloride **1**, 312
iodamide,
  metformin hydrochloride **1**, 312
iodipamide meglumine,
  metformin hydrochloride **1**, 312
iodoquinol,
  metformin hydrochloride **1**, 312
iodoxamine meglumine,
  metformin hydrochloride **1**, 312
iopamidol,
  metformin hydrochloride **1**, 312
iopanoic acid,
  metformin hydrochloride **1**, 312
iopodic acid,

# Index

metformin hydrochloride **1**, 312
iopydol,
   metformin hydrochloride **1**, 312
iopydone,
   metformin hydrochloride **1**, 312
iothalamate meglumine,
   metformin hydrochloride **1**, 312
iothalamate sodium,
   metformin hydrochloride **1**, 312
iotrolan,
   metformin hydrochloride **1**, 312
ioversol,
   metformin hydrochloride **1**, 312
ioxaglate meglumine,
   metformin hydrochloride **1**, 312
ioxaglate sodium,
   metformin hydrochloride **1**, 312
ipodate calcium,
   metformin hydrochloride **1**, 312
ipodate sodium,
   metformin hydrochloride **1**, 312
iron peptonized,
   demeclocycline hydrochloride, 212
   doxycycline hydrochloride, 212
   lymecycline, 212
   methacycline hydrochloride, 212
   minocycline hydrochloride, 212
   minocycline hydrochloride pellets, 212
   oxytetracycline, 212
   tetracycline, 212
isocarboxazid,
   alfentanil hydrochloride, 15
   amphetamine, 191–192
   anileridine, 15
   apraclonidine hydrochloride **1**, 388
   benzphetamine hydrochloride, 191–192
   brimonidine tartrate, ophthalmic **1**, 388
   buprenorphine hydrochloride, 15
   bupropion hydrochloride **1**, 388
   citalopram hydrobromide **1**, 144–145
   codeine, 15
   dexfenfluramine hydrochloride, 159–160
   dextroamphetamine, 159–160
   dextromethorphan hbr, 15
   diethylpropion hydrochloride, 159–160
   difenoxin hydrochloride, 15
   dihydrocodeine bitartrate, 15
   diphenoxylate hydrochloride, 15
   dopamine hydrochloride, 159–160
   entacapone **1**, 388
   ephedrine, 159–160
   etafedrine hydrochloride, 159–160
   fenfluramine hydrochloride, 159–160
   fluoxetine hydrochloride, 144–145
   fluvoxamine maleate, 144–145
   hydrocodone bitartrate, 15
   hydromorphone hydrochloride, 15
   indoramin **1**, 388
   isometheptene, 159–160
   levodopa, 157–158
   levorphanol tartrate, 15
   mazindol, 159–160
   meperidine hydrochloride, 15
   mephentermine sulfate, 159–160
   meptazinol, 15
   metaraminol bitartrate, 159–160
   methamphetamine hydrochloride, 159–160
   methylphenidate hydrochloride, 159–160
   nalbuphine hydrochloride, 15
   naphazoline hydrochloride, 159–160
   nefazodone hydrochloride **1**, 388
   opium, 15
   oxycodone, 15
   oxymetazoline hydrochloride, 159–160
   oxymorphone hydrochloride, 15
   paroxetine hydrochloride, 144–145
   phendimetrazine tartrate, 159–160
   phenmetrazine hydrochloride, 159–160
   phenoperidine hydrochloride, 15
   phentermine hydrochloride, 159–160
   phenylephrine, 159–160
   phenylpropanolamine, 159–160
   pseudoephedrine, 159–160
   rizatriptan benzoate **1**, 388
   sertraline hydrochloride, 144–145
   sibutramine hydrochloride monohyd **1**, 388
   sufentanil citrate, 15
   sumatriptan, nasal **1**, 388
   sumatriptan succinate **1**, 388
   sumatriptan succinate, oral **1**, 388
   tetrahydrozoline hydrochloride, 159–160
   tolcapone **1**, 388
   venlafaxine hydrochloride, 144–145
   xylometazoline hydrochloride, 159–160
   zolmitriptan **1**, 388
isoconazole nitrate,
   fosphenytoin sodium, injectable, 121–122
   lovastatin **1**, 388
   mizolastine **1**, 388
   phenytoin, 121–122
   simvastatin **1**, 388
isoetharine,
   chloroform, 28
   enflurane, 28
   halothane, 28

# Index

isoflurane,
  methoxyflurane, 28
  metoprolol tartrate, 267
  timolol maleate, oral, 267
isoflurane,
  amikacin sulfate, 27
  epinephrine, 28
  gentamicin sulfate, 27
  kanamycin sulfate, injectable, 27
  kanamycin sulfate, oral, 27
  streptomycin sulfate, 27
  succinylcholine chloride **2**, 37
  tobramycin, 27
isometheptene,
  chloroform, 28
  enflurane, 28
  furazolidone, 159–160
  halothane, 28
  isocarboxazid, 159–160
  linezolid, 159–160
  moclobemide, 159–160
  pargyline hydrochloride, 159–160
  phenelzine sulfate, 159–160
  procarbazine hydrochloride, 159–160
  tranylcypromine sulfate, 159–160
isoniazid,
  acetaminophen **3**, 2
  aluminum hydroxide **3**, 195
  carbamazepine **2**, 106
  chlorzoxazone **3**, 195
  diazepam **3**, 241
  disulfiram **3**, 195
  enflurane **3**, 26
  ethosuximide **3**, 111–112
  insulin **3**, 177
  meperidine hydrochloride **3**, 196
  phenytoin **2**, 124
  prednisolone **3**, 196
  propranolol hydrochloride **3**, 196
  pyridoxine hydrochloride **3**, 196–197
  rifampin **2**, 197
  stavudine **3**, 197
  theophylline **3**, 348
  valproic acid **3**, 135
  warfarin **3**, 89–90
isopropamide iodide,
  digoxin, 287
isoproterenol,
  aminophylline **3**, 338
  chloroform, 28
  enflurane, 28
  epinephrine, 28
  ether, 28
  flecainide acetate **2**, 53
  halothane, 28
  methoxyflurane, 28
isosorbide dinitrate,
  sildenafil citrate **1**, 388
isosorbide dinitrate, sublingual,
  disopyramide phosphate **2**, 49–50

  sildenafil citrate **1**, 388
isosorbide mononitrate,
  sildenafil citrate **1**, 388
isotretinoin,
  carbamazepine **3**, 106
itraconazole,
  cyclosporine, 199–200
  fosphenytoin sodium, injectable, 121–122
  phenytoin, 121–122
  simvastatin **1**, 388
  terfenadine, 201–202
itraconazole, oral,
  alprazolam **1**, 388
  astemizole **1**, 388
  atorvastatin calcium **1**, 388
  buspirone hydrochloride **3**, 197–198
  cisapride **1**, 388
  cyclosporine, 199–200
  didanosine **2**, 198
  digoxin **2**, 283–284
  felodipine **3**, 51–52
  fosphenytoin sodium, injectable, 121–122
  haloperidol **3**, 244
  lovastatin **1**, 388
  phenytoin, 121–122
  pimozide **1**, 388
  quinidine **1**, 388
  sertindole **1**, 388
  simvastatin **1**, 388
  terfenadine, 201–202
  triazolam **1**, 388
ivermectin,
  acenocoumarol **3**, 70

# K

kanamycin sulfate, injectable,
  alcuronium chloride, 41
  ampicillin sodium, 192
  atracurium besylate, 41
  benethamine penicillin, 192
  bumetanide, 198
  bumetanide, injectable, 198
  carbenicillin disodium, 192
  cefprozil, 192
  ceftibuten dihyrate, 192
  cefuroxime, 192
  cephalexin, 192
  cephalothin sodium, 192
  doxacurium chloride, 41
  enflurane, 27
  ethacrynic acid, 198
  ethacrynic acid, injectable, 198
  ether, 27
  furosemide, 198
  furosemide, injectable, 198
  gallamine triethiodide, 41
  halothane, 27
  isoflurane, 27

# Index

methoxyflurane, 27
metocurine iodide, 41
mivacurium chloride, 41
moxalactam disodium, 192
nitrous oxide, 27
pancuronium bromide, 41
penicillin G, 192
penicillin G benzathine, 192
penicillin G procaine, 192
penicillin V, 192
pipecuronium bromide, 41
piretanide, 198
rapacuronium bromide, 41
rocuronium bromide, 41
succinylcholine chloride, 41
temocillin sodium, 192
ticarcillin disodium, 192
torsemide, injectable, 198
torsemide, oral, 198
tubocurarine chloride, 41
vecuronium bromide, 41
kanamycin sulfate, oral,
  alcuronium chloride, 41
  ampicillin sodium, 192
  atracurium besylate, 41
  benethamine penicillin, 192
  bumetanide, 198
  bumetanide, injectable, 198
  carbenicillin disodium, 192
  cefprozil, 192
  ceftibuten dihyrate, 192
  cefuroxime, 192
  cephalexin, 192
  cephalothin sodium, 192
  doxacurium chloride, 41
  enflurane, 27
  ethacrynic acid **1**, 198
  ethacrynic acid, injectable, 198
  ether, 27
  furosemide, 198
  furosemide, injectable, 198
  gallamine triethiodide, 41
  halothane, 27
  isoflurane, 27
  methoxyflurane, 27
  metocurine iodide, 41
  mivacurium chloride, 41
  moxalactam disodium, 192
  nitrous oxide, 27
  pancuronium bromide, 41
  penicillin G, 192
  penicillin G benzathine, 192
  penicillin G procaine, 192
  penicillin V, 192
  pipecuronium bromide, 41
  piretanide, 198
  rapacuronium bromide, 41
  rocuronium bromide, 41
  succinylcholine chloride, 41
  temocillin sodium, 192
  ticarcillin disodium, 192
  torsemide, injectable, 198
  torsemide, oral, 198
  tubocurarine chloride, 41
  vecuronium bromide, 41
kaolin,
  attapulgite, 211–212
  chloroquine **3**, 185
  demeclocycline hydrochloride, 211–212
  digoxin **2**, 284
  doxycycline hydrochloride, 211–212
  lincomycin hydrochloride **1**, 202
  lymecycline, 211–212
  methacycline hydrochloride, 211–212
  minocycline hydrochloride, 211–212
  minocycline hydrochloride pellets, 211–212
  oxytetracycline, 211–212
  tetracycline, 211–212
kava,
  alprazolam **3**, 231
ketamine hydrochloride,
  aminophylline **3**, 338
  diazepam **2**, 29
  halothane **2**, 29
  thyroid strong **3**, 30
  tubocurarine chloride **2**, 41
ketoconazole, oral,
  alcohol, ethyl–oral/injectable **3**, 319
  alprazolam **1**, 388
  aluminum hydroxide **2**, 198–199
  astemizole, 201–202
  carbamazepine **3**, 106–107
  chlordiazepoxide **3**, 258
  cimetidine, oral **2**, 199
  cisapride **1**, 388
  cyclosporine **1**, 199–200
  dofetilide **1**, 388
  fosphenytoin sodium, injectable, 121–122
  indinavir sulfate **1**, 388
  lovastatin **1**, 388
  magnesium hydroxide **2**, 198–199
  methylprednisolone **2**, 200
  mizolastine **1**, 388
  omeprazole **2**, 200
  phenytoin, 121–122
  quinidine **2**, 63–64
  rifampin **2**, 200–201
  sertindole **1**, 388
  simvastatin **1**, 388
  sirolimus **1**, 388
  sucralfate **3**, 201
  terfenadine **1**, 201–202
  theophylline **3**, 349
  toremifene **1**, 388
  triazolam **1**, 388
ketoprofen,
  ketorolac tromethamine **1**, 388
  ketorolac tromethamine, injectable

# Index

**1**, 388
methotrexate **2**, 223–224
ketorolac tromethamine,
  acemetacin **1**, 388
  aloxiprin **1**, 388
  aspirin **1**, 388
  calcium carbaspirin **1**, 388
  diclofenac **1**, 388
  etodolac **1**, 388
  fenbufen **1**, 388
  fenoprofen calcium **1**, 388
  flurbiprofen **1**, 388
  ibuprofen **1**, 388
  indomethacin **1**, 388
  indomethacin sodium trihyd,
    injectable **1**, 388
  ketoprofen **1**, 388
  meclofenamate sodium **1**, 388
  mefenamic acid **1**, 388
  nabumetone **1**, 388
  naproxen **1**, 388
  oxaprozin **1**, 388
  oxyphenbutazone **1**, 388
  phenylbutazone **1**, 388
  piroxicam **1**, 388
  probenecid **1**, 388
  sulindac **1**, 388
  tiaprofenic acid **1**, 388
  tolfenamic acid **1**, 388
  tolmetin sodium **1**, 388
ketorolac tromethamine, injectable,
  acemetacin **1**, 388
  aloxiprin **1**, 388
  aspirin **1**, 388
  diclofenac **1**, 388
  etodolac **1**, 388
  fenbufen **1**, 388
  fenoprofen calcium **1**, 388
  flurbiprofen **1**, 388
  ibuprofen **1**, 388
  indomethacin **1**, 388
  indomethacin sodium trihyd,
    injectable **1**, 388
  ketoprofen **1**, 388
  meclofenamate sodium **1**, 388
  mefenamic acid **1**, 388
  nabumetone **1**, 388
  naproxen **1**, 388
  oxaprozin **1**, 388
  oxyphenbutazone **1**, 388
  phenylbutazone **1**, 388
  piroxicam **1**, 388
  probenecid **1**, 388
  sulindac **1**, 388
  tiaprofenic acid **1**, 388
  tolfenamic acid **1**, 388
  tolmetin sodium **1**, 388
khat,
  ampicillin sodium **3**, 180
kyushin,
  digoxin **3**, 284

## L

labetalol hydrochloride,
  arbutamine hydrochloride **1**, 388
  cimetidine, oral, 266
  cimetidine hydrochloride,
    injectable, 266
  glutethimide **3**, 261
  halothane **2**, 261
  insulin, 311
lamotrigine,
  acetaminophen **3**, 112
  rifampin **3**, 112–113
  valproic acid **3**, 113
lercanidipine hydrochloride,
  cyclosporine, 47–48
  quinidine, 65–66
leucovorin calcium,
  methotrexate **1**, 224
  methotrexate sodium, injectable,
    224
levobunolol hydrochloride,
  ophthalmic,
  arbutamine hydrochloride **1**, 388
levodopa,
  aluminum hydroxide **3**, 368
  chlorpromazine hydrochloride **3**,
    234
  diazepam **3**, 241
  domperidone **3**, 369
  ferrous sulfate **2**, 369
  furazolidone, 157–158
  imipramine **3**, 148
  isocarboxazid, 157–158
  linezolid, 157–158
  magnesium hydroxide **3**, 368
  methyldopa **3**, 174
  metoclopramide hydrochloride **3**,
    375–376
  mirtazapine **3**, 150–151
  moclobemide, 157–158
  papaverine hydrochloride **3**,
    369–370
  pargyline hydrochloride, 157–158
  phenelzine sulfate **1**, 157–158
  phenytoin **3**, 125
  procarbazine hydrochloride,
    157–158
  pyridoxine hydrochloride **1**, 334
  tranylcypromine sulfate, 157–158
  trihexyphenidyl hydrochloride **4**,
    370
levodopa, comb w/ benserazide,
  orphenadrine citrate **3**, 369
levodopa, comb w/ carbidopa,
  domperidone **3**, 369
  linezolid, 157–158
levomethadyl acetate hydrochloride,
  naltrexone hydrochloride **1**, 388
levorphanol tartrate,
  isocarboxazid, 15
  naltrexone hydrochloride **1**, 388

# Index

pargyline hydrochloride, 15
phenelzine sulfate, 15
selegiline hydrochloride, 15
tranylcypromine sulfate, 15
levothyroxine sodium,
  acenocoumarol, 100
  aminophylline **3**, 338
  anisindione, 100
  calcium carbonate, oral **3**, 370
  chloroquine **3**, 185
  coumarin, 100
  dicumarol, 100
  ferrous sulfate **3**, 370–371
  lovastatin **3**, 371
  phenytoin **3**, 125
  sucralfate **3**, 371
  warfarin, 100
lidocaine hydrochloride,
local–injectable,
  arbutamine hydrochloride **1**, 388
  cimetidine, oral, 54
  cimetidine hydrochloride,
    injectable, 54
  grepafloxacin hydrochloride **1**, 388
lidocaine hydrochloride, systemic,
  amiodarone hydrochloride **2**,
    46–47
  amprenavir **1**, 388
  arbutamine hydrochloride **1**, 388
  cimetidine, oral **1**, 54
  cimetidine hydrochloride,
    injectable, 54
  grepafloxacin hydrochloride **1**, 388
  phenobarbital **3**, 54
  procainamide hydrochloride **3**, 55
  propranolol hydrochloride **2**, 55
  succinylcholine chloride **2**, 37–38
lincomycin hydrochloride,
  erythromycin **3**, 202
  kaolin **1**, 202
linezolid,
  dextromethorphan hbr, 15
  fluoxetine hydrochloride **1**, 388
  isometheptene, 159–160
  levodopa, 157–158
  levodopa, comb w/ carbidopa,
    157–158
  meperidine hydrochloride, 15
  mephentermine sulfate, 159–160
  methamphetamine hydrochloride,
    159–160
  methylphenidate hydrochloride,
    159–160
  phendimetrazine tartrate, 159–160
  phenmetrazine hydrochloride,
    159–160
liothyronine sodium,
  acenocoumarol, 100
  coumarin, 100
  dicumarol, 100
  imipramine **2**, 148

warfarin, 100
lithium,
  acetazolamide **1**, 245–246
  acyclovir sodium, injectable **3**, 246
  alcohol, ethyl–oral/injectable **3**, 246
  bendroflumethiazide, 247
  benzthiazide, 247
  brinzolamide, ophthalmic, 245–246
  bumetanide, 247
  bumetanide, injectable, 247
  carbamazepine **2**, 246–247
  chlorothiazide **1**, 247
  chlorpromazine hydrochloride **2**,
    235
  chlorthalidone, 247
  cisplatin **3**, 247
  cyclopenthiazide, 247
  cyclothiazide, 247
  diazepam **3**, 247–248
  dichlorphenamide, 245–246
  disodium hydrogen citrate,
    245–246
  dorzolamide hydrochloride,
    245–246
  enalapril maleate **2**, 248
  ethacrynic acid, 247
  ethacrynic acid, injectable, 247
  flumethiazide, 247
  fluoxetine hydrochloride **2**, 248
  furosemide, 247
  furosemide, injectable, 247
  haloperidol **2**, 248–249
  hydrochlorothiazide, 247
  hydroflumethiazide, 247
  imipramine **3**, 148–149
  indapamide, 247
  indomethacin **2**, 249
  losartan potassium **3**, 250
  mazindol **2**, 250
  methazolamide, 245–246
  methyclothiazide, 247
  methyldopa **2**, 250
  metolazone, 247
  metoprolol tartrate **2**, 251
  metronidazole, oral/vaginal **2**, 251
  norepinephrine bitartrate **3**, 251
  pancuronium bromide **3**, 34
  phenytoin **3**, 251–252
  piretanide, 247
  polythiazide, 247
  potassium citrate, 245–246
  potassium iodide **2**, 252
  psyllium **3**, 249–250
  quinethazone, 247
  sodium acetate, 245–246
  sodium bicarbonate, 245–246
  sodium bicarbonate, injectable,
    245–246
  sodium citrate, 245–246
  sodium lactate, 245–246
  tetracycline **2**, 252

# Index

theophylline **2**, 252–253
thioridazine hydrochloride **2**, 253
torsemide, injectable, 247
torsemide, oral, 247
trichlormethiazide, 247
tromethamine, 245–246
verapamil hydrochloride **2**, 253–254
xipamide, 247
lofexidine hydrochloride,
  nebivolol hydrochloride, 167
  propranolol hydrochloride, 167
lomefloxacin hydrochloride,
  warfarin, 93
lomustine,
  theophylline **3**, 221
lorazepam,
  probenecid **3**, 254
losartan potassium,
  lithium **3**, 250
  rifampin **2**, 172–173
lovastatin,
  azithromycin, 373
  butoconazole nitrate **1**, 388
  clarithromycin, 373
  clotrimazole **1**, 388
  cyclosporine **2**, 372
  diltiazem hydrochloride **2**, 372–373
  econazole nitrate **1**, 388
  erythromycin **1**, 373
  erythromycin estolate, 373
  erythromycin ethylsuccinate, 373
  erythromycin glucepate, 373
  erythromycin lactobionate, 373
  erythromycin stearate, 373
  fenticonazole nitrate **1**, 388
  fluconazole **1**, 388
  gemfibrozil **2**, 373–374
  grapefruit juice **1**, 374
  isoconazole nitrate **1**, 388
  itraconazole, oral **1**, 388
  ketoconazole, oral **1**, 388
  levothyroxine sodium **3**, 371
  mibefradil dihydrochloride **1**, 388
  miconazole nitrate **1**, 388
  niacin, vitamin B3 **2**, 374
  oxiconazole nitrate **1**, 388
  terconazole **1**, 388
  tioconazole **1**, 388
  warfarin **2**, 90
loxapine,
  guanethidine, 169
  sumatriptan succinate, injectable **3**, 254
lymecycline,
  alcuronium chloride, 41
  attapulgite, 211–212
  calcium lactobionate, oral, 211–212
  carbonyl iron, 212
  deferiprone, 212
  digoxin, 289
  digoxin capsule, stabilized, 289
  doxacurium chloride, 41
  ferric ammonium citrate, 212
  ferrous citrate, 212
  ferrous fumarate, 212
  ferrous gluconate, 212
  ferrous glycine sulfate, 212
  ferrous hydroxide polymaltose, 212
  ferrous ions, salt unspecified, 212
  ferrous succinate, 212
  ferrous sulfate, 212
  gallamine triethiodide, 41
  iron peptonized, 212
  kaolin, 211–212
  magaldrate, 211–212
  metocurine iodide, 41
  minocycline hydrochloride pellets, 289
  mivacurium chloride, 41
  pancuronium bromide, 41
  pipecuronium bromide, 41
  rapacuronium bromide, 41
  rocuronium bromide, 41
  succinylcholine chloride, 41
  tubocurarine chloride, 41
  vecuronium bromide, 41

## M

magaldrate,
  demeclocycline hydrochloride, 211–212
  doxycycline hydrochloride, 211–212
  lymecycline, 211–212
  methacycline hydrochloride, 211–212
  minocycline hydrochloride, 211–212
  minocycline hydrochloride pellets, 211–212
  oxytetracycline, 211–212
  tetracycline, 211–212
  ticlopidine hydrochloride **3**, 74–75
magnesium, salt unspecified,
  tetracycline, 211–212
magnesium aspartate,
  tetracycline, 211–212
magnesium carbonate,
  captopril **3**, 163
  demeclocycline hydrochloride, 211–212
  doxycycline hydrochloride, 211–212
  ferrous sulfate **3**, 329
  methacycline hydrochloride, 211–212
  oxytetracycline, 211–212
  tetracycline, 211–212
magnesium chloride, oral,
  demeclocycline hydrochloride, 211–212
  doxycycline hydrochloride, 211–212
  methacycline hydrochloride, 211–212

# Index

oxytetracycline, 211–212
tetracycline, 211–212
magnesium citrate,
   tetracycline, 211–212
magnesium glucoheptonate,
   tetracycline, 211–212
magnesium gluconate,
   tetracycline, 211–212
magnesium hydroxide,
   aspirin **2**, 7
   captopril **3**, 163
   chlorpromazine hydrochloride **3**, 232–233
   cimetidine, oral **3**, 358
   ciprofloxacin hydrochloride **2**, 186
   clorazepate dipotassium **3**, 236
   demeclocycline hydrochloride, 211–212
   digoxin **2**, 276–277
   doxycycline hydrochloride, 211–212
   ferrous sulfate **3**, 329
   ketoconazole, oral **2**, 198–199
   levodopa **3**, 368
   methacycline hydrochloride, 211–212
   mexiletine hydrochloride **3**, 55
   misoprostol **3**, 376–377
   oxytetracycline, 211–212
   penicillamine **3**, 379
   sodium polystyrene sulfonate **2**, 375
   tetracycline, 211–212
   theophylline **3**, 342
   ticlopidine hydrochloride **3**, 74–75
   warfarin **4**, 90
magnesium lactate,
   tetracycline, 211–212
magnesium oxide,
   demeclocycline hydrochloride, 211–212
   doxycycline hydrochloride, 211–212
   methacycline hydrochloride, 211–212
   oxytetracycline, 211–212
   tetracycline, 211–212
magnesium salicylate,
   demeclocycline hydrochloride, 211–212
   methotrexate, 222
   methotrexate sodium, injectable, 222
magnesium sulfate,
   demeclocycline hydrochloride, 211–212
   doxycycline hydrochloride, 211–212
   methacycline hydrochloride, 211–212
   nifedipine **3**, 59
   oxytetracycline, 211–212
   tetracycline, 211–212
magnesium sulfate, injectable,
   vecuronium bromide **2**, 43
magnesium trisilicate,
   demeclocycline hydrochloride, 211–212
   digoxin **2**, 276–277
   doxycycline hydrochloride, 211–212
   methacycline hydrochloride, 211–212
   nitrofurantoin **3**, 204
   oxytetracycline, 211–212
   phenytoin **3**, 114
   tetracycline, 211–212
maprotiline hydrochloride,
   guanadrel sulfate, 169
   guanethidine, 169
marijuana,
   fluoxetine hydrochloride **2**, 144
   nortriptyline hydrochloride **2**, 152
mazindol,
   bethanidine sulphate **2**, 163
   chloroform, 28
   enflurane, 28
   furazolidone, 191–192
   halothane, 28
   isocarboxazid, 159–160
   lithium **2**, 250
   methoxyflurane, 28
   metoprolol tartrate, 267
   nebivolol hydrochloride, 267
   pargyline hydrochloride, 191–192
   phenelzine sulfate, 191–192
   procarbazine hydrochloride, 191–192
   propranolol hydrochloride, 267
   timolol maleate, ophthalmic, 267
   timolol maleate, oral, 267
   tranylcypromine sulfate, 159–160
mecillinam,
   gentamicin sulfate, 192
meclofenamate sodium,
   ketorolac tromethamine **1**, 388
   ketorolac tromethamine, injectable **1**, 388
medroxyprogesterone acetate,
   aminoglutethimide **3**, 375
mefenamic acid,
   ketorolac tromethamine **1**, 388
   ketorolac tromethamine, injectable **1**, 388
mefloquine hydrochloride,
   halofantrine hydrochloride **1**, 388
meglumine iotroxiate,
   metformin hydrochloride **1**, 312
melatonin,
   fluvoxamine maleate **3**, 145
melphalan,
   cyclosporine **2**, 221
menadiol sodium diphosphate, vitamin K4,
   acenocoumarol, 95
   anisindione, 95

# Index

coumarin, 95
dicumarol, 95
phenindione, 95
warfarin, 95
menadione,
  acenocoumarol, 95
  anisindione, 95
  coumarin, 95
  dicumarol, 95
  phenindione, 95
  warfarin, 95
mepenzolate bromide,
  digoxin, 287
meperidine hydrochloride,
  chlorpromazine hydrochloride **2**, 15
  furazolidone, 15
  isocarboxazid, 15
  isoniazid **3**, 196
  linezolid, 15
  moclobemide, 15
  naltrexone hydrochloride **1**, 388
  pargyline hydrochloride, 15
  phenelzine sulfate **1**, 15
  phenobarbital **3**, 15–16
  phenytoin **3**, 16
  procarbazine hydrochloride, 15
  ritonavir **1**, 388
  selegiline hydrochloride, 15
  tranylcypromine sulfate, 15
mephentermine sulfate,
  chloroform, 28
  enflurane, 28
  furazolidone, 191–192
  halothane, 28
  isocarboxazid, 159–160
  linezolid, 159–160
  methoxyflurane, 28
  moclobemide, 159–160
  pargyline hydrochloride, 159–160
  phenelzine sulfate, 159–160
  procarbazine hydrochloride, 159–160
  tranylcypromine sulfate, 159–160
mephenytoin,
  cimetidine, oral, 117–118
  cimetidine hydrochloride, injectable, 117–118
  disulfiram, 120
  fluconazole, 121–122
  ranitidine hydrochloride, injectable, 117–118
  ranitidine hydrochloride, oral, 117–118
mephobarbital,
  acenocoumarol, 94
  coumarin, 94
  dicumarol, 94
  warfarin, 94
meprobamate,
  alcohol, ethyl–oral/injectable **2**, 321

imipramine **3**, 321–322
warfarin **3**, 90–91
meptazinol,
  isocarboxazid, 15
  naltrexone hydrochloride **1**, 388
  pargyline hydrochloride, 15
  phenelzine sulfate, 15
  selegiline hydrochloride, 15
  tranylcypromine sulfate, 15
mequitazine,
  guanethidine, 169
mercaptopurine,
  allopurinol **1**, 221–222
mesalamine, oral,
  digoxin **3**, 277
  rifampin **4**, 207–208
mesoridazine besylate,
  cabergoline **1**, 388
  cisapride **1**, 388
  grepafloxacin hydrochloride **1**, 388
  guanethidine, 169
  halofantrine hydrochloride **1**, 388
  pergolide mesylate **1**, 388
  pimozide **1**, 388
mestranol,
  rifampin, 209
metaproterenol sulfate,
  chloroform, 28
  enflurane, 28
  halothane, 28
  methoxyflurane, 28
  metoprolol tartrate, 267
  timolol maleate, oral, 267
metaraminol bitartrate,
  chloroform, 28
  enflurane, 28
  furazolidone, 159–160
  halothane, 28
  isocarboxazid, 159–160
  methoxyflurane, 28
  metoprolol tartrate, 267
  nebivolol hydrochloride, 267
  pargyline hydrochloride, 159–160
  phenelzine sulfate, 159–160
  procarbazine hydrochloride, 159–160
  propranolol hydrochloride, 267
  timolol maleate, ophthalmic, 267
  timolol maleate, oral, 267
  tranylcypromine sulfate, 159–160
metformin hydrochloride,
  calcium iodate **1**, 312
  diatrizoate meglumine **1**, 312
  diatrizoate sodium **1**, 312
  dofetilide **2**, 388
  iocetamic acid **1**, 312
  iodamide **1**, 312
  iodipamide meglumine **1**, 312
  iodoquinol **1**, 312
  iodoxamine meglumine **1**, 312
  iopamidol **1**, 312

# Index

iopanoic acid **1**, 312
iopodic acid **1**, 312
iopydol **1**, 312
iopydone **1**, 312
iothalamate meglumine **1**, 312
iothalamate sodium **1**, 312
iotrolan **1**, 312
ioversol **1**, 312
ioxaglate meglumine **1**, 312
ioxaglate sodium **1**, 312
ipodate calcium **1**, 312
ipodate sodium **1**, 312
meglumine iotroxiate **1**, 312
metrizamide **1**, 312
propyliodine **1**, 312
radioactive iodine–131 **1**, 312
tyropanoate sodium **1**, 312
methacycline hydrochloride,
  alcuronium chloride, 41
  aluminum carbonate, basic, 211–212
  aluminum hydroxide, 211–212
  aluminum oxide, 211–212
  aluminum phosphate, 211–212
  attapulgite, 211–212
  bismuth subsalicylate, 211–212
  calcium, oral salt unspecified, 211–212
  calcium acetate, 211–212
  calcium ascorbate, 211–212
  calcium carbonate, oral, 211–212
  calcium chloride, oral, 211–212
  calcium citrate, oral, 211–212
  calcium glubionate, oral, 211–212
  calcium glucoheptonate, 211–212
  calcium gluconate, oral, 211–212
  calcium glycerophosphate, oral, 211–212
  calcium iodate, 211–212
  calcium lactate, oral, 211–212
  calcium lactate gluconate, 211–212
  calcium lactobionate, oral, 211–212
  calcium phosphate, oral, 211–212
  carbonyl iron, 212
  digoxin, 289
  digoxin capsule, stabilized, 289
  dihydroxyaluminum, 211–212
  doxacurium chloride, 41
  ferric ammonium citrate, 212
  ferrous citrate, 212
  ferrous fumarate, 212
  ferrous gluconate, 212
  ferrous glycine sulfate, 212
  ferrous hydroxide polymaltose, 212
  ferrous ions, salt unspecified, 212
  ferrous succinate, 212
  ferrous sulfate, 212
  gallamine triethiodide, 41
  iron peptonized, 212
  kaolin, 211–212
  magaldrate, 211–212
  magnesium carbonate, 211–212
  magnesium chloride, oral, 211–212
  magnesium hydroxide, 211–212
  magnesium oxide, 211–212
  magnesium sulfate, 211–212
  magnesium trisilicate, 211–212
  metocurine iodide, 41
  mivacurium chloride, 41
  pancuronium bromide, 41
  pipecuronium bromide, 41
  rapacuronium bromide, 41
  rocuronium bromide, 41
  succinylcholine chloride, 41
  sucralfate, 211–212
  tubocurarine chloride, 41
  vecuronium bromide, 41
methadone hydrochloride,
  ammonium chloride **3**, 16
  diazepam **3**, 16–17
  didanosine **3**, 17
  naltrexone hydrochloride **1**, 388
  nevirapine **2**, 17
  rifampin **2**, 18
methamphetamine hydrochloride,
  chloroform, 28
  enflurane, 28
  furazolidone, 191–192
  halothane, 28
  isocarboxazid, 159–160
  linezolid, 159–160
  methoxyflurane, 28
  moclobemide, 159–160
  pargyline hydrochloride, 159–160
  phenelzine sulfate, 159–160
  procarbazine hydrochloride, 159–160
  tranylcypromine sulfate, 159–160
methandrostenolone,
  acenocoumarol, 91
  coumarin, 91
  dicumarol, 91
  oxyphenbutazone **3**, 20–21
  phenindione, 91
  warfarin, 91
methantheline bromide,
  digoxin, 287
metharbital,
  acenocoumarol, 94
  coumarin, 94
  dicumarol, 94
  warfarin, 94
methazolamide,
  lithium, 245–246
methdilazine,
  cabergoline **1**, 388
  cisapride **1**, 388
  grepafloxacin hydrochloride **1**, 388
  guanethidine, 169
  halofantrine hydrochloride **1**, 388
  pergolide mesylate **1**, 388
  pimozide **1**, 388

# Index

methenamine,
  sulfacytine **1**, 388
  sulfadiazine **1**, 388
  sulfadoxine **1**, 388
  sulfamerazine **1**, 388
  sulfamethazine **1**, 388
  sulfamethoxazole **1**, 388
  sulfapyridine **1**, 388
  sulfasalazine **1**, 388
  sulfisoxazole **1**, 388
methicillin sodium,
  amikacin sulfate, 192
  gentamicin sulfate, 192
  neomycin sulfate, oral, 192
  netilmicin, 192
  tobramycin, 192
methimazole,
  theophylline **3**, 349
methohexital sodium,
  acenocoumarol, 94
  coumarin, 94
  dicumarol, 94
  warfarin, 94
methotrexate,
  alcohol, ethyl–oral/injectable **3**, 222
  aloxiprin, 222
  asparaginase, e. coli derived **1**, 388
  aspirin **1**, 222
  azapropazone dihydrate **1**, 388
  calcium carbaspirin, 222
  choline salicylate, 222
  cisplatin **2**, 222–223
  cyclophosphamide **3**, 218–219
  cytarabine **3**, 223
  diflunisal, 222
  etretinate **2**, 223
  hydrochlorothiazide **3**, 218
  ketoprofen **2**, 223–224
  leucovorin calcium **1**, 224
  magnesium salicylate, 222
  neomycin sulfate, oral **2**, 224
  phenytoin **2**, 116
  piperacillin sodium **2**, 225
  probenecid **1**, 225
  procarbazine hydrochloride **2**, 226
  proguanil hydrochloride, 226
  salicylamide, 222
  salsalate, 222
  sodium bicarbonate **3**, 226
  sodium salicylate, 222
  sodium thiosalicylate, 222
  sulfacytine, 226
  sulfadiazine, 226
  sulfadoxine, 226
  sulfamerazine, 226
  sulfamethazine, 226
  sulfamethizole, 226
  sulfamethoxazole **1**, 226
  sulfapyridine, 226
  sulfasalazine, 226
  sulfisoxazole, 226
  trimethoprim **1**, 226
  zonisamide, 226
methotrexate sodium, injectable,
  aloxiprin, 222
  asparaginase, e. coli derived **1**, 388
  aspirin, 222
  azapropazone dihydrate **1**, 388
  calcium carbaspirin, 222
  choline salicylate, 222
  cytarabine **3**, 223
  diflunisal, 222
  leucovorin calcium, 224
  magnesium salicylate, 222
  omeprazole **2**, 225
  piperacillin sodium **2**, 225
  probenecid, 225
  proguanil hydrochloride, 226
  salicylamide, 222
  salsalate, 222
  sodium salicylate, 222
  sodium thiosalicylate, 222
  sulfacytine, 226
  sulfadiazine, 226
  sulfadoxine, 226
  sulfamerazine, 226
  sulfamethazine, 226
  sulfamethizole, 226
  sulfamethoxazole, 226
  sulfapyridine, 226
  sulfasalazine, 226
  sulfisoxazole, 226
  trimethoprim, 226
  zonisamide, 226
methotrimeprazine,
  guanethidine, 169
methoxamine hydrochloride,
  chloroform, 28
  enflurane, 28
  halothane, 28
  methoxyflurane, 28
  metoprolol tartrate, 267
  nebivolol hydrochloride, 267
  propranolol hydrochloride, 267
  timolol maleate, ophthalmic, 267
  timolol maleate, oral, 267
methoxsalen,
  caffeine **3**, 340
  phenytoin **2**, 125
methoxyflurane,
  albuterol sulfate, 28
  amikacin sulfate, 27
  amphetamine, 28
  arbutamine hydrochloride, 28
  bacitracin, 27
  benzphetamine hydrochloride, 28
  bitolterol mesylate, 28
  clindamycin, 27
  clindamycin phosphate, injectable, 27

# Index

colistin sulfate, 27
dexfenfluramine hydrochloride, 28
dextroamphetamine, 28
diethylpropion hydrochloride, 28
dobutamine hydrochloride, 28
dopamine hydrochloride, 28
ephedrine, 28
epinephrine, 28
etafedrine hydrochloride, 28
ethylnorepinephrine hydrochloride, 28
fenfluramine hydrochloride, 28
fenoterol hydrobromide, 28
formoterol fumarate, inhl, 28
gentamicin sulfate, 27
isoetharine, 28
isoproterenol, 28
kanamycin sulfate, injectable, 27
kanamycin sulfate, oral, 27
mazindol, 28
mephentermine sulfate, 28
metaproterenol sulfate, 28
metaraminol bitartrate, 28
methamphetamine hydrochloride, 28
methoxamine hydrochloride, 28
methylphenidate hydrochloride, 28
neomycin sulfate, injectable, 27
neomycin sulfate, oral, 27
norepinephrine bitartrate, 28
phendimetrazine tartrate, 28
phenmetrazine hydrochloride, 28
phentermine hydrochloride, 28
phenylephrine, 28
phenylpropanolamine, 28
pirbuterol acetate, 28
polymyxin B sulfate, 27
polymyxin B sulfate, vaccine use, 27
procaterol hydrochloride, 28
pseudoephedrine, 28
rimiterol hydrobromide, 28
salmeterol xinafoate, 28
secobarbital **2**, 30
streptomycin sulfate, 27
terbutaline sulfate, 28
tetracycline **2**, 30
tobramycin, 27
methscopolamine bromide,
 digoxin, 287
methscopolamine nitrate,
 digoxin, 287
methyclothiazide,
 lithium, 247
methyldopa,
 amitriptyline hydrochloride **3**, 173
 digoxin **3**, 284–285
 ferrous sulfate **2**, 173
 haloperidol **3**, 174
 levodopa **3**, 174
 lithium **2**, 250
 norepinephrine bitartrate **2**, 174
 pargyline hydrochloride **3**, 153–154
 phenobarbital **4**, 175
 phenoxybenzamine hydrochloride **3**, 175
 propranolol hydrochloride **2**, 175
 tolbutamide **3**, 314
methylergonovine maleate,
 efavirenz **1**, 388
 indinavir sulfate **1**, 388
 rizatriptan benzoate **1**, 388
 saquinavir **1**, 388
 sumatriptan, nasal **1**, 388
 sumatriptan succinate **1**, 388
 sumatriptan succinate, injectable **1**, 388
 sumatriptan succinate, oral **1**, 388
 zolmitriptan **1**, 388
methylphenidate hydrochloride,
 carbamazepine **3**, 107
 chloroform, 28
 dicumarol **3**, 71–72
 enflurane, 28
 furazolidone, 191–192
 halothane, 28
 isocarboxazid, 159–160
 linezolid, 159–160
 methoxyflurane, 28
 moclobemide, 159–160
 pargyline hydrochloride, 159–160
 phenelzine sulfate, 159–160
 phenytoin **3**, 125–126
 procarbazine hydrochloride, 159–160
 tranylcypromine sulfate, 159–160
 valproic acid **3**, 135
methylprednisolone,
 aspirin **2**, 9
 ketoconazole, oral **2**, 200
 pyridostigmine **3**, 381
 troleandomycin **2**, 213–214
methyltestosterone,
 acenocoumarol, 91
 anisindione, 91
 coumarin, 91
 cyclosporine **2**, 362
 dicumarol, 91
 imipramine **3**, 149
 warfarin **1**, 91
methyprylon,
 acenocoumarol, 87
 coumarin, 87
 dicumarol, 87
 warfarin, 87
methysergide maleate,
 efavirenz **1**, 388
 indinavir sulfate **1**, 388
 rizatriptan benzoate **1**, 388
 saquinavir **1**, 388
 sumatriptan, nasal **1**, 388
 sumatriptan succinate **1**, 388

# Index

sumatriptan succinate, injectable **1**, 388
sumatriptan succinate, oral **1**, 388
zolmitriptan **1**, 388
metipranolol hydrochloride, ophthalmic,
  arbutamine hydrochloride **1**, 388
metoclopramide hydrochloride,
  alcohol, ethyl–oral/injectable **3**, 319
  atropine **3**, 375
  carbamazepine **3**, 107
  chlorothiazide **3**, 293
  cimetidine, oral **3**, 359
  cyclosporine **2**, 362–363
  digoxin **2**, 285
  levodopa **3**, 375–376
  mexiletine hydrochloride **3**, 56
  morphine **3**, 19–20
  quinidine **3**, 64
  succinylcholine chloride **3**, 38
metocurine iodide,
  amikacin sulfate, 41
  bacitracin, 41
  colistin sulfate, 41
  demeclocycline hydrochloride, 41
  doxycycline hydrochloride, 41
  doxycycline hyclate, injectable, 41
  gentamicin sulfate, 41
  kanamycin sulfate, injectable, 41
  kanamycin sulfate, oral, 41
  lymecycline, 41
  methacycline hydrochloride, 41
  minocycline, injectable, 41
  minocycline hydrochloride, 41
  minocycline hydrochloride pellets, 41
  neomycin sulfate, injectable, 41
  neomycin sulfate, oral, 41
  netilmicin, 41
  oxytetracycline, 41
  oxytetracycline, injectable, 41
  paromomycin sulfate, 41
  phenytoin **2**, 31
  polymyxin B sulfate, 41
  polymyxin B sulfate, vaccine use, 41
  rolitetracycline, injectable, 41
  streptomycin sulfate, 41
  tetracycline, 41
  tetracycline hydrochloride, injectable, 41
  tobramycin, 41
metolazone,
  lithium, 247
metoprolol tartrate,
  amiodarone hydrochloride **2**, 262
  arbutamine hydrochloride **1**, 388
  bitolterol mesylate, 267
  cimetidine, oral, 266
  cimetidine hydrochloride, injectable, 266
  clonidine hydrochloride, 167
  clonidine hydrochloride, transdermal, 167
  dexfenfluramine hydrochloride, 267
  dopamine hydrochloride, 267
  etafedrine hydrochloride, 267
  ethylnorepinephrine hydrochloride, 267
  fenoterol hydrobromide, 267
  formoterol fumarate, inhl, 267
  hormonal contraceptive **3**, 262
  isoetharine, 267
  lithium **2**, 251
  mazindol, 267
  metaproterenol sulfate, 267
  metaraminol bitartrate, 267
  methoxamine hydrochloride, 267
  pentobarbital sodium **2**, 262–263
  pirbuterol acetate, 267
  procaterol hydrochloride, 267
  rifampin **2**, 263
  rimiterol hydrobromide, 267
  salmeterol xinafoate, 267
  terbutaline sulfate, 267
metrizamide,
  metformin hydrochloride **1**, 312
metronidazole, injectable,
  astemizole **1**, 388
  cimetidine, oral **3**, 203
  cyclosporine **3**, 376
  fluorouracil **2**, 220
metronidazole, oral/vaginal,
  alcohol, ethyl–oral/injectable **2**, 319–320
  astemizole **1**, 388
  carbamazepine **2**, 107–108
  chloroquine **2**, 202–203
  cyclosporine **3**, 376
  disulfiram **2**, 203
  fluorouracil **2**, 220
  lithium **2**, 251
  phenobarbital **2**, 203–204
  phenytoin **3**, 126
  tacrolimus **3**, 384–385
  warfarin **2**, 91–92
metyrapone,
  phenytoin **3**, 376
mexiletine hydrochloride,
  aluminum hydroxide **3**, 55
  ammonium chloride **3**, 56
  atropine **3**, 56
  digoxin **4**, 285
  grepafloxacin hydrochloride **1**, 388
  magnesium hydroxide **3**, 55
  metoclopramide hydrochloride **3**, 56
  phenytoin **3**, 56–57
  rifampin **3**, 57
  theophylline **2**, 349–350
  tobacco **3**, 57
mezlocillin sodium,

# Index

amikacin sulfate, 192
gentamicin sulfate, 192
netilmicin, 192
tobramycin, 192
mibefradil dihydrochloride,
  astemizole **1**, 388
  cisapride **1**, 388
  lovastatin **1**, 388
  simvastatin **1**, 388
  terfenadine **1**, 388
miconazole nitrate,
  astemizole **1**, 388
  cisapride **1**, 388
  cyclosporine, 199–200
  fosphenytoin sodium, injectable, 121–122
  lovastatin **1**, 388
  mizolastine **1**, 388
  phenytoin, 121–122
  simvastatin **1**, 388
  tobramycin **3**, 213
midazolam hydrochloride,
  amprenavir **1**, 388
  efavirenz **1**, 388
  erythromycin **2**, 254–255
  indinavir sulfate **1**, 388
  nelfinavir mesylate **1**, 388
  ritonavir **1**, 388
  saquinavir **1**, 388
  thiopental sodium **3**, 255
miglitol,
  amylase **1**, 388
  charcoal **1**, 388
  pancreatin **1**, 388
minocycline, injectable,
  alcuronium chloride, 41
  digoxin, 289
  digoxin capsule, stabilized, 289
  doxacurium chloride, 41
  gallamine triethiodide, 41
  metocurine iodide, 41
  mivacurium chloride, 41
  pancuronium bromide, 41
  pipecuronium bromide, 41
  rapacuronium bromide, 41
  rocuronium bromide, 41
  succinylcholine chloride, 41
  tubocurarine chloride, 41
  vecuronium bromide, 41
minocycline hydrochloride,
  alcuronium chloride, 41
  attapulgite, 211–212
  calcium lactobionate, oral, 211–212
  carbonyl iron, 212
  digoxin, 289
  digoxin capsule, stabilized, 289
  doxacurium chloride, 41
  ferric ammonium citrate, 212
  ferrous citrate, 212
  ferrous fumarate, 212
  ferrous gluconate, 212
  ferrous glycine sulfate, 212
  ferrous hydroxide polymaltose, 212
  ferrous ions, salt unspecified, 212
  ferrous succinate, 212
  ferrous sulfate, 212
  gallamine triethiodide, 41
  iron peptonized, 212
  kaolin, 211–212
  magaldrate, 211–212
  metocurine iodide, 41
  mivacurium chloride, 41
  pancuronium bromide, 41
  pipecuronium bromide, 41
  rapacuronium bromide, 41
  rocuronium bromide, 41
  succinylcholine chloride, 41
  tubocurarine chloride, 41
  vecuronium bromide, 41
minocycline hydrochloride pellets,
  alcuronium chloride, 41
  attapulgite, 211–212
  calcium lactobionate, oral, 211–212
  carbonyl iron, 212
  digoxin, 289
  doxacurium chloride, 41
  ferric ammonium citrate, 212
  ferrous citrate, 212
  ferrous fumarate, 212
  ferrous gluconate, 212
  ferrous glycine sulfate, 212
  ferrous hydroxide polymaltose, 212
  ferrous ions, salt unspecified, 212
  ferrous succinate, 212
  ferrous sulfate, 212
  gallamine triethiodide, 41
  iron peptonized, 212
  kaolin, 211–212
  lymecycline, 289
  magaldrate, 211–212
  metocurine iodide, 41
  mivacurium chloride, 41
  pancuronium bromide, 41
  pipecuronium bromide, 41
  rapacuronium bromide, 41
  rocuronium bromide, 41
  succinylcholine chloride, 41
  tubocurarine chloride, 41
  vecuronium bromide, 41
minoxidil,
  guanethidine **2**, 170–171
mirtazapine,
  cisapride **1**, 388
  clonidine hydrochloride **2**, 166
  levodopa **3**, 150–151
  sertraline hydrochloride **3**, 151
misoprostol,
  aluminum hydroxide **3**, 376–377
  magnesium hydroxide **3**, 376–377
  phenylbutazone **3**, 21–22
  propranolol hydrochloride **3**, 270
mitomycin,

# Index

etoposide **3**, 227
vinblastine sulfate **2**, 227
mitotane,
  spironolactone **3**, 227
  warfarin **2**, 92
mivacurium chloride,
  amikacin sulfate, 41
  bacitracin, 41
  colistin sulfate, 41
  demeclocycline hydrochloride, 41
  doxycycline hydrochloride, 41
  doxycycline hyclate, injectable, 41
  gentamicin sulfate, 41
  kanamycin sulfate, injectable, 41
  kanamycin sulfate, oral, 41
  lymecycline, 41
  methacycline hydrochloride, 41
  minocycline, injectable, 41
  minocycline hydrochloride, 41
  minocycline hydrochloride pellets, 41
  neomycin sulfate, injectable, 41
  neomycin sulfate, oral, 41
  netilmicin, 41
  oxytetracycline, 41
  oxytetracycline, injectable, 41
  paromomycin sulfate, 41
  polymyxin B sulfate, 41
  polymyxin B sulfate, vaccine use, 41
  rolitetracycline, injectable, 41
  streptomycin sulfate, 41
  tetracycline, 41
  tetracycline hydrochloride, injectable, 41
  tobramycin, 41
mizolastine,
  amiodarone hydrochloride **1**, 388
  azithromycin **1**, 388
  butoconazole nitrate **1**, 388
  clarithromycin **1**, 388
  clotrimazole **1**, 388
  dirithromycin **1**, 388
  disopyramide phosphate **1**, 388
  econazole nitrate **1**, 388
  erythromycin **1**, 388
  erythromycin estolate **1**, 388
  erythromycin ethylsuccinate **1**, 388
  erythromycin gluceptate **1**, 388
  erythromycin lactobionate **1**, 388
  erythromycin stearate **1**, 388
  fenticonazole nitrate **1**, 388
  flecainide acetate **1**, 388
  fluconazole **1**, 388
  ibutilide fumarate **1**, 388
  isoconazole nitrate **1**, 388
  ketoconazole, oral **1**, 388
  miconazole nitrate **1**, 388
  oxiconazole nitrate **1**, 388
  procainamide hydrochloride **1**, 388
  quinidine **1**, 388
  sotalol hydrochloride **1**, 388
  spiramycin **1**, 388
  sulfamethoxazole–trimethoprim **1**, 388
  terconazole **1**, 388
  tioconazole **1**, 388
  troleandomycin **1**, 388
moclobemide,
  apraclonidine hydrochloride **1**, 388
  benzphetamine hydrochloride, 159–160
  brimonidine tartrate, ophthalmic **1**, 388
  bupropion hydrochloride **1**, 388
  citalopram hydrobromide, 144–145
  dexfenfluramine hydrochloride, 159–160
  dextroamphetamine, 159–160
  dextromethorphan hbr, 15
  diethylpropion hydrochloride, 159–160
  dopamine hydrochloride, 159–160
  entacapone **1**, 388
  ephedrine, 159–160
  fenfluramine hydrochloride, 159–160
  fluoxetine hydrochloride, 144–145
  fluvoxamine maleate, 144–145
  indoramin **1**, 388
  isometheptene, 159–160
  levodopa, 157–158
  meperidine hydrochloride, 15
  mephentermine sulfate, 159–160
  methamphetamine hydrochloride, 159–160
  methylphenidate hydrochloride, 159–160
  nefazodone hydrochloride **1**, 388
  phendimetrazine tartrate, 159–160
  phenmetrazine hydrochloride, 159–160
  phenylpropanolamine, 159–160
  pseudoephedrine, 159–160
  rizatriptan benzoate **1**, 388
  sertraline hydrochloride **1**, 388
  sibutramine hydrochloride monohyd **1**, 388
  sumatriptan, nasal **1**, 388
  sumatriptan succinate **1**, 388
  sumatriptan succinate, injectable **1**, 388
  sumatriptan succinate, oral **1**, 388
  venlafaxine hydrochloride, 144–145
  zolmitriptan **1**, 388
monosulfiram,
  alcohol, ethyl–oral/injectable, 318
moricizine hydrochloride,
  cimetidine, oral **3**, 57–58
  digoxin **4**, 285
  halofantrine hydrochloride **1**, 388
  theophylline **2**, 350

## Index

warfarin **2**, 92
morphine,
   amitriptyline hydrochloride **3**, 18
   cimetidine, oral **2**, 18–19
   cyclosporine **2**, 19
   metoclopramide hydrochloride **3**, 19–20
   naltrexone hydrochloride **1**, 388
   thiopental sodium **2**, 40
   tubocurarine chloride **2**, 42
moxalactam disodium,
   amikacin sulfate, 192
   gentamicin sulfate, 192
   kanamycin sulfate, injectable, 192
   kanamycin sulfate, oral, 192
   neomycin sulfate, injectable, 192
   neomycin sulfate, oral, 192
   netilmicin, 192
   paromomycin sulfate, 192
   streptomycin sulfate, 192
   tobramycin, 192
moxifloxacin hydrochloride, oral,
   amiodarone hydrochloride **1**, 388
   bretylium tosylate **1**, 388
   disopyramide phosphate **1**, 388
   ibutilide fumarate **1**, 388
   procainamide hydrochloride **1**, 388
   quinidine **1**, 388
   sotalol hydrochloride **1**, 388
   thioridazine hydrochloride **1**, 388
mycophenolate mofetil,
   cyclosporine **3**, 377

## N

nabumetone,
   ketorolac tromethamine **1**, 388
   ketorolac tromethamine, injectable **1**, 388
nadolol,
   arbutamine hydrochloride **1**, 388
   clonidine hydrochloride, 167
   clonidine hydrochloride, transdermal, 167
   epinephrine, 267
   insulin, 311
   phenelzine sulfate **3**, 263
nafcillin sodium,
   amikacin sulfate, 192
   cyclosporine **2**, 363
   gentamicin sulfate, 192
   netilmicin, 192
   tobramycin, 192
   warfarin **2**, 92–93
nalbuphine hydrochloride,
   furazolidone, 15
   isocarboxazid, 15
   naltrexone hydrochloride **1**, 388
   pargyline hydrochloride, 15
   phenelzine sulfate, 15
   selegiline hydrochloride, 15
   tranylcypromine sulfate, 15

nalidixic acid,
   acenocoumarol, 93
   anisindione, 93
   coumarin, 93
   dicumarol, 93
   warfarin **1**, 93
naloxone hydrochloride,
   captopril **3**, 165
   clonidine hydrochloride **3**, 167
naltrexone hydrochloride,
   alfentanil hydrochloride **1**, 388
   anileridine **1**, 388
   buprenorphine hydrochloride **1**, 388
   butorphanol tartrate **1**, 388
   codeine **1**, 388
   dextromoramide **1**, 388
   dezocine **1**, 388
   diamorphine hydrochloride **1**, 388
   difenoxin hydrochloride **1**, 388
   dihydrocodeine bitartrate **1**, 388
   diphenoxylate hydrochloride **1**, 388
   ethoheptazine citrate **1**, 388
   fentanyl citrate **1**, 388
   hydrocodone bitartrate **1**, 388
   hydromorphone hydrochloride **1**, 388
   levomethadyl acetate hydrochloride **1**, 388
   levorphanol tartrate **1**, 388
   meperidine hydrochloride **1**, 388
   meptazinol **1**, 388
   methadone hydrochloride **1**, 388
   morphine **1**, 388
   nalbuphine hydrochloride **1**, 388
   opium **1**, 388
   oxycodone **1**, 388
   oxymorphone hydrochloride **1**, 388
   pentazocine **1**, 388
   phenoperidine hydrochloride **1**, 388
   propoxyphene **1**, 388
   remifentanil hydrochloride **1**, 388
   sufentanil citrate **1**, 388
naphazoline hydrochloride,
   furazolidone, 159–160
   isocarboxazid, 159–160
   pargyline hydrochloride, 159–160
   phenelzine sulfate, 159–160
   tranylcypromine sulfate, 159–160
naproxen,
   alendronate sodium **2**, 20
   cholestyramine **3**, 20
   gold sodium thiomalate **2**, 12
   ketorolac tromethamine **1**, 388
   ketorolac tromethamine, injectable **1**, 388
   valproic acid **3**, 131
naratriptan hydrochloride,
   rizatriptan benzoate **1**, 388

# Index

sumatriptan, nasal **1**, 388
sumatriptan succinate **1**, 388
sumatriptan succinate, injectable **1**, 388
sumatriptan succinate, oral **1**, 388
zolmitriptan **1**, 388
nebivolol hydrochloride,
  arbutamine hydrochloride **1**, 388
  cimetidine, oral, 266
  cimetidine hydrochloride, injectable, 266
  clonidine hydrochloride, 167
  clonidine hydrochloride, transdermal, 167
  dexfenfluramine hydrochloride, 267
  dobutamine hydrochloride, 267
  dopamine hydrochloride, 267
  epinephrine, 267
  etafedrine hydrochloride, 267
  insulin, 311
  lofexidine hydrochloride, 167
  mazindol, 267
  metaraminol bitartrate, 267
  methoxamine hydrochloride, 267
nefazodone hydrochloride,
  astemizole **1**, 388
  cisapride **1**, 388
  furazolidone **1**, 388
  isocarboxazid **1**, 388
  moclobemide **1**, 388
  pargyline hydrochloride **1**, 388
  phenelzine sulfate **1**, 388
  procarbazine hydrochloride **1**, 388
  selegiline hydrochloride **1**, 388
  simvastatin **3**, 383
  tacrolimus **2**, 385
  terfenadine **1**, 388
  tranylcypromine sulfate **1**, 388
  trazodone hydrochloride **3**, 386–387
  triazolam **1**, 388
nelfinavir mesylate,
  astemizole **1**, 388
  cisapride **1**, 388
  midazolam hydrochloride **1**, 388
  rifampin **1**, 388
  rifapentine **1**, 388
  sildenafil citrate **1**, 388
  terfenadine **1**, 388
  triazolam **1**, 388
neomycin sulfate, injectable,
  alcuronium chloride, 41
  ampicillin sodium, 192
  atracurium besylate, 41
  benethamine penicillin, 192
  bumetanide, 198
  bumetanide, injectable, 198
  carbenicillin disodium, 192
  cefprozil, 192
  ceftibuten dihyrate, 192
  cefuroxime, 192
  cephalexin, 192
  cephalothin sodium, 192
  doxacurium chloride, 41
  ethacrynic acid, 198
  ethacrynic acid, injectable, 198
  ether, 27
  furosemide, 198
  furosemide, injectable, 198
  gallamine triethiodide, 41
  halothane, 27
  methoxyflurane, 27
  metocurine iodide, 41
  mivacurium chloride, 41
  moxalactam disodium, 192
  nitrous oxide, 27
  pancuronium bromide, 41
  penicillin G, 192
  penicillin G benzathine, 192
  penicillin G procaine, 192
  penicillin V, 192
  pipecuronium bromide, 41
  piretanide, 198
  rapacuronium bromide, 41
  rocuronium bromide, 41
  succinylcholine chloride, 41
  temocillin sodium, 192
  ticarcillin disodium, 192
  torsemide, injectable, 198
  tubocurarine chloride, 41
  vecuronium bromide, 41
neomycin sulfate, oral,
  alcuronium chloride, 41
  ampicillin sodium, 192
  atracurium besylate, 41
  benethamine penicillin, 192
  bumetanide, 198
  bumetanide, injectable, 198
  carbenicillin disodium, 192
  cefprozil, 192
  ceftibuten dihyrate, 192
  cefuroxime, 192
  cephalexin, 192
  cephalothin sodium, 192
  digoxin **2**, 286
  doxacurium chloride, 41
  ethacrynic acid, 198
  ethacrynic acid, injectable, 198
  ether **1**, 27
  furosemide, 198
  furosemide, injectable, 198
  gallamine triethiodide, 41
  halothane, 27
  methicillin sodium, 192
  methotrexate **2**, 224
  methoxyflurane, 27
  metocurine iodide, 41
  mivacurium chloride, 41
  moxalactam disodium, 192
  nitrous oxide, 27
  pancuronium bromide, 41
  penicillin G, 192

# Index

penicillin G benzathine, 192
penicillin G procaine, 192
penicillin V, 192
pipecuronium bromide, 41
piretanide, 198
rapacuronium bromide, 41
rocuronium bromide, 41
succinylcholine chloride, 41
temocillin sodium, 192
ticarcillin disodium, 192
torsemide, injectable, 198
torsemide, oral, 198
tubocurarine chloride, 41
vecuronium bromide, 41
vitamin A **3**, 335
vitamin A, prenatal multivitamin use **3**, 335
warfarin **3**, 93
neostigmine,
  succinylcholine chloride **2**, 38
netilmicin,
  alcuronium chloride, 41
  amoxicillin, 192
  ampicillin sodium, 192
  atracurium besylate, 41
  azlocillin sodium, 192
  bacampicillin hydrochloride, 192
  benethamine penicillin, 192
  bumetanide, 198
  bumetanide, injectable, 198
  carbenicillin disodium, 192
  cefprozil, 192
  ceftibuten dihyrate, 192
  cefuroxime, 192
  cephalexin, 192
  cephalothin sodium, 192
  cloxacillin sodium, 192
  cyclacillin, 192
  dicloxacillin, 192
  doxacurium chloride, 41
  ethacrynic acid, 198
  ethacrynic acid, injectable, 198
  flucloxacillin, 192
  furosemide, 198
  furosemide, injectable, 198
  gallamine triethiodide, 41
  methicillin sodium, 192
  metocurine iodide, 41
  mezlocillin sodium, 192
  mivacurium chloride, 41
  moxalactam disodium, 192
  nafcillin sodium, 192
  oxacillin sodium, 192
  pancuronium bromide, 41
  penicillin G, 192
  penicillin G benzathine, 192
  penicillin G procaine, 192
  penicillin V, 192
  pipecuronium bromide, 41
  piperacillin sodium, 192
  piretanide, 198
  rapacuronium bromide, 41
  rocuronium bromide, 41
  succinylcholine chloride, 41
  temocillin sodium, 192
  ticarcillin disodium, 192
  torsemide, injectable, 198
  torsemide, oral, 198
  tubocurarine chloride, 41
  vecuronium bromide, 41
nevirapine,
  hormonal contraceptive **1**, 388
  hormonal contraceptive, low dose **1**, 388
  indinavir sulfate **1**, 388
  methadone hydrochloride **2**, 17
  ritonavir **1**, 388
  saquinavir **1**, 388
niacin, vitamin B3,
  aspirin **3**, 334
  lovastatin **2**, 374
  sulfinpyrazone **3**, 24
niacinamide (nicotinamide),
  carbamazepine **3**, 108
nicardipine hydrochloride,
  cyclosporine, 47–48
  quinidine, 65–66
nicardipine hydrochloride, injectable,
  cyclosporine, 47–48
  quinidine, 65–66
nifedipine,
  alcohol, ethyl–oral/injectable **3**, 58
  cimetidine, oral **2**, 58
  cyclosporine, 47–48
  digoxin, 290
  digoxin capsule, stabilized, 290
  fluoxetine hydrochloride **3**, 58–59
  halothane **3**, 59
  magnesium sulfate **3**, 59
  phenytoin **2**, 126
  quinidine, 65–66
  tacrolimus **3**, 385
nimodipine,
  quinidine, 65–66
nisoldipine,
  cyclosporine, 47–48
nitric oxide, inhalation,
  alcohol, ethyl–oral/injectable **2**, 31
nitrofurantoin,
  magnesium trisilicate **3**, 204
  phenytoin **3**, 126
  probenecid **3**, 204
  propantheline bromide **3**, 205
nitroglycerin,
  alteplase, recombinant **2**, 357
  aspirin **3**, 9
  dihydroergotamine mesylate **2**, 365
  heparin **2**, 74
  indomethacin **3**, 14
  pancuronium bromide **3**, 34
  sildenafil citrate **1**, 388

# Index

nitroglycerin, sublingual,
  imipramine **2**, 149
  pancuronium bromide **3**, 34
  sildenafil citrate **1**, 388
nitroprusside sodium,
  captopril **3**, 175–176
  esmolol hydrochloride **3**, 177–178
nitrous oxide,
  amikacin sulfate, 27
  clindamycin, 27
  clindamycin phosphate, injectable, 27
  colistin sulfate, 27
  gentamicin sulfate, 27
  kanamycin sulfate, injectable, 27
  kanamycin sulfate, oral, 27
  neomycin sulfate, injectable, 27
  neomycin sulfate, oral, 27
  polymyxin B sulfate, 27
  polymyxin B sulfate, vaccine use, 27
  streptomycin sulfate, 27
  tobramycin, 27
nizatidine,
  charcoal **3**, 377
norepinephrine bitartrate,
  chloroform, 28
  enflurane, 28
  epinephrine, 28
  ether, 28
  halothane, 28
  lithium **3**, 251
  methoxyflurane, 28
  methyldopa **2**, 174
  timolol maleate, ophthalmic, 267
norfloxacin,
  acenocoumarol, 93
  anisindione, 93
  coumarin, 93
  dicumarol, 93
  sucralfate **2**, 205
  warfarin, 93
nortriptyline hydrochloride,
  amprenavir **1**, 388
  arbutamine hydrochloride **1**, 388
  charcoal **3**, 151
  fluoxetine hydrochloride **2**, 151–152
  guanadrel sulfate, 169
  guanethidine, 169
  halofantrine hydrochloride **1**, 388
  marijuana **2**, 152
  phenobarbital **3**, 152–153
  rifampin **3**, 153
  terbinafine hydrochloride **2**, 153
  warfarin **4**, 93–94

## O

octreotide acetate,
  cyclosporine **2**, 377–378
ofloxacin,
  warfarin, 93
ofloxacin, injectable,
  warfarin, 93
olanzapine,
  fluvoxamine maleate **3**, 255
omeprazole,
  clarithromycin **3**, 378
  cyanocobalamin, vitamin B12 **3**, 328
  cyclosporine **2**, 378
  diazepam **3**, 241
  indinavir sulfate **3**, 368
  ketoconazole, oral **2**, 200
  methotrexate sodium, injectable **2**, 225
  phenytoin **2**, 127
  theophylline **4**, 350
  warfarin **3**, 94
opipramol,
  guanadrel sulfate, 169
  guanethidine, 169
opium,
  isocarboxazid, 15
  naltrexone hydrochloride **1**, 388
  pargyline hydrochloride, 15
  phenelzine sulfate, 15
  selegiline hydrochloride, 15
  tranylcypromine sulfate, 15
orphenadrine citrate,
  benserazide **3**, 369
  levodopa, comb w/ benserazide **3**, 369
  propoxyphene **4**, 23–24
oxacillin sodium,
  amikacin sulfate, 192
  gentamicin sulfate, 192
  netilmicin, 192
  tobramycin, 192
oxandrolone,
  acenocoumarol, 91
  coumarin, 91
  dicumarol, 91
  warfarin, 91
oxaprozin,
  ketorolac tromethamine **1**, 388
  ketorolac tromethamine, injectable **1**, 388
oxazepam,
  diflunisal **3**, 256
oxiconazole nitrate,
  cyclosporine, 199–200
  fosphenytoin sodium, injectable, 121–122
  lovastatin **1**, 388
  mizolastine **1**, 388
  phenytoin, 121–122
  simvastatin **1**, 388
oxprenolol,
  arbutamine hydrochloride **1**, 388
  epinephrine, 267
  insulin, 311
oxtriphylline,

# Index

cimetidine, oral, 344
cimetidine hydrochloride,
   injectable, 344
erythromycin, 346
erythromycin estolate, 346
erythromycin ethylsuccinate, 346
erythromycin gluceptate, 346
erythromycin lactobionate, 346
erythromycin stearate, 346
halothane, 337
tobacco, 354
oxybutynin chloride,
   clomipramine hydrochloride **3**, 379
   digoxin, 287
oxycodone,
   isocarboxazid, 15
   naltrexone hydrochloride **1**, 388
   pargyline hydrochloride, 15
   phenelzine sulfate, 15
   selegiline hydrochloride, 15
   tranylcypromine sulfate, 15
oxymetazoline hydrochloride,
   furazolidone, 159–160
   isocarboxazid, 159–160
   pargyline hydrochloride, 159–160
   phenelzine sulfate, 159–160
   tranylcypromine sulfate, 159–160
oxymetholone,
   acenocoumarol, 91
   anisindione, 91
   coumarin, 91
   dicumarol, 91
   phenindione, 91
   warfarin, 91
oxymorphone hydrochloride,
   isocarboxazid, 15
   naltrexone hydrochloride **1**, 388
   pargyline hydrochloride, 15
   phenelzine sulfate, 15
   selegiline hydrochloride, 15
   tranylcypromine sulfate, 15
oxypertine,
   guanethidine, 169
oxyphenbutazone,
   acenocoumarol, 94–95
   acetohexamide, 314–315
   anisindione, 94–95
   chlorpropamide, 314–315
   coumarin, 94–95
   dicumarol, 94–95
   gliclazide, 314–315
   glimepiride, 314–315
   gliquidone, 314–315
   ketorolac tromethamine **1**, 388
   ketorolac tromethamine, injectable **1**, 388
   methandrostenolone **3**, 20–21
   tolazamide, 314–315
   tolbutamide, 314–315
   warfarin, 94–95
oxyphencyclimine hydrochloride,
   digoxin, 287
oxytetracycline,
   alcuronium chloride, 41
   aluminum carbonate, basic, 211–212
   aluminum hydroxide, 211–212
   aluminum oxide, 211–212
   aluminum phosphate, 211–212
   attapulgite, 211–212
   bismuth subsalicylate, 211–212
   calcium, oral salt unspecified, 211–212
   calcium acetate, 211–212
   calcium ascorbate, 211–212
   calcium carbonate, oral, 211–212
   calcium chloride, oral, 211–212
   calcium citrate, oral, 211–212
   calcium glubionate, oral, 211–212
   calcium glucoheptonate, 211–212
   calcium gluconate, oral, 211–212
   calcium glycerophosphate, oral, 211–212
   calcium iodate, 211–212
   calcium lactate, oral, 211–212
   calcium lactate gluconate, 211–212
   calcium lactobionate, oral, 211–212
   calcium phosphate, oral, 211–212
   carbonyl iron, 212
   digoxin, 289
   digoxin capsule, stabilized, 289
   dihydroxyaluminum, 211–212
   doxacurium chloride, 41
   ether, 27
   ferric ammonium citrate, 212
   ferrous citrate, 212
   ferrous fumarate, 212
   ferrous gluconate, 212
   ferrous glycine sulfate, 212
   ferrous hydroxide polymaltose, 212
   ferrous ions, salt unspecified, 212
   ferrous succinate, 212
   ferrous sulfate, 212
   gallamine triethiodide, 41
   insulin **2**, 310
   iron peptonized, 212
   kaolin, 211–212
   magaldrate, 211–212
   magnesium carbonate, 211–212
   magnesium chloride, oral, 211–212
   magnesium hydroxide, 211–212
   magnesium oxide, 211–212
   magnesium sulfate, 211–212
   magnesium trisilicate, 211–212
   metocurine iodide, 41
   mivacurium chloride, 41
   pancuronium bromide, 41
   pipecuronium bromide, 41
   rapacuronium bromide, 41
   rocuronium bromide, 41
   succinylcholine chloride, 41
   sucralfate, 211–212

# Index

tubocurarine chloride, 41
vecuronium bromide, 41
oxytetracycline, injectable,
alcuronium chloride, 41
digoxin, 289
digoxin capsule, stabilized, 289
doxacurium chloride, 41
ether, 27
gallamine triethiodide, 41
metocurine iodide, 41
mivacurium chloride, 41
pancuronium bromide, 41
pipecuronium bromide, 41
rapacuronium bromide, 41
rocuronium bromide, 41
succinylcholine chloride, 41
tubocurarine chloride, 41
vecuronium bromide, 41

## P

paclitaxel,
cisplatin **2**, 227–228
pancreatin,
miglitol **1**, 388
pancuronium bromide,
amikacin sulfate, 41
aminophylline **2**, 31
azathioprine sodium **3**, 32
bacitracin, 41
carbamazepine **3**, 32
clindamycin **2**, 32
clindamycin phosphate, injectable **2**, 32
colistin sulfate, 41
cyclosporine **2**, 33
demeclocycline hydrochloride, 41
doxycycline hydrochloride, 41
doxycycline hyclate, injectable, 41
furosemide **3**, 33
gentamicin sulfate, 41
hydrocortisone, oral/systemic **3**, 33–34
hydrocortisone acet, injectable **3**, 33–34
hydrocortisone sodium phos **3**, 33–34
hydrocortisone sodium succinate **3**, 33–34
kanamycin sulfate, injectable, 41
kanamycin sulfate, oral, 41
lithium **3**, 34
lymecycline, 41
methacycline hydrochloride, 41
minocycline, injectable, 41
minocycline hydrochloride, 41
minocycline hydrochloride pellets, 41
neomycin sulfate, injectable, 41
neomycin sulfate, oral, 41
netilmicin, 41
nitroglycerin **3**, 34
nitroglycerin, sublingual **3**, 34
oxytetracycline, 41
oxytetracycline, injectable, 41
paromomycin sulfate, 41
polymyxin B sulfate, 41
polymyxin B sulfate, vaccine use, 41
streptomycin sulfate, 41
tetracycline, 41
tobramycin, 41
triethylene thiophosphoramide **3**, 34–35
papaverine hydrochloride,
levodopa **3**, 369–370
para–aminobenzoic acid,
procainamide hydrochloride **3**, 60
pargyline hydrochloride,
alfentanil hydrochloride, 15
amphetamine, 191–192
anileridine, 15
apraclonidine hydrochloride **1**, 388
benzphetamine hydrochloride, 159–160
brimonidine tartrate, ophthalmic **1**, 388
buprenorphine hydrochloride, 15
bupropion hydrochloride **1**, 388
butorphanol tartrate, 15
citalopram hydrobromide **1**, 144–145
codeine, 15
dexfenfluramine hydrochloride, 159–160
dextroamphetamine, 159–160
dextromethorphan hbr, 15
diethylpropion hydrochloride, 159–160
difenoxin hydrochloride, 15
dihydrocodeine bitartrate, 15
diphenoxylate hydrochloride, 15
dopamine hydrochloride, 159–160
entacapone **1**, 388
ephedrine, 159–160
etafedrine hydrochloride, 159–160
fenfluramine hydrochloride, 159–160
fentanyl citrate, 15
fluoxetine hydrochloride, 144–145
fluvoxamine maleate, 144–145
hydrocodone bitartrate, 15
hydromorphone hydrochloride, 15
indoramin **1**, 388
isometheptene, 159–160
levodopa, 157–158
levorphanol tartrate, 15
mazindol, 191–192
meperidine hydrochloride, 15
mephentermine sulfate, 159–160
meptazinol, 15
metaraminol bitartrate, 159–160
methamphetamine hydrochloride,

# Index

159–160
methyldopa **3**, 153–154
methylphenidate hydrochloride, 159–160
nalbuphine hydrochloride, 15
naphazoline hydrochloride, 159–160
nefazodone hydrochloride **1**, 388
opium, 15
oxycodone, 15
oxymetazoline hydrochloride, 159–160
oxymorphone hydrochloride, 15
paroxetine hydrochloride, 144–145
phendimetrazine tartrate, 159–160
phenmetrazine hydrochloride, 159–160
phenoperidine hydrochloride, 15
phentermine hydrochloride, 191–192
phenylephrine, 159–160
phenylpropanolamine, 159–160
pseudoephedrine, 159–160
remifentanil hydrochloride, 15
rizatriptan benzoate **1**, 388
sertraline hydrochloride **1**, 388
sibutramine hydrochloride monohyd **1**, 388
sufentanil citrate, 15
sumatriptan, nasal **1**, 388
sumatriptan succinate **1**, 388
sumatriptan succinate, oral **1**, 388
tetrahydrozoline hydrochloride, 159–160
tolcapone **1**, 388
venlafaxine hydrochloride, 144–145
xylometazoline hydrochloride, 159–160
zolmitriptan **1**, 388
paricalcitol,
alfacalcidol **1**, 388
calcifediol **1**, 388
calcipotriene **1**, 388
calcitriol **1**, 388
cholecalciferol, vitamin D3 **1**, 388
dihydrotachysterol **1**, 388
ergocalciferol, vitamin D2 **1**, 388
phosphorus **1**, 388
potassium biphosphate **1**, 388
potassium glycerophosphate, oral **1**, 388
potassium phosphate **1**, 388
sodium biphosphate **1**, 388
sodium phosphate, oral **1**, 388
vitamin D1, 388
vitamin D2, prenatal multivitamin use **1**, 388
vitamin D3, prenatal multivitamin use **1**, 388
paromomycin sulfate,
alcuronium chloride, 41
ampicillin sodium, 192
atracurium besylate, 41
benethamine penicillin, 192
carbenicillin disodium, 192
cefprozil, 192
ceftibuten dihyrate, 192
cefuroxime, 192
cephalexin, 192
cephalothin sodium, 192
doxacurium chloride, 41
gallamine triethiodide, 41
metocurine iodide, 41
mivacurium chloride, 41
moxalactam disodium, 192
pancuronium bromide, 41
penicillin G, 192
penicillin G benzathine, 192
penicillin G procaine, 192
penicillin V, 192
pipecuronium bromide, 41
rapacuronium bromide, 41
rocuronium bromide, 41
succinylcholine chloride, 41
temocillin sodium, 192
ticarcillin disodium, 192
tubocurarine chloride, 41
vecuronium bromide, 41
paroxetine hydrochloride,
astemizole **1**, 388
cimetidine, oral **3**, 154
dextromethorphan hbr **2**, 154–155
donepezil hydrochloride **2**, 140–141
hypericum **3**, 155
interferon alfa-2a **3**, 155–156
isocarboxazid, 144–145
pargyline hydrochloride, 144–145
phenelzine sulfate, 144–145
selegiline hydrochloride, 144–145
thioridazine hydrochloride **1**, 388
tranylcypromine sulfate, 144–145
zolpidem tartrate **3**, 156
penbutolol sulfate,
arbutamine hydrochloride **1**, 388
clonidine hydrochloride, 167
clonidine hydrochloride, transdermal, 167
epinephrine, 267
insulin, 311
penicillamine,
aluminum hydroxide **3**, 379
chloroquine **3**, 379
digoxin **2**, 286
ferrous sulfate **2**, 329–330
indomethacin **3**, 380
magnesium hydroxide **3**, 379
probenecid **3**, 22
penicillin G,
amikacin sulfate, 192
aspirin **3**, 205
chloramphenicol **4**, 205–206

# Index

chlortetracycline hydrochloride **2**, 206
erythromycin **3**, 206
gentamicin sulfate, 192
kanamycin sulfate, injectable, 192
kanamycin sulfate, oral, 192
neomycin sulfate, injectable, 192
neomycin sulfate, oral, 192
netilmicin, 192
paromomycin sulfate, 192
probenecid **3**, 206–207
streptomycin sulfate, 192
tobramycin, 192

penicillin G benzathine,
amikacin sulfate, 192
gentamicin sulfate, 192
kanamycin sulfate, injectable, 192
kanamycin sulfate, oral, 192
neomycin sulfate, injectable, 192
neomycin sulfate, oral, 192
netilmicin, 192
paromomycin sulfate, 192
streptomycin sulfate, 192
tobramycin, 192

penicillin G procaine,
amikacin sulfate, 192
gentamicin sulfate, 192
kanamycin sulfate, injectable, 192
kanamycin sulfate, oral, 192
neomycin sulfate, injectable, 192
neomycin sulfate, oral, 192
netilmicin, 192
paromomycin sulfate, 192
streptomycin sulfate, 192
tobramycin, 192

penicillin V,
amikacin sulfate, 192
gentamicin sulfate, 192
guar gum **3**, 207
kanamycin sulfate, injectable, 192
kanamycin sulfate, oral, 192
neomycin sulfate, injectable, 192
neomycin sulfate, oral, 192
netilmicin, 192
paromomycin sulfate, 192
streptomycin sulfate, 192
tobramycin, 192

pentaerythritol tetranitrate,
sildenafil citrate **1**, 388

pentamidine isethionate,
grepafloxacin hydrochloride **1**, 388

pentamidine isethionate, inhalation,
grepafloxacin hydrochloride **1**, 388

pentazocine,
naltrexone hydrochloride **1**, 388
phenelzine sulfate, 15
selegiline hydrochloride, 15
tranylcypromine sulfate, 15

pentobarbital sodium,
acenocoumarol, 94
anisindione, 94
coumarin, 94
dicumarol, 94
metoprolol tartrate **2**, 262–263
warfarin, 94

pentoxifylline,
cimetidine, oral, 344
cimetidine hydrochloride, injectable, 344

pergolide mesylate,
acetophenazine maleate **1**, 388
benperidol **1**, 388
chlorpromazine hydrochloride **1**, 388
chlorprothixene **1**, 388
efavirenz **1**, 388
flupenthixol decanoate, injectable **1**, 388
flupenthixol dihydrochloride, oral **1**, 388
fluphenazine **1**, 388
haloperidol **1**, 388
indinavir sulfate **1**, 388
mesoridazine besylate **1**, 388
methdilazine **1**, 388
perphenazine **1**, 388
prochlorperazine **1**, 388
promethazine **1**, 388
propiomazine hydrochloride **1**, 388
rizatriptan benzoate **1**, 388
saquinavir **1**, 388
sumatriptan succinate **1**, 388
sumatriptan succinate, injectable **1**, 388
sumatriptan succinate, oral **1**, 388
thiethylperazine maleate **1**, 388
thioridazine hydrochloride **1**, 388
thiothixene **1**, 388
trifluoperazine hydrochloride **1**, 388
trifluperidol hydrochloride **1**, 388
triflupromazine hydrochloride **1**, 388
trimeprazine tartrate **1**, 388

pericyazine,
cabergoline **1**, 388
cisapride **1**, 388
grepafloxacin hydrochloride **1**, 388
guanethidine, 169
halofantrine hydrochloride **1**, 388
pimozide **1**, 388

perphenazine,
cabergoline **1**, 388
disulfiram **3**, 256
guanethidine, 169
halofantrine hydrochloride **1**, 388
pergolide mesylate **1**, 388

phendimetrazine tartrate,
chloroform, 28
enflurane, 28
furazolidone, 191–192
halothane, 28

# Index

isocarboxazid, 159–160
linezolid, 159–160
methoxyflurane, 28
moclobemide, 159–160
pargyline hydrochloride, 159–160
phenelzine sulfate, 159–160
procarbazine hydrochloride, 159–160
tranylcypromine sulfate, 159–160
phenelzine sulfate,
  alfentanil hydrochloride, 15
  amphetamine, 191–192
  anileridine, 15
  apraclonidine hydrochloride **1**, 388
  benzphetamine hydrochloride, 159–160
  brimonidine tartrate, ophthalmic **1**, 388
  buprenorphine hydrochloride, 15
  bupropion hydrochloride **1**, 388
  buspirone hydrochloride **3**, 156
  butorphanol tartrate, 15
  citalopram hydrobromide **1**, 144–145
  clonazepam **3**, 156–157
  codeine, 15
  dexfenfluramine hydrochloride, 159–160
  dextroamphetamine, 159–160
  dextromethorphan hbr, 15
  diethylpropion hydrochloride, 159–160
  difenoxin hydrochloride, 15
  dihydrocodeine bitartrate, 15
  diphenoxylate hydrochloride, 15
  dopamine hydrochloride, 159–160
  entacapone **1**, 388
  ephedrine, 159–160
  etafedrine hydrochloride, 159–160
  fenfluramine hydrochloride, 159–160
  fentanyl citrate, 15
  fluoxetine hydrochloride, 144–145
  fluvoxamine maleate, 144–145
  ginseng **3**, 157
  guanethidine **2**, 171
  hydrocodone bitartrate, 15
  hydromorphone hydrochloride, 15
  indoramin **1**, 388
  insulin **2**, 310–311
  isometheptene, 159–160
  levodopa **1**, 157–158
  levorphanol tartrate, 15
  mazindol, 191–192
  meperidine hydrochloride **1**, 15
  mephentermine sulfate, 159–160
  meptazinol, 15
  metaraminol bitartrate, 159–160
  methamphetamine hydrochloride, 159–160
  methylphenidate hydrochloride, 159–160
  nadolol **3**, 263
  nalbuphine hydrochloride, 15
  naphazoline hydrochloride, 159–160
  nefazodone hydrochloride **1**, 388
  opium, 15
  oxycodone, 15
  oxymetazoline hydrochloride, 159–160
  oxymorphone hydrochloride, 15
  paroxetine hydrochloride, 144–145
  pentazocine, 15
  phendimetrazine tartrate, 159–160
  phenmetrazine hydrochloride, 159–160
  phenoperidine hydrochloride, 15
  phentermine hydrochloride, 159–160
  phenylephrine, 159–160
  phenylpropanolamine, 159–160
  propoxyphene, 15
  pseudoephedrine, 159–160
  remifentanil hydrochloride, 15
  rizatriptan benzoate **1**, 388
  sertraline hydrochloride, 144–145
  sibutramine hydrochloride monohyd **1**, 388
  sufentanil citrate, 15
  sulfisoxazole **3**, 158
  sumatriptan, nasal **1**, 388
  sumatriptan succinate **1**, 388
  sumatriptan succinate, oral **1**, 388
  tetrahydrozoline hydrochloride, 159–160
  tolcapone **1**, 388
  venlafaxine hydrochloride, 144–145
  xylometazoline hydrochloride, 159–160
  zolmitriptan **1**, 388
phenindione,
  aloxiprin, 77
  barbital, 94
  bezafibrate, 81
  butobarbitone, 94
  calcium carbaspirin, 77
  cimetidine, oral, 80
  cimetidine hydrochloride, injectable, 80
  ciprofibrate, 81
  danazol, 91
  fenofibrate, micronized, 81
  gemfibrozil, 81
  haloperidol **3**, 74
  menadiol sodium diphosphate, vitamin K4, 95
  menadione, 95
  methandrostenolone, 91
  oxymetholone, 91
  phytonadione, vitamin K1, 95
  rifabutin, 97

# Index

stanozolol, 91
toremifene **1**, 388
phenmetrazine hydrochloride,
  chloroform, 28
  enflurane, 28
  furazolidone, 191–192
  halothane, 28
  isocarboxazid, 159–160
  linezolid, 159–160
  methoxyflurane, 28
  moclobemide, 159–160
  pargyline hydrochloride, 159–160
  phenelzine sulfate, 159–160
  procarbazine hydrochloride, 159–160
  tranylcypromine sulfate, 159–160
phenobarbital,
  acenocoumarol, 94
  acetaminophen **3**, 3
  alcohol, ethyl–oral/injectable **2**, 322
  anisindione, 94
  carbamazepine **3**, 108–109
  charcoal **3**, 322
  chloramphenicol **3**, 184
  chlorcyclizine hydrochloride **3**, 322–323
  chlorpromazine hydrochloride **3**, 235
  cimetidine, oral **3**, 323
  coumarin, 94
  cyclosporine **2**, 323
  dexamethasone **2**, 323–324
  dicumarol, 94
  digitoxin **2**, 275–276
  doxorubicin hydrochloride **3**, 219
  doxycycline hydrochloride **2**, 189
  felbamate **3**, 324
  fenoprofen calcium **3**, 11
  griseofulvin **3**, 194
  guanfacine hydrochloride **3**, 172
  hormonal contraceptive **2**, 324
  hormonal contraceptive, low–dose **2**, 324
  lidocaine hydrochloride, systemic **3**, 54
  meperidine hydrochloride **3**, 15–16
  methyldopa **4**, 175
  metronidazole, oral/vaginal **2**, 203–204
  nortriptyline hydrochloride **3**, 152–153
  phenytoin **3**, 127
  pyridoxine hydrochloride **3**, 324–325
  quinidine **2**, 64
  theophylline **2**, 350–351
  valproic acid **2**, 113
  verapamil hydrochloride **3**, 66–67
  warfarin **1**, 94
phenoperidine hydrochloride,
  isocarboxazid, 15
  naltrexone hydrochloride **1**, 388
  pargyline hydrochloride, 15
  phenelzine sulfate, 15
  selegiline hydrochloride, 15
  tranylcypromine sulfate, 15
phenoxybenzamine hydrochloride,
  alfuzosin hydrochloride **1**, 388
  methyldopa **3**, 175
phentermine hydrochloride,
  chloroform, 28
  dexfenfluramine hydrochloride **1**, 388
  enflurane, 28
  fenfluramine hydrochloride **1**, 388
  furazolidone, 191–192
  halothane, 28
  isocarboxazid, 159–160
  methoxyflurane, 28
  pargyline hydrochloride, 191–192
  phenelzine sulfate, 159–160
  procarbazine hydrochloride, 159–160
  tranylcypromine sulfate, 159–160
phentolamine,
  alfuzosin hydrochloride **1**, 388
phenylbutazone,
  acenocoumarol, 94–95
  acetohexamide, 314–315
  anisindione, 94–95
  charcoal **3**, 21
  chlorpropamide, 314–315
  coumarin, 94–95
  desipramine hydrochloride **3**, 21
  dicumarol, 94–95
  digitoxin **3**, 276
  gliclazide, 314–315
  glimepiride, 314–315
  gliquidone, 314–315
  ketorolac tromethamine **1**, 388
  ketorolac tromethamine, injectable **1**, 388
  misoprostol **3**, 21–22
  phenytoin **2**, 127–128
  tolazamide, 314–315
  tolbutamide **1**, 314–315
  warfarin **1**, 94–95
phenylephrine,
  chloroform, 28
  enflurane, 28
  furazolidone, 159–160
  guanethidine **2**, 171
  halothane, 28
  isocarboxazid, 159–160
  methoxyflurane, 28
  pargyline hydrochloride, 159–160
  phenelzine sulfate, 159–160
  procarbazine hydrochloride, 159–160
  timolol maleate, ophthalmic, 267
  tranylcypromine sulfate, 159–160
phenylpropanolamine,

# Index

caffeine **3**, 341
chloroform, 28
enflurane, 28
furazolidone, 191–192
halothane, 28
indomethacin **2**, 14
isocarboxazid, 159–160
methoxyflurane, 28
moclobemide, 159–160
pargyline hydrochloride, 159–160
phenelzine sulfate, 159–160
procarbazine hydrochloride, 159–160
thioridazine hydrochloride **2**, 233
tranylcypromine sulfate **1**, 159–160
phenytoin,
  acetaminophen **3**, 3
  acetazolamide **4**, 113–114
  alcohol, ethyl-oral/injectable **2**, 114
  allopurinol **2**, 114
  aluminum hydroxide **3**, 114
  amiodarone hydrochloride **2**, 115
  aspirin **4**, 115
  azapropazone dihydrate **1**, 388
  butoconazole nitrate, 121–122
  carbamazepine **3**, 115
  carmustine **2**, 116
  charcoal **2**, 116
  chloramphenicol **2**, 116
  chlorpheniramine **2**, 117
  chlorpromazine hydrochloride **3**, 117
  cimetidine, oral **1**, 117–118
  cimetidine hydrochloride, injectable, 117–118
  ciprofloxacin hydrochloride **2**, 118
  ciprofloxacin hydrochloride, injectable **2**, 118
  clarithromycin **3**, 118
  clotrimazole, 121–122
  cyclosporine **2**, 119
  dexamethasone **2**, 119
  diazepam **3**, 119–120
  diazoxide, oral **2**, 120
  dicumarol **2**, 72
  digitalis **2**, 274
  disopyramide phosphate **2**, 50
  disulfiram **1**, 120
  dopamine hydrochloride **1**, 120–121
  doxycycline hydrochloride **2**, 189
  econazole nitrate, 121–122
  ergocalciferol, vitamin D2 **2**, 328
  ethosuximide **3**, 121
  felbamate **2**, 121
  fenticonazole nitrate, 121–122
  fluconazole **1**, 121–122
  fluoxetine hydrochloride **2**, 122
  folic acid **2**, 122
  furosemide **3**, 297
  grepafloxacin hydrochloride **1**, 388
  halothane **3**, 28–29
  hormonal contraceptive **3**, 123
  ibuprofen **2**, 123
  imipramine **3**, 124
  influenza virus vaccine, split virion **3**, 124
  insulin **3**, 311
  isoconazole nitrate, 121–122
  isoniazid **2**, 124
  itraconazole, 121–122
  itraconazole, oral, 121–122
  ketoconazole, oral, 121–122
  levodopa **3**, 125
  levothyroxine sodium **3**, 125
  lithium **3**, 251–252
  magnesium trisilicate **3**, 114
  meperidine hydrochloride **3**, 16
  methotrexate **2**, 116
  methoxsalen **2**, 125
  methylphenidate hydrochloride **3**, 125–126
  metocurine iodide **2**, 31
  metronidazole, oral/vaginal **3**, 126
  metyrapone **3**, 376
  mexiletine hydrochloride **3**, 56–57
  miconazole nitrate, 121–122
  nifedipine **2**, 126
  nitrofurantoin **3**, 126
  omeprazole **2**, 127
  oxiconazole nitrate, 121–122
  phenobarbital **3**, 127
  phenylbutazone **2**, 127–128
  primidone **2**, 131
  pyridoxine hydrochloride **3**, 128
  quinidine **2**, 64
  ranitidine hydrochloride, injectable, 117–118
  ranitidine hydrochloride, oral, 117–118
  rifampin **2**, 128
  sucralfate **2**, 128–129
  sulfamethizole **2**, 129
  terconazole, 121–122
  theophylline **2**, 351
  ticlopidine hydrochloride **3**, 129
  tioconazole, 121–122
  trazodone hydrochloride **3**, 129–130
  trimethoprim **2**, 130
  valproic acid **2**, 130
  vinblastine sulfate **2**, 116
  vitamin D2, prenatal multivitamin use **2**, 328
phosphorus,
  paricalcitol **1**, 388
phytonadione, vitamin K1,
  acenocoumarol, 95
  anisindione, 95
  coumarin, 95
  dicumarol, 95
  phenindione, 95

# Index

pimozide,
- warfarin **1**, 95
- pimozide,
  - acetophenazine maleate **1**, 388
  - amiodarone hydrochloride **1**, 388
  - amitriptyline hydrochloride **1**, 388
  - azithromycin **1**, 388
  - bretylium tosylate **1**, 388
  - clarithromycin **1**, 388
  - desipramine hydrochloride **1**, 388
  - dirithromycin **1**, 388
  - disopyramide phosphate **1**, 388
  - doxepin hydrochloride **1**, 388
  - encainide hydrochloride **1**, 388
  - erythromycin **1**, 388
  - erythromycin estolate **1**, 388
  - erythromycin ethylsuccinate **1**, 388
  - erythromycin gluceptate **1**, 388
  - erythromycin lactobionate **1**, 388
  - erythromycin stearate **1**, 388
  - flecainide acetate **1**, 388
  - fluoxetine hydrochloride **3**, 256–257
  - ibutilide fumarate **1**, 388
  - imipramine **1**, 388
  - indecainide hydrochloride **1**, 388
  - itraconazole, oral **1**, 388
  - mesoridazine besylate **1**, 388
  - methdilazine **1**, 388
  - pericyazine **1**, 388
  - procainamide hydrochloride **1**, 388
  - promazine hydrochloride **1**, 388
  - promethazine **1**, 388
  - propafenone hydrochloride **1**, 388
  - propiomazine hydrochloride **1**, 388
  - ritonavir **1**, 388
  - sotalol hydrochloride **1**, 388
  - sulfisoxazole **3**, 158
  - thiethylperazine maleate **1**, 388
  - thioproperazine mesylate **1**, 388
  - thioridazine hydrochloride **1**, 388
  - triflupromazine hydrochloride **1**, 388
  - trimeprazine tartrate **1**, 388
  - trimethoprim **3**, 158
  - trimipramine maleate **1**, 388

pindolol,
- arbutamine hydrochloride **1**, 388
- clonidine hydrochloride, 167
- clonidine hydrochloride, transdermal, 167
- epinephrine, 267
- insulin, 311
- thioridazine hydrochloride **1**, 388

pipecuronium bromide,
- amikacin sulfate, 41
- bacitracin, 41
- colistin sulfate, 41
- demeclocycline hydrochloride, 41
- doxycycline hydrochloride, 41
- doxycycline hyclate, injectable, 41
- gentamicin sulfate, 41
- kanamycin sulfate, injectable, 41
- kanamycin sulfate, oral, 41
- lymecycline, 41
- methacycline hydrochloride, 41
- minocycline, injectable, 41
- minocycline hydrochloride, 41
- minocycline hydrochloride pellets, 41
- neomycin sulfate, injectable, 41
- neomycin sulfate, oral, 41
- netilmicin, 41
- oxytetracycline, 41
- oxytetracycline, injectable, 41
- paromomycin sulfate, 41
- polymyxin B sulfate, 41
- polymyxin B sulfate, vaccine use, 41
- rolitetracycline, injectable, 41
- streptomycin sulfate, 41
- tetracycline, 41
- tetracycline hydrochloride, injectable, 41
- tobramycin, 41

piperacetazine,
- cisapride **1**, 388
- grepafloxacin hydrochloride **1**, 388
- guanethidine, 169
- halofantrine hydrochloride **1**, 388

piperacillin sodium,
- amikacin sulfate, 192
- gentamicin sulfate, 192
- methotrexate **2**, 225
- methotrexate sodium, injectable **2**, 225
- netilmicin, 192
- tobramycin, 192
- vecuronium bromide **2**, 43–44

piperazine,
- chlorpromazine hydrochloride **3**, 235

pirbuterol acetate,
- chloroform, 28
- enflurane, 28
- halothane, 28
- methoxyflurane, 28
- metoprolol tartrate, 267
- timolol maleate, oral, 267

pirenzepine dihydrochloride,
- digoxin, 287

piretanide,
- amikacin sulfate, 198
- gentamicin sulfate, 198
- kanamycin sulfate, injectable, 198
- kanamycin sulfate, oral, 198
- lithium, 247
- neomycin sulfate, injectable, 198
- neomycin sulfate, oral, 198
- netilmicin, 198
- streptomycin sulfate, 198
- tobramycin, 198

piroxicam,

# Index

ketorolac trometamine **1**, 388
ketorolac trometamine, injectable **1**, 388
ritonavir **1**, 388
polyestradiol phosphate,
  rifampin, 209
polymyxin B sulfate,
  alcuronium chloride, 41
  doxacurium chloride, 41
  enflurane, 27
  ether, 27
  gallamine triethiodide, 41
  gentamicin sulfate **2**, 193
  halothane, 27
  methoxyflurane, 27
  metocurine iodide, 41
  mivacurium chloride, 41
  nitrous oxide, 27
  pancuronium bromide, 41
  pipecuronium bromide, 41
  prochlorperazine **2**, 207
  rapacuronium bromide, 41
  rocuronium bromide, 41
  succinylcholine chloride, 41
  tubocurarine chloride, 41
  vecuronium bromide, 41
polymyxin B sulfate, vaccine use,
  alcuronium chloride, 41
  doxacurium chloride, 41
  enflurane, 27
  ether, 27
  gallamine triethiodide, 41
  halothane, 27
  methoxyflurane, 27
  metocurine iodide, 41
  mivacurium chloride, 41
  nitrous oxide, 27
  pancuronium bromide, 41
  pipecuronium bromide, 41
  rapacuronium bromide, 41
  rocuronium bromide, 41
  succinylcholine chloride, 41
  tubocurarine chloride, 41
  vecuronium bromide, 41
polythiazide,
  lithium, 247
potassium, salt unspecified,
  amiloride hydrochloride, 299
  potassium canrenoate, 299
  spironolactone, 299
  triamterene, 299
potassium acetate,
  amiloride hydrochloride, 299
  potassium canrenoate, 299
  spironolactone, 299
  triamterene, 299
potassium aminobenzoate,
  sulfacytine **1**, 388
  sulfadiazine **1**, 388
  sulfadoxine **1**, 388
  sulfamerazine **1**, 388

sulfamethazine **1**, 388
sulfamethizole **1**, 388
sulfamethoxazole **1**, 388
sulfapyridine **1**, 388
sulfasalazine **1**, 388
sulfisoxazole **1**, 388
potassium bicarbonate,
  amiloride hydrochloride, 299
  potassium canrenoate, 299
  spironolactone, 299
  triamterene, 299
potassium biphosphate,
  amiloride hydrochloride, 299
  paricalcitol **1**, 388
  potassium canrenoate, 299
  spironolactone, 299
  triamterene, 299
potassium canrenoate,
  potassium, salt unspecified, 299
  potassium acetate, 299
  potassium bicarbonate, 299
  potassium biphosphate, 299
  potassium chloride, 299
  potassium citrate, 299
  potassium gluconate, 299
  potassium glycerophosphate, oral, 299
  potassium iodide, 299
  potassium iodide, prenatal multivitamin use, 299
  potassium perchlorate, 299
  potassium phosphate, 299
  potassium salicylate, 299
potassium chloride,
  amiloride hydrochloride, 299
  captopril **3**, 165
  potassium canrenoate, 299
  spironolactone **1**, 299
  triamterene, 299
potassium citrate,
  amiloride hydrochloride, 299
  lithium, 245–246
  potassium canrenoate, 299
  spironolactone, 299
  triamterene, 299
potassium gluconate,
  amiloride hydrochloride, 299
  potassium canrenoate, 299
  spironolactone, 299
  triamterene, 299
potassium glycerophosphate, oral,
  amiloride hydrochloride, 299
  paricalcitol **1**, 388
  potassium canrenoate, 299
  spironolactone, 299
  triamterene, 299
potassium iodide,
  amiloride hydrochloride, 299
  lithium **2**, 252
  potassium canrenoate, 299
  spironolactone, 299

# Index

triamterene, 299
potassium iodide, prenatal multivitamin use,
  amiloride hydrochloride, 299
  potassium canrenoate, 299
  spironolactone, 299
  triamterene, 299
potassium perchlorate,
  amiloride hydrochloride, 299
  potassium canrenoate, 299
  spironolactone, 299
  triamterene, 299
potassium phosphate,
  amiloride hydrochloride, 299
  paricalcitol **1**, 388
  potassium canrenoate, 299
  spironolactone, 299
  triamterene, 299
potassium salicylate,
  amiloride hydrochloride, 299
  potassium canrenoate, 299
  spironolactone, 299
  triamterene, 299
pravastatin sodium,
  propranolol hydrochloride **3**, 270
praziquantel,
  cimetidine, oral **3**, 359
  cimetidine hydrochloride, injectable **3**, 359
prazosin hydrochloride,
  digoxin **2**, 286
  indomethacin **2**, 176
  propranolol hydrochloride **2**, 176
  verapamil hydrochloride **3**, 176
prednisolone,
  cyclosporine **2**, 380
  glycyrrhiza, (licorice) inert **3**, 380
  glycyrrhiza, (licorice) noninert **3**, 380
  hormonal contraceptive **2**, 380–381
  isoniazid **3**, 196
  rifampin **2**, 209
prednisone,
  aluminum hydroxide **3**, 381
  cyclophosphamide **3**, 219
  digoxin **2**, 278–279
  timolol maleate, ophthalmic **2**, 272
primidone,
  acenocoumarol, 94
  acetazolamide **3**, 130
  clonazepam **4**, 111
  coumarin, 94
  dicumarol, 94
  phenytoin **2**, 131
  warfarin, 94
probenecid,
  acyclovir, oral **3**, 180
  allopurinol **3**, 6
  bumetanide **3**, 297
  captopril **3**, 165–166
  cephalothin sodium **2**, 182–183
  chlorothiazide **3**, 294
  chlorpropamide **3**, 304
  clofibrate **3**, 22
  dyphylline **2**, 341
  furosemide **3**, 297
  indomethacin **2**, 14
  ketorolac tromethamine **1**, 388
  ketorolac tromethamine, injectable **1**, 388
  lorazepam **3**, 254
  methotrexate **1**, 225
  methotrexate sodium, injectable, 225
  nitrofurantoin **3**, 204
  penicillamine **3**, 22
  penicillin G **3**, 206–207
  rifampin **4**, 210
  sulfinpyrazone **4**, 24
  thiopental sodium **3**, 40
  zidovudine **2**, 215
probucol,
  cyclosporine **2**, 381
procainamide hydrochloride,
  alcohol, ethyl–oral/injectable **3**, 59–60
  amiodarone hydrochloride **2**, 60
  astemizole **1**, 388
  cimetidine, oral **2**, 60
  cisapride **1**, 388
  grepafloxacin hydrochloride **1**, 388
  halofantrine hydrochloride **1**, 388
  lidocaine hydrochloride, systemic **3**, 55
  mizolastine **1**, 388
  moxifloxacin hydrochloride, oral **1**, 388
  para–aminobenzoic acid **3**, 60
  pimozide **1**, 388
  propranolol hydrochloride **3**, 61
  quinidine **3**, 61
  sotalol hydrochloride **1**, 388
  sparfloxacin **1**, 388
  succinylcholine chloride **3**, 38–39
  trimethoprim **3**, 61
procarbazine hydrochloride,
  amphetamine, 191–192
  benzphetamine hydrochloride, 159–160
  brimonidine tartrate, ophthalmic **1**, 388
  bupropion hydrochloride **1**, 388
  dexfenfluramine hydrochloride, 159–160
  dextroamphetamine, 159–160
  diethylpropion hydrochloride, 159–160
  digoxin **2**, 278–279
  dopamine hydrochloride, 159–160
  entacapone **1**, 388
  ephedrine, 159–160

## Index

etafedrine hydrochloride, 159–160
fenfluramine hydrochloride, 159–160
fluoxetine hydrochloride, 144–145
fluvoxamine maleate, 144–145
indoramin **1**, 388
isometheptene, 159–160
levodopa, 157–158
mazindol, 191–192
meperidine hydrochloride, 15
mephentermine sulfate, 159–160
metaraminol bitartrate, 159–160
methamphetamine hydrochloride, 159–160
methotrexate **2**, 226
methylphenidate hydrochloride, 159–160
nefazodone hydrochloride **1**, 388
phendimetrazine tartrate, 159–160
phenmetrazine hydrochloride, 159–160
phentermine hydrochloride, 159–160
phenylephrine, 159–160
phenylpropanolamine, 159–160
pseudoephedrine, 159–160
rizatriptan benzoate **1**, 388
sertraline hydrochloride **1**, 388
sibutramine hydrochloride monohyd **1**, 388
sumatriptan, nasal **1**, 388
sumatriptan succinate **1**, 388
sumatriptan succinate, oral **1**, 388
tolcapone **1**, 388
venlafaxine hydrochloride, 144–145
procaterol hydrochloride,
  chloroform, 28
  enflurane, 28
  halothane, 28
  methoxyflurane, 28
  metoprolol tartrate, 267
  timolol maleate, oral, 267
prochlorperazine,
  cabergoline **1**, 388
  guanethidine, 169
  halofantrine hydrochloride **1**, 388
  pergolide mesylate **1**, 388
  polymyxin B sulfate **2**, 207
procyclidine hydrochloride,
  digoxin, 287
proguanil hydrochloride,
  methotrexate, 226
  methotrexate sodium, injectable, 226
  warfarin, 98
promazine hydrochloride,
  cabergoline **1**, 388
  charcoal **3**, 257
  cisapride **1**, 388
  grepafloxacin hydrochloride **1**, 388
  guanethidine, 169

halofantrine hydrochloride **1**, 388
pimozide **1**, 388
succinylcholine chloride **2**, 39
promethazine,
  cabergoline **1**, 388
  cisapride **1**, 388
  grepafloxacin hydrochloride **1**, 388
  guanethidine, 169
  halofantrine hydrochloride **1**, 388
  pergolide mesylate **1**, 388
  pimozide **1**, 388
propafenone hydrochloride,
  astemizole **1**, 388
  cyclosporine **2**, 61–62
  digoxin **2**, 286–287
  digoxin capsule, stabilized **2**, 286–287
  fluoxetine hydrochloride **2**, 62
  grepafloxacin hydrochloride **1**, 388
  halofantrine hydrochloride **1**, 388
  pimozide **1**, 388
  quinidine **2**, 62
  ritonavir **1**, 388
  theophylline **2**, 351
  warfarin **2**, 95–96
propantheline bromide,
  atenolol **3**, 260
  chlorothiazide **3**, 294
  cimetidine, oral **3**, 359
  deslanoside, 287
  digitalis, 287
  digitoxin, 287
  digoxin **1**, 287
  nitrofurantoin **3**, 205
propiomazine hydrochloride,
  cabergoline **1**, 388
  cisapride **1**, 388
  grepafloxacin hydrochloride **1**, 388
  halofantrine hydrochloride **1**, 388
  pergolide mesylate **1**, 388
  pimozide **1**, 388
propofol,
  aminophylline **3**, 35
  diazepam **3**, 35
propoxyphene,
  alcohol, ethyl–oral/injectable **2**, 22–23
  amphetamine **3**, 23
  carbamazepine **2**, 109
  charcoal **3**, 23
  doxepin hydrochloride **3**, 141
  naltrexone hydrochloride **1**, 388
  orphenadrine citrate **4**, 23–24
  phenelzine sulfate, 15
  ritonavir **1**, 388
  selegiline hydrochloride, 15
  warfarin **2**, 96
propranolol hydrochloride,
  acetaminophen **3**, 3–4
  alcohol, ethyl–oral/injectable **3**, 263
  allergenic extract **3**, 264

# Index

aluminum hydroxide **3**, 264
aminoglutethimide **3**, 264
arbutamine hydrochloride **1**, 388
aspirin **3**, 264–265
chlorpheniramine **4**, 265
chlorpromazine hydrochloride **2**, 265
cholestyramine **3**, 265–266
cimetidine, oral **1**, 266
cimetidine hydrochloride, injectable, 266
clonidine hydrochloride **1**, 167
clonidine hydrochloride, transdermal, 167
cocaine hydrochloride **2**, 266
desipramine hydrochloride **3**, 266
dexfenfluramine hydrochloride, 267
diatrizoate sodium **3**, 267
diazepam **3**, 242
dobutamine hydrochloride, 267
dopamine hydrochloride, 267
epinephrine **1**, 267
ergotamine tartrate **3**, 267–268
etafedrine hydrochloride, 267
fentanyl citrate **3**, 11–12
flecainide acetate **3**, 268
fluoxetine hydrochloride **2**, 268
furosemide **2**, 269
hydralazine hydrochloride **3**, 269
indomethacin **2**, 269
insulin **1**, 311
isoniazid **3**, 196
lidocaine hydrochloride, systemic **2**, 55
lofexidine hydrochloride, 167
mazindol, 267
metaraminol bitartrate, 267
methoxamine hydrochloride, 267
methyldopa **2**, 175
misoprostol **3**, 270
pravastatin sodium **3**, 270
prazosin hydrochloride **2**, 176
procainamide hydrochloride **3**, 61
quinidine **3**, 270
rizatriptan benzoate **1**, 388
theophylline **2**, 351–352
thioridazine hydrochloride **1**, 388
thyroid strong **2**, 271
tobacco **2**, 271
tranylcypromine sulfate **4**, 160
tubocurarine chloride **2**, 42
verapamil hydrochloride **2**, 67
warfarin **2**, 96
propyliodone,
  metformin hydrochloride **1**, 312
propylthiouracil,
  warfarin, 100
protriptyline hydrochloride,
  amprenavir **1**, 388
  arbutamine hydrochloride **1**, 388
  guanadrel sulfate, 169
  guanethidine, 169
  halofantrine hydrochloride **1**, 388
pseudoephedrine,
  chloroform, 28
  enflurane, 28
  furazolidone, 191–192
  halothane, 28
  isocarboxazid, 159–160
  methoxyflurane, 28
  moclobemide, 159–160
  pargyline hydrochloride, 159–160
  phenelzine sulfate, 159–160
  procarbazine hydrochloride, 159–160
  tranylcypromine sulfate, 159–160
psyllium,
  digoxin **3**, 287
  lithium **3**, 249–250
pyrantel pamoate,
  theophylline **2**, 352
pyridostigmine,
  methylprednisolone **3**, 381
pyridoxine hydrochloride,
  altretamine **1**, 388
  isoniazid **3**, 196–197
  levodopa **1**, 334
  phenobarbital **3**, 324–325
  phenytoin **3**, 128

## Q

quetiapine fumarate,
  sparfloxacin **1**, 388
  thioridazine hydrochloride **1**, 388
quinestrol,
  rifampin, 209
quinethazone,
  lithium, 247
quinidine,
  aluminum hydroxide **3**, 65
  amiodarone hydrochloride **1**, 62–63
  amprenavir **1**, 388
  arbutamine hydrochloride **1**, 388
  astemizole **1**, 388
  cimetidine, oral **2**, 63
  cisapride **1**, 388
  codeine **2**, 10
  desipramine hydrochloride **3**, 140
  digitoxin, 287–288
  digoxin **1**, 287–288
  digoxin capsule, stabilized, 287–288
  diltiazem hydrochloride, 65–66
  diphenoxylate hydrochloride **3**, 63
  disopyramide phosphate **3**, 50
  grapefruit juice **3**, 332–333
  grepafloxacin hydrochloride **1**, 388
  halofantrine hydrochloride **1**, 388
  itraconazole, oral **1**, 388
  ketoconazole, oral **2**, 63–64
  lercanidipine hydrochloride, 65–66

## Index

metoclopramide hydrochloride **3**, 64
mizolastine **1**, 388
moxifloxacin hydrochloride, oral **1**, 388
nicardipine hydrochloride, 65–66
nicardipine hydrochloride, injectable, 65–66
nifedipine, 65–66
nimodipine, 65–66
phenobarbital **2**, 64
phenytoin **2**, 64
procainamide hydrochloride **3**, 61
propafenone hydrochloride **2**, 62
propranolol hydrochloride **3**, 270
reserpine **3**, 65
rifampin **2**, 65
ritonavir **1**, 388
sertindole **1**, 388
sparfloxacin **1**, 388
tubocurarine chloride **2**, 42–43
verapamil hydrochloride **1**, 65–66
verapamil hydrochloride, sustained-release, 65–66
verapamil hydrochloride pellets, 65–66
warfarin **2**, 96–97
quinine,
astemizole **1**, 388
cyclosporine **2**, 363–364
flecainide acetate **3**, 53–54
terfenadine **1**, 388

## R

radioactive iodine–131,
metformin hydrochloride **1**, 312
ranitidine hydrochloride, injectable,
ethotoin, 117–118
fosphenytoin sodium, injectable, 117–118
mephenytoin, 117–118
phenytoin, 117–118
warfarin, 80
ranitidine hydrochloride, oral,
acetaminophen **3**, 4
ethotoin, 117–118
fosphenytoin sodium, injectable, 117–118
mephenytoin, 117–118
phenytoin, 117–118
sucralfate **3**, 382
warfarin, 80
rapacuronium bromide,
amikacin sulfate, 41
bacitracin, 41
colistin sulfate, 41
demeclocycline hydrochloride, 41
doxycycline hydrochloride, 41
doxycycline hyclate, injectable, 41
gentamicin sulfate, 41
kanamycin sulfate, injectable, 41
kanamycin sulfate, oral, 41
lymecycline, 41
methacycline hydrochloride, 41
minocycline, injectable, 41
minocycline hydrochloride, 41
minocycline hydrochloride pellets, 41
neomycin sulfate, injectable, 41
neomycin sulfate, oral, 41
netilmicin, 41
oxytetracycline, 41
oxytetracycline, injectable, 41
paromomycin sulfate, 41
polymyxin B sulfate, 41
polymyxin B sulfate, vaccine use, 41
rolitetracycline, injectable, 41
streptomycin sulfate, 41
tetracycline, 41
tetracycline hydrochloride, injectable, 41
tobramycin, 41
remifentanil hydrochloride,
naltrexone hydrochloride **1**, 388
pargyline hydrochloride, 15
phenelzine sulfate, 15
selegiline hydrochloride, 15
tranylcypromine sulfate, 15
reserpine,
digitalis **3**, 274–275
ephedrine **2**, 177
halothane **3**, 177
imipramine **3**, 149
quinidine **3**, 65
thiopental sodium **2**, 40
reviparin sodium,
sodium salicylate, 77
ribavirin,
zidovudine **1**, 387
rifabutin,
acenocoumarol, 97
anisindione, 97
coumarin, 97
cyclosporine, 209
dicumarol, 97
digitoxin, 276
digoxin, 276
estradiol, 209
estradiol, transdermal, 209
ethinyl estradiol, 209
hormonal contraceptive, 209
hormonal contraceptive, low-dose, 209
phenindione, 97
ritonavir **1**, 388
saquinavir **1**, 388
warfarin, 97
rifampin,
acenocoumarol, 97
amiodarone hydrochloride **2**, 208
amprenavir **1**, 388

# Index

anisindione, 97
buspirone hydrochloride **3**, 208
chloramphenicol **2**, 184
chlorotrianisene, 209
clofibrate **3**, 208
clonidine hydrochloride **4**, 167
clozapine **2**, 239
conjugated estrogens, 209
coumarin, 97
cyclosporine **1**, 209
dapsone **3**, 188
deslanoside, 276
diazepam **3**, 242
dicumarol, 97
diethylstilbestrol, 209
digitalis, 276
digitoxin **1**, 276
digoxin, 276
digoxin capsule, stabilized, 276
disopyramide phosphate **3**, 50–51
enalapril maleate **3**, 168
esterified estrogens, 209
estradiol, 209
estradiol, transdermal, 209
estriol, 209
estrogen, 209
estrone, 209
estropipate, 209
ethinyl estradiol, 209
glyburide **3**, 306–307
haloperidol **2**, 244–245
halothane **2**, 29
hexobarbital **3**, 321
hormonal contraceptive **1**, 209
hormonal contraceptive, low–dose, 209
indinavir sulfate **1**, 388
isoniazid **2**, 197
ketoconazole, oral **2**, 200–201
lamotrigine **3**, 112–113
losartan potassium **2**, 172–173
mesalamine, oral **4**, 207–208
mestranol, 209
methadone hydrochloride **2**, 18
metoprolol tartrate **2**, 263
mexiletine hydrochloride **3**, 57
nelfinavir mesylate **1**, 388
nortriptyline hydrochloride **3**, 153
phenytoin **2**, 128
polyestradiol phosphate, 209
prednisolone **2**, 209
probenecid **4**, 210
quinestrol, 209
quinidine **2**, 65
saquinavir **1**, 388
sertraline hydrochloride **3**, 159
sirolimus **1**, 388
tacrolimus **2**, 386
theophylline **2**, 352
verapamil hydrochloride **2**, 67
warfarin **1**, 97

zidovudine **2**, 388
zolpidem tartrate **2**, 325
rifapentine,
  indinavir sulfate **1**, 388
  nelfinavir mesylate **1**, 388
  ritonavir **1**, 388
  saquinavir **1**, 388
rimiterol hydrobromide,
  chloroform, 28
  enflurane, 28
  halothane, 28
  methoxyflurane, 28
  metoprolol tartrate, 267
  timolol maleate, oral, 267
ritodrine hydrochloride,
  bupivacaine hydrochloride **2**, 26
  glycopyrrolate **2**, 366
ritonavir,
  alprazolam **1**, 388
  amiodarone hydrochloride **1**, 388
  astemizole **1**, 388
  bepridil hydrochloride **1**, 388
  bupropion hydrochloride **1**, 388
  buspirone hydrochloride **3**, 232
  cisapride **1**, 388
  clorazepate dipotassium **1**, 388
  clozapine **1**, 388
  desipramine hydrochloride **2**, 382
  diazepam **1**, 388
  dihydroergotamine mesylate **1**, 388
  encainide hydrochloride **1**, 388
  ergotamine tartrate **1**, 388
  estazolam **1**, 388
  flecainide acetate **1**, 388
  flurazepam hydrochloride **1**, 388
  meperidine hydrochloride **1**, 388
  midazolam hydrochloride **1**, 388
  nevirapine **1**, 388
  pimozide **1**, 388
  piroxicam **1**, 388
  propafenone hydrochloride **1**, 388
  propoxyphene **1**, 388
  quinidine **1**, 388
  rifabutin **1**, 388
  rifapentine **1**, 388
  sildenafil citrate **1**, 388
  terfenadine **1**, 388
  triazolam **1**, 388
  zolpidem tartrate **1**, 388
rizatriptan benzoate,
  bromocriptine mesylate **1**, 388
  cabergoline **1**, 388
  dihydroergotamine mesylate **1**, 388
  dihydroergotamine mesylate, inhl **1**, 388
  ergoloid mesylates **1**, 388
  ergonovine maleate **1**, 388
  ergotamine tartrate **1**, 388
  furazolidone **1**, 388
  hypericum **1**, 388
  isocarboxazid **1**, 388

## Index

methylergonovine maleate **1**, 388
methysergide maleate **1**, 388
moclobemide **1**, 388
naratriptan hydrochloride **1**, 388
pargyline hydrochloride **1**, 388
pergolide mesylate **1**, 388
phenelzine sulfate **1**, 388
procarbazine hydrochloride **1**, 388
propranolol hydrochloride **1**, 388
sumatriptan, nasal **1**, 388
sumatriptan succinate **1**, 388
sumatriptan succinate, injectable **1**, 388
sumatriptan succinate, oral **1**, 388
tranylcypromine sulfate **1**, 388
zolmitriptan **1**, 388
rocuronium bromide,
amikacin sulfate, 41
bacitracin, 41
colistin sulfate, 41
demeclocycline hydrochloride, 41
doxycycline hydrochloride, 41
doxycycline hyclate, injectable, 41
gentamicin sulfate, 41
kanamycin sulfate, injectable, 41
kanamycin sulfate, oral, 41
lymecycline, 41
methacycline hydrochloride, 41
minocycline, injectable, 41
minocycline hydrochloride, 41
minocycline hydrochloride pellets, 41
neomycin sulfate, injectable, 41
neomycin sulfate, oral, 41
netilmicin, 41
oxytetracycline, 41
oxytetracycline, injectable, 41
paromomycin sulfate, 41
polymyxin B sulfate, 41
polymyxin B sulfate, vaccine use, 41
rolitetracycline, injectable, 41
streptomycin sulfate, 41
tetracycline, 41
tetracycline hydrochloride, injectable, 41
tobramycin, 41
rolitetracycline, injectable,
alcuronium chloride, 41
digoxin, 289
digoxin capsule, stabilized, 289
ether, 27
gallamine triethiodide, 41
metocurine iodide, 41
mivacurium chloride, 41
pipecuronium bromide, 41
rapacuronium bromide, 41
rocuronium bromide, 41
succinylcholine chloride, 41
tubocurarine chloride, 41
vecuronium bromide, 41

## S

s–adneosylmethionine,
clomipramine hydrochloride **3**, 158
salicylamide,
methotrexate, 222
methotrexate sodium, injectable, 222
salmeterol xinafoate,
chloroform, 28
enflurane, 28
halothane, 28
methoxyflurane, 28
metoprolol tartrate, 267
timolol maleate, oral, 267
salsalate,
methotrexate, 222
methotrexate sodium, injectable, 222
saquinavir,
astemizole **1**, 388
bromocriptine mesylate **1**, 388
cabergoline **1**, 388
cisapride **1**, 388
dihydroergotamine mesylate **1**, 388
dihydroergotamine mesylate, inhl **1**, 388
efavirenz **1**, 388
ergoloid mesylates **1**, 388
ergonovine maleate **1**, 388
ergotamine tartrate **1**, 388
garlic **2**, 330
grapefruit juice **2**, 333
methylergonovine maleate **1**, 388
methysergide maleate **1**, 388
midazolam hydrochloride **1**, 388
nevirapine **1**, 388
pergolide mesylate **1**, 388
rifabutin **1**, 388
rifampin **1**, 388
rifapentine **1**, 388
sildenafil citrate **1**, 388
terfenadine **1**, 388
triazolam **1**, 388
scopolamine, ophthalmic,
digoxin, 287
scopolamine, systemic,
digoxin, 287
secobarbital,
acenocoumarol, 94
anisindione, 94
coumarin, 94
dicumarol, 94
methoxyflurane **2**, 30
warfarin, 94
selegiline hydrochloride,
alfentanil hydrochloride, 15
anileridine, 15
brimonidine tartrate, ophthalmic **1**, 388
buprenorphine hydrochloride, 15
bupropion hydrochloride **1**, 388

# Index

butorphanol tartrate, 15
citalopram hydrobromide **1**, 144–145
codeine, 15
dexfenfluramine hydrochloride, 159–160
dextromethorphan hbr, 15
dezocine, 15
difenoxin hydrochloride, 15
dihydrocodeine bitartrate, 15
diphenoxylate hydrochloride, 15
fentanyl citrate, 15
fluoxetine hydrochloride, 144–145
fluvoxamine maleate, 144–145
hormonal contraceptive **3**, 382–383
hormonal contraceptive, low–dose **3**, 382–383
hydrocodone bitartrate, 15
hydromorphone hydrochloride, 15
levorphanol tartrate, 15
meperidine hydrochloride, 15
meptazinol, 15
nalbuphine hydrochloride, 15
nefazodone hydrochloride **1**, 388
opium, 15
oxycodone, 15
oxymorphone hydrochloride, 15
paroxetine hydrochloride, 144–145
pentazocine, 15
phenoperidine hydrochloride, 15
propoxyphene, 15
remifentanil hydrochloride, 15
sertraline hydrochloride, 144–145
sibutramine hydrochloride monohyd **1**, 388
sufentanil citrate, 15
sumatriptan, nasal **1**, 388
sumatriptan succinate **1**, 388
sumatriptan succinate, oral **1**, 388
venlafaxine hydrochloride, 144–145
sertindole,
  itraconazole, oral **1**, 388
  ketoconazole, oral **1**, 388
  quinidine **1**, 388
sertraline hydrochloride,
  astemizole **1**, 388
  furazolidone **1**, 388
  grapefruit juice **3**, 333
  isocarboxazid, 144–145
  mirtazapine **3**, 151
  moclobemide **1**, 388
  pargyline hydrochloride **1**, 388
  phenelzine sulfate, 144–145
  procarbazine hydrochloride **1**, 388
  rifampin **3**, 159
  selegiline hydrochloride, 144–145
  tranylcypromine sulfate **1**, 388
sevoflurane,
  epinephrine, 28
sibutramine hydrochloride monohyd,
  furazolidone **1**, 388
  hypericum **1**, 388
  isocarboxazid **1**, 388
  moclobemide **1**, 388
  pargyline hydrochloride **1**, 388
  phenelzine sulfate **1**, 388
  procarbazine hydrochloride **1**, 388
  selegiline hydrochloride **1**, 388
  tranylcypromine sulfate **1**, 388
sildenafil citrate,
  amprenavir **1**, 388
  amyl nitrite **1**, 388
  erythrityl tetranitrate **1**, 388
  indinavir sulfate **1**, 388
  isosorbide dinitrate **1**, 388
  isosorbide dinitrate, sublingual **1**, 388
  isosorbide mononitrate **1**, 388
  nelfinavir mesylate **1**, 388
  nitroglycerin **1**, 388
  nitroglycerin, sublingual **1**, 388
  pentaerythritol tetranitrate **1**, 388
  ritonavir **1**, 388
  saquinavir **1**, 388
simvastatin,
  butoconazole nitrate **1**, 388
  clarithromycin, 373
  clotrimazole **1**, 388
  econazole nitrate **1**, 388
  erythromycin, 373
  erythromycin estolate, 373
  erythromycin ethylsuccinate, 373
  erythromycin glucepate, 373
  erythromycin lactobionate, 373
  erythromycin stearate, 373
  fenticonazole nitrate **1**, 388
  fluconazole **1**, 388
  grapefruit juice, 374
  isoconazole nitrate **1**, 388
  itraconazole **1**, 388
  itraconazole, oral **1**, 388
  ketoconazole, oral **1**, 388
  mibefradil dihydrochloride **1**, 388
  miconazole nitrate **1**, 388
  nefazodone hydrochloride **3**, 383
  oxiconazole nitrate **1**, 388
  terconazole **1**, 388
  tioconazole **1**, 388
  troleandomycin, 373
sirolimus,
  ketoconazole, oral **1**, 388
  rifampin **1**, 388
sodium acetate,
  lithium, 245–246
sodium bicarbonate,
  amphetamine **3**, 358
  flecainide acetate **2**, 54
  lithium, 245–246
  methotrexate **3**, 226
  tetracycline **4**, 213
sodium bicarbonate, injectable,

# Index

lithium, 245–246
sodium biphosphate,
  paricalcitol **1**, 388
sodium citrate,
  lithium, 245–246
sodium lactate,
  lithium, 245–246
sodium phosphate, oral,
  paricalcitol **1**, 388
sodium polystyrene sulfonate,
  magnesium hydroxide **2**, 375
sodium salicylate,
  acenocoumarol, 77
  anisindione, 77
  ardeparin sodium, 77
  certoparin, 77
  coumarin, 77
  dalteparin sodium, 77
  dicumarol, 77
  enoxaparin sodium, 77
  heparin, 77
  methotrexate, 222
  methotrexate sodium, injectable, 222
  reviparin sodium, 77
  tinzaparin sodium, 77
  warfarin, 77
sodium thiosalicylate,
  methotrexate, 222
  methotrexate sodium, injectable, 222
sotalol hydrochloride,
  amiodarone hydrochloride **1**, 388
  arbutamine hydrochloride **1**, 388
  astemizole **1**, 388
  bretylium tosylate **1**, 388
  cisapride **1**, 388
  disopyramide phosphate **1**, 388
  epinephrine, 267
  grepafloxacin hydrochloride **1**, 388
  halofantrine hydrochloride **1**, 388
  ibutilide fumarate **1**, 388
  insulin, 311
  mizolastine **1**, 388
  moxifloxacin hydrochloride, oral **1**, 388
  pimozide **1**, 388
  procainamide hydrochloride **1**, 388
  sparfloxacin **1**, 388
  thioridazine hydrochloride **1**, 388
sparfloxacin,
  amiodarone hydrochloride **1**, 388
  astemizole **1**, 388
  bepridil hydrochloride **1**, 388
  cisapride **1**, 388
  disopyramide phosphate **1**, 388
  ibutilide fumarate **1**, 388
  procainamide hydrochloride **1**, 388
  quetiapine fumarate **1**, 388
  quinidine **1**, 388
  sotalol hydrochloride **1**, 388
  sulfamethoxazole–trimethoprim **1**, 388
  terfenadine **1**, 388
  thioridazine hydrochloride **1**, 388
spiramycin,
  astemizole, 191
  mizolastine **1**, 388
  terfenadine, 191
spironolactone,
  aspirin **3**, 298
  captopril **3**, 298–299
  cholestyramine **2**, 178
  digoxin **2**, 288
  mitotane **3**, 227
  potassium, salt unspecified, 299
  potassium acetate, 299
  potassium bicarbonate, 299
  potassium biphosphate, 299
  potassium chloride **1**, 299
  potassium citrate, 299
  potassium gluconate, 299
  potassium glycerophosphate, oral, 299
  potassium iodide, 299
  potassium iodide, prenatal multivitamin use, 299
  potassium perchlorate, 299
  potassium phosphate, 299
  potassium salicylate, 299
  warfarin **3**, 97
stanozolol,
  acenocoumarol, 91
  coumarin, 91
  dicumarol, 91
  phenindione, 91
  warfarin, 91
stavudine,
  isoniazid **3**, 197
streptomycin sulfate,
  alcuronium chloride, 41
  ampicillin sodium, 192
  atracurium besylate, 41
  benethamine penicillin, 192
  bumetanide, 198
  bumetanide, injectable, 198
  carbenicillin disodium, 192
  cefprozil, 192
  ceftibuten dihyrate, 192
  cefuroxime, 192
  cephalexin, 192
  cephalothin sodium, 192
  doxacurium chloride, 41
  enflurane, 27
  ethacrynic acid, 198
  ethacrynic acid, injectable, 198
  ether, 27
  furosemide, 198
  furosemide, injectable, 198
  gallamine triethiodide, 41
  halothane, 27
  isoflurane, 27

# Index

methoxyflurane, 27
metocurine iodide, 41
mivacurium chloride, 41
moxalactam disodium, 192
nitrous oxide, 27
pancuronium bromide, 41
penicillin G, 192
penicillin G benzathine, 192
penicillin G procaine, 192
penicillin V, 192
pipecuronium bromide, 41
piretanide, 198
rapacuronium bromide, 41
rocuronium bromide, 41
succinylcholine chloride, 41
temocillin sodium, 192
ticarcillin disodium, 192
torsemide, injectable, 198
torsemide, oral, 198
tubocurarine chloride, 41
vecuronium bromide, 41
streptomycin sulfate, vaccine use,
  ceftibuten dihyrate, 192
succinylcholine chloride,
  amikacin sulfate, 41
  bacitracin, 41
  cimetidine, oral **2**, 35–36
  colistin sulfate, 41
  cyclophosphamide **2**, 36
  demeclocycline hydrochloride, 41
  dexpanthenol **4**, 36
  diethylstilbestrol **2**, 36–37
  digoxin **2**, 288
  doxycycline hydrochloride, 41
  doxycycline hyclate, injectable, 41
  echothiophate iodide **2**, 37
  gentamicin sulfate, 41
  isoflurane **2**, 37
  kanamycin sulfate, injectable, 41
  kanamycin sulfate, oral, 41
  lidocaine hydrochloride, systemic
    **2**, 37–38
  lymecycline, 41
  methacycline hydrochloride, 41
  metoclopramide hydrochloride **3**,
    38
  minocycline, injectable, 41
  minocycline hydrochloride, 41
  minocycline hydrochloride pellets,
    41
  neomycin sulfate, injectable, 41
  neomycin sulfate, oral, 41
  neostigmine **2**, 38
  netilmicin, 41
  oxytetracycline, 41
  oxytetracycline, injectable, 41
  paromomycin sulfate, 41
  polymyxin B sulfate, 41
  polymyxin B sulfate, vaccine use, 41
  procainamide hydrochloride **3**,
    38–39
  promazine hydrochloride **2**, 39
  rolitetracycline, injectable, 41
  streptomycin sulfate, 41
  tetracycline, 41
  tetracycline hydrochloride,
    injectable, 41
  thiopental sodium **2**, 39
  tobramycin, 41
  trimethaphan camsylate **2**, 39–40
sucralfate,
  chlorpropamide **4**, 304
  demeclocycline hydrochloride,
    211–212
  doxycycline hydrochloride, 211–212
  ketoconazole, oral **3**, 201
  levothyroxine sodium **3**, 371
  methacycline hydrochloride,
    211–212
  norfloxacin **2**, 205
  oxytetracycline, 211–212
  phenytoin **2**, 128–129
  ranitidine hydrochloride, oral **3**, 382
  tetracycline, 211–212
  theophylline **3**, 352–353
  warfarin **3**, 97–98
sufentanil citrate,
  isocarboxazid, 15
  naltrexone hydrochloride **1**, 388
  pargyline hydrochloride, 15
  phenelzine sulfate, 15
  selegiline hydrochloride, 15
  tranylcypromine sulfate, 15
sulfacytine,
  methenamine **1**, 388
  methotrexate, 226
  methotrexate sodium, injectable,
    226
  potassium aminobenzoate **1**, 388
  warfarin, 98
sulfadiazine,
  cyclosporine **2**, 210
  methenamine **1**, 388
  methotrexate, 226
  methotrexate sodium, injectable,
    226
  potassium aminobenzoate **1**, 388
  warfarin, 98
sulfadoxine,
  methenamine **1**, 388
  methotrexate, 226
  methotrexate sodium, injectable,
    226
  potassium aminobenzoate **1**, 388
  warfarin, 98
sulfamerazine,
  methenamine **1**, 388
  methotrexate, 226
  methotrexate sodium, injectable,
    226
  potassium aminobenzoate **1**, 388
  warfarin, 98

# Index

sulfamethazine,
  methenamine **1**, 388
  methotrexate, 226
  methotrexate sodium, injectable, 226
  potassium aminobenzoate **1**, 388
  warfarin, 98
sulfamethizole,
  methotrexate, 226
  methotrexate sodium, injectable, 226
  phenytoin **2**, 129
  potassium aminobenzoate **1**, 388
  tolbutamide **2**, 315
  warfarin, 98
sulfamethoxazole,
  methenamine **1**, 388
  methotrexate **1**, 226
  methotrexate sodium, injectable, 226
  potassium aminobenzoate **1**, 388
  warfarin **1**, 98
sulfamethoxazole–trimethoprim,
  astemizole **1**, 388
  cisapride **1**, 388
  dofetilide **1**, 388
  grepafloxacin hydrochloride **1**, 388
  mizolastine **1**, 388
  sparfloxacin **1**, 388
sulfapyridine,
  methenamine **1**, 388
  methotrexate, 226
  methotrexate sodium, injectable, 226
  potassium aminobenzoate **1**, 388
  warfarin, 98
sulfasalazine,
  ampicillin sodium **3**, 211
  digoxin **2**, 288
  folic acid **3**, 330
  methenamine **1**, 388
  methotrexate, 226
  methotrexate sodium, injectable, 226
  potassium aminobenzoate **1**, 388
  warfarin, 98
sulfinpyrazone,
  acetaminophen **3**, 4
  aspirin **2**, 24
  niacin, vitamin B3 **3**, 24
  probenecid **4**, 24
  verapamil hydrochloride **3**, 68
  warfarin **1**, 98
sulfisoxazole,
  methenamine **1**, 388
  methotrexate, 226
  methotrexate sodium, injectable, 226
  phenelzine sulfate **3**, 158
  pimozide **3**, 158
  potassium aminobenzoate **1**, 388

thiopental sodium **2**, 41
warfarin, 98
sulindac,
  ketorolac tromethamine **1**, 388
  ketorolac tromethamine, injectable **1**, 388
sumatriptan, nasal,
  dihydroergotamine mesylate **1**, 388
  ergoloid mesylates **1**, 388
  ergonovine maleate **1**, 388
  ergotamine tartrate **1**, 388
  furazolidone **1**, 388
  isocarboxazid **1**, 388
  methylergonovine maleate **1**, 388
  methysergide maleate **1**, 388
  moclobemide **1**, 388
  naratriptan hydrochloride **1**, 388
  pargyline hydrochloride **1**, 388
  phenelzine sulfate **1**, 388
  procarbazine hydrochloride **1**, 388
  rizatriptan benzoate **1**, 388
  selegiline hydrochloride **1**, 388
  thioridazine hydrochloride **1**, 388
  tranylcypromine sulfate **1**, 388
  zolmitriptan **1**, 388
sumatriptan succinate,
  cabergoline **1**, 388
  dihydroergotamine mesylate **1**, 388
  dihydroergotamine mesylate, inhl **1**, 388
  ergoloid mesylates **1**, 388
  ergonovine maleate **1**, 388
  ergotamine tartrate **1**, 388
  furazolidone **1**, 388
  isocarboxazid **1**, 388
  methylergonovine maleate **1**, 388
  methysergide maleate **1**, 388
  moclobemide **1**, 388
  naratriptan hydrochloride **1**, 388
  pargyline hydrochloride **1**, 388
  pergolide mesylate **1**, 388
  phenelzine sulfate **1**, 388
  procarbazine hydrochloride **1**, 388
  rizatriptan benzoate **1**, 388
  selegiline hydrochloride **1**, 388
  tranylcypromine sulfate **1**, 388
  zolmitriptan **1**, 388
sumatriptan succinate, injectable,
  cabergoline **1**, 388
  dihydroergotamine mesylate **1**, 388
  dihydroergotamine mesylate, inhl **1**, 388
  ergoloid mesylates **1**, 388
  ergonovine maleate **1**, 388
  ergotamine tartrate **1**, 388
  loxapine **1**, 254
  methylergonovine maleate **1**, 388
  methysergide maleate **1**, 388
  moclobemide **1**, 388
  naratriptan hydrochloride **1**, 388
  pergolide mesylate **1**, 388

# Index

rizatriptan benzoate **1**, 388
thioridazine hydrochloride **1**, 388
zolmitriptan **1**, 388
sumatriptan succinate, oral,
  cabergoline **1**, 388
  dihydroergotamine mesylate **1**, 388
  dihydroergotamine mesylate, inhl **1**, 388
  ergoloid mesylates **1**, 388
  ergonovine maleate **1**, 388
  ergotamine tartrate **1**, 388
  furazolidone **1**, 388
  isocarboxazid **1**, 388
  methylergonovine maleate **1**, 388
  methysergide maleate **1**, 388
  moclobemide **1**, 388
  naratriptan hydrochloride **1**, 388
  pargyline hydrochloride **1**, 388
  pergolide mesylate **1**, 388
  phenelzine sulfate **1**, 388
  procarbazine hydrochloride **1**, 388
  rizatriptan benzoate **1**, 388
  selegiline hydrochloride **1**, 388
  thioridazine hydrochloride **1**, 388
  tranylcypromine sulfate **1**, 388
  zolmitriptan **1**, 388

# T

tacrine hydrochloride,
  aminophylline **2**, 339
  fluvoxamine maleate **2**, 145–146
  haloperidol **2**, 245
  hormonal contraceptive **3**, 383
tacrolimus,
  erythromycin **2**, 383–384
  fluconazole **2**, 384
  grapefruit juice **1**, 388
  metronidazole, oral/vaginal **3**, 384–385
  nefazodone hydrochloride **2**, 385
  nifedipine **3**, 385
  rifampin **2**, 386
  theophylline **3**, 353
talbutal,
  acenocoumarol, 94
  coumarin, 94
  dicumarol, 94
  warfarin, 94
tamoxifen citrate,
  warfarin **2**, 98–99
temafloxacin hydrochloride,
  warfarin, 93
temazepam,
  diphenhydramine **2**, 257
temocillin sodium,
  amikacin sulfate, 192
  gentamicin sulfate, 192
  kanamycin sulfate, injectable, 192
  kanamycin sulfate, oral, 192
  neomycin sulfate, injectable, 192
  neomycin sulfate, oral, 192
  netilmicin, 192
  paromomycin sulfate, 192
  streptomycin sulfate, 192
  tobramycin, 192
terbinafine hydrochloride,
  aminophylline **2**, 339–340
  cyclosporine **2**, 211
  nortriptyline hydrochloride **2**, 153
  warfarin **2**, 99
terbutaline sulfate,
  chloroform, 28
  enflurane, 28
  epinephrine, 28
  ether, 28
  halothane, 28
  methoxyflurane, 28
  metoprolol tartrate, 267
  timolol maleate, oral, 267
terconazole,
  cyclosporine, 199–200
  fosphenytoin sodium, injectable, 121–122
  lovastatin **1**, 388
  mizolastine **1**, 388
  phenytoin, 121–122
  simvastatin **1**, 388
terfenadine,
  acetaminophen **2**, 5
  amprenavir **1**, 388
  astemizole **1**, 388
  carbamazepine **3**, 109
  cisapride **1**, 388
  clarithromycin, 191
  efavirenz **1**, 388
  erythromycin **2**, 191
  erythromycin estolate, 191
  erythromycin ethylsuccinate, 191
  erythromycin gluceptate, 191
  erythromycin lactobionate, 191
  erythromycin stearate, 191
  fluconazole **1**, 388
  fluvoxamine maleate **1**, 388
  grapefruit juice **2**, 333–334
  grepafloxacin hydrochloride **1**, 388
  halofantrine hydrochloride **1**, 388
  indinavir sulfate **1**, 388
  itraconazole, 201–202
  itraconazole, oral, 201–202
  ketoconazole, oral **1**, 201–202
  mibefradil dihydrochloride **1**, 388
  nefazodone hydrochloride **1**, 388
  nelfinavir mesylate **1**, 388
  quinine **1**, 388
  ritonavir **1**, 388
  saquinavir **1**, 388
  sparfloxacin **1**, 388
  spiramycin, 191
  troleandomycin, 191
  zileuton **1**, 388
terodiline hydrochloride,
  cisapride **1**, 388

# Index

tertatolol hydrochloride,
  arbutamine hydrochloride **1**, 388
  clonidine hydrochloride, 167
  clonidine hydrochloride,
    transdermal, 167
  epinephrine, 267
  insulin, 311
testosterone,
  vecuronium bromide **3**, 44
tetracycline,
  alcuronium chloride, 41
  aluminum carbonate, basic,
    211–212
  aluminum hydroxide **1**, 211–212
  aluminum oxide, 211–212
  aluminum phosphate, 211–212
  attapulgite, 211–212
  bismuth subsalicylate, 211–212
  calcium, oral salt unspecified,
    211–212
  calcium acetate, 211–212
  calcium ascorbate, 211–212
  calcium carbonate, oral, 211–212
  calcium chloride, oral, 211–212
  calcium citrate, oral, 211–212
  calcium glubionate, oral, 211–212
  calcium glucoheptonate, 211–212
  calcium gluconate, oral, 211–212
  calcium glycerophosphate, oral,
    211–212
  calcium iodate, 211–212
  calcium lactate, oral, 211–212
  calcium lactate gluconate, 211–212
  calcium lactobionate, oral, 211–212
  calcium phosphate, oral, 211–212
  carbonyl iron, 212
  cimetidine, oral **3**, 212
  dicalcium phosphate, 211–212
  digoxin **1**, 289
  digoxin capsule, stabilized, 289
  dihydroxyaluminum, 211–212
  doxacurium chloride, 41
  ether, 27
  ferric ammonium citrate, 212
  ferrous citrate, 212
  ferrous fumarate, 212
  ferrous gluconate, 212
  ferrous glycine sulfate, 212
  ferrous hydroxide polymaltose, 212
  ferrous ions, salt unspecified, 212
  ferrous succinate, 212
  ferrous sulfate **1**, 212
  gallamine triethiodide, 41
  hormonal contraceptive **2**, 212
  iron peptonized, 212
  kaolin, 211–212
  lithium **2**, 252
  magaldrate, 211–212
  magnesium, salt unspecified,
    211–212
  magnesium aspartate, 211–212
  magnesium carbonate, 211–212
  magnesium chloride, oral, 211–212
  magnesium citrate, 211–212
  magnesium glucoheptonate,
    211–212
  magnesium gluconate, 211–212
  magnesium hydroxide, 211–212
  magnesium lactate, 211–212
  magnesium oxide, 211–212
  magnesium sulfate, 211–212
  magnesium trisilicate, 211–212
  methoxyflurane **2**, 30
  metocurine iodide, 41
  mivacurium chloride, 41
  pancuronium bromide, 41
  pipecuronium bromide, 41
  rapacuronium bromide, 41
  rocuronium bromide, 41
  sodium bicarbonate **4**, 213
  succinylcholine chloride, 41
  sucralfate, 211–212
  theophylline **3**, 353
  thimerosal, ophthalmic **3**, 213
  tubocurarine chloride, 41
  vecuronium bromide, 41
  warfarin **3**, 99
tetracycline hydrochloride, injectable,
  alcuronium chloride, 41
  digoxin, 289
  digoxin capsule, stabilized, 289
  ether, 27
  gallamine triethiodide, 41
  metocurine iodide, 41
  mivacurium chloride, 41
  pipecuronium bromide, 41
  rapacuronium bromide, 41
  rocuronium bromide, 41
  succinylcholine chloride, 41
  tubocurarine chloride, 41
  vecuronium bromide, 41
tetrahydrozoline hydrochloride,
  furazolidone, 159–160
  isocarboxazid, 159–160
  pargyline hydrochloride, 159–160
  phenelzine sulfate, 159–160
  tranylcypromine sulfate, 159–160
theophylline,
  allopurinol **2**, 341–342
  aluminum hydroxide **3**, 342
  aminoglutethimide **3**, 342
  caffeine **2**, 342–343
  carbamazepine **2**, 343
  cefaclor **3**, 343
  charcoal **1**, 343–344
  cimetidine, oral **1**, 344
  cimetidine hydrochloride,
    injectable, 344
  ciprofloxacin hydrochloride **2**,
    344–345
  clarithromycin, 346
  dipyridamole, injectable **2**, 345

# Index

disulfiram **2**, 345–346
erythromycin **1**, 346
erythromycin estolate, 346
erythromycin ethylsuccinate, 346
erythromycin gluceptate, 346
erythromycin lactobionate, 346
erythromycin stearate, 346
fluvoxamine maleate **3**, 347
furosemide **2**, 347
halothane, 337
hydrocortisone, oral/systemic **3**, 347
hydrocortisone acet, injectable **3**, 347
hydrocortisone sodium phos **3**, 347
hydrocortisone sodium succinate **3**, 347
hypericum **3**, 347–348
influenza virus vaccine, split virion **3**, 348
influenza virus vaccine, whole virion **3**, 348
isoniazid **3**, 348
ketoconazole, oral **3**, 349
lithium **2**, 252–253
lomustine **3**, 221
magnesium hydroxide **3**, 342
methimazole **3**, 349
mexiletine hydrochloride **2**, 349–350
moricizine hydrochloride **2**, 350
omeprazole **4**, 350
phenobarbital **2**, 350–351
phenytoin **2**, 351
propafenone hydrochloride **2**, 351
propranolol hydrochloride **2**, 351–352
pyrantel pamoate **2**, 352
rifampin **2**, 352
sucralfate **3**, 352–353
tacrolimus **3**, 353
tetracycline **3**, 353
ticlopidine hydrochloride **2**, 353–354
tobacco **1**, 354
troleandomycin, 346
verapamil hydrochloride **2**, 354
vidarabine **3**, 354–355
thiabendazole,
aminophylline **2**, 340
thiamylal sodium,
acenocoumarol, 94
coumarin, 94
dicumarol, 94
warfarin, 94
thiethylperazine maleate,
cabergoline **1**, 388
cisapride **1**, 388
grepafloxacin hydrochloride **1**, 388
guanethidine, 169
halofantrine hydrochloride **1**, 388
pergolide mesylate **1**, 388
pimozide **1**, 388
thimerosal, ophthalmic,
tetracycline **3**, 213
thiopental sodium,
acenocoumarol, 94
coumarin, 94
dicumarol, 94
midazolam hydrochloride **3**, 255
morphine **2**, 40
probenecid **3**, 40
reserpine **2**, 40
succinylcholine chloride **2**, 39
sulfisoxazole **2**, 41
warfarin, 94
thioproperazine mesylate,
cisapride **1**, 388
grepafloxacin hydrochloride **1**, 388
guanethidine, 169
halofantrine hydrochloride **1**, 388
pimozide **1**, 388
thioridazine hydrochloride,
amitriptyline hydrochloride **1**, 388
bromocriptine mesylate **2**, 257
cabergoline **1**, 388
cisapride **1**, 388
desipramine hydrochloride **1**, 140
dofetilide **1**, 388
doxepin hydrochloride **1**, 388
fluoxetine hydrochloride **1**, 388
fluvoxamine maleate **1**, 388
fosphenytoin sodium, injectable **1**, 388
grepafloxacin hydrochloride **1**, 388
guanethidine, 169
halofantrine hydrochloride **1**, 388
imipramine **1**, 388
lithium **2**, 253
moxifloxacin hydrochloride, oral **1**, 388
paroxetine hydrochloride **1**, 388
pergolide mesylate **1**, 388
phenylpropanolamine **2**, 233
pimozide **1**, 388
pindolol **1**, 388
propranolol hydrochloride **1**, 388
quetiapine fumarate **1**, 388
sotalol hydrochloride **1**, 388
sparfloxacin **1**, 388
sumatriptan, nasal **1**, 388
sumatriptan succinate, injectable **1**, 388
sumatriptan succinate, oral **1**, 388
thiothixene,
cabergoline **1**, 388
guanethidine, 169
pergolide mesylate **1**, 388
thiram, topical,
alcohol, ethyl–oral/injectable, 318
thyroglobulin,

# Index

acenocoumarol, 100
  coumarin, 100
  dicumarol, 100
  warfarin, 100
thyroid desiccated,
  acenocoumarol, 100
  anisindione, 100
  coumarin, 100
  dicumarol, 100
  insulin **2**, 311–312
  warfarin **1**, 100
thyroid strong,
  acenocoumarol, 100
  anisindione, 100
  cholestyramine **2**, 386
  coumarin, 100
  dicumarol, 100
  digoxin **2**, 289
  ketamine hydrochloride **3**, 30
  propranolol hydrochloride **2**, 271
  warfarin, 100
tiaprofenic acid,
  ketorolac tromethamine **1**, 388
  ketorolac tromethamine, injectable **1**, 388
ticarcillin disodium,
  amikacin sulfate, 192
  gentamicin sulfate, 192
  kanamycin sulfate, injectable, 192
  kanamycin sulfate, oral, 192
  neomycin sulfate, injectable, 192
  neomycin sulfate, oral, 192
  netilmicin, 192
  paromomycin sulfate, 192
  streptomycin sulfate, 192
  tobramycin, 192
ticlopidine hydrochloride,
  aluminum hydroxide **3**, 74–75
  carbamazepine **2**, 109–110
  cyclosporine **2**, 75
  magaldrate **3**, 74–75
  magnesium hydroxide **3**, 74–75
  phenytoin **2**, 129
  theophylline **2**, 353–354
timolol maleate, ophthalmic,
  acetazolamide **3**, 271
  arbutamine hydrochloride **1**, 388
  dexfenfluramine hydrochloride, 267
  dobutamine hydrochloride, 267
  dopamine hydrochloride, 267
  epinephrine, 267
  etafedrine hydrochloride, 267
  insulin, 311
  mazindol, 267
  metaraminol bitartrate, 267
  methoxamine hydrochloride, 267
  norepinephrine bitartrate, 267
  phenylephrine, 267
  prednisone **2**, 272
timolol maleate, oral,
  albuterol sulfate, 267
  arbutamine hydrochloride **1**, 388
  bitolterol mesylate, 267
  clonidine hydrochloride, 167
  clonidine hydrochloride, transdermal, 167
  dexfenfluramine hydrochloride, 267
  dobutamine hydrochloride, 267
  dopamine hydrochloride, 267
  epinephrine, 267
  etafedrine hydrochloride, 267
  ethylnorepinephrine hydrochloride, 267
  fenoterol hydrobromide, 267
  formoterol fumarate, inhl, 267
  insulin, 311
  isoetharine, 267
  mazindol, 267
  metaproterenol sulfate, 267
  metaraminol bitartrate, 267
  methoxamine hydrochloride, 267
  pirbuterol acetate, 267
  procaterol hydrochloride, 267
  rimiterol hydrobromide, 267
  salmeterol xinafoate, 267
  terbutaline sulfate, 267
tinzaparin sodium,
  sodium salicylate, 77
tioconazole,
  cyclosporine, 199–200
  fosphenytoin sodium, injectable, 121–122
  lovastatin **1**, 388
  mizolastine **1**, 388
  phenytoin, 121–122
  simvastatin **1**, 388
tirofiban hydrochloride,
  eptifibatide **1**, 388
tobacco,
  aminophylline, 354
  chlorpromazine hydrochloride **3**, 236
  diazepam **3**, 243
  gold sodium thiomalate **3**, 12
  heparin **3**, 74
  imipramine **3**, 150
  insulin **3**, 312
  mexiletine hydrochloride **3**, 57
  oxtriphylline, 354
  propranolol hydrochloride **2**, 271
  theophylline **1**, 354
  warfarin **4**, 100
tobramycin,
  alcuronium chloride, 41
  amoxicillin, 192
  ampicillin sodium, 192
  azlocillin sodium, 192
  bacampicillin hydrochloride, 192
  benethamine penicillin, 192
  bumetanide, 198
  bumetanide, injectable, 198
  carbenicillin disodium, 192

# Index

cefaclor, 192
cefadroxil monohydrate, 192
cefamandole nafate, 192
cefazolin sodium, 192
cefdinir, 192
cefepime hydrochloride, 192
cefmetazole sodium, 192
cefonicid sodium, 192
cefoperazone sodium, 192
ceforanide, 192
cefotaxime sodium, 192
cefotetan disodium, 192
cefoxitin sodium, 192
cefpirome sulfate, 192
cefpodoxime proxetil, 192
cefprozil, 192
ceftazidime, 192
ceftibuten dihyrate, 192
ceftizoxime sodium, 192
ceftriaxone sodium, 192
cefuroxime, 192
cephalexin, 192
cephalothin sodium, 192
cephapirin sodium, 192
cephradine, 192
cloxacillin sodium, 192
cyclacillin, 192
dicloxacillin, 192
doxacurium chloride, 41
enflurane, 27
ethacrynic acid, 198
ethacrynic acid, injectable, 198
ether, 27
flucloxacillin, 192
furosemide, 198
furosemide, injectable, 198
gallamine triethiodide, 41
halothane, 27
isoflurane, 27
methicillin sodium, 192
methoxyflurane, 27
metocurine iodide, 41
mezlocillin sodium, 192
miconazole nitrate **3**, 213
mivacurium chloride, 41
moxalactam disodium, 192
nafcillin sodium, 192
nitrous oxide, 27
oxacillin sodium, 192
pancuronium bromide, 41
penicillin G, 192
penicillin G benzathine, 192
penicillin G procaine, 192
penicillin V, 192
pipecuronium bromide, 41
piperacillin sodium, 192
piretanide, 198
rapacuronium bromide, 41
rocuronium bromide, 41
succinylcholine chloride, 41
temocillin sodium, 192

ticarcillin disodium, 192
torsemide, injectable, 198
torsemide, oral, 198
tubocurarine chloride, 41
vecuronium bromide, 41
tocopherol, vitamin E,
  warfarin **2**, 102
tolazamide,
  alcohol, ethyl–oral/injectable, 302
  doxepin hydrochloride **2**, 312–313
  feprazone, 314–315
  oxyphenbutazone, 314–315
  phenylbutazone, 314–315
tolbutamide,
  alcohol, ethyl–oral/injectable, 302
  chloramphenicol **2**, 313
  diazoxide, oral **3**, 313
  dicumarol **2**, 313–314
  digoxin **3**, 289
  feprazone, 314–315
  fluconazole **3**, 314
  methyldopa **3**, 314
  oxyphenbutazone, 314–315
  phenylbutazone **1**, 314–315
  sulfamethizole **2**, 315
tolcapone,
  furazolidone **1**, 388
  hypericum **1**, 388
  isocarboxazid **1**, 388
  pargyline hydrochloride **1**, 388
  phenelzine sulfate **1**, 388
  procarbazine hydrochloride **1**, 388
  tranylcypromine sulfate **1**, 388
tolfenamic acid,
  ketorolac tromethamine **1**, 388
  ketorolac tromethamine, injectable
    **1**, 388
tolmetin sodium,
  ketorolac tromethamine **1**, 388
  ketorolac tromethamine, injectable
    **1**, 388
tolterodine tartrate,
  warfarin **2**, 100–101
toremifene,
  acenocoumarol **1**, 388
  anisindione **1**, 388
  dicumarol **1**, 388
  erythromycin **1**, 388
  erythromycin estolate **1**, 388
  erythromycin ethylsuccinate **1**, 388
  erythromycin gluceptate **1**, 388
  erythromycin lactobionate **1**, 388
  erythromycin stearate **1**, 388
  ketoconazole, oral **1**, 388
  phenindione **1**, 388
  troleandomycin **1**, 388
  warfarin **1**, 388
torsemide, injectable,
  amikacin sulfate, 198
  gentamicin sulfate, 198
  kanamycin sulfate, injectable, 198

## Index

kanamycin sulfate, oral, 198
lithium, 247
neomycin sulfate, injectable, 198
neomycin sulfate, oral, 198
netilmicin, 198
streptomycin sulfate, 198
tobramycin, 198
torsemide, oral,
  amikacin sulfate, 198
  gentamicin sulfate, 198
  kanamycin sulfate, injectable, 198
  kanamycin sulfate, oral, 198
  lithium, 247
  neomycin sulfate, oral, 198
  netilmicin, 198
  streptomycin sulfate, 198
  tobramycin, 198
tranylcypromine sulfate,
  alfentanil hydrochloride, 15
  amobarbital **3**, 320
  amphetamine, 191–192
  anileridine, 15
  apraclonidine hydrochloride **1**, 388
  atracurium besylate **3**, 159
  benzphetamine hydrochloride, 159–160
  brimonidine tartrate, ophthalmic **1**, 388
  buprenorphine hydrochloride, 15
  bupropion hydrochloride **1**, 388
  butorphanol tartrate, 15
  citalopram hydrobromide, 144–145
  codeine, 15
  dexfenfluramine hydrochloride, 159–160
  dextroamphetamine, 159–160
  dextromethorphan hbr, 15
  diethylpropion hydrochloride, 159–160
  difenoxin hydrochloride, 15
  dihydrocodeine bitartrate, 15
  diphenoxylate hydrochloride, 15
  dopamine hydrochloride, 159–160
  entacapone **1**, 388
  ephedrine, 159–160
  etafedrine hydrochloride, 159–160
  fenfluramine hydrochloride, 159–160
  fentanyl citrate, 15
  fluoxetine hydrochloride **1**, 144–145
  fluvoxamine maleate, 144–145
  hydrocodone bitartrate, 15
  hydromorphone hydrochloride, 15
  imipramine **2**, 150
  indoramin **1**, 388
  isometheptene, 159–160
  levodopa, 157–158
  levorphanol tartrate, 15
  mazindol, 159–160
  meperidine hydrochloride, 15
  mephentermine sulfate, 159–160
  meptazinol, 15
  metaraminol bitartrate, 159–160
  methamphetamine hydrochloride, 159–160
  methylphenidate hydrochloride, 159–160
  nalbuphine hydrochloride, 15
  naphazoline hydrochloride, 159–160
  nefazodone hydrochloride **1**, 388
  opium, 15
  oxycodone, 15
  oxymetazoline hydrochloride, 159–160
  oxymorphone hydrochloride, 15
  paroxetine hydrochloride, 144–145
  pentazocine, 15
  phendimetrazine tartrate, 159–160
  phenmetrazine hydrochloride, 159–160
  phenoperidine hydrochloride, 15
  phentermine hydrochloride, 159–160
  phenylephrine, 159–160
  phenylpropanolamine **1**, 159–160
  propranolol hydrochloride **4**, 160
  pseudoephedrine, 159–160
  remifentanil hydrochloride, 15
  rizatriptan benzoate **1**, 388
  sertraline hydrochloride **1**, 388
  sibutramine hydrochloride monohyd **1**, 388
  sufentanil citrate, 15
  sumatriptan, nasal **1**, 388
  sumatriptan succinate **1**, 388
  sumatriptan succinate, oral **1**, 388
  tetrahydrozoline hydrochloride, 159–160
  tolcapone **1**, 388
  tryptophan **3**, 160
  venlafaxine hydrochloride, 144–145
  xylometazoline hydrochloride, 159–160
  zolmitriptan **1**, 388
trastuzumab,
  cyclophosphamide **1**, 388
  daunorubicin citrate liposome **1**, 388
  daunorubicin hydrochloride **1**, 388
  doxorubicin hydrochloride **1**, 388
  doxorubicin hydrochloride liposome **1**, 388
  epirubicin hydrochloride **1**, 388
  idarubicin hydrochloride **1**, 388
  warfarin **2**, 101
trazodone hydrochloride,
  carbamazepine **3**, 110
  digoxin **3**, 289–290
  fluoxetine hydrochloride **3**, 160
  ginkgo biloba **3**, 161
  nefazodone hydrochloride **3**,

# Index

386–387
phenytoin **3**, 129–130
warfarin **3**, 101
triamterene,
  amantadine hydrochloride **3**, 298
  cimetidine, oral **3**, 299
  dofetilide **2**, 388
  indomethacin **2**, 299
  potassium, salt unspecified, 299
  potassium acetate, 299
  potassium bicarbonate, 299
  potassium biphosphate, 299
  potassium chloride, 299
  potassium citrate, 299
  potassium gluconate, 299
  potassium glycerophosphate, oral, 299
  potassium iodide, 299
  potassium iodide, prenatal multivitamin use, 299
  potassium perchlorate, 299
  potassium phosphate, 299
  potassium salicylate, 299
triazolam,
  amprenavir **1**, 388
  efavirenz **1**, 388
  indinavir sulfate **1**, 388
  itraconazole, oral **1**, 388
  ketoconazole, oral **1**, 388
  nefazodone hydrochloride **1**, 388
  nelfinavir mesylate **1**, 388
  ritonavir **1**, 388
  saquinavir **1**, 388
trichlormethiazide,
  diazoxide, oral **3**, 300
  lithium, 247
tridihexethyl chloride,
  digoxin, 287
triethylene thiophosphoramide,
  pancuronium bromide **3**, 34–35
trifluoperazine hydrochloride,
  cabergoline **1**, 388
  guanethidine, 169
  halofantrine hydrochloride **1**, 388
  pergolide mesylate **1**, 388
trifluperidol hydrochloride,
  cabergoline **1**, 388
  pergolide mesylate **1**, 388
triflupromazine hydrochloride,
  cabergoline **1**, 388
  cisapride **1**, 388
  grepafloxacin hydrochloride **1**, 388
  guanethidine, 169
  halofantrine hydrochloride **1**, 388
  pergolide mesylate **1**, 388
  pimozide **1**, 388
trihexyphenidyl hydrochloride,
  digoxin, 287
  levodopa **4**, 370
trimeprazine tartrate,
  cabergoline **1**, 388
  cisapride **1**, 388
  grepafloxacin hydrochloride **1**, 388
  guanethidine, 169
  halofantrine hydrochloride **1**, 388
  pergolide mesylate **1**, 388
  pimozide **1**, 388
trimethaphan camsylate,
  succinylcholine chloride **2**, 39–40
trimethoprim,
  cyclosporine **3**, 210
  dapsone **3**, 188–189
  digoxin **3**, 290
  dofetilide **1**, 388
  hormonal contraceptive **3**, 210–211
  methotrexate **1**, 226
  methotrexate sodium, injectable, 226
  phenytoin **2**, 130
  pimozide **3**, 158
  procainamide hydrochloride **3**, 61
  warfarin, 98
trimipramine maleate,
  amprenavir **1**, 388
  arbutamine hydrochloride **1**, 388
  cisapride **1**, 388
  grepafloxacin hydrochloride **1**, 388
  guanethidine, 169
  halofantrine hydrochloride **1**, 388
  pimozide **1**, 388
troglitazone,
  warfarin **3**, 102
troleandomycin,
  astemizole, 191
  carbamazepine, 105
  cisapride **1**, 388
  cyclosporine, 190
  hormonal contraceptive **2**, 214
  methylprednisolone **2**, 213–214
  mizolastine **1**, 388
  simvastatin, 373
  terfenadine, 191
  theophylline, 346
  toremifene **1**, 388
  warfarin, 83
tromethamine,
  lithium, 245–246
tryptophan,
  fluoxetine hydrochloride **3**, 145
  tranylcypromine sulfate **3**, 160
tubocurarine chloride,
  amikacin sulfate, 41
  bacitracin, 41
  colistin sulfate, 41
  demeclocycline hydrochloride, 41
  doxycycline hydrochloride, 41
  doxycycline hyclate, injectable, 41
  gentamicin sulfate **1**, 41
  kanamycin sulfate, injectable, 41
  kanamycin sulfate, oral, 41
  ketamine hydrochloride **2**, 41
  lymecycline, 41

# Index

methacycline hydrochloride, 41
minocycline, injectable, 41
minocycline hydrochloride, 41
minocycline hydrochloride pellets, 41
morphine **2**, 42
neomycin sulfate, injectable, 41
neomycin sulfate, oral, 41
netilmicin, 41
oxytetracycline, 41
oxytetracycline, injectable, 41
paromomycin sulfate, 41
polymyxin B sulfate, 41
polymyxin B sulfate, vaccine use, 41
propranolol hydrochloride **2**, 42
quinidine **2**, 42–43
rolitetracycline, injectable, 41
streptomycin sulfate, 41
tetracycline, 41
tetracycline hydrochloride, injectable, 41
tobramycin, 41
tyropanoate sodium,
  metformin hydrochloride **1**, 312

## V

valproic acid,
  aluminum hydroxide **3**, 132
  amitriptyline hydrochloride **3**, 132
  aspirin **2**, 132–133
  carbamazepine **2**, 133
  chlorpromazine hydrochloride **3**, 133
  cimetidine, oral **3**, 131
  clonazepam **3**, 133–134
  erythromycin **2**, 134
  erythromycin ethylsuccinate **2**, 134
  ethosuximide **3**, 112
  felbamate **2**, 134
  fluoxetine hydrochloride **3**, 134–135
  isoniazid **3**, 135
  lamotrigine **3**, 113
  methylphenidate hydrochloride **3**, 135
  naproxen **3**, 131
  phenobarbital **2**, 113
  phenytoin **2**, 130
vancomycin hydrochloride,
  gentamicin sulfate **3**, 193
vecuronium bromide,
  amikacin sulfate, 41
  bacitracin, 41
  colistin sulfate, 41
  dantrolene sodium **3**, 43
  demeclocycline hydrochloride, 41
  doxycycline hydrochloride, 41
  doxycycline hyclate, injectable, 41
  gentamicin sulfate, 41
  kanamycin sulfate, injectable, 41
  kanamycin sulfate, oral, 41
  lymecycline, 41
  magnesium sulfate, injectable **2**, 43
  methacycline hydrochloride, 41
  minocycline, injectable, 41
  minocycline hydrochloride, 41
  minocycline hydrochloride pellets, 41
  neomycin sulfate, injectable, 41
  neomycin sulfate, oral, 41
  netilmicin, 41
  oxytetracycline, 41
  oxytetracycline, injectable, 41
  paromomycin sulfate, 41
  piperacillin sodium **2**, 43–44
  polymyxin B sulfate, 41
  polymyxin B sulfate, vaccine use, 41
  rolitetracycline, injectable, 41
  streptomycin sulfate, 41
  testosterone **3**, 44
  tetracycline, 41
  tetracycline hydrochloride, injectable, 41
  tobramycin, 41
  verapamil hydrochloride **2**, 44
venlafaxine hydrochloride,
  cimetidine, oral **3**, 161
  dexfenfluramine hydrochloride, 159–160
  furazolidone, 144–145
  isocarboxazid, 144–145
  moclobemide, 144–145
  pargyline hydrochloride, 144–145
  phenelzine sulfate, 144–145
  procarbazine hydrochloride, 144–145
  selegiline hydrochloride, 144–145
  tranylcypromine sulfate, 144–145
verapamil hydrochloride,
  calcium gluconate, oral **2**, 66
  carbamazepine **2**, 110
  cyclosporine, 47–48
  dantrolene sodium **2**, 66
  digitoxin, 290
  digoxin **1**, 290
  digoxin capsule, stabilized, 290
  dofetilide **1**, 388
  etomidate **3**, 27
  lithium **2**, 253–254
  phenobarbital **3**, 66–67
  prazosin hydrochloride **3**, 176
  propranolol hydrochloride **2**, 67
  quinidine **1**, 65–66
  rifampin **2**, 67
  sulfinpyrazone **3**, 68
  theophylline **2**, 354
  vecuronium bromide **2**, 44
verapamil hydrochloride, sustained-release,

# Index

cyclosporine, 47–48
digitoxin, 290
digoxin, 290
digoxin capsule, stabilized, 290
dofetilide **1**, 388
quinidine, 65–66
verapamil hydrochloride pellets,
  cyclosporine, 47–48
  digitoxin, 290
  digoxin, 290
  digoxin capsule, stabilized, 290
  dofetilide **1**, 388
  quinidine, 65–66
vidarabine,
  allopurinol **2**, 214
  theophylline **3**, 354–355
vinblastine sulfate,
  erythromycin **3**, 228
  mitomycin **2**, 227
  phenytoin **2**, 116
vincristine sulfate,
  carbamazepine **2**, 229
  digoxin **2**, 278–279
vindesine sulfate,
  warfarin **3**, 84
vitamin A,
  neomycin sulfate, oral **3**, 335
vitamin A, prenatal multivitamin use,
  neomycin sulfate, oral **3**, 335
vitamin D,
  paricalcitol **1**, 388
vitamin D2, prenatal multivitamin use,
  paricalcitol **1**, 388
  phenytoin **2**, 328
vitamin D3, prenatal multivitamin use,
  aluminum hydroxide **2**, 327
  paricalcitol **1**, 388

## W

warfarin,
  acarbose **2**, 75
  acetaminophen **3**, 76
  alcohol, ethyl–oral/injectable **3**, 76
  allopurinol, 70–71
  aloxiprin, 77
  aminoglutethimide, 87
  amiodarone hydrochloride **1**, 76–77
  amobarbital, 94
  aprobarbital, 94
  ascorbic acid, vitamin C **4**, 77
  aspirin **1**, 77
  azapropazone dihydrate **1**, 388
  azathioprine sodium **2**, 78
  azithromycin, 83
  barbital, 94
  bezafibrate, 81
  butabarbital sodium, 94
  butalbital, 94
  butobarbitone, 94
  calcium carbaspirin, 77
  calcium carbimide, 82–83
  cefamandole nafate **2**, 78
  chloral hydrate **2**, 78–79
  chlordiazepoxide **4**, 79
  chlorthalidone **3**, 79
  cholestyramine **2**, 79–80
  cimetidine, oral **1**, 80
  cimetidine hydrochloride, injectable, 80
  cinoxacin, 93
  ciprofloxacin hydrochloride, 93
  ciprofloxacin hydrochloride, injectable, 93
  cisapride **2**, 80
  clarithromycin, 83
  clofibrate **1**, 81
  cyclosporine **2**, 81
  danazol, 91
  danshen **2**, 81
  dextrothyroxine sodium, 100
  diazoxide, oral **3**, 82
  diflunisal, 77
  diphenhydramine **4**, 82
  dirithromycin, 83
  disopyramide phosphate **3**, 82
  disulfiram **1**, 82–83
  dong quai **3**, 83
  enoxacin, 93
  erythromycin **1**, 83
  erythromycin estolate, 83
  erythromycin ethylsuccinate, 83
  erythromycin glucepate, 83
  erythromycin lactobionate, 83
  erythromycin stearate, 83
  ethacrynic acid **2**, 84
  ethchlorvynol **2**, 84
  ethylestrenol, 91
  etoposide **3**, 84
  etretinate **2**, 85
  felbamate **2**, 85
  fenofibrate, micronized, 81
  feprazone, 94–95
  flosequinan, 93
  fluconazole **2**, 85–86
  fluoxetine hydrochloride **3**, 86
  fluoxymesterone, 91
  gemfibrozil, 81
  ginkgo biloba **3**, 86
  ginseng **3**, 87
  glucagon **1**, 87
  glucagon, recombinant, 87
  glutethimide **1**, 87
  griseofulvin **2**, 88
  ibuprofen **2**, 88
  ifosfamide **2**, 88–89
  indomethacin **2**, 89
  influenza virus vaccine, split virion **3**, 89
  isoniazid **3**, 89–90
  levothyroxine sodium, 100
  liothyronine sodium, 100

# Index

lomefloxacin hydrochloride, 93
lovastatin **2**, 90
magnesium hydroxide **4**, 90
menadiol sodium diphosphate, vitamin K4, 95
menadione, 95
mephobarbital, 94
meprobamate **3**, 90–91
methandrostenolone, 91
metharbital, 94
methohexital sodium, 94
methyltestosterone **1**, 91
methyprylon, 87
metronidazole, oral/vaginal **2**, 91–92
mitotane **2**, 92
moricizine hydrochloride **2**, 92
nafcillin sodium **2**, 92–93
nalidixic acid **1**, 93
neomycin sulfate, oral **3**, 93
norfloxacin, 93
nortriptyline hydrochloride **4**, 93–94
ofloxacin, 93
ofloxacin, injectable, 93
omeprazole **3**, 94
oxandrolone, 91
oxymetholone, 91
oxyphenbutazone, 94–95
pentobarbital sodium, 94
phenobarbital **1**, 94
phenylbutazone **1**, 94–95
phytonadione, vitamin K1 **1**, 95
primidone, 94
proguanil hydrochloride, 98
propafenone hydrochloride **2**, 95–96
propoxyphene **2**, 96
propranolol hydrochloride **2**, 96
propylthiouracil, 100
quinidine **2**, 96–97
ranitidine hydrochloride, injectable, 80
ranitidine hydrochloride, oral, 80
rifabutin, 97
rifampin **1**, 97
secobarbital, 94
sodium salicylate, 77
spironolactone **3**, 97
stanozolol, 91
sucralfate **3**, 97–98
sulfacytine, 98
sulfadiazine, 98
sulfadoxine, 98
sulfamerazine, 98
sulfamethazine, 98
sulfamethizole, 98
sulfamethoxazole **1**, 98
sulfapyridine, 98
sulfasalazine, 98
sulfinpyrazone **1**, 98
sulfisoxazole, 98
talbutal, 94
tamoxifen citrate **2**, 98–99
temafloxacin hydrochloride, 93
terbinafine hydrochloride **2**, 99
tetracycline **3**, 99
thiamylal sodium, 94
thiopental sodium, 94
thyroglobulin, 100
thyroid desiccated **1**, 100
thyroid strong, 100
tobacco **4**, 100
tocopherol, vitamin E **2**, 102
tolterodine tartrate **2**, 100–101
toremifene **1**, 388
trastuzumab **2**, 101
trazodone hydrochloride **3**, 101
trimethoprim, 98
troglitazone **3**, 102
troleandomycin, 83
vindesine sulfate **3**, 84
watercress,
  chlorzoxazone **3**, 335
  dexbrompheniramine maleate **3**, 335

## X

xipamide,
  lithium, 247
xylometazoline hydrochloride,
  furazolidone, 159–160
  isocarboxazid, 159–160
  pargyline hydrochloride, 159–160
  phenelzine sulfate, 159–160
  tranylcypromine sulfate, 159–160

## Z

zidovudine,
  acetaminophen **3**, 214
  acyclovir, oral **3**, 215
  atovaquone **2**, 387
  probenecid **2**, 215
  ribavirin **1**, 387
  rifampin **2**, 388
zileuton,
  astemizole **1**, 388
  terfenadine **1**, 388
zolmitriptan,
  dihydroergotamine mesylate **1**, 388
  ergoloid mesylates **1**, 388
  ergonovine maleate **1**, 388
  ergotamine tartrate **1**, 388
  isocarboxazid **1**, 388
  methylergonovine maleate **1**, 388
  methysergide maleate **1**, 388
  moclobemide **1**, 388
  naratriptan hydrochloride **1**, 388
  pargyline hydrochloride **1**, 388
  phenelzine sulfate **1**, 388

# Index

rizatriptan benzoate **1**, 388
sumatriptan, nasal **1**, 388
sumatriptan succinate **1**, 388
sumatriptan succinate, injectable
  **1**, 388
sumatriptan succinate, oral **1**, 388
tranylcypromine sulfate **1**, 388
zolpidem tartrate,
  paroxetine hydrochloride **3**, 156
  rifampin **2**, 325
  ritonavir **1**, 388
zonisamide,
  methotrexate, 226
  methotrexate sodium, injectable,
    226
zuclopenthixol,
  guanethidine, 169

# AHFS*first*™ - Web Edition

*Electronic drug reference from the first names in drug information.*

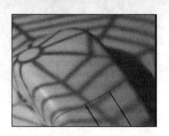

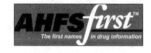

### Comprehensive
The first names in drug information have combined the two most comprehensive drug references available today into one easy-to-use software product. AHFS*first* provides access to information on over 100,000 drug products from First DataBank's National Drug Data File ® (NDDF) and American Society of Health-System Pharmacists (ASHP) AHFS Drug Information monographs.

### Easy Access
Extensive searching features and tiered navigation allow you to pinpoint the precise information needs or delve deeper into a drug topic. Simultaneous multi-drug interaction screening as well as product identification searches are easily performed within the software.

### Affordable
AHFS*first* is the first choice in value too. Nothing else even comes close for in-depth, up-to-date drug information at such an affordab price.

Call **800.428.4495** today and ask about a *FREE* 90 day trial of AHFS*first* - web edition!

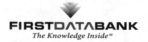

© 2001, First DataBank Inc.

# Our drug content has taken millions of hits.

## Successfully.

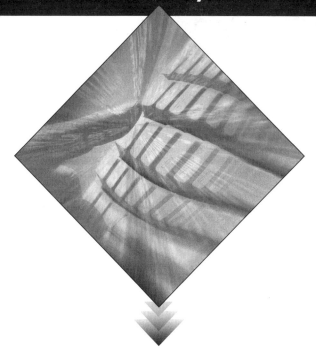

**First DataBank content has withstood the test of time.** Our drug content has been challenged–daily–by physicians, pharmacists and other medical professionals for over two decades. Consistently, it has hit the mark for accurate, comprehensive coverage of drugs.

Today, First DataBank provides the knowledge inside thousands of hospital and retail pharmacy systems nationwide.

Our core product, NDDF Plus™, is the industry's most trusted and widely used source of up-to-date drug information. It delivers descriptive, clinical and pricing information for every drug approved by the FDA–plus clinical decision-support and patient-education information. For details, contact First DataBank or your information system vendor today. Call **1-800-428-4495**, or visit our website at www.firstdatabank.com.

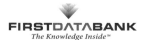

**FIRSTDATABANK**
*The Knowledge Inside℠*

© 2001, First DataBank Inc.

*For pharmacists:*

# One of the most valuable features of your drug information.
# *Timeliness.*

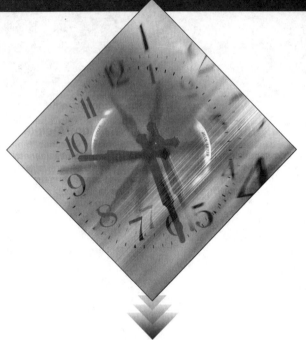

**With First DataBank's drug information integrated into your pharmacy system, you can be sure it's up to date.** So you never have to worry about its shelf life.

And since our comprehensive drug information has been time-tested for accuracy in pharmacy systems for over two decades, you know it's reliable. Today, it's the knowledge inside systems in thousands of retail pharmacies and hospitals nationwide. Plus it delivers clinical decision-support for professionals, and patient information for consumers.

To keep you up with the times, we've recently expanded coverage of alternative therapy agents in our knowledge bases–including herbals, nutraceuticals and dietary supplements. And our patient-education materials are being brought into effective compliance with the FDA's Keystone Action Plan. For details, contact First DataBank or your pharmacy system vendor today. **Call 1-800-428-4495**, or visit our website at www.firstdatabank.com.

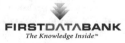

© 2001, First DataBank Inc.